# The Unofficial Guide to Passing OSCEs:

Candidate Briefings, Patient Briefings and Mark Schemes

EDITION
# 2

# The Unofficial Guide to Passing OSCEs:

## Candidate Briefings, Patient Briefings and Mark Schemes

### Series Editor

Zeshan Qureshi, BM, BSc (Hons), MSc, MRCPCH, FAcadMEd, MRCPS(Glasg)
Paediatric Registrar
London Deanery
United Kingdom

### Editors

Emily Hotton, MBChB (Dist), BSc (Hons) PhD, MRCOG
Women's and Children's Research
Southmead Hospital;
Translational Health Sciences
University of Bristol, Bristol
United Kingdom

Sammie Mak, MBChB
Junior Doctor
NHS England, Manchester
United Kingdom

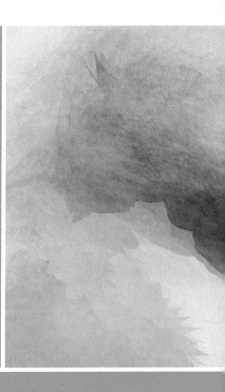

ELSEVIER

ELSEVIER

© 2024 Elsevier Limited. All rights reserved.

First edition © 2013. Published by Zeshan Qureshi.

---

**Notices**

Practitioners and researchers must always rely on their own experience and knowledge in evaluating and using any information, methods, compounds or experiments described herein. Because of rapid advances in the medical sciences, in particular, independent verification of diagnoses and drug dosages should be made. To the fullest extent of the law, no responsibility is assumed by Elsevier, authors, editors or contributors for any injury and/or damage to persons or property as a matter of products liability, negligence or otherwise, or from any use or operation of any methods, products, instructions, or ideas contained in the material herein.

---

ISBN: 978-0-323-93188-5

*Content Strategist*: Jeremy Bowes
*Content Project Manager*: Shubham Dixit
*Design*: Miles Hitchen
*Marketing Manager*: Deborah Watkins

Printed in India by Thomson Press (India) Limited.

Last digit is the print number: 9 8 7 6 5 4 3 2 1

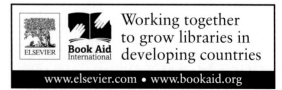

# Series Editor Foreword

The Unofficial Guide to Medicine is not just about helping students study, it is also about allowing those that learn to take back control of their own education. Since its inception, it has been driven by the voices of students, and through this, democratised the process of medical education, blurring the line between learners and teachers.

Medical education is an evolving process, and the latest iteration of our titles has been rewritten to bring them up to date with modern curriculums, after extensive deliberation and consultation. We have kept the series up to date, incorporating new guidelines and perspectives from a wide range of students, junior doctors, and senior clinicians. There is greater consistency across the titles, more illustrations, and through these and other changes, I hope the books will now be even better study aids.

These books though are a process of continual improvement. By reading this book, I hope that you not only get through your exams but also consider contributing to a future edition. You may be a student now, but you are also the future of medical education.

I wish you all the best with your future career and any upcoming exams.

**Zeshan Qureshi**
November 2022

# Introduction

*The Unofficial Guide to Passing OSCEs: Candidate Briefings, Patient Briefings and Mark Schemes* is a perfect supplement to *The Unofficial Guide to Passing OSCEs.* This updated second edition book contains all of the scenarios from *The Unofficial Guide to Passing OSCEs* (2nd edition) along with mark schemes so that medical students can apply the knowledge that they gain to realistic OSCE stations. Each mark scheme has been carefully curated to include the justification and thinking process behind the examiner so that the candidate can really grasp and understand why the mark has been given. The huge breadth of scenarios means that a broad range of specialities and areas are covered, as well as additional practical procedures and prescribing stations that are expected to be performed by junior doctors and trainees. Written by recently qualified foundation doctors, with review by senior clinicians, we have ensured that all procedures follow current guidelines, wherever possible.

In addition, at the end of all mark schemes, there are ten newly associated questions per station, to challenge you further and to make you think about common follow-up questions that may be asked on that topic. This should encourage you to think outside the box and gain a deep understanding of the subject area. The aim is to give you a concise collection of scenarios and mark schemes so that you can practise with and we hope this book will prove to be a handy study companion for your undergraduate and postgraduate training.

This book is useful for self-assessment, developing your knowledge with peers and as a guide to studying for your OSCE exams. The included mark schemes will offer guidance for group study sessions with the opportunity to mark your colleagues.

With this textbook, we hope you will become more confident and competent in both examinations and clinical practices.

Good luck with your future career and any upcoming exams.

**Emily Hotton, Sammie Mak and Zeshan Qureshi**
January 2023

# Contributors

**Lauren Franklin, Medical Student**
School of Medicine, Keele University, Staffordshire,
United Kingdom

**Lisa Kirk, MBChB, MRCOG, PG Cert**
Southmead Hospital, Bristol, United Kingdom

**Ashvin Kuri, MSc**
Barts and The London School of Medicine and
Dentistry, Queen Mary University of London

**Megan McGlone, MBChB, BSc**
Glasgow Royal Infirmary, NHS Greater Glasgow and
Clyde, Glasgow, United Kingdom

**Hui-Ling Ong, MbChB, BHSc**
Yeovil District Hospital, Yeovil, United Kingdom;
University of Glasgow, Glasgow, United Kingdom

**Ronan Pilkington**
North West Deanery - Lancashire Teaching Hospitals
NHS Foundation Trust

**Danielle Pollitt-Walmsley, BSc Human Neuroscience
(Hons)**
The University of Birmingham, Birmingham, United
Kingdom

**Ella Quintela, BMBS**
Department of Anaesthesia, Sheffield Teaching
Hospitals Trust; School of Health and Related
Research, University of Sheffield, United Kingdom

# Acknowledgements

We would like to acknowledge the work of medical students and clinicians of the first edition: Lizzie Casselden, Chris Gee, Matt Harris, Katherine Lattey, Chris Moseley, Sabrina Qureshi, Mark Rodrigues and Matt Wood.

# Contents

# History Taking

1

## Outline

## Station 1.1   Tiredness

### Doctor Briefing

You are a junior doctor in primary care and have been asked to see Yvonne Paisley, a 48-year-old woman, who has presented feeling tired all the time. She has noticed a significant amount of unintentional weight loss, and her partner reports that she seems paler than usual. Additionally, she has felt some lumps in her neck. Please take a history from Mrs Paisley, present your findings and formulate an appropriate management plan.

### Patient Briefing

This is your first visit to the doctor. You recall feeling unwell for several weeks and have noticed unintentional weight loss of around 8 kg over the last 3 months. On questioning you have noticed painless swellings in your neck and axilla, which seem to be getting slightly larger.

Your partner has reported that you have been having night sweats as well as some breathlessness on exertion. These do not seem that dramatic to you, as they have been present for several months and are not getting worse.

If specifically asked, there is a family history of cancer but you are unsure of the exact diagnosis.

You are concerned because you don't know what is causing the weight loss but you are worried you may have cancer.

### Mark Scheme for Examiner

#### Introduction

| | | | | | | |
|---|---|---|---|---|---|---|
| Cleans hands, introduces self, confirms patient identity and gains consent for history taking | | | | | | |
| Establishes current patient knowledge and concerns | | | | | | |

## History of Presenting Complaint

| Question | Justification | Answer | Thoughts | | | | |
|---|---|---|---|---|---|---|---|
| When did you first notice that you were more tired than normal? | This helps to determine if this is acute or chronic. Rarely tiredness secondary to anaemia or malignancy is acute | 'A few months' | A bit more worried, since more chronic sounding | | | | |
| Have you noticed any other new symptoms? Anything else that is concerning to you? | A patient may be tired due to life stressors; however, you need to rule out red flags for something more sinister | 'I have noticed some weight loss and sometimes I get really hot at night, sort of sweaty' | Unintentional weight loss as well as night sweats are red flags for malignancy. You need to explore further to determine any other signs of a sinister presentation | | | | |
| How much weight do you think you have lost? Have you made a conscious effort to lose weight? | You need to check whether this weight loss was intentional or unintentional. Some patients weigh themselves (quantitative) whereas others will report trousers becoming looser (qualitative) | 'I have lost around 8 kg in 3 months without really trying' | | | | | |
| Have you noticed any lightheadedness, breathlessness or palpitations? | May potentially be a result of anaemia and malignancy. Remember these symptoms can also suggest a cardiovascular issue | 'No' | Sounds like the patient is systemically well. If you were concerned you could enquire further regarding fevers, jaundice and itching | | | | |
| Have you noticed any abnormal bleeding or bruising? | Bleeding disorders are common in malignancy. Be sure to ask about haematuria and haemoptysis as well as prolonged bleeding or bruising after trauma | 'No' | No additional concerns | | | | |
| Have you come across any new noticeable lumps? | This is checking for enlarged lymph nodes | 'Yes, I have noticed some small painless lumps in my neck and armpit' | This indicates that the patient may have lymphoma | | | | |

## Past Medical History

| | | | | | | | |
|---|---|---|---|---|---|---|---|
| Have you ever had these symptoms before? | Checking that these are not recurring symptoms allows you to explore the past medical history | 'No, never' | No additional concerns | | | | |
| Have you had any recent illnesses or infections? | Haematological patients are more susceptible to infections as they become immunocompromised to common and opportunistic organisms | 'I have had a recent cold, which is funny considering it is the summer. It has lingered on for a while' | An indication that this patient may be immunocompromised | | | | |

## Drug History

| Question | Justification | Answer | Thoughts | | | | | |
|---|---|---|---|---|---|---|---|---|
| Are you on any medication at the moment, or have any allergies? | Unlikely to be on any medication but important to check, as people may not disclose their whole medical history. You must always check for allergies | 'No medications and no allergies' | No additional concerns | | | | | |
| Have you ever been on a drug that could affect your bleeding, such as aspirin or warfarin? | If you need to consider a specific drug, always ask about it directly. The patient may have recently stopped taking it. These drugs can have an effect on bleeding | 'No. I have never taken those medications' | No additional concerns | | | | | |
| Have you had all your immunisations? | Very important to check, especially in a younger patient. Recent vaccinations (especially live) can be potentially harmful to an immunocompromised patient | 'Yes, a long time ago now' | No additional concerns | | | | | |

## Family History

| Question | Justification | Answer | Thoughts | | | | | |
|---|---|---|---|---|---|---|---|---|
| Are there any diseases that run in the family, including any cancers? | Important always to check for relevant heritable conditions | 'My grandmother and aunt both died of cancer, but I don't know which one' | Possible concern; however, you have no further information to go on at the moment | | | | | |

## Social and Travel History

| Question | Justification | Answer | Thoughts | | | | | |
|---|---|---|---|---|---|---|---|---|
| Who is currently at home? Are you working? | Find out if there are any social concerns or if wider support is needed | 'I live with my husband and work full-time in a restaurant' | No additional concerns | | | | | |
| Do you smoke? | Find out a patient's wider risk factors | 'No, I have never smoked' | No additional concerns | | | | | |
| What is your average weekly alcohol consumption? | Find out a patient's wider risk factors as well as exploring causes for symptom changes | 'I only have around 4 units a week' | Patient not disclosing any further concerns at present | | | | | |
| Have you recently travelled abroad? | Ensure no tropical infections as a cause of the patient's symptoms | 'No, not for several years' | No additional concerns | | | | | |

## Systems Review

| Question | Justification | Answer | Thoughts | | | | | |
|---|---|---|---|---|---|---|---|---|
| Just to check, have you had any problems with bladder or bowel function? | Find out if there are any wider concerns that have not arisen yet | 'No, they have been normal' | No additional concerns | | | | | |

## Systems Review

| Question | Justification | Answer | Thoughts | | | | |
|---|---|---|---|---|---|---|---|
| Have you had any fever or fatigue? | It is essential to ask about B symptoms to rule out certain causes, such as infection | 'No' | No additional concerns | | | | |

## Finishing the Consultation

| | | | | | | | |
|---|---|---|---|---|---|---|---|
| Is there anything that I've missed, or anything that you are particularly concerned about? | May identify useful information that has been missed. Will also help when framing communication with the patient | 'I'm just really keen to find out what is going on and causing me to feel so unwell' | Take the time to explain what will happen from here | | | | |
| Do you have any questions for me at the moment? | | | | | | | |

## Present Your Findings

Mrs Paisley is a 48-year-old woman who presents with a 3-month history of unexplained weight loss. On questioning she also describes new neck lumps and fatigue. She has no medical history and is not taking any medication currently. She has a viral illness at the moment which she feels she is unable to get rid of.

My main differential would be lymphoma but I would like to investigate for anaemia of chronic disease.

I am going to take several blood tests from Mrs Paisley, including full blood count (FBC), urea and electrolytes U&Es, coagulation, lactate dehydrogenase and a blood film and gain consent for human immunodeficiency virus (HIV) testing. I would like to arrange a chest X-ray and lymph node biopsy.

## General Points

| | | | | | |
|---|---|---|---|---|---|
| Polite to patient | | | | | |
| Maintains good eye contact | | | | | |
| Appropriate use of open and closed questions | | | | | |
| No or limited use of medical jargon | | | | | |

## ❓ QUESTIONS FROM THE EXAMINER

### What is the name of the pathognomonic cell that is seen on microscopy in Hodgkin's disease?

The Reed–Sternberg cell, which is a giant cell, and visible on microscopy.

### Broadly classify the causes of anaemia.

Increased blood loss or red-cell breakdown, defective (dietary) or inadequate (marrow failure) production of red blood cells. It is also acceptable to classify anaemia histologically in terms of the mean corpuscular volume (MCV) – low, high or normal MCV.

### List some common causes of iron-deficiency anaemia.

The common causes stem from gastrointestinal (GI) blood loss and include peptic ulceration, cancer anywhere in the GI tract, drugs such as aspirin, non-steroidal anti-inflammatory drugs (NSAIDs) or anticoagulants, and hereditary diseases such as angiodysplasia and hereditary haemorrhagic telangiectasia.

## What do you understand by the terms lymphoproliferative disorder and myeloproliferative disorder?

In lymphoproliferative disorder there are excessive quantities of lymphocytes. There are two main groups of lymphocytes, B cells and T cells.

Myeloproliferative disorders are a group of heterogeneous disorders where bone marrow precursor cells develop in excessive quantities or are forced out of the bone marrow by fibrous tissue.

## What are hypersegmented neutrophils? What conditions might they occur in?

A hypersegmented neutrophil is one with increased number of lobes. As a neutrophil matures, the number of lobes it has increases; however, this is usually to three or four.

Hypersegmented neutrophils are commonly seen in megaloblastic anaemia and in folate or vitamin $B_{12}$ deficiency.

## What is the difference between leukaemia and lymphoma?

Leukaemias and lymphomas are both types of cancer. Leukaemia cancers start in the bone marrow. Lymphoma is cancer of the lymphatic system.

## What is the difference between acute and chronic leukaemia? What age groups do they affect?

In acute leukaemia the abnormal blast cells rapidly increase in number and remain very immature. The disease gets worse rapidly. It can affect both children and adults, although it is commonly seen in children and young adults.

In chronic leukaemia the abnormal blast cells are present but tend to be more mature. The disease gets worse more slowly. It can affect both children and adults, although is more commonly seen in adults over the age of 50.

## How are the lymphomas broadly classified?

There are several ways that lymphomas can be commonly classified, typically either as Hodgkin's or non-Hodgkin's, or alternatively as B- or T-cell lymphoma.

## How would you investigate microcytic anaemia?

Initial investigations should include: FBC, clotting screen, liver function tests (LFTs) and a blood film. Further investigations depend on the underlying cause. This can include endoscopy (to exclude upper GI bleed) or abdominal ultrasound scan (to exclude intra-abdominal bleeding).

## How would you investigate macrocytic anaemia?

Initial investigations should include FBC, clotting screen, vitamin $B_{12}$ and folate levels. Further investigations depend on the underlying causes. This can include tissue transglutaminase (to rule out Crohn's disease), anti-intrinsic factor (to rule out pernicious anaemia) and bone marrow aspiration.

## Station 1.2    Weight Loss

### Doctor Briefing

You are a junior doctor in primary care and have been asked to see Aysha Patel, a 64-year-old woman, who has presented with weight loss. She has lost 13 kg over the last 6 weeks and is very concerned by this. She has a history of hypertension, angina and gastro-oesophageal reflux disease (GORD). Please take a history from Mrs Patel, present your findings and formulate an appropriate management plan.

### Patient Briefing

You are a 64-year-old woman visiting your doctor. You have noticed a significant weight loss of 13 kg over the last 6 weeks. You have not been trying to lose weight. Your family has noticed that your face is looking skinnier and sallow.

You have been a bit constipated. You have not had any fever symptoms. You do not have night sweats. You have been more fatigued than usual and have taken several sick days from work for exhaustion.

You previously smoked one pack of cigarettes a day for 20 years, but quit after being diagnosed with type 2 diabetes when you were 44. You also have high blood pressure, angina and GORD.

Your father died aged 49 from pancreatic cancer. Your paternal grandmother died aged 51 from pancreatic cancer. Your mother is still alive, aged 85.

You take metformin, amlodipine, aspirin and lansoprazole and have a glyceryl trinitrate (GTN) spray for when needed. Your diet is balanced but you have noticed a reduction in appetite recently. You are widowed and live alone. You have not been travelling recently (>3 years).

You are very concerned by this sudden drop in weight and are worried that there is something seriously wrong.

### Mark Scheme for Examiner

| Introduction | | | | | | |
|---|---|---|---|---|---|---|
| Cleans hands, introduces self, confirms patient identity and gains consent for history taking | | | | | | |
| Establishes current patient knowledge and concerns | | | | | | |

**History of Presenting Complaint**

| Question | Justification | Answer | Thoughts | | | |
|---|---|---|---|---|---|---|
| How much weight have you lost and over what period of time has this occurred? What is your normal body weight? | It is important to ascertain the precise amount of weight loss and what percentage this is relative to the patient's usual body weight. This will inform the severity of weight loss and may give diagnostic clues | '13 kg over the last 6 weeks. I'm normally 66 kg' | This amount of weight loss requires further investigation | | | |
| Have you been intentionally trying to lose weight? | Ascertaining if this weight loss is intentional is important as it may offer an immediate explanation for the weight loss | 'No' | This suggests there may be an underlying pathology responsible for the weight loss | | | |
| Have you noticed any changes in appetite? | Changes in appetite can help distinguish between different potential differential diagnoses for sudden rapid weight loss | 'I've been less hungry than usual' | This reduction in appetite helps to order potential differential diagnoses | | | |
| Do you have a fever, or have you had any fever symptoms recently? | Certain pathological causes of weight loss are associated with fever, such as HIV or tuberculosis | 'No' | Suggests infectious causes are less likely | | | |

## History of Presenting Complaint

| Question | Justification | Answer | Thoughts | | | | |
|---|---|---|---|---|---|---|---|
| Have you noticed any changes in bowel habits or changes to your stool as regards consistency or a particular smell? | Bowel habit changes occur with various causes of weight loss. For example, malabsorption is associated with steatorrhoea | 'I've been a bit constipated' | This may increase clinical suspicion of a malignancy of the abdomen | | | | |
| Have you noticed you've been more tired than usual? | Fatigue is associated with various causes of weight loss. Malabsorption, HIV, malignancy and depression can all present with fatigue | 'Yes. I've had to take some sick days off work' | Owing to the range of potential differential diagnoses presenting with fatigue, more exploration is required | | | | |
| Have you been having any night sweats? | Night sweats can be associated with tuberculosis and some malignancies, such as lymphoma | 'No' | No additional concerns | | | | |
| Have you noticed any changes in your urinary habits? | Some causes of weight loss can also be associated with urinary habit changes, such as polyuria in diabetes | 'No' | No additional concerns | | | | |

## Past Medical History

| Question | Justification | Answer | Thoughts | | | | |
|---|---|---|---|---|---|---|---|
| Do you have chronic medical conditions? | Some medical conditions may explain the patient's sudden weight loss | 'I have had type 2 diabetes for 20 years, but this is well controlled. I also have high blood pressure, angina and GORD' | Diabetes mellitus can cause weight loss; however, given the length of time since the diagnosis and the good control, this is a less likely explanation for her sudden weight loss | | | | |
| Do you have any history of cancer? | An existing diagnosis of a malignancy could suggest this weight loss presentation is associated with further metastatic spread. A previous diagnosis of malignancy could suggest recurrence | 'No' | No additional concerns | | | | |
| Have you had any recent surgery or any operations in the past? | Surgery can lead to malabsorption as a complication | 'No' | No additional concerns | | | | |

## Drug History

| Question | Justification | Answer | Thoughts | | | | |
|---|---|---|---|---|---|---|---|
| Are you on any regular medications for any conditions? | Important to check for contraindications in the potential management plan, or if certain medications may be causing iatrogenic effects explaining the symptoms | 'I take amlodipine, metformin, aspirin and lansoprazole' | Metformin can be an appetite suppressant, though the patient has been on this medication for a long time | | | | |

**Drug History**

| Question | Justification | Answer | Thoughts | | | | |
|---|---|---|---|---|---|---|---|
| Do you take any herbal supplements or vitamins? | Always ask. Various herbal and alternative treatments can have potentially harmful systemic side effects | 'No' | No additional concerns | | | | |
| Do you have any allergies? | Important for potential management plans | 'No' | No additional concerns | | | | |

**Family History**

| Question | Justification | Answer | Thoughts | | | | |
|---|---|---|---|---|---|---|---|
| Is there a history of cancer in your family? | Family history of malignancy may render malignancy a more likely differential diagnosis, particularly if the cancer is known to have a strong heritable component | 'My dad and grandad passed away from pancreatic cancer when they were pretty young' | Significant immediate family history of a malignancy is a very important risk factor | | | | |
| Do you have any family history of infections such as tuberculosis? | This is more significant for immediate family with whom the patient may be in close contact. Tuberculosis is an important cause of weight loss that requires exclusion | 'No' | Less likely to be an infectious cause or tuberculosis | | | | |

**Social and Travel History**

| Question | Justification | Answer | Thoughts | | | | |
|---|---|---|---|---|---|---|---|
| Do you currently live with anyone? | Always important to ascertain home support network for management plans | 'I live alone' | Important to ensure patient feels supported and is independent in her activities of daily living | | | | |
| How is your diet? | Poor diet and nutritional deficiencies may cause weight loss | 'It's well balanced' | No additional concerns | | | | |
| Do you drink alcohol? | Excess alcohol consumption is a risk factor for some malignancies | 'No' | No additional concerns | | | | |
| Do you smoke? | Smoking is a risk factor for various causes of weight loss, including malignancy | 'I used to but quit after I was diagnosed with diabetes. I smoked a pack a day for 20 years' | 20-pack-year smoking history increases risk of malignancy | | | | |
| Do you take any recreational drugs? | Recreational drug use can have important implications for management plan | 'No' | No additional concerns | | | | |
| Have you recently travelled abroad? | Some tropical infections can cause chronic GI infection and weight loss | 'No.' | No additional concerns | | | | |

## Systems Review

| Question | Justification | Answer | Thoughts | | | | | |
|---|---|---|---|---|---|---|---|---|
| Have you had any nausea or vomiting? | Nausea and vomiting can be associated with infectious causes of weight loss | 'No' | No additional concerns | | | | | |
| Have you had any difficulties swallowing? | Swallowing difficulties can explain reduced intake and reduced appetite | 'No' | No additional concerns | | | | | |
| Have you had any breathlessness? | Conditions that cause breathlessness can cause weight loss. This can be because of difficulty eating owing to the breathlessness, or reduced appetite | 'No' | No additional concerns | | | | | |
| Have you had any heat intolerance, palpitations or noticed a tremor? | Important to ask about symptoms of hyperthyroidism as this can cause weight loss | 'No' | No additional concerns | | | | | |
| How is your mood? | Important to ask about mood and if necessary to follow up by asking about the cardinal symptoms of depression, as depression can cause appetite changes that can lead to weight loss | 'It's good. I'm generally pretty happy' | No additional concerns | | | | | |

## Finishing the Consultation

| | | | | | | | | |
|---|---|---|---|---|---|---|---|---|
| Is there anything that I've missed, or anything that you are particularly concerned about? | May identify useful information that has been missed. Will also help when framing communication with the patient | 'I think that's all' | Take the time to explain what will happen from here | | | | | |
| Do you have any questions for me at the moment? | | | | | | | | |

## Present Your Findings

Mrs Patel is a 64-year-old woman who has presented with rapid weight loss, loss of appetite and changes in bowel habit over the last 8 weeks. She has unintentionally lost 13 kg over the last 6 weeks and has been constipated. She does not have any symptoms of fever, nausea or vomiting and has not recently been travelling. She has hypertension, type 2 diabetes, angina and GORD. Two family members have died due to pancreatic cancer.

My main differential diagnosis would be a malignancy of the abdomen, specifically pancreatic cancer. I would also consider malabsorption, or infectious causes such as tuberculosis.

I would like to investigate with a computed tomography (CT) abdomen scan and run blood tests to look for malignancy markers, such as CA19-9

| General Points | | | | |
|---|---|---|---|---|
| Polite to patient | | | | |
| Maintains good eye contact | | | | |
| Appropriate use of open and closed questions | | | | |
| No or limited use of medical jargon | | | | |

## ❓ QUESTIONS FROM THE EXAMINER

### What are the major risk factors for developing pancreatic cancer?

Age, lifestyle factors (including smoking, alcohol use, diet, obesity) and genetic factors (Peutz–Jeghers syndrome, *PALB2*, *BRCA1/2* and *FAMM* genes) can all be involved in the development of family cancer syndromes.

### What is the prognosis of pancreatic cancer?

Pancreatic cancer has a very poor prognosis. The 5-year survival is very low, at ~5–10%. A key reason for this is the late stage of presentation of many patients as symptoms can be silent in earlier stages of disease.

### What is TNM staging?

TNM staging varies between cancers, as cancer development follows different patterns in different cancers. Generally, T refers to tumour size and progression (Tis, 1, 2, 3, 4), N refers to lymph node involvement (0, 1, 2) and M refers to the presence/absence of metastasis in a binary manner (0, 1).

### What is the relationship between pancreatitis and pancreatic cancer?

Chronic pancreatitis is associated with a two- to threefold increase in risk of pancreatic cancer.

### What is the UK national screening programme for bowel cancer?

All individuals aged 60–74, living in England, and registered with a general practitioner (GP), are automatically sent a bowel cancer screening kit every 2 years. The kit is a faecal immunochemical test.

### What body mass index (BMI) is usually considered the cut-off for anorexia nervosa?

<17.5.

### What are some common chemotherapy drugs used to treat pancreatic cancer?

Oxiplatin, fluorouracil and folinic acid.

### Give three types of imaging that may be used to help diagnose pancreatic cancer.

Magnetic resonance imaging (MRI), CT (positron emission tomography (PET) CT) and endoscopic ultrasound scan.

### Name three potential causes of pancreatitis.

Abdominal surgery, gallstones, hypercalcaemia, hypertriglyceridaemia, infections and cystic fibrosis.

### Discuss the blood supply to the pancreas.

The head of the pancreas is supplied by the superior and inferior pancreaticoduodenal arteries, while the splenic artery supplies the left body and tail of the pancreas. The head of the pancreas drains into the superior mesenteric and portal veins, while the body and neck of the pancreas drain into the splenic vein.

## Station 1.3   Chest Pain

### Doctor Briefing

You are a junior doctor working in the emergency department (ED) and you have been asked to see Amy Jones. She is a 60-year-old woman who presented with a 2-h history of central chest pain, shortness of breath and sweating. Please take a history, present your findings and formulate an appropriate management plan.

### Patient Briefing

You are a 60-year-old woman attending the ED as you have been having intermittent central chest pain accompanied by shortness of breath and sweating. The pain feels like a central crushing pain, and you also feel this in your neck, left arm and shoulders. You recall feeling chest pain after climbing the stairs in your house or after walking to the supermarket. This pain subsides after resting for several minutes. During these episodes you also feel breathless and sometimes nauseous.

Upon specific questioning about past medical history, you report that you have hypertension which is reasonably well controlled on amlodipine.

Upon specific questioning about family history, you report that your mother is alive and well, aged 84, but your father passed away from a sudden heart attack aged 60.

Upon specific questioning about smoking and alcohol use, you mention you have smoked 20 cigarettes a day for 20 years but do not drink alcohol.

You are very concerned as you have never had these symptoms before, and you would like to understand what is causing them.

### Mark Scheme for Examiner

#### Introduction

| | | | | | |
|---|---|---|---|---|---|
| Cleans hands, introduces self, confirms patient identity and gains consent for history taking | | | | | |
| Establishes current patient knowledge and concerns | | | | | |

#### History of Presenting Complaint

| Question | Justification | Answer | Thoughts | | |
|---|---|---|---|---|---|
| Have you ever had episodes like this before? | If the patient has had this pain investigated previously, that information can be useful for diagnosis | 'Never' | This is new-onset intermittent chest pain suggesting a new pathology | | |
| Could you tell me/point to where the pain is felt during these episodes? | Ascertaining the specific site of pain gives indications as to the cause. For example, central crushing pain is suggestive of myocardial infarction (MI), whereas retrosternal pain may suggest GORD, biliary colic or MI as well | 'I feel it in my chest (points to centre of chest)' | Central chest pain radiating to the described locations is suggestive of acute coronary syndrome (ACS) | | |
| Does anything in particular trigger the pain? | Pain after exertion is more suggestive of angina pectoris. Pain on lying down may suggest pericarditis | 'It usually comes on after walking up the stairs or going to the supermarket' | Onset of chest pain on exertion is indicative of angina pectoris | | |

## History of Presenting Complaint

| Question | Justification | Answer | Thoughts | | | | | |
|---|---|---|---|---|---|---|---|---|
| Could you describe the nature/character of the pain? | Different characters suggest different diagnoses | 'Crushing pain' | Character of pain is highly variable so whilst it supports current thinking, in and of itself it is not indicative of a particular diagnosis | | | | | |
| Do you feel pain anywhere other than the chest during these episodes? | Where pain radiates gives clues to diagnosis. For example, radiation to the back may suggest aortic dissection | 'Left arm, neck and shoulders' | Consistent with ACS. Starting to build a more typical picture of angina pectoris | | | | | |
| Do you have any other symptoms during these episodes? (Ask about breathlessness, nausea, fever, syncope, sweating) | Associated symptoms during episodes again give indications to diagnosis. Palpitations may suggest electrophysiological issues or fever may suggest pericarditis | 'I get quite breathless and a bit nauseous, but they both subside' | Additional symptoms that are in keeping with a variety of conditions therefore need more information. | | | | | |
| How long do the episodes last? | Continuous versus intermittent gives clues to pathology. MIs are typically continuous pain, whereas angina pectoris comes and goes in cycles of exertion and rest | 'As long as I'm walking around' | Walking or exercise seems to bring on the pain. | | | | | |
| How long have you been having these episodes? | Ascertaining the initial onset of these episodes is important in order to recognise how long the patient has been living with these symptoms | 'Several months now' | Ongoing problem that is not self resolving is concerning. | | | | | |
| Does anything make the pain worse? | Exacerbating factors such as lying flat may suggest pericarditis. Or worse on inspiration may suggest pulmonary embolism (PE) | 'Exercise, I suppose' | Exercise is a possible exacerbating factor of the underlying cause. | | | | | |
| Does anything make the pain better? | In angina, rest/GTN spray often makes the pain better. In MI typically there is little that improves the pain | 'After I've sat down for a few minutes I feel better' | Less likely to be an MI. | | | | | |
| On a scale of 1–10, how severe would you say the pain is during the episodes? | Gives an indication of the severity of the pathology | '8' | Clearly a very debilitating symptom | | | | | |

## Past Medical History

| Question | Justification | Answer | Thoughts | | | | | |
|---|---|---|---|---|---|---|---|---|
| Do you have any history of heart disease? | Previous ischaemic heart disease predisposes to various cardiac sequelae | 'No' | No additional concerns | | | | | |

**Past Medical History**

| Question | Justification | Answer | Thoughts | | | | |
|---|---|---|---|---|---|---|---|
| Do you have hypertension or high cholesterol? | Hypertension and hypercholesterolaemia are both risk factors for heart disease | 'I have high blood pressure, not sure about cholesterol' | Hypertension is a risk factor for ischamic heart disease | | | | |
| Do you have any history of acid reflux or swallowing problems? | Whilst these may be lower down the differential list by this stage, they are still important differentials for chest pain | 'Not that I know of' | No additional concerns | | | | |
| Do you have any other chronic medical conditions? | Comorbidities have implications for both diagnosis and management of heart disease | 'No' | No additional concerns | | | | |
| Have you ever had any surgical operations? | Previous heart operations could give clues to the diagnosis | 'I had my appendix out when I was a teenager' | No additional concerns | | | | |

**Drug History**

| Question | Justification | Answer | Thoughts | | | | |
|---|---|---|---|---|---|---|---|
| Are you on any regular medications? | Important to check for contraindications in potential management plan, or to check if certain medications may be causing iatrogenic effects explaining the symptoms | 'Just amlodipine' | Need to check adequate control of blood pressure | | | | |
| Do you have any allergies? | Always ask. Important for potential management plans | 'Shellfish and peanuts' | No additional concerns | | | | |

**Family History**

| Question | Justification | Answer | Thoughts | | | | |
|---|---|---|---|---|---|---|---|
| Has anyone in your family suffered from heart or cardiovascular disease? Do you have any siblings and has anyone passed away under the age of 50? | Family history of heart disease is a significant risk factor for heart disease. Family history of deaths of first-degree relatives under the age of 50 is significant to the medical history | 'My father died from a heart attack aged 60. I don't have any siblings. I'm not aware of anyone dying at a young age.' | Significant immediate family history is an important risk factor | | | | |
| Do you have any family history of other medical conditions? | Other hereditary medical conditions may impact management plans or reveal other possible risk factors for heart disease | 'Mum has type 2 diabetes' | No additional concerns | | | | |

## Social and Travel History

| Question | Justification | Answer | Thoughts | | | | | |
|---|---|---|---|---|---|---|---|---|
| Do you currently live with anyone? | Always important to ascertain home support network for management plans | 'I live with my husband' | Support system in place at home if necessary, for management plan | | | | | |
| Have you had any difficulties at work? | Gives insight into the extent of disability that the condition may be causing | 'I'm retired' | No additional concerns | | | | | |
| Do you drink alcohol? | Excess alcohol consumption is a risk factor for heart disease | 'No' | No additional concerns | | | | | |
| Do you smoke? | Smoking is a risk factor for heart disease | 'Yes. 20 a day for over 20 years' | Significant smoking history is a risk factor for ischaemic heart disease | | | | | |
| How is your diet? | Poor diet is a risk factor for high cholesterol, obesity and cardiovascular disease generally | 'It's OK, but I am overweight' | Lifestyle advice should be given | | | | | |

## Systems Review

| Question | Justification | Answer | Thoughts | | | | | |
|---|---|---|---|---|---|---|---|---|
| Does the pain ever come on after eating food or drinking? | Important to exclude GORD | 'No' | No additional concerns | | | | | |
| Do you ever get short of breath after low levels of exercise? | Important to exclude respiratory problems either concurrently with cardiovascular problems, or on their own | 'No' | No additional concerns | | | | | |
| Just to check, have you had any problems with bladder or bowel function? | Find out if there are any wider concerns that have not arisen yet | 'No, they have been normal' | No additional concerns | | | | | |
| Have you had any recent night sweats, fever, weight loss or fatigue? | It is essential to ask about B symptoms to rule out certain causes, such as infection | 'No' | No additional concerns | | | | | |

## Finishing the Consultation

| Question | Justification | Answer | Thoughts | | | | | |
|---|---|---|---|---|---|---|---|---|
| Is there anything that I've missed, or anything that you are particularly concerned about? | May identify useful information that has been missed. Will also help when framing communication with the patient | 'I think that's all' | Take the time to explain what will happen from here | | | | | |
| Do you have any questions for me at the moment? | | | | | | | | |

**Present Your Findings**

Mrs Jones is a 60-year-old woman who presents with intermittent chest pain and breathlessness that is brought on by exertion. The pain is central and crushing and radiates to the left arm, neck and shoulders. The episodes are relieved after resting for several minutes after exertion. She has some breathlessness and nausea during the episodes, and she describes the pain as 8/10 during the episodes.

My main differential would be stable angina pectoris. It would be useful to rule out unstable angina, MI or GORD.

I would like to take a collateral history and discuss pharmacological and lifestyle management with Mrs Jones. Pharmacological management could include GTN, nicorandil or ivabradine, whilst lifestyle management includes exercise, dietary advice and cessation of smoking. I would also like to arrange for several investigations, including an electrocardiogram (ECG) and exercise ECG

**General Points**

Polite to patient

Maintains good eye contact

Appropriate use of open and closed questions

No or limited use of medical jargon

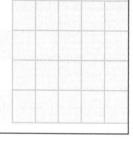

## ❓ QUESTIONS FROM THE EXAMINER

### What are the three key features of angina?

- Constricting or heavy discomfort to the chest, jaw, neck, shoulders or arms
- Symptoms brought on by exertion
- Symptoms relieved within 5 min by rest or GTN

### What is Prinzmetal angina?

Also termed vasospastic angina, variant angina or angina inversa. It occurs due to coronary artery spasm, and typically the chest pain occurs during rest. Probable triggers include recreational drug use (cocaine, marijuana, smoking, stress, exposure to cold weather, amphetamines), hypomagnesaemia and artery instrumentation (for example, during angiography)

### Give two common side effects of GTN.

- Headaches
- Hypotension
- Flushing or redness of skin
- Dizziness
- Nausea or vomiting

### What is the mechanism of action of ivabradine?

It lowers heart rate by selectively and specifically inhibiting the 'funny current' ($I_f$ pacemaker current). The current is a mixed sodium–potassium inward current that controls spontaneous diastolic depolarisation in the sinoatrial node.

### What is the mechanism of action of nicorandil?

It is a dual-action potassium channel opener, promoting $K^+$ efflux and inhibiting voltage-gated calcium channels.

### Give three non-pharmacological interventions to consider in the treatment of angina.

- Cessation of smoking
- Exercise
- Dietary advice

**What is the standard dose of aspirin to give as secondary prevention for cardiovascular disease?**

75 mg daily.

**Give three precipitants other than exercise that may cause an episode of angina.**

- Cold weather
- Heavy meals
- Emotion

**With regards to the fundamental pathology, what is the difference in the occluding thrombus in a non-ST elevation MI (NSTEMI) compared with an ST elevation MI (STEMI)?**

In an NSTEMI, the thrombus is subocclusive (or occasionally transiently occlusive), whereas in a STEMI, the thrombus is completely occlusive.

**Give two examples of functional imaging for angina.**

Myocardial perfusion scintigraphy and stress echocardiography (echocardiogram during exercise or dobutamine infusion).

## Station 1.4   Palpitations

### Doctor Briefing

You are a junior doctor working in the ED and are asked to see Jane Porter, a 29-year-old woman, who has presented with palpitations. She has had a number of previous similar episodes, lasting a few minutes each time. Please take a history from Miss Porter, present your findings and formulate an appropriate management plan.

### Patient Briefing

You are a 29-year-old woman attending the ED. You present with episodes of 'fluttering in your chest'. The episodes occur a couple of times a day, and each of the episodes lasts for around 5 min. The episodes are accompanied by some shortness of breath, chest discomfort and sweating.

Upon specific questioning about exacerbating factors for the episodes, say that they tend to start at particularly stressful times during the workday.

Upon specific questioning about past medical history, you report that you have asthma and previously had moderate depression for 3 years.

Upon specific questioning about family history, you report your mother and father are both alive and well and there is no history of cardiovascular history in the family; however, your sister has asthma.

Upon specific questioning about smoking and alcohol use, you mention you have never smoked but drink several times a week with colleagues. Your diet is healthy and balanced.

You are concerned, as these symptoms have come on suddenly.

### Mark Scheme for Examiner

#### Introduction

| | | | | |
|---|---|---|---|---|
| Cleans hands, introduces self, confirms patient identity and gains consent for history taking | | | | |
| Establishes current patient knowledge and concerns | | | | |

#### History of Presenting Complaint

| Question | Justification | Answer | Thoughts | | | |
|---|---|---|---|---|---|---|
| When did you start having these episodes? | Important to discover if this is a long-standing or recent symptom, as this gives a clue to the duration of the underlying pathology | 'A month ago' | Likely to be a more recent underlying cause | | | |
| Have you ever had episodes like this before? | If the patient has had these symptoms investigated previously, that information can be useful for diagnosis | 'Other than the last month, never' | New onset – will need thorough history to discover cause | | | |
| Does anything specifically bring on the episodes? | Triggers can give a clue to the diagnosis. For example, alcohol and caffeine use can cause palpitations | 'Usually on days when work is more stressful' | Suggests anxiety may be an underlying cause of the palpitations | | | |
| Does anything make them better or worse? | Certain exacerbating and relieving factors give clues to the diagnosis. For example, if vagal manoeuvres improve the symptoms, then paroxysmal supraventricular tachycardia is a potential diagnosis | 'Not really' | No additional concerns | | | |

## History of Presenting Complaint

| Question | Justification | Answer | Thoughts | | | | |
|---|---|---|---|---|---|---|---|
| Could you use your hand to tap out the rhythm of the palpitations? | Determining the rate and rhythm of the palpitations can give clues to the diagnosis. For example, skipped beats suggest 'ectopic beats' | (Tap a regular, tachycardic rhythm) | The regular tapping potentially rules out certain diagnoses. However, it is insufficient on its own to give a clue to the diagnosis | | | | |
| How long does each episode usually last? | Duration gives clues to diagnosis. For example, short durations may be indicative of supraventricular tachycardia, whilst episodes that come and go gradually may suggest anxiety | 'A couple of minutes' | No additional concerns | | | | |
| How many times a day do you have these episodes? | Important to ascertain the severity and how debilitating the symptoms are to everyday life | 'A few times a day, but only on a handful of days in the month' | Irregular nature suggests there may be a specific trigger | | | | |
| Do you experience any other symptoms during the episodes? Specific questioning about syncope, breathlessness, abdominal discomfort and nausea | Associated symptoms are key in this history owing to the wide range of potential causes. Breathlessness and syncope are more indicative of cardiac causes, whilst abdominal pain may suggest phaeochromocytoma | 'I feel a bit breathless, but nothing else' | This fits with the current thinking of anxiety. However, a more detailed history is necessary | | | | |

## Past Medical History

| Question | Justification | Answer | Thoughts | | | | |
|---|---|---|---|---|---|---|---|
| Do you have any existing heart conditions? | A known heart condition could explain the current palpitations; for example, a diagnosis of Wolff–Parkinson–White (WPW) syndrome | 'No' | No additional concerns | | | | |
| Have you ever had any thyroid illnesses? | Hyperthyroidism is a potential cause of palpitations | 'No' | No additional concerns | | | | |
| Do you have any other chronic medical conditions? | Comorbidities have implications for both diagnosis and management of the condition | 'No' | No additional concerns | | | | |
| Have you ever had any surgical operations? | Previous heart operations could give clues to the diagnosis | 'I had an operation for a broken leg when I was 10' | No additional concerns | | | | |

## Drug History

| Question | Justification | Answer | Thoughts | | | | | |
|---|---|---|---|---|---|---|---|---|
| Are you on any regular medications for any conditions? | Important to check for contraindications in the potential management plan, or to check if certain medications may be causing iatrogenic effects explaining the symptoms. Very rarely there are iatrogenic causes of palpitations from asthma medications, such as theophylline | 'I take the combined oral contraceptive pill' | No additional concerns | | | | | |
| Do you take any herbal supplements or vitamins? | Various herbal and alternative treatments can have potentially harmful systemic side effects | 'No' | No additional concerns | | | | | |
| Do you have any allergies? | Important for potential management plans | 'Peanuts' | No additional concerns | | | | | |

## Family History

| Question | Justification | Answer | Thoughts | | | | | |
|---|---|---|---|---|---|---|---|---|
| Has anyone in your family suffered from heart or cardiovascular disease, or have a heart condition? Do you have any siblings and has anyone passed away under the age of 50? | Family history of heart disease is a significant risk factor for heart disease. Family history of deaths of first-degree relatives under the age of 50 is significant to the medical history. In particular, sudden death is important to see if there is a history of cardiomyopathy or supraventricular tachycardia | Both my parents are alive and healthy. I have a sister who is well. I don't think anyone in my family has heart disease' | The lack of cardiac family history suggests it is less likely to be a hereditary underlying cause | | | | | |
| Do you have any family history of other medical conditions? | Other hereditary medical conditions may impact management plans or reveal other possible risk factors for the underlying pathology | 'Both my parents are healthy. My sister has asthma' | No additional concerns | | | | | |

## Social and Travel History

| Question | Justification | Answer | Thoughts | | | | | |
|---|---|---|---|---|---|---|---|---|
| Do you currently live with anyone? | Always important to ascertain home support network for management plans | 'I live with my partner and children' | Support system in place at home if necessary, for management plan | | | | | |
| Are you currently employed? | An insight into the work and potential work stresses is particularly relevant to this history. Palpitations can be precipitated by anxiety | 'Yes, I work as an investment banker in a big city firm' | Her job is likely to be stressful. Important to discuss further any specific stresses as triggers | | | | | |

## Social and Travel History

| Question | Justification | Answer | Thoughts | | | | |
|---|---|---|---|---|---|---|---|
| Do you drink alcohol? | Heavy or chronic alcohol consumption can precipitate palpitations | 'I have a couple of pints after work but nothing more' | Potential trigger to consider in the management plan | | | | |
| Do you drink caffeinated beverages? | Caffeine can precipitate palpitations. This is not only coffee; it includes energy drinks! | 'I have one coffee every morning and sometimes a Red Bull in the evening if I'm working late' | Potential trigger to consider in the management plan | | | | |
| Do you smoke? | Smoking is a risk factor for a range of conditions that could be causing the palpitations, including heart disease | 'No' | No additional concerns | | | | |
| Do you take any recreational drugs? | Recreational drug use such as cocaine and amphetamines can precipitate palpitations and cardiac conditions | 'No' | No additional concerns | | | | |

## Systems Review

| | | | | | | | |
|---|---|---|---|---|---|---|---|
| Have you had any abdominal discomfort or nausea? | Checking for abdominal causes of palpitations such as phaeochromocytomas | 'No' | No additional concerns | | | | |
| Have you noticed any recent hair loss, or have you been feeling particularly warm or cold recently? | Checking for thyroid causes of palpitations such as thyrotoxicosis | 'No' | No additional concerns | | | | |
| Just to check, have you had any problems with bladder or bowel function? | Find out if there are any wider concerns that have not arisen yet | 'No, they have been normal' | No additional concerns | | | | |
| Have you had any recent night sweats, fever, weight loss or fatigue? | It is essential to ask about B symptoms to rule out certain causes, such as infection | 'No' | No additional concerns | | | | |

## Finishing the Consultation

| | | | | | | | |
|---|---|---|---|---|---|---|---|
| Is there anything that I've missed, or anything that you are particularly concerned about? | May identify useful information that has been missed. Will also help when framing communication with the patient | 'I think that's all' | Take the time to explain what will happen from here | | | | |
| Do you have any questions for me at the moment? | | | | | | | |

### Present Your Findings

Miss Porter is a 29-year-old woman who presents with palpitations. The episodes occur a few times a day but not every day. The episodes last a couple of minutes each time, are regular, and there are no specific exacerbating or relieving factors. During the episodes she has some breathlessness but no syncope or abdominal discomfort.

My main differential would be palpitations caused by anxiety. It is also possible that caffeine and alcohol use are specific triggers of the episodes. I would like to rule out any cardiac or thyroid causes of the episodes.

I would like to take a collateral history and discuss pharmacological and lifestyle management with Miss Porter. Pharmacological management could include anxiolytic medications, although this should be referred to psychiatry for a more complete assessment. Lifestyle management includes avoiding potential triggers including caffeine and alcohol use. I would also like to arrange for several investigations to rule out other causes of the palpitations, including a 12-lead ECG and thyroid function tests

### General Points

| | | | |
|---|---|---|---|
| Polite to patient | | | |
| Maintains good eye contact | | | |
| Appropriate use of open and closed questions | | | |
| No or limited use of medical jargon | | | |

## ❓ QUESTIONS FROM THE EXAMINER

### Name three non-cardiac causes of palpitations.

Phaeochromocytoma, thyrotoxicosis and anxiety.

### Give two lifestyle management strategies you would give to a patient with palpitations.

Avoid caffeinated beverages (including coffee and energy drinks), alcohol and recreational drug use.

### What is WPW syndrome?

WPW is a pre-excitation syndrome involving an accessory pathway between the atria and ventricles. This results in an inappropriately fast impulse conduction between the atria and ventricles. On an ECG, WPW will often show a short PR interval and can show a delta wave and broad QRS complex.

### What is the mechanism of action of flecainide?

Flecainide is a class 1c antiarrhythmic. It blocks the Nav1.5 sodium cannel in the heart, reducing excitability.

### What is the mechanism of action of amiodarone?

Amiodarone is a class III antiarrhythmic. It blocks voltage-gated potassium channels (KCNH2) and voltage-gated calcium channels (CACNA2D2), therefore prolonging the repolarisation phase of the cardiac action potential.

### What is the difference between first- and second-degree atrioventricular block?

In first-degree atrioventricular block, there is a consistently prolonged PR interval. In second-degree atrioventricular block, the PR prolongation increases with every beat, until a whole complex is dropped.

### Give three recreational drugs that can precipitate palpitations.

Cocaine, amphetamines and ecstasy.

**What are the two main classes of ectopic (heart) beats?**

Premature atrial contraction and premature ventricular contraction.

**Why is family history of sudden death particularly important to look out for in a patient presenting with palpitations?**

Sudden arrhythmic death syndrome in the family history may be hereditary, as are certain cardiomyopathies, such as hypertrophic cardiomyopathy.

**The class 1a antiarrhythmics include quinidine and procainamide. What causes the common side effects of these drugs and how do they manifest?**

Anticholinergic effects can occur with class 1a antiarrhythmics. This can include tachycardia, blurred vision and dry mouth.

## Station 1.5  Cough

### Doctor Briefing

You are a junior doctor in primary care and have been asked to see Gerald Gordon, a 60-year-old man, who has presented with a 3-day history of a productive cough and has been finding it increasingly difficult to sleep and get around his house. He is a lifelong cigarette smoker. Please take a history from Mr Gordon, present your findings and formulate an appropriate management plan.

### Patient Briefing

You are a 60-year-old man visiting your doctor. You have noticed a worsening productive cough over the last 3 days that is accompanied by sharp chest pain when you breathe in. You bring up green phlegm when you cough (no blood), and nothing makes the cough better or worse. The pain is partially relieved by taking shallow breaths, but this makes you cough more. You have developed a fever and feel generally unwell.

You have known chronic obstructive pulmonary disease (COPD) for which you take salbutamol, tiotropium and Fostair. You also have hypertension and chronic kidney disease (CKD) and take ramipril and vitamin D tablets. Your COPD is usually well controlled, and you have never required hospital admission or ventilation support. You have not been in hospital recently, and have never had an operation. You have no known drug allergies.

You have no significant family history. You are a retired engineer and live with your son who doesn't have any similar symptoms. You used to smoke around 30 a day for about 20 years and drink around 4 pints of beer each weekend.

You are concerned about the pain in your chest.

### Mark Scheme for Examiner

#### Introduction

| | | | | |
|---|---|---|---|---|
| Cleans hands, introduces self, confirms patient identity and gains consent for history taking | | | | |
| Establishes current patient knowledge and concerns | | | | |

#### History of Presenting Complaint

| Question | Justification | Answer | Thoughts | | | |
|---|---|---|---|---|---|---|
| When did the cough start? | This helps to determine if this is acute or chronic | 'Three days ago' | Acute causes should be excluded | | | |
| Is the cough productive? If so, what colour is the sputum? | Green sputum may indicate an infective cause. Pink or red sputum may indicate blood is present, and prompt towards cardiac causes or a PE | 'Yes, green sputum' | May be indicative of an infective cause | | | |
| Have you had any episodes of coughing up blood? Have you unintentionally lost weight in the last few months? | It is important to ask directly about red-flag symptoms | 'No' | Reduced concern regarding malignancy | | | |
| Do you have any chest pain currently? | Cardiac causes such as heart failure, and respiratory causes (including PE and pneumonia) may be associated with chest pain. Malignancy is more likely to be painless | 'Yes, I get stabbing chest pain going through to my back' | Reduced concern regarding malignancy. Pain needs exploring further | | | |

## History of Presenting Complaint

| Question | Justification | Answer | Thoughts | | | | | |
|---|---|---|---|---|---|---|---|---|
| Does anything make the pain better or worse? | Pleuritic pain may be exacerbated by inhalation. Cardiac pain may be induced by increasing activity | 'It is worse when I cough and breathe in. Nothing makes it better' | The patient is describing pleuritic chest pain | | | | | |
| Do you have a fever? | The patient may have systemic features on an infection | 'Yes' | Likely to be an infective cause | | | | | |
| Have you noticed a wheeze? | Asthma and COPD may present with a wheeze | 'Yes, sometimes when I breathe out' | It is important to check the patient's past medical history | | | | | |
| Are you currently short of breath? | A COPD exacerbation, infection or cardiac causes may be associated with shortness of breath. It is important to assess severity and for respiratory failure | 'More than usual' | Assess for respiratory failure and if the patient needs more urgent treatment | | | | | |

## Past Medical History

| | | | | | | | | |
|---|---|---|---|---|---|---|---|---|
| Do you have any other medical problems? | The patient may have a previously diagnosed condition that may explain the symptoms | 'I have COPD, hypertension and CKD' | The patient may be experiencing an exacerbation of COPD | | | | | |
| Have you had any recent operations? | PE may be associated with recent surgery. The patient may have a hospital-acquired infection, which is likely to be from different organisms to those in the community | 'No' | No additional concerns | | | | | |
| Have you ever been admitted to hospital or required ventilation support for COPD? | It is important to assess the severity of the patient's conditions | 'No' | No additional concerns | | | | | |
| Do you have rescue packs at home for your COPD? | It is important to assess what treatment the patient has already tried | 'Yes, with steroids and antibiotics, but I haven't used any recently' | The patient hasn't yet taken any treatment for a COPD exacerbation | | | | | |

## Drug History

| | | | | | | | | |
|---|---|---|---|---|---|---|---|---|
| Are you currently taking any medication, or have any allergies? | This may indicate the severity of the patient's known medical conditions. Always ask about allergies as this may impact on management plans | 'Ramipril, salbutamol, tiotropium, Fostair and vitamin D. I have no allergies' | Note that the patient's COPD is controlled on second-line treatment | | | | | |

## Drug History

| Question | Justification | Answer | Thoughts | | | | |
|---|---|---|---|---|---|---|---|
| Are you prescribed oxygen for COPD? | This may indicate the severity of the patient's known medical conditions. It may further provide information as to whether the patient retains carbon dioxide | 'No' | No additional concerns | | | | |

## Family History

| Question | Justification | Answer | Thoughts | | | | |
|---|---|---|---|---|---|---|---|
| Are there any medical conditions which run in the family, including cancers and cardiovascular or respiratory disease? | Always check for relevant heritable conditions | 'Mum has type 2 diabetes' | No additional concerns. The patient's blood glucose levels can be screened | | | | |

## Social and Travel History

| Question | Justification | Answer | Thoughts | | | | |
|---|---|---|---|---|---|---|---|
| Do you currently live with anyone? Do they have similar symptoms? | If there is an infective cause, other household members may have similar symptoms | 'I live with my son, but he doesn't have any symptoms' | Other household members do not have infective symptoms | | | | |
| Have you travelled anywhere recently? | Infective organisms may differ depending on where the patient has travelled | 'No' | No additional concerns | | | | |
| Are you currently working? | Occupational causes of respiratory disease should be excluded, such as asbestosis and interstitial lung disease | 'I'm a retired engineer' | No additional concerns | | | | |
| Do you smoke? | Smoking is a risk factor for lung cancer and COPD | 'I used to smoke around 30 a day for about 20 years' | The patient has increased risk for COPD and lung cancer | | | | |
| What is your average weekly alcohol consumption? | It is important to assess the patient's wider cardiovascular risk factors | 'Around 4 pints on the weekend' | No additional concerns | | | | |

## Systems Review

| Question | Justification | Answer | Thoughts | | | | |
|---|---|---|---|---|---|---|---|
| Just to check, have you had any problems with bladder or bowel function? | Find out if there are any wider concerns that have not arisen yet | 'No, they have been normal' | No additional concerns | | | | |
| Have you had any recent night sweats, fever, weight loss or fatigue? | It is essential to ask about B symptoms to rule out certain causes, such as infection | 'No' | No additional concerns | | | | |

### Finishing the Consultation

| Question | Justification | Answer | Thoughts | | | | |
|---|---|---|---|---|---|---|---|
| Is there anything that I've missed, or anything that you are particularly concerned about? | May identify useful information that has been missed. Will also help when framing communication with the patient | 'I am just in a lot of pain and want help' | Take the time to explain what will happen from here | | | | |
| Do you have any questions for me at the moment? | | | | | | | |

### Present Your Findings

Mr Gordon is a 62-year-old man who presented with a 3-day history of a productive cough with green sputum on a background of known COPD maintained with salbutamol, Fostair and tiotropium. He described an associated pleuritic chest pain and fever. The patient has no red-flag symptoms for malignancy. He has a 20-pack-year smoking history and no relevant family or occupational history.

My main differential is an infective exacerbation of COPD. My differential diagnoses include community-acquired pneumonia and congestive heart failure.

I would like to do a respiratory and cardiovascular system examination on Mr Gordon. I will also take sputum cultures, conduct an arterial blood gas and perform a chest X-ray

### General Points

| | | | | |
|---|---|---|---|---|
| Polite to patient | | | | |
| Maintains good eye contact | | | | |
| Appropriate use of open and closed questions | | | | |
| No or limited use of medical jargon | | | | |

## ❓ QUESTIONS FROM THE EXAMINER

### What is the mechanism of action of penicillin?

Penicillin kills bacteria through binding the beta-lactam ring to DD-transpeptidase, preventing new cell wall formation. This causes the bacteria cell to die.

### What is the mechanism of action of ceftriaxone?

Ceftriaxone irreversibly inhibits bacterial cell wall synthesis. It binds to transpeptidases, similar to penicillin.

### Give three potential complications of pneumonia.

Pleurisy, pleural effusions, empyema, lung abscess and sepsis.

### In paediatric patients, what is the main symptom that distinguishes severity of pneumonia?

Extent of tachypnoea.

### What is the principle of a non-rebreather mask?

A non-rebreather mask fully covers the patient's nose and mouth with a seal. When the patient inhales, he breathes in the pure oxygen within the bag attached to the mask. Exhaled air is removed from the mask through a one-way valve, preventing re-inhalation of exhaled air. Typically, oxygen is delivered at a rate of 15 L/min using this mask.

## What is the principle of a Venturi mask?

The Venturi mask allows a known oxygen concentration to be delivered to patients at a prespecified $Fio_2$. There are various holes in the mask that allow exhaled air to be released easily, preventing rebreathing of exhaled air.

## In what group of patients should a follow-up chest X-ray be taken following the resolution of pneumonia?

Persistent symptoms, smoker and age >50 years.

## What is Bernoulli's principle?

Bernoulli's principle is rooted in fluid dynamics. Effectively, it describes the inverse relationship between pressure and speed at a point in a fluid. Higher-pressure regions within a fluid have a lower speed, whilst lower-pressure regions have a higher fluid speed.

## Which group of antivirals could be used to treat viral pneumonia?

Neuraminidase inhibitors.

## What might be seen on physical examination of a patient with pneumonia?

Tachypnoea, low oxygen saturations, low blood pressure, tachycardia, pyrexia and crackles on stethoscope auscultation of the chest.

## Station 1.6   Shortness of Breath

### Doctor Briefing

You are a junior doctor on the acute medical take and have been asked to see Sophie Stark, a 59-year-old woman, who was referred by her primary care doctor with a 3-day history of worsening shortness of breath. This is associated with a productive cough, wheeze and difficulty walking up the stairs. Please take a history from Mrs Stark, present your findings and formulate an appropriate management plan.

### Patient Briefing

You are a 59-year-old woman who has been referred to hospital by your primary care doctor after you had noticed worsening breathlessness over the last few days. It occurs after very mild exercise (<100 m of walking and walking upstairs).

You have a past medical history of hypertension and asthma. Using your reliever inhaler improves the breathlessness, but it then worsens again after an hour. You have also had a productive cough over the same period and have sounded wheezy. You have been ill for the last few days with a fever. You have not coughed up any blood.

You take amlodipine to control your hypertension, and your blue inhaler when you really need it. You do not take any other medications. Your mother had asthma which was poorly controlled throughout her life. You have no other significant family history.

You were a smoker for 10 years during your 20s, smoking a pack of 20 cigarettes every day. You drink alcohol socially and do not take recreational drugs. Your diet is relatively balanced. You live with your partner at home.

You are concerned as the breathlessness is making it difficult to carry out normal activities of daily living.

### Mark Scheme for Examiner

#### Introduction

| | | | | |
|---|---|---|---|---|
| Cleans hands, introduces self, confirms patient identity and gains consent for history taking | | | | |
| Establishes current patient knowledge and concerns | | | | |

#### History of Presenting Complaint

| Question | Justification | Answer | Thoughts | | | | |
|---|---|---|---|---|---|---|---|
| How long have you had the breathlessness? | Gives an indication as to whether the shortness of breath is an acute or chronic problem | 'The last few days, but it has got worse today' | This is a new-onset problem, suggesting a gradual onset with an acute phase of worsening | | | | |
| Is the breathlessness constant or does it come and go? | Establishing if the problem is chronic or intermittent has important implications for diagnosis. For example, constant acute breathlessness may suggest an asthma attack or panic attack, whilst intermittent breathlessness may be associated with a particular exacerbating factor such as exercise in angina | 'I'm constantly more breathless than usual. Some things make it better and worse though' | Need to explore the relieving and exacerbating factors more | | | | |
| What sort of activities or actions make the breathlessness better or worse? | Certain exacerbating and relieving factors can point clearly to specific diagnoses. For example, if lying flat makes it worse and using multiple pillows to sleep helps, this may point towards heart failure | 'Walking makes it worse; rest and my inhaler make it better' | This suggests asthma may be the more likely differential diagnosis | | | | |

## History of Presenting Complaint

| Question | Justification | Answer | Thoughts | | | | |
|---|---|---|---|---|---|---|---|
| Have you noticed any changes in your exercise tolerance? | Gives insight into the severity of the problem. It is important to qualify the patient's description (distance of walking before stopping or breathlessness) | 'I get tired after about 100 m of walking. Before I could run 5 K' | This suggests the patient has had a deterioration in exercise tolerance | | | | |
| Do you have a cough? | Coughs are commonly associated with shortness of breath and must be enquired about | 'I have a cough and sometimes sound wheezy with it' | A wheeze is in keeping with asthma. Asthma can also present with a cough, but this is non-specific | | | | |
| Are you bringing anything up when you cough? If so, is there blood in it? | Productive cough may suggest bronchitis or infection. Non-productive cough may suggest asthma or allergies. Always establish if there is haemoptysis | 'I've been bringing up some mucus. There's no blood' | More reassuring that there is no haemoptysis | | | | |

## Past Medical History

| | | | | | | | |
|---|---|---|---|---|---|---|---|
| Do you have any chronic medical conditions? | Comorbidities have implications for diagnosis and management. Established diagnoses of respiratory disease may explain the patient's presentation. Various cardiac problems can also cause breathlessness | 'I have asthma and high blood pressure' | This makes an asthma attack a more likely diagnosis. However, the problem has occurred over several days, which perhaps suggests this is a general worsening of asthma preceding an attack | | | | |
| Have you had any recent surgery or been immobile for a long period of time, such as on a long-haul flight? | Surgery and prolonged immobility are risk factors for PE which could cause breathlessness | 'No' | No additional concerns | | | | |

## Drug History

| | | | | | | | |
|---|---|---|---|---|---|---|---|
| Are you on any regular medications? | Important to check for contraindications in potential management plan, or to check if certain medications may be causing iatrogenic effects explaining the symptoms. In known asthmatics, it is also important to check inhaler technique, if used | 'I take blood pressure tablets – amlodipine daily. I also use my blue inhaler when I really need it and have been using it a few times a day over the last few days' | Increased use of the reliever inhaler suggests this is significantly worsening | | | | |
| Do you have any allergies? | Always ask regarding drug allergies | 'No' | No additional concerns | | | | |

**Family History**

| Question | Justification | Answer | Thoughts | | | | | |
|---|---|---|---|---|---|---|---|---|
| Do you have any family history of medical conditions, specifically asthma or COPD? | Family history of asthma is a predisposing factor for asthma. It is less relevant here, as the patient has already received a diagnosis, but the severity of the family member's asthma is important | 'My mum had asthma which was poorly controlled. Nothing else in the family' | Significant immediate family history of poorly controlled asthma | | | | | |
| Has anyone in your family had any heart problems? | Family history of heart problems increasing the risk of heart disease | 'No' | No additional concerns | | | | | |

**Social and Travel History**

| | | | | | | | | |
|---|---|---|---|---|---|---|---|---|
| Do you currently live with anyone? | Always important to ascertain home support network for management plans | 'I live with my partner' | Support system in place at home | | | | | |
| Do you work? | Establish any occupation risk factors for current breathlessness. Also gives insight into the extent of disability that the condition may be causing | 'I'm a receptionist, but I haven't been able to work the last few days' | No occupation risks identified but symptoms are causing significant problems | | | | | |
| Do you drink alcohol? | Always important to document alcohol consumption | 'Just socially, a couple of glasses of wine on the weekend' | No additional concerns | | | | | |
| Do you smoke? | Smoking may exacerbate asthma and cause asthma attacks | 'I used to, but quit when I was 30 as it made my asthma worse' | No additional concerns | | | | | |
| Do you have any pets at home? | Pets can cause allergic reactions which can cause breathlessness, or worsen asthma | 'No' | No additional concerns | | | | | |
| Do you take any recreational drugs? | Recreational drug use could be a risk factor for an asthma attack. For example, smoking marijuana may precipitate an asthma attack | 'No' | No additional concerns | | | | | |

**Systems Review**

| | | | | | | | | |
|---|---|---|---|---|---|---|---|---|
| Have you had any recent night sweats, fever, weight loss or fatigue? | Enquire specifically about fevers as this suggests recent illness that could precipitate various causes of breathlessness | 'Yes. I've had the flu for a few days' | Fever may be the trigger for worsening of asthma | | | | | |

## Systems Review

| Question | Justification | Answer | Thoughts | | | | |
|---|---|---|---|---|---|---|---|
| Have you noticed any leg swelling? | This may suggest a deep venous thromboembolism (DVT) or heart failure | 'No' | No additional concerns | | | | |
| Have you had any chest pain or palpitations? | Palpitations and chest pain may suggest a cardiac cause of breathlessness | 'No' | No additional concerns | | | | |
| Just to check, have you had any problems with bladder or bowel function? | Find out if there are any wider concerns that have not arisen yet | 'No, they have been normal' | No additional concerns | | | | |

## Finishing the Consultation

| | | | | | | | |
|---|---|---|---|---|---|---|---|
| Is there anything that I've missed, or anything that you are particularly concerned about? | May identify useful information that has been missed. Will also help when framing communication with the patient | 'I think that's all' | Take the time to explain what will happen from here | | | | |
| Do you have any questions for me at the moment? | | | | | | | |

## Present Your Findings

Sophie Stark is a 59-year-old woman who presents with worsening breathlessness over the last few days, especially today. She has found it difficult to carry out normal activities of daily living, including walking. Rest and her salbutamol inhaler relieve the breathlessness. In addition, she has had a productive cough and flu-like symptoms. She is known to have asthma and hypertension, which is well controlled on amlodipine.

My main diagnosis would be an asthma exacerbation secondary to a concurrent viral illness, which has developed into a more serious acute asthma attack over the last day. My differential diagnoses would include ACS and angina pectoris.

I would like to perform a full cardiovascular and respiratory system examination. I would then like to do a peak flow assessment and an ECG and commence the asthma attack management pathway

## General Points

Polite to patient

Maintains good eye contact

Appropriate use of open and closed questions

No or limited use of medical jargon

## ❓ QUESTIONS FROM THE EXAMINER

### How many lobes does each lung have?

The right lung has three lobes and the left lung has two lobes.

### What are the key fissures within each lung?

In the right lung, there is an oblique fissure and a horizontal fissure, whilst in the left lung there is only an oblique fissure.

### Both lungs have three surfaces, each facing a different part of the thorax. What are the names of these surfaces?

Mediastinal, diaphragmatic and costal surface.

### Give a genetic cause of COPD.

Alpha-1 antitrypsin deficiency, which makes up ~1% of all cases of COPD.

### Name the structures enclosed within the lung root.

The bronchus, two pulmonary veins and one pulmonary artery, the pulmonary plexus of nerves and lymphatic vessels, as well as bronchial vessels.

### What is the parasympathetic and sympathetic nerve supply to the lungs?

Parasympathetic supply is derived from the vagus nerve. Sympathetic supply is derived from the sympathetic trunks.

### After spirometry and an initial clinical evaluation for COPD, patients should have other investigations to exclude other pathologies and assess prognosis. What are these three assessments?

Chest radiograph, FBC and BMI.

### Give some examples of short-acting and long-acting bronchodilator inhalers.

Examples of short-acting bronchodilator inhalers include beta-2 agonist inhalers (salbutamol, terbutaline) and antimuscarinic inhalers (ipratropium). Examples of long-acting bronchodilator inhalers include beta-2 agonist inhalers (salmeterol, formoterol, indacaterol) and antimuscarinic inhalers (tiotropium, glycopyronium, aclidinium).

### When are steroids often required in the management of COPD?

During acute flare-ups/exacerbations of COPD.

### What is the mechanism of action of theophylline?

Theophylline is a competitive inhibitor of the type 3 and 4 phosphodiesterase inhibitor. Normally, this enzyme breaks down cyclic adenosine monophosphate in smooth-muscle cells, which causes signalling cascades preventing bronchodilation. The prevention of this breakdown will result in a higher degree of bronchodilation.

## Station 1.7   Abdominal Pain

### Doctor Briefing

You are a junior doctor in the ED and are asked to see Sophie Angelman, a 23-year-old female, who has presented with abdominal pain. The pain started this morning but has now moved to the right side and become more severe. Please take a history from Sophie, present your findings and formulate an appropriate management plan.

### Patient Briefing

You are a 23-year-old woman presenting to the ED. You began to have tummy pain this morning, which is worsening. You have no symptoms of fever, nausea, vomiting or pain in any other part of your body. You have not noticed any changes in bowel habit. The pain is located in the middle/lower right of your tummy. Nothing has made the pain better or worse. You have not noticed any changes in appetite.

On specific questioning, you have noticed some light vaginal bleeding. You are concerned as it is out of timing with your usual menstrual cycle. You have never had an episode like this previously.

You are a non-smoker and drink alcohol socially. You do not take recreational drugs and keep very physically active.

On specific questioning, you had unprotected sexual intercourse after going to a party about 6 weeks ago. You have not had any sexual health check-ups in the last year. Two years ago, you had a diagnosis of pelvic inflammatory disease secondary to a chlamydia infection, which was treated with antibiotics at the time.

You do not have a history of any other medical conditions (nor are there any in the family) and do not take any regular medications.

You are worried that you have got appendicitis and will need surgery.

### Mark Scheme for Examiner

#### Introduction

| | | | |
|---|---|---|---|
| Cleans hands, introduces self, confirms patient identity and gains consent for history taking | | | |
| Establishes current patient knowledge and concerns | | | |

#### History of Presenting Complaint

| Question | Justification | Answer | Thoughts | | | |
|---|---|---|---|---|---|---|
| Could you point to where the pain is felt during these episodes? | Ascertaining the specific site of pain may give clues towards the diagnosis. For example, epigastric pain may suggest gastritis, right-upper-quadrant pain may suggest cholecystitis, or right iliac fossa pain may suggest appendicitis | 'I feel it in my middle and lower right tummy' | Right iliac fossa and lumbar pain could suggest appendicitis or pathology of the reproductive system, amongst others | | | |
| When did the pain start? | The onset of pain could indicate the underlying pathology and whether this is an acute or chronic problem | 'Pain began this morning and is worsening' | This is an acute presentation and suggests new-onset pathology | | | |
| Could you describe the character of the pain? | Different characters may suggest different diagnoses. For example, sharp pain may suggest appendicitis | 'It started dull, but is now getting sharper and more severe' | Character of pain is highly variable so although it may help in the context of further information, it does not lead to an obvious differential at this stage | | | |

## History of Presenting Complaint

| Question | Justification | Answer | Thoughts | | | | | |
|---|---|---|---|---|---|---|---|---|
| Do you feel pain anywhere other than the right tummy? | If there is referred pain, it may indicate particular diagnoses. For example, shoulder tip pain may be felt in an ectopic pregnancy | 'No' | No additional concerns | | | | | |
| Does anything make the pain better or worse? | Exacerbating and relieving factors are important in abdominal pain histories. For example, lying on one's back may exacerbate pancreatitis, whilst leaning forwards may be relieving | 'No, it's just getting worse' | The pathology may be progressing acutely | | | | | |
| On a scale of 1–10, how severe would you say the pain is during the episodes? | Gives an indication as to the severity of the pathology | '7' | Clearly a very concerning and debilitating symptom | | | | | |
| Do you have any other symptoms at the moment? | Associated symptoms give indications to diagnosis | 'I have had a bit of vaginal bleeding since this morning' | Consider a pathology of the reproductive system | | | | | |
| Is this vaginal bleeding out of timing with your normal menstrual cycle? When was your last period? | Important to ascertain if this is in keeping with her normal menstrual cycle. Intermenstrual bleeding is more concerning with her presentation | 'Yes. I missed my last period and I'm halfway through this cycle' | This should prompt you to consider a gynaecological problem | | | | | |
| How heavy is the bleeding? | Ascertaining heaviness of bleeding is important for the diagnosis. For example, heavy intermenstrual bleeding could suggest malignancy, whilst lighter bleeding outside the menstrual cycle could be spotting from implantation in early pregnancy | 'It's a bit lighter than my normal periods' | In itself this does not particularly help to order differentials but is useful to know | | | | | |

## Past Medical History

| Question | Justification | Answer | Thoughts | | | | | |
|---|---|---|---|---|---|---|---|---|
| Do you have any medical conditions? | Comorbidities have implications for both diagnosis and management | 'No' | No additional concerns | | | | | |

## Past Medical History

| Question | Justification | Answer | Thoughts | | | | | |
|---|---|---|---|---|---|---|---|---|
| Specifically, have you had any previous gynaecological problems? | Previous diagnoses may help in ordering differentials. For example, previous ectopic pregnancies increase the risk of another. Or, if the patient has had previous pelvic surgeries or untreated infections, there may be adhesions or scarring that could make certain differentials more/less likely | 'I had pelvic inflammatory disease after a chlamydia infection a couple of years ago' | Pelvic inflammatory disease can increase the risks of subsequent ectopic pregnancies | | | | | |
| Have you had any previous surgeries for these problems or otherwise before? | Gynaecological surgeries can increase the risk of certain conditions. For example, pelvic surgery can result in patients having adhesions | 'No' | No additional concerns | | | | | |
| Have you ever had any pregnancies or miscarriages? | Obstetric history is relevant to her presentation | 'No' | No additional concerns | | | | | |

## Drug History

| Question | Justification | Answer | Thoughts | | | | | |
|---|---|---|---|---|---|---|---|---|
| Are you on any regular medications for anything? | Important to check for contraindications in potential management plan, or to check if certain medications may be causing iatrogenic effects explaining the symptoms | 'No' | No additional concerns | | | | | |
| Do you have any allergies? | Important for potential management plans | 'No' | No additional concerns | | | | | |

## Family History

| Question | Justification | Answer | Thoughts | | | | | |
|---|---|---|---|---|---|---|---|---|
| Do you have any family history of medical conditions? | Other hereditary medical conditions may impact management plans or reveal other possible risk factors for her presentation | 'Not that I know' | No additional concerns | | | | | |
| Has anyone in your family had a bleeding disorder? | Considering her per vaginam (PV) bleeding, it is also important to consider an undiagnosed bleeding disorder | 'No' | No additional concerns | | | | | |

## Social and Travel History

| Question | Justification | Answer | Thoughts | | | | | |
|---|---|---|---|---|---|---|---|---|
| Do you drink alcohol? | Important to get an overview of patient's general lifestyle | 'Recreationally. A few small glasses of wine on the weekend' | No additional concerns | | | | | |

## Social and Travel History

| Question | Justification | Answer | Thoughts | | | | |
|---|---|---|---|---|---|---|---|
| Do you smoke? | It is important to explore wider risk factors. | 'No.' | No additional concerns | | | | |
| 'Are you sexually active and if so, have you had unprotected sex recently? | Important to consider if she could be pregnant, as an ectopic pregnancy is high on the differentials | 'Yes. About 6 weeks ago' | Suggests she could be pregnant, but needs confirmation with a pregnancy test | | | | |

## Systems Review

| | | | | | | | |
|---|---|---|---|---|---|---|---|
| Just to check, have you had any problems with bladder or bowel function? | Find out if there are any wider concerns that have not arisen yet | 'No, they have been normal' | No additional concerns | | | | |
| Have you had any recent night sweats, fever, weight loss or fatigue? | It is essential to ask about B symptoms to rule out certain causes, such as infection or malignancies. A fever could suggest infection which may be a sign of conditions such as pelvic inflammatory disease | 'No' | No additional concerns | | | | |
| Have you noticed any changes to your menstrual cycle recently? | Important to take a menstrual history, particularly in the context of a presentation with abdominal pain and intermenstrual bleeding | 'I missed my last period but otherwise no' | No additional concerns | | | | |

## Finishing the Consultation

| | | | | | | | |
|---|---|---|---|---|---|---|---|
| Is there anything that I've missed, or anything that you are particularly concerned about? | May identify useful information that has been missed. Will also help when framing communication with the patient | 'I think that's all' | Take the time to explain what will happen from here | | | | |
| Do you have any questions for me at the moment? | | | | | | | |

## Present Your Findings

Miss Angelman is a 23-year-old woman who presented with right-sided pain in the iliac fossa and lumbar quadrants, and intermenstrual PV bleeding. The PV bleeding is not particularly heavy. She has no history of gynaecological or abdominal disease and no significant family history. She has not had any changes in bowel or urinary habits, nor has she been vomiting. She has recently had sexual intercourse without contraception and missed her last period.

My main differential would be an ectopic pregnancy. I would also consider a sexually transmitted infection, pyelonephritis or nephrolithiasis.

I would like to do a full abdominal and gynaecological examination. Then, I would do a urine pregnancy test and take bloods including FBCs, LFTs, amylase, U&Es and beta-HCG.

| General Points | | | | |
|---|---|---|---|---|
| Polite to patient | | | | |
| Maintains good eye contact | | | | |
| Appropriate use of open and closed questions | | | | |
| No or limited use of medical jargon | | | | |

## ❓ QUESTIONS FROM THE EXAMINER

### What is the significance of McBurney's point and where is it located?

McBurney's point is at base of the appendix and, if tender, is a sign of appendicitis. Specifically, it is located two-thirds of the distance from the navel to the right anterior superior iliac spine.

### What are the nine quadrants of the abdomen termed?

Right iliac, suprapubic/hypogastric, left iliac, right lumbar, umbilical, left lumbar, right hypochondrium, epigastric and left hypochondrium region.

### What is the physiological basis of abdominal guarding?

Guarding is the tensing of abdominal muscles on palpation. It can be a sign of protection of inflamed organs within the abdomen.

### At what spinal level does the coeliac trunk branch from the aorta?

T12.

### What are the branches of the coeliac trunk?

Left gastric, splenic and common hepatic artery.

### What is the innervation to the external and internal oblique muscles?

Both the external and internal obliques are innervated by the thoracoabdominal nerves (T7–T11) and subcostal nerve (T12). Additionally, the internal oblique is innervated by branches of the lumbar plexus.

### What are the differences between a midline, paramedian and Kocher incision?

A midline incision is made through the linea alba. A paramedian incision is done laterally to the linea alba. A Kocher incision is done inferolaterally, from the inferior aspect of the xiphoid process towards the right costal margin.

### What are the bony attachments of the rectus abdominis?

It originates from the crest of the pubis and inserts into both the costal cartilage of ribs 5–7 and the xiphoid process.

### What is the physiological basis of rebound tenderness?

Rebound tenderness is pain when removing pressure of palpation, rather than when providing initial pressure. It typically suggests some irritation of the parietal peritoneum when moved/stretched, which may occur in appendicitis or ulcerative colitis.

### What is Murphy's sign?

Murphy's sign is elicited by firmly pressing at the costal margin in the right upper quadrant while the patient is breathing in deeply. A positive Murphy's sign is if the patient experiences pain and catches her breath as the gallbladder descends to where the examiner's hand is located. This suggests acute cholecystitis.

## Station 1.8   Dysphagia

### Doctor Briefing

You are a junior doctor in primary care and have been asked to see Melody Jones, a 72-year-old woman, who has had difficulty swallowing over the last 2 months. She is finding it difficult to swallow both solid foods and liquids. She has also lost 7 kg in weight. Please take a history, present your findings and formulate an appropriate management plan.

### Patient Briefing

You are visiting your doctor, as you have been struggling to swallow both solids and liquids for the past 2 months. You have struggled with reflux for the past 20 years, for which you take omeprazole and antacids. On questioning, you have pain at the bottom of your sternum, where it feels as though food is 'getting stuck'. You have also experienced regurgitation but not noticed any neck swellings or changes in your voice.

You are concerned as you have lost 7 kg of weight unintentionally in the last 2 months, as your current symptoms have 'put you off eating'. You have been trying to quit smoking but are still currently smoking around 10 cigarettes a day and have done so for the past 50 years.

You are worried you have caused your current symptoms through smoking.

### Mark Scheme for Examiner

#### Introduction

Cleans hands, introduces self, confirms patient identity and gains consent for history taking

Establishes current patient knowledge and concerns

#### History of Presenting Complaint

| Question | Justification | Answer | Thoughts | | | | |
|---|---|---|---|---|---|---|---|
| When did you first notice that you were having difficulty swallowing? | This helps to determine if this is acute or chronic | 'Around 2 months ago' | The patient is describing a more chronic progression | | | | |
| Did you experience any trauma prior to the onset of symptoms? | It is important to assess if trauma preceded symptoms | 'No' | No additional concerns | | | | |
| Are you unable to swallow both solids and liquids? | It is important to clarify what the patient is describing by 'difficulties swallowing' | 'Yes, I am unable to swallow either' | This suggests a larger obstruction, or motility disorder | | | | |
| Were you unable to swallow both solids and liquids initially? | Obstructive causes of dysphagia often present with difficulty swallowing liquids, then solids. Motility disorders often present with difficulty swallowing both liquids and solids initially | 'Liquids then solids' | Indicative of an obstructive disorder | | | | |
| Have you experienced any vomiting or regurgitation? | An obstruction or stricture may cause regurgitation | 'Yes' | | | | | |

## History of Presenting Complaint

| Question | Justification | Answer | Thoughts | | | | | |
|---|---|---|---|---|---|---|---|---|
| Do you experience any pain on swallowing? | Pain may indicate ulceration or spasm | 'Yes, behind my breastbone' | Pain is most commonly associated with oesophagitis. However, the patient could be describing pain caused by reflux | | | | | |
| Where does it feel like the food gets stuck? | This allows assessment of the level of obstruction or motility disruption | 'At the bottom of my breastbone' | The patient is describing the retrosternal region, suggesting oesophageal dysphagia | | | | | |
| Have you lost any weight unintentionally over the last 2 months? | Unintentional weight loss is a red flag for malignancy | 'About 7 kg over the last 2 months' | Increased concern, as the patient has described significant unintentional weight loss | | | | | |
| Is the difficulty swallowing consistent or intermittent? | Diffuse oesophageal spasm is associated with intermittent swallowing difficulties | 'Constant' | Symptoms are not consistent with diffuse oesophageal spasm | | | | | |
| Have you experienced heartburn or indigestion? | Dyspepsia may be associated with an oesophageal stricture | 'Yes, frequently' | Symptoms are consistent with an oesophageal stricture | | | | | |
| Have you noticed any swellings in your neck or gurgling sounds on swallowing? | Such symptoms may be indicative of a pharyngeal pouch | 'No' | Symptoms are not indicative of a pharyngeal pouch | | | | | |
| Have you noticed any changes in your voice? | Oesophageal malignancy may be associated with a hoarse voice | 'No' | No additional concerns | | | | | |

## Past Medical History

| Question | Justification | Answer | Thoughts | | | | | |
|---|---|---|---|---|---|---|---|---|
| Do you have any known medical conditions? | GORD may precipitate benign oesophageal strictures, or oesophagitis | 'I have had reflux for over 20 years' | This should be explored further | | | | | |
| Have you been diagnosed with any neurological diseases such as previous strokes, Parkinson's disease or myasthenia gravis? | Such disorders may impede the mechanism of swallowing | 'No' | No additional concerns | | | | | |

## Drug History

| Question | Justification | Answer | Thoughts | | | | | |
|---|---|---|---|---|---|---|---|---|
| Are you currently on any medication, or have any allergies? | It is important to exclude drug-induced dysphasia, which may be caused by neuroleptics, or chemotherapy agents.<br>NSAIDs and steroids increase risk of oesophagitis.<br>You must always check for allergies | 'Omeprazole, Rennie and ibuprofen. No allergies' | The patient has already disclosed a past medical history of reflux.<br>NSAID use may increase the risk of oesophagitis | | | | | |
| Have you ever taken a drug that could affect your bleeding, such as aspirin or warfarin? | The patient may have recently stopped taking it. These drugs can have an effect on bleeding | 'Never' | No additional concerns | | | | | |

## Family History

| Question | Justification | Answer | Thoughts | | | | | |
|---|---|---|---|---|---|---|---|---|
| Are there any diseases that run in the family, including any cancers? | Important always to check for relevant heritable conditions | 'My father and uncle also had reflux' | This may be important and should be further investigated | | | | | |

## Social and Travel History

| Question | Justification | Answer | Thoughts | | | | | |
|---|---|---|---|---|---|---|---|---|
| Who is currently at home? Are you working? | Find out if there are any social concerns or if wider support is needed | 'I live in an assisted-living home, and am a retired nurse' | No current social concerns | | | | | |
| Do you smoke? | Smoking is a risk factor for GORD and oesophageal malignancy | 'I have smoked around 10 a day for 50 years' | The patient has around 25 pack years, increasing the risk of oesophageal malignancy and GORD | | | | | |
| What is your average weekly alcohol consumption? | Find out a patient's wider risk factors as well as exploring causes for symptom changes | 'I have two glasses of wine an evening' | The patient is drinking over the recommended units, which may contribute to reflux symptoms | | | | | |

## Systems Review

| Question | Justification | Answer | Thoughts | | | | | |
|---|---|---|---|---|---|---|---|---|
| Just to check, have you had any problems with bladder or bowel function? | Find out if there are any wider concerns that have not arisen yet | 'No, they have been normal' | No additional concerns | | | | | |
| Have you had any recent night sweats, fever, weight loss or fatigue? | It is essential to ask about B symptoms to rule out certain causes, such as infection | 'No' | No additional concerns | | | | | |

**Finishing the Consultation**

| Question | Justification | Answer | Thoughts | | | | |
|---|---|---|---|---|---|---|---|
| Is there anything that I've missed, or anything you are concerned about? | May identify useful information that has been missed | 'I am worried about losing so much weight' | Take the time to explain what will happen from here | | | | |
| Do you have any questions? | | | | | | | |

**Present Your Findings**

Mrs Jones is a 72-year-old woman with a 20-year history of reflux treated with omeprazole and antacids, who has presented with a 2-month history of dysphagia of both solids and liquids simultaneously. The patient also has retrosternal pain and is experiencing regurgitation. Mrs Jones has further lost 7 kg of weight unintentionally in the last 2 months. Mrs Jones has 25 pack-years and drinks around 30 units a week.

My main differential would be oesophageal stricture, but I would also like to investigate for achalasia and oesophageal cancer due to the patient's smoking history and age.

I am going to take several blood tests from Mrs Jones, including FBC. I would also like to arrange an endoscopy with biopsy

**General Points**

| | | | |
|---|---|---|---|
| Polite to patient | | | |
| Maintains good eye contact | | | |
| Appropriate use of open and closed questions | | | |
| No or limited use of medical jargon | | | |

## ❓ QUESTIONS FROM THE EXAMINER

### What is bulbar palsy, and which cranial nerves are involved?

Bulbar palsy is a lower motor neurone lesion most commonly caused by a brainstem stroke or tumour. Cranial nerves IX, X and XII are affected.

### What is pseudobulbar palsy, and which cranial nerves are involved?

Pseudobulbar palsy is an upper motor neurone lesion affecting the corticobulbar tracts bilaterally. Causes include: trauma, stroke, tumour and neurological diseases such as Parkinson's disease. Cranial nerves IX, X and XII are affected.

### Which members of a multidisciplinary team may be involved in the management of a patient with bulbar or pseudobulbar palsy?

The speech and language therapy team may review to assist with swallowing symptoms.

### Describe the normal histological appearance of the endothelium through the GI tract.

The mouth to the oesophageal–gastric junction is lined with simple squamous epithelium. From the oesophageal–gastric junction to the anus is lined with simple columnar epithelium. The anus is lined with stratified columnar epithelium.

### Describe the histological changes that occur in GORD.

In GORD, the transition from simple squamous epithelium to simple columnar epithelium occurs superior to the oesophageal–gastric junction. Due to the presence of acid, the simple squamous epithelium superior to the oesophageal–gastric junction transitions into simple columnar epithelium.

### List the risk factors for GORD.

Alcohol, smoking, hiatus hernia, pregnancy and obesity.

### What management may be offered in GORD?

Lifestyle advice, including weight loss, avoiding trigger meals, eating 3–4 h before lying down, smoking cessation, reducing alcohol consumption. A 4–8-week course of proton pump inhibitors, e.g. omeprazole or lansoprazole, can also be prescribed. Second-line would be histamine 2 receptor antagonists, e.g. ranitidine.

### What are the four types of hiatus hernia?

Sliding, rolling, combination of sliding and rolling, and additional abdominal organs protruding into thorax.

### Describe the difference between a sliding and rolling hiatus hernia.

A sliding hiatus hernia occurs when the stomach slides through the diaphragm and the gastro-oesophageal junction protrudes into the thorax. Alternatively, a rolling hiatus hernia describes the fundus of the stomach folding and passing through the oesophageal hiatus in the diaphragm.

### What surgical intervention may be used to treat a hiatus hernia?

Laparoscopic fundoplication. This procedure involves wrapping the fundus of the stomach around the oesophagus to create a sphincter.

## Station 1.9   Nausea and Vomiting

### Doctor Briefing

You are a junior doctor in primary care and have been asked to see Jack Fawn, a 28-year-old man, who presented with a 2-day history of nausea and vomiting. He feels generally unwell and is struggling to hold down any food. Please take a history from Jack, present your findings and formulate an appropriate management plan.

### Patient Briefing

You are a 28-year-old man who is presenting with a 2-day history of vomiting. You have vomited several times (7–8 times) in the last 2 days. The vomiting is bloody (bright red in colour) and began 2 days ago. Each vomit is about 2–3 cups in volume. You are struggling to keep food and drink down, but eating does not trigger the vomiting. You also have central tummy pain that is burning in character and radiates all the way through to your back. You have also noticed changes in your stools as they are black and tarry in colour and have an unusual smell.

Four years ago, you had a motorbike accident which required a knee operation and left you with knee pain. You manage this knee pain with ibuprofen. You have taken ibuprofen at double the recommended dose daily for about 4 years. You have no other significant medical problems. You have no allergies.

You smoke two packs of cigarettes a day and have done so for about 10 years. You do not drink alcohol and take no recreational drugs. You are very physically active and live with some friends as flatmates. You have not recently been travelling, nor come into contact with anyone who has had similar symptoms.

You are concerned as the pain is getting worse and the vomit is still bright red in colour.

### Mark Scheme for Examiner

#### Introduction

Cleans hands, introduces self, confirms patient identity and gains consent for history taking

Establishes current patient knowledge and concerns

#### History of Presenting Complaint

| Question | Justification | Answer | Thoughts | | | | | |
|---|---|---|---|---|---|---|---|---|
| When did the vomiting start? | Ascertaining onset will indicate whether this is an acute or chronic problem | 'About 2 days ago' | Suggests it is a new-onset problem | | | | | |
| Did anything trigger the first episode? | Important to establish if there is an obvious trigger to the vomiting. For example, a clear source of food poisoning | 'Nothing that I can think of' | Suggests there is no immediately obvious cause | | | | | |
| How many times have you vomited since your symptoms began? | Frequency gives an indication of severity of symptoms | '7–8 times' | In 2 days, this is a high frequency | | | | | |
| Does anything in particular trigger the vomiting? | Establishing patterns and if it is associated with eating or taking medications is important. For example, nausea and vomiting after eating may be associated with gastroparesis | 'Not that I can think of' | No clear trigger | | | | | |

**History of Presenting Complaint**

| Question | Justification | Answer | Thoughts | | | | |
|---|---|---|---|---|---|---|---|
| What is the content of the vomit? Is there a particular colour, does it appear bloody or is there an unusual smell? | Establishing the character of the vomitus is important to the diagnosis. For example, faeculant vomiting may suggest bowel obstruction. Fresh blood in the vomit may suggest an upper GI bleed | 'It is bloody, bright red. There's no real smell' | There should be high clinical suspicion for haematemesis from this description, which suggests an upper GI bleed as the differential diagnosis | | | | |
| In each vomiting episode, what is the volume of vomit? You can give your answer in terms of cups | Important to avoid qualifiers such as lots or little, as this is very subjective | 'Maybe 2–3 cups' | If this is haematemesis and there is significant blood in each vomit, there should be a concern about the haemodynamic stability of the patient | | | | |
| Are you able to eat and drink and keep anything down? | Important to establish if the patient's nutritional needs are being met and if the patient may be clinically dehydrated | 'I can sometimes keep it down between vomits, but sometimes struggle' | Suggests the patient may be meeting nutritional needs, but given the frequency and volume of vomits, this requires exploration | | | | |
| Have you had any other symptoms alongside the vomiting? | Associated symptoms can give key clues to the diagnosis. For example, colicky abdominal pain and distension may suggest bowel obstruction, severe abdominal pain may suggest an acute abdomen, or a headache with aura and visual disturbance may suggest a migraine | 'I have central tummy pain that goes to the back. My bowel habits have also changed' | Epigastric abdominal pain fits with the existing clinical suspicion of an upper GI bleed. Important to characterise the abdominal pain and the changes in bowel habits fully | | | | |
| Have you noticed any changes in bowel habits? Have your stools been an unusual colour or smell? | Bowel habit changes are associated with various causes of vomiting. For example, absolute constipation is associated with bowel obstruction. Diarrhoea is associated with gastroenteritis, whilst upper GI bleeds may be associated with melaena | 'My stools have been black and tarry and smelt weird' | This description suggests the patient has melaena. This fits with the clinical suspicion of an upper GI bleed | | | | |
| Have you had any fever or felt unwell? | Infectious causes of vomiting must be considered, such as gastroenteritis | 'No' | No additional concerns | | | | |

**Past Medical History**

| | | | | | | | |
|---|---|---|---|---|---|---|---|
| Do you have any chronic medical conditions? | Chronic medical conditions can sometimes have complications that result in vomiting | 'I have chronic pain in my knee' | Important to establish how the patient is managing the knee pain as NSAIDs increase the risk of bleeding | | | | |

**Past Medical History**

| Question | Justification | Answer | Thoughts | | | | | |
|---|---|---|---|---|---|---|---|---|
| Have you ever had any surgical operations? | Previous abdominal surgeries could result in complications that may cause vomiting. Furthermore, recent surgical operations can affect management plans, as the patient may be put on various medications postoperatively | 'I had a knee operation 4 years ago after a motorbike accident' | No additional concerns | | | | | |

**Drug History**

| Question | Justification | Answer | Thoughts | | | | | |
|---|---|---|---|---|---|---|---|---|
| Are you on any regular medications for any conditions? | Important to check for contraindications in potential management plan, or to check if certain medications may be causing iatrogenic effects explaining the symptoms | 'I take ibuprofen every day' | Long-term use of NSAIDs can cause peptic ulcers which are a cause of upper GI bleeds | | | | | |
| Do you have any allergies? | Always ask. Important for potential management plans | 'No' | No additional concerns | | | | | |

**Family History**

| Question | Justification | Answer | Thoughts | | | | | |
|---|---|---|---|---|---|---|---|---|
| Has anyone in your family had any significant tummy problems? | Family history of GI disease or disorders of metabolism needs to be elicited | 'No' | No additional concerns | | | | | |
| Do you have any family history of other medical conditions? | Other hereditary medical conditions may impact management plans or reveal other possible risk factors for the patient's presentation | 'No' | No additional concerns | | | | | |

**Social and Travel History**

| Question | Justification | Answer | Thoughts | | | | | |
|---|---|---|---|---|---|---|---|---|
| Do you currently live with anyone? | Always important to ascertain home support network for management plans | 'I live with my flatmates who are good friends of mine' | Support system in place at home if necessary, for management plan | | | | | |
| Have you had any difficulties at work? | Gives insight into the extent of disability that the condition may be causing | 'I'm an engineer but I've had to take some time off work because of this problem.' | No additional concerns | | | | | |
| Do you drink alcohol? | Withdrawal after alcohol dependency can cause vomiting. Acute intoxication can cause vomiting, as can hangovers | 'No' | No additional concerns | | | | | |
| Do you smoke? | Tobacco smoking is also a known risk factor for peptic ulcer development | 'Yes. Two packs a day for 10 years' | Significant history of smoking of 20 pack years | | | | | |

### Social and Travel History

| Question | Justification | Answer | Thoughts | | | | | |
|---|---|---|---|---|---|---|---|---|
| Have you recently travelled abroad? | Tropical infections can cause GI disease that could cause vomiting | 'No' | No additional concerns | | | | | |
| Have you recently eaten at any new or unusual food places? | Important to check for possible sources of food poisoning | 'No' | No additional concerns | | | | | |
| Have you come into contact with anyone who has had similar symptoms to you? | Certain infectious causes of this presentation may be transmitted between infected individuals | 'No' | No additional concerns | | | | | |

### Systems Review

| Question | Justification | Answer | Thoughts | | | | | |
|---|---|---|---|---|---|---|---|---|
| Have you noticed any other changes to your tummy other than the pain? Any bloating? | Important to check for abdominal distension, as this may suggest a bowel obstruction | 'No' | No additional concerns | | | | | |
| Have you had any headaches? | Important to check for migraine as the cause for the patient's nausea and vomiting | 'No' | No additional concerns | | | | | |
| Have you had any vertigo? | Vertigo is associated with labyrinthitis which may cause nausea and vomiting | 'No' | No additional concerns | | | | | |
| Have you had any recent night sweats, fever, weight loss or fatigue? | It is essential to ask about B symptoms to rule out certain causes, such as infection | 'No' | No additional concerns | | | | | |

### Finishing the Consultation

| Question | Justification | Answer | Thoughts | | | | | |
|---|---|---|---|---|---|---|---|---|
| Is there anything that I've missed, or anything that you are particularly concerned about? | May identify useful information that has been missed. Will also help when framing communication with the patient | 'I think that's all' | Take the time to explain what will happen from here | | | | | |
| Do you have any questions for me at the moment? | | | | | | | | |

### Present Your Findings

Jack Fawn is a 28-year-old man, presenting with nausea and vomiting over the last 2 days. He has vomited 7–8 times in 2 days and each time vomits about 2–3 cups in volume. The vomit contains fresh blood. He also has epigastric abdominal pain which radiates to the back and melaena. He has taken ibuprofen regularly for 4 years. He has not been travelling recently and has not eaten anything unusual. He has no fever and no relevant family history.

My main differential would be an upper GI bleed secondary to a peptic ulcer. I would also consider infectious causes of the presentation.

I would like to do a full abdominal examination of Jack and have him referred for an urgent diagnostic endoscopy

| General Points | | | | |
|---|---|---|---|---|
| Polite to patient | | | | |
| Maintains good eye contact | | | | |
| Appropriate use of open and closed questions | | | | |
| No or limited use of medical jargon | | | | |

## ❓ QUESTIONS FROM THE EXAMINER

### What is false hypoglycaemia?

Patients with consistently high glucose levels may experience symptoms of hypoglycaemia at a higher level than someone with good glycaemic control.

### How might excessive alcohol intake cause hypoglycaemia?

Alcohol contains ethanol, which is metabolised to acetaldehyde by alcohol dehydrogenase to produce acetate. During these processes, $NAD^+$ is converted to NADH. $NAD^+$ is necessary in gluconeogenesis, therefore excessive alcohol intake can reduce the amount of available $NAD^+$ for gluconeogenesis, potentially precipitating hypoglycaemia.

### What is hypoglycaemic unawareness and what is its prevalence?

Loss of early-warning signs of hypoglycaemia, which is seen in approximately 25% of patients with type 1 diabetes.

### What are the two major ketone bodies involved in the pathogenesis of diabetic ketoacidosis (DKA)?

3-hydroxybutyric acid (3-OH-butyric acid) and acetoacetic acid (acetone).

### What is the effect of insulin on ketosis?

Insulin will terminate ketosis instantaneously. This is because it allows glucose to enter cells and be used.

### What is the definition of significant hyperglycaemia?

Random blood glucose level greater than 11 mmol/L.

### Why are urea and creatinine frequently raised in DKA?

The dehydration that occurs in DKA leads to reduced renal function.

### Elevated capillary blood glucose is a key feature of DKA. However, sometimes this level may be lower than expected for the diagnosis on admission. Why might this be?

Euglycaemic ketosis, alcoholic ketosis or sometimes the patient may have been given a bit of insulin before arrival.

### Fluid therapy is a key part of DKA management. What are the initial three fluids usually given in DKA?

1 L 0.9% saline stat, 1 L/h 0.9% saline and 1 L/2 h + 20 mmol potassium chloride (KCl).

### What is the major complication of DKA and in which age group does it kill most people?

Cerebral oedema; children are most commonly affected children; it is the most common cause of death from DKA.

## Station 1.10    Diarrhoea

### Doctor Briefing

You are a junior doctor in primary care and have been asked to see Danielle Sanderson, a 60-year-old woman, who has been experiencing severe abdominal pain and diarrhoea for the past 4 days. She was recently discharged from hospital following an appendectomy. Please take a history from Mrs Sanderson, present your findings and formulate an appropriate management plan.

### Patient Briefing

You are a 60-year-old woman and have been having severe abdominal pain and diarrhoea for the last 4 days. The pain is located on the lower left side of your abdomen. Nothing seems to make the pain better or worse.

You are passing stools about five times a day. You sometimes wake up at night needing to empty your bowels. You do not have bowel incontinence. The stools are soft and have blood within them. You have not been vomiting. You have a raised body temperature and no other pain elsewhere in your body. You have not had any recent unintentional weight loss.

You were recently discharged from hospital following an appendicectomy. When you were having scans in the hospital, the doctor mentioned you had some sort of 'pouch' disease in the tummy, but you did not follow and were more concerned about the appendicitis. Volunteer this information when the examinee asks about any chronic medical conditions.

You have no other chronic medical conditions. Your father had diverticular disease, but there is no other significant family medical history. You are on your last day of antibiotics after your appendectomy and take no other regular medications.

You are a non-smoker, drink alcohol socially and do not take any recreational drugs. You are physically active but have a raised BMI and your diet is not balanced. You eat lots of protein and fats but little fibre and vegetables. You have not been travelling recently. You live with your partner at home.

You are concerned, as the diarrhoea is not getting any better.

### Mark Scheme for Examiner

#### Introduction

| | | | | |
|---|---|---|---|---|
| Cleans hands, introduces self, confirms patient identity and gains consent for history taking | | | | |
| Establishes current patient knowledge and concerns | | | | |

#### History of Presenting Complaint

| Question | Justification | Answer | Thoughts | | | | |
|---|---|---|---|---|---|---|---|
| When did the diarrhoea begin? | Important to ascertain if this is an acute or chronic diarrhoea | 'The day after I was discharged from the hospital. So about 3 days ago' | This is a new-onset problem, suggesting an acute cause | | | | |
| How many times a day are you having bowel movements? | Important to quantify the number of bowel movements and volume of stool | 'Five times a day' | This fits the clinical definition of 3+ bowel movements/day. However, it is also important to ensure you enquire about the normal number of bowel movements for the patient | | | | |
| Do you wake up at night to open your bowels? | This gives insight into the severity of the condition and can give clues to the diagnosis | 'Sometimes' | Suggests the problem is severe | | | | |

**History of Presenting Complaint**

| Question | Justification | Answer | Thoughts | | | | |
|---|---|---|---|---|---|---|---|
| Have you ever accidentally opened your bowels without intending to? | Important to ascertain if the patient has bowel incontinence. Bowel incontinence can be caused by inflammatory bowel disease, irritable-bowel syndrome or post-surgery damage to the muscles/nerves that supply the bowels | 'No' | No bowel incontinence helps order potential differential diagnoses | | | | |
| What is the consistency of the stools? | Important to establish the character of the stool. Consistency can be compared with the Bristol stool chart, which can give clues to the diagnosis | 'Soft' | Soft stools point to a range of potential differential diagnoses, so further exploration is required | | | | |
| What colour are the stools? Is there any blood within them? | Colour gives clues to the diagnosis. For example, black, tarry stools may suggest melaena which could be indicative of an upper GI bleed. Fresh blood in the stools may suggest inflammatory bowel disease or diverticular disease | 'They are brown but have fresh bright red blood in them' | Bloody diarrhoea is a clearer sign to help order differentials. Inflammatory bowel disease of diverticular disease may be likely diagnoses, but other causes need to be considered | | | | |
| Does anything make the diarrhoea better or worse? | Exacerbating and relieving factors of the diarrhoea may give clues to the diagnosis. For example, worsening on eating gluten may suggest coeliac disease | 'No' | Unlikely to be coeliac disease | | | | |
| Do you have any other symptoms? | Associated symptoms are important to consider. For example, gastroenteritis may be associated with cramping abdominal pain and vomiting, whilst colorectal cancer may be associated with weight loss | 'I have some pain in the bottom left of my tummy' | Left iliac fossa pain may suggest this is more likely to be diverticular disease | | | | |
| Have you had any nausea or vomiting? | Nausea and vomiting are associated with a range of conditions that can cause diarrhoea, including gastroenteritis | 'No' | Less likely to be gastroenteritis | | | | |
| Have you had a fever? | Fevers are associated with a range of conditions that can cause diarrhoea, particularly infectious causes | 'A little bit' | May suggest an infective cause is more likely. However, infection can also precipitate worsening of other causes of diarrhoea, so this must also be considered | | | | |
| Have you had any unintentional weight loss? | Unintentional weight loss is associated with malignancy such as colorectal cancer and must be considered, particularly given the patient's age | 'No' | Less likely to be a malignancy | | | | |

## Past Medical History

| Question | Justification | Answer | Thoughts | | | | |
|----------|---------------|--------|----------|--|--|--|--|
| Have you ever had these episodes of diarrhoea before? | Past episodes of diarrhoea may fit with the relapsing remitting disease course of certain GI diseases such as inflammatory bowel disease | 'No' | This is a new-onset acute diarrhoea | | | | |
| Do you have any chronic medical conditions? | Could explain the cause of the patient's symptoms | 'No, but when I was in hospital, the doctor mentioned I may have some pouch disease in my tummy?' | This sounds like it may be diverticular disease which was picked up whilst the patient was in hospital recently | | | | |
| Have you had any surgical operations previously? | History of abdominal surgery may increase the risk of certain conditions. In particular, recent surgery may render hospital-acquired gastroenteritis a key differential diagnosis | 'I had my appendix out a few days ago, but other than that, nothing' | The recent surgery makes a hospital-acquired infection a more prominent differential. However, given the patient mentioned she may have diverticular disease, diverticulitis would also present in a similar way | | | | |

## Drug History

| Question | Justification | Answer | Thoughts | | | | |
|----------|---------------|--------|----------|--|--|--|--|
| Are you on any regular medications for any conditions? | Important to check for contraindications in potential management plan. In particular, it is important to ask about recent antibiotics in relation to hospital-acquired infections such as *Clostridium difficile* | 'I'm on my last day of antibiotics after my operation. I take no other medications' | Recent surgery makes an infective cause more likely, particularly hospital-acquired infections such as *Clostridium difficile* | | | | |
| Do you have any allergies? | Always ask. Important for potential management plans | 'No' | No additional concerns | | | | |

## Family History

| Question | Justification | Answer | Thoughts | | | | |
|----------|---------------|--------|----------|--|--|--|--|
| Does anyone in your family have any tummy problems? | Family history of abdominal problems such as inflammatory bowel disease, coeliac disease or malignancy is relevant owing to the heritable component of these diseases. Important to avoid jargon in questions | 'My dad had diverticular disease' | Significant immediate family history of diverticular disease is an important risk factor | | | | |
| Do you have a family history of any other medical conditions? | Other hereditary medical conditions may impact management plans or reveal other possible risk factors for the patient's presentation | 'No' | No additional concerns | | | | |

## Social and Travel History

| Question | Justification | Answer | Thoughts | | | | |
|---|---|---|---|---|---|---|---|
| Do you currently live with anyone? | Always important to ascertain home support network for management plans | 'I live with my husband' | Support system in place at home, if necessary, for management plan | | | | |
| Do you drink alcohol? | Alcohol-related problems such as chronic pancreatitis can cause diarrhoea | 'Socially. A glass or two at the weekend.' | No additional concerns | | | | |
| Do you smoke? | Always important to document smoking history | 'No' | No additional concerns | | | | |
| How is your diet? | Diet is highly relevant to this history. Certain foods can trigger conditions such as coeliac disease. Low-fibre diets can be a risk factor for diverticular disease | 'It's not great. I don't eat much fruit, vegetables or fibre' | Low-fibre diet is a risk factor for diverticular disease | | | | |
| Have you recently been travelling? | Recent travel may suggest certain infective causes of diarrhoea are more likely, such as 'traveller's diarrhoea' | 'No' | No additional concerns | | | | |
| Do you take any recreational drugs? | Always important to document recreational drug use | 'No' | No additional concerns | | | | |

## Systems Review

| Question | Justification | Answer | Thoughts | | | | |
|---|---|---|---|---|---|---|---|
| Have you noticed any problems with your eyes? | Some conditions such as Crohn's disease can cause eye problems, including episcleritis | 'No' | No additional concerns | | | | |
| Have you noticed any joint pains? | Arthritis is an extraintestinal problem associated with inflammatory bowel disease | 'No' | No additional concerns | | | | |

## Finishing the Consultation

| Question | Justification | Answer | Thoughts | | | | |
|---|---|---|---|---|---|---|---|
| Is there anything that I've missed, or anything that you are particularly concerned about? | May identify useful information that has been missed. Will also help when framing communication with the patient | 'I think that's all' | Take the time to explain what will happen from here | | | | |
| Do you have any questions for me at the moment? | | | | | | | |

**Present Your Findings**

Mrs Sanderson is a 60-year-old woman who has presented with a 4-day history of severe abdominal pain localised to the left iliac fossa and diarrhoea. She describes the diarrhoea as bloody and is passing stools five times a day. She reports a fever but does not have any further systemic problems. She has recently had an appendectomy for which she is completing a course of antibiotics. She has a possible diagnosis of diverticular disease and has a family history of diverticular disease.

My main differential would be diverticulitis. I would like to rule out hospital-acquired infection such as *Clostridium difficile* and would also consider malignancy such as colorectal cancer.

I would like to perform an abdominal examination on Mrs Sanderson. I would then like to take bloods, cultures and lactate level to rule out an infective source, as well as possibly arranging a CT scan after discussing with a senior

**General Points**

Polite to patient

Maintains good eye contact

Appropriate use of open and closed questions

No or limited use of medical jargon

## ❓ QUESTIONS FROM THE EXAMINER

### What are the compositions of oral rehydration solution?

Water, salt (NaCl), trisodium citrate dihydrate, KCl and anhydrous glucose.

### Why was the standard osmolarity of oral rehydration solution reduced by the World Health Organization (WHO) several years ago?

Numerous clinical trials showed that reduced osmolarity reduces vomiting, need for intravenous therapy and stool volume in children with diarrhoea.

### What is the mechanism of action of clarithyromycin?

Clarithryomycin is a macrolide antibiotic that inhibits bacterial protein synthesis by binding to the bacterial 50S ribosomal subunit, inhibiting peptidyl transferase activity and interfering with amino acid translocation.

### What are some of the causative viral organisms underlying gastroenteritis?

Rotavirus, noroviruses and adenoviruses.

### What are some of the causative parasites underlying gastroenteritis?

Cryptosporidiosis, Entamoeba histolytica and Giardia intestinalis.

### What characterises haemolytic uraemic syndrome and what is the mortality rate of this complication?

Haemolytic uraemic syndrome begins with bloody diarrhoea, followed by acute kidney injury, thrombocytopenia and microangiopathic haemolytic anaemia, about a week after the onset of diarrhoea. The mortality rate is 3–5%.

### What is the structure of the rotavirus vaccination programme in England?

Vaccination given at 8 and 12 weeks.

### What classification of vaccine is rotavirus?

Live attenuated vaccine.

## Name two indications of loperamide.

(Acute and chronic) diarrhoea, faecal incontinence and bowel colic pain in palliative care.

## What is the Bristol Stool Scale?

It is s a diagnostic medical tool designed to classify human faeces into different categories.

## Station 1.11    Oliguria

### Doctor Briefing

You have been asked to review 72-year-old Mr Kaur during your ward cover shift. He was admitted under the medical team yesterday following a fall. The nursing staff are concerned, as he has passed very little urine since admission. Please take a history from Mr Kaur, present your findings and formulate an appropriate management plan.

### Patient Briefing

You are a 72-year-old man who was admitted to a hospital ward yesterday following a fall. Since your admission you have passed very little urine.

You have some swelling in your lower legs which has become more noticeable over the last month. You have also been feeling tired and weaker over the last 2 months, and you get fatigued from even small activities. You do not have any pain and have not noticed any changes in your bowel habits.

You have long-standing hypertension which is poorly controlled. You take amlodipine and losartan, but your blood pressure is still consistently over 140/90 mmHg. You have no other significant medical conditions and do not take any other regular medications. You have never had any heart problems.

You have no significant family history of medical conditions. You do not have any family. Your parents passed away in their 80s, one from breast cancer and the other from a heart attack.

You are a non-smoker and drink alcohol socially. You do not take any recreational drugs. You are retired, live by yourself at home and generally keep physically active. Your diet is normally balanced, but you are overweight.

You are concerned that you might have a kidney infection.

### Mark Scheme for Examiner

#### Introduction

| | | | | |
|---|---|---|---|---|
| Cleans hands, introduces self, confirms patient identity and gains consent for history taking | | | | |
| Establishes current patient knowledge and concerns | | | | |

#### History of Presenting Complaint

| Question | Justification | Answer | Thoughts | | | |
|---|---|---|---|---|---|---|
| Have you noticed that you've not been passing water as much recently? | Establish how much insight the patient has regarding his reduced urine output | 'Yes' | Worth exploring oliguria and other associated symptoms | | | |
| Have you felt unwell in yourself or had any other concerns? | Explore any associated symptoms | 'I've actually been a bit concerned about swelling in both my legs' | More information on this is required | | | |
| How long have you had the swelling in your legs? Is it the same on both sides and could you tell me the distribution of swelling? | Important to establish if this is an acute or chronic swelling. Acute swelling could be the result of recent trauma or secondary to a DVT. By contrast, chronic swelling is more likely to be secondary to heart failure or kidney disease | 'I noticed it about a month ago, and it's getting bigger. It's the same on both sides and goes up from my ankles to near my knees' | Suggests this is not an acute pathology and its bilateral nature perhaps suggests it is less likely to be oedema secondary to an injury | | | |

## History of Presenting Complaint

| Question | Justification | Answer | Thoughts | | | | |
|---|---|---|---|---|---|---|---|
| Did anything in particular trigger the swelling? | It is important to know of any triggers of the event, for example, an injury | 'Not that I can think of' | Suggests this is perhaps a manifestation of an underlying pathology rather than a singular injury | | | | |
| Do you have any pain or tenderness associated with the swelling? | Pain associated with the swelling may suggest an inflammatory process at the site of swelling | 'No' | Starting to suspect a peripheral oedema | | | | |
| Have you noticed any other symptoms whilst you've had the oedema, such as chest pain? | Associated symptoms could give clues to the diagnosis. For example, chest pain may suggest a cardiac pathology, whilst fatigue could suggest anaemia secondary to kidney disease | 'I've felt more tired than usual and a bit weak generally. No chest pain' | The lack of chest pain renders a cardiac pathology less likely. The weakness and fatigue may suggest anaemia | | | | |
| How long have you had this tiredness and weakness? | The length of the fatigue will indicate if this overlaps with the oedema and indicates if this is a new-onset or longer-standing problem | 'A couple of months' | The long-standing fatigue is in keeping with a potential anaemia | | | | |
| Could you give me an example of some activities you find tiring that didn't trouble you before? | Important to note that tiredness and weakness are very generalised symptoms that could even be a feature of low mood/depression. It's important to gauge the impact this is having on activities of daily living | 'I can only walk for a few hundred metres before getting pretty tired' | Exertional fatigue still fits with anaemia | | | | |

## Past Medical History

| Question | Justification | Answer | Thoughts | | | | |
|---|---|---|---|---|---|---|---|
| Do you have any chronic medical conditions? | Important to know in case these symptoms are a manifestation of an existing underlying diagnosis – such as peripheral oedema secondary to known congestive heart failure | 'I have had high blood pressure for about 20 years' | Hypertension is a risk factor for a range of conditions that could cause this presentation, including ACS and CKD | | | | |
| How do you control your blood pressure? | Important to understand if the blood pressure is well controlled. Poorly controlled hypertension is a significant risk factor and can be a precipitant for acute events | 'I take amlodipine and losartan. It's not well controlled, though' | Poorly controlled hypertension could be a risk factor for a range of conditions, as above | | | | |
| Do you have any history of kidney or heart problems? | Specifically ask these questions, as they are both key differential diagnoses for this patient's presentation | 'Not that I know of' | No additional concerns | | | | |

## Drug History

| Question | Justification | Answer | Thoughts | | | | | |
|---|---|---|---|---|---|---|---|---|
| Are you on any regular medications for any conditions? | Important to check for contraindications in potential management plan. Also note that as kidney disease is a key differential, this will need to be considered with regard to pharmacological management plan (drug excretion capacity) | 'Just amlodipine and losartan' | Need to check adequate control of blood pressure | | | | | |
| Do you have any allergies? | Always ask. Important for potential management plans | 'No' | No additional concerns | | | | | |

## Family History

| Question | Justification | Answer | Thoughts | | | | | |
|---|---|---|---|---|---|---|---|---|
| Is there any history of heart disease in your family? | Family history of heart disease is a significant risk factor for heart disease | 'My father died from a heart attack in his 80s' | Significant immediate family history is an important risk factor; however, important to note age of father (80s) | | | | | |
| Is there any history of kidney disease in your family? | Family history of kidney disease may give clues to the diagnosis | 'No' | No additional concerns | | | | | |
| Do you have any family history of other medical conditions? | Other hereditary medical conditions may impact management plans or reveal other possible risk factors for the diagnosis | 'No' | No additional concerns | | | | | |

## Social and Travel History

| Question | Justification | Answer | Thoughts | | | | | |
|---|---|---|---|---|---|---|---|---|
| Do you currently live with anyone? | Always important to ascertain home support network for management plans | 'I live alone' | Consider support systems at home and if he requires assistance as part of his management plan | | | | | |
| Have you had any difficulties at work? | Gives insight into the extent of disability that the condition may be causing | 'I'm retired' | No additional concerns | | | | | |
| Do you drink alcohol? | Excess alcohol consumption is a risk factor for heart and kidney disease | 'No' | No additional concerns | | | | | |
| Do you smoke? | Smoking is a risk factor for heart and kidney disease | 'No' | No additional concerns | | | | | |
| How is your diet? | Poor diet is a risk factor for cardiovascular disease, including worsening hypertension, which can cause CKD | 'It's OK, but I'm a bit overweight' | Raised BMI is a risk factor for cardiovascular disease, which could also cause/worsen CKD (hypertension) | | | | | |

**Systems Review**

| Question | Justification | Answer | Thoughts | | | | | | |
|---|---|---|---|---|---|---|---|---|---|
| Do you feel particularly hot or cold, or feel like you have a fever? | Could suggest infection which may be a sign of an evolving inflammatory process at the site of swelling | 'No' | No additional concerns | | | | | | |
| Have you noticed any changes in your urinary habits? | Urinary habits may be altered in kidney disease | 'I don't seem to be going as much' | No additional concerns | | | | | | |
| Do you ever get short of breath after low levels of exercise? | It is important to explore potential respiratory problems which occur either concurrently with cardiovascular problems, or on their own | 'No' | No additional concerns | | | | | | |
| Just to check, have you had any problems with bladder or bowel function? | Find out if there are any wider concerns that have not arisen yet | 'No, they have been normal' | No additional concerns | | | | | | |
| Have you had any recent night sweats, fever, weight loss or fatigue? | It is essential to ask about B symptoms to rule out certain causes, such as infection | 'No' | No additional concerns | | | | | | |

**Finishing the Consultation**

| Question | Justification | Answer | Thoughts | | | | | |
|---|---|---|---|---|---|---|---|---|
| Is there anything that I've missed, or anything that you are particularly concerned about? | May identify useful information that has been missed. Will also help when framing communication with the patient | 'I think that's all' | Take the time to explain what will happen from here | | | | | |
| Do you have any questions for me at the moment? | | | | | | | | |

**Present Your Findings**

Mr Kaur is a 72-year-old man who presented with a fall and was noted to have oliguria. On further probing his history revealed bilateral lower-leg oedema, fatigue and generalised weakness. He has no other systemic symptoms. He has poorly controlled hypertension, for which he takes amlodipine and losartan, but does not achieve adequate control. He has no other relevant medical conditions. He has no significant family history.

My main differential for Mr Kaur would be CKD secondary to long-standing hypertension. The fatigue and generalised weakness may be due to anaemia secondary to this CKD. Based on his presentation, I would also consider congestive heart failure as an important differential diagnosis.

I would like to do an abdominal and chest examination on Mr Kaur. I would like to order urea and electrolytes for renal function, FBCs to look for anaemia, LFTs for baseline and ECG and echocardiogram for cardiac function

| General Points | | | | |
|---|---|---|---|---|
| Polite to patient | | | | |
| Maintains good eye contact | | | | |
| Appropriate use of open and closed questions | | | | |
| No or limited use of medical jargon | | | | |

## ❓ QUESTIONS FROM THE EXAMINER

### Name four causes of CKD.

Diabetes mellitus (most common), glomerulonephritis, hypertension, chronic pyelonephritis and renal vascular disease.

### Name some symptoms of uraemia.

Nausea, vomiting, pruritus, muscle cramps, hyperventilation and uraemic frost.

### What is the pathophysiology of anaemia in CKD?

Patients CKD can develop anaemia, owing to the critical role of the kidneys in producing erythropoietin (EPO). Interstitial fibroblasts in the kidneys produce EPO, which stimulates red blood cell production. In CKD, this physiological process can be disrupted, leading to less EPO production and, subsequently, anaemia.

### What are potential complications of peritoneal dialysis?

Infection (peritonitis, exit-site infection), membrane failure, encapsulating peritoneal sclerosis and peritoneal leak.

### What are the indications for dialysis in acute kidney injury?

Critically unwell, severe hyperkalaemia >6.5 mmol/L, significant acidosis, uraemic complications (encephalopathy, pericarditis).

### Where in the nephron does furosemide act?

Furosemide is a loop diuretic. It blocks the sodium/potassium/chloride symporter in the thick ascending limb of the loop of Henle.

### What is the pathophysiology underlying volume overload in CKD?

Reduced sodium reabsorption in the kidneys leads to reduced fluid excretion.

### What is the pathophysiology underlying renal osteodystrophy in CKD?

Reduced phosphate excretion from the kidneys results in hyperphosphataemia. Concurrently, reduced vitamin D activation by 1-alpha hydroxylase in the kidney can result in hypocalcaemia. Both hyperphosphataemia and hypocalcaemia result in increased parathyroid hormone secretion from the parathyroid glands, which can lead to renal osteodystrophy.

### What is the specific mechanism of action of angiotensin-converting enzyme (ACE) inhibitors on the kidney?

It causes efferent arteriole dilation which decreases filtration pressure.

### Which dialysis technique requires an arteriovenous fistula?

Haemodialysis.

## Station 1.12   Headache

### Doctor Briefing

You are the junior doctor on call and have been asked to review Anna Hart, a 25-year-old patient, who has presented to the ED with a new and severe headache. Please take a history from Mrs Hart, present your findings and formulate an appropriate management plan.

### Patient Briefing

You are a 25-year woman who has presented to the ED with a severe headache. It affects the right side of the head only and has never occurred before. The headache was preceded by bright-coloured lights appearing in your vision and blurring of the edges of your visual field. This lasted around 15 min before a severe headache began. The headache has lasted around 6 h so far and has not subsided, despite use of paracetamol.

On specific questioning about exacerbating and relieving factors, you reveal that you could not stay in the waiting room of the ED, as the lights were too bright and there was too much noise, which made the headache worse. Sitting in the quiet and dark bathroom has helped to an extent.

There is no history of recent head trauma or problems with your nerves or brain, but your mother has suffered from migraines all her life.

You are generally fit and well. You drink two cups of coffee a day and have a stressful job as a banker in the city. You drink alcohol socially and take no recreational drugs.

You are concerned as the headache is very debilitating.

### Mark Scheme for Examiner

#### Introduction

| | | | |
|---|---|---|---|
| Cleans hands, introduces self, confirms patient identity and gains consent for history taking | | | |
| Establishes current patient knowledge and concerns | | | |

#### History of Presenting Complaint

| Question | Justification | Answer | Thoughts | |
|---|---|---|---|---|
| Could you point to where you feel the headache? | Establishing the site of the headache is crucial. It gives clues to the differential diagnoses. For example, migraines are commonly unilateral, whereas tension headaches are commonly 'around the whole head' | (Point to whole left side of forehead and head) | Unilateral headache reduces the likelihood of certain differentials, such as tension headache | |
| Have you ever had this headache before? | If the patient has had the headache investigated previously, it may give clues to diagnosis. Also gives insight to how debilitating the condition is to daily life | 'Never' | It is new-onset, suggesting a new underlying aetiology or trigger | |
| When did this headache begin? | Ascertaining the duration of the headache gives insight into potential diagnosis. For example, migraines can last up to 72 h, whereas tension headaches are typically shorter | 'About 6 h ago' | The relatively long-standing duration of this headache suggests the pathology is less likely to be a tension headache. The fact that it was not instantly severe also suggests it is unlikely to be a subarachnoid haemorrhage | |

## History of Presenting Complaint

| Question | Justification | Answer | Thoughts | | | | |
|---|---|---|---|---|---|---|---|
| Could you describe the headache? | This gives an indication of severity and character. For example, descriptions such as 'stabbing' in the distribution of the trigeminal nerve may suggest a trigeminal neuralgia | 'Throbbing' | Throbbing character, coupled with the preceding elements of the history, suggests migraine should be a significant differential | | | | |
| Do you feel a similar pain in other parts of your body? | Assessing radiation of the headache gives clues to diagnosis. Key areas to note are radiation to face, eye or neck | 'Not really' | No additional concerns | | | | |
| Do you have any other symptoms at the moment? | Key associated symptoms include nausea and vomiting, watering of eyes/nasal congestion and scalp tenderness. Neck stiffness, rash, fever and photophobia should also be assessed | 'I've thrown up a few times and feel nauseous' | Diagnosis of migraine becoming more likely | | | | |
| Does anything make the headache better or worse? | Key exacerbating factors to monitor include changes on lying down/coughing or photophobia. Key relieving factors to note are relief when patient sits in a quiet/dark room or sleeps | 'Sitting in the quiet bathroom helped. Nothing else has worked' | No additional concerns | | | | |
| Could you rate the severity of the pain on a scale of 1–10? | Severity gives a clue to diagnosis. Cluster headaches are profoundly painful, whereas tension headaches may be less painful. Subjective but important question | '8' | Severity suggests it may lack the intensity of a thunderclap headache/cluster headache | | | | |

## Past Medical History

| Question | Justification | Answer | Thoughts | | | | |
|---|---|---|---|---|---|---|---|
| Do you have a history of any brain or nervous system conditions? | Certain central nervous system conditions are associated with headaches, such as neurovascular conditions | 'No' | Diagnosis is likely to be novel and unrelated to existing disease | | | | |
| Have you recently had any head injuries or concussions? | Recent head trauma can cause temporal episodes of headache | 'No' | Diagnosis unlikely to be related to head trauma | | | | |
| Do you have any other chronic medical conditions? | Comorbidities have implications for both diagnosis and management of headaches | 'No' | No additional concerns | | | | |
| Have you ever had any surgical operations? | Previous neurosurgical operations could be the cause of temporal headaches | 'I had a tibia fracture repaired as a teenager' | No additional concerns | | | | |

## Drug History

| Question | Justification | Answer | Thoughts | | | | | |
|---|---|---|---|---|---|---|---|---|
| Are you on any regular medications for any conditions? | Important to check for contraindications in potential management plan, or to check if certain medications may be causing iatrogenic effects explaining the symptoms | 'No' | No additional concerns | | | | | |
| Do you have any allergies? | Always ask. Important for potential management plans | 'No' | No additional concerns | | | | | |

## Family History

| Question | Justification | Answer | Thoughts | | | | | |
|---|---|---|---|---|---|---|---|---|
| Has anyone in your family suffered from headaches or brain diseases? Do you have any siblings and has anyone passed away under the age of 50? | Family history of headaches gives a clue to diagnosis. Whilst there are very few monogenic causes of headaches, research suggests that there are genetic causes underlying a range of conditions that cause headaches, including migraine. Death of family members <50 may suggest a familial risk of subarachnoid haemorrhage and is always an important part of the family history | 'My mum has had migraines since she was a teenager' 'I don't have any siblings and no one has died before 50.' | Possibly more indicative of migraine, but genetic factors only confer part of the risk of developing migraines | | | | | |
| Do you have any family history of other medical conditions? | Other hereditary medical conditions may impact management plans or reveal other possible risk factors for headaches | 'Dad has type 2 diabetes' | No additional concerns | | | | | |

## Social and Travel History

| Question | Justification | Answer | Thoughts | | | | | |
|---|---|---|---|---|---|---|---|---|
| Do you currently live with anyone? | Always important to ascertain home support network for management plans | 'I live with my partner and two children' | Support system in place at home if necessary, for management plan | | | | | |
| Have you had any difficulties at work? | Gives insight into the extent of disability that the condition may be causing. Further, stress at work can be a trigger for migraines | 'Work is a bit stressful at the moment' | Note that stress could be a trigger for the patient's symptoms | | | | | |
| Do you drink alcohol? Do you smoke? Do you take any recreational drugs? Do you drink caffeinated coffee? | Alcohol, recreational drugs, caffeine and smoking are all potential triggers for migraine onset | 'I drink socially, have never smoked and don't take recreational drugs. I drink two cups of coffee a day' | Note that alcohol and caffeine could be triggers for the patient's condition | | | | | |

**Systems Review**

| Question | Justification | Answer | Thoughts | | | | | | |
|---|---|---|---|---|---|---|---|---|---|
| How is your sleep currently? | Sleep deprivation may explain the patient's symptoms | 'I sleep well' | No additional concerns | | | | | | |
| Have you been feeling very hot or cold, or been running a temperature? | Fever is associated with meningitis, which needs urgent treatment | 'No' | No additional concerns | | | | | | |
| Just to check, have you had any problems with bladder or bowel function? | Find out if there are any wider concerns that have not arisen yet | 'No, they have been normal' | No additional concerns | | | | | | |
| Have you had any recent night sweats, fever, weight loss or fatigue? | It is essential to ask about B symptoms to rule out certain causes, such as infection | 'No' | No additional concerns | | | | | | |

**Finishing the Consultation**

| | | | | | | | | | |
|---|---|---|---|---|---|---|---|---|---|
| Is there anything that I've missed, or anything that you are particularly concerned about? | May identify useful information that has been missed. Will also help when framing communication with the patient | 'I think that's all' | Take the time to explain what will happen from here | | | | | | |
| Do you have any questions for me at the moment? | | | | | | | | | |

**Present Your Findings**

Mrs Hart is a 25-year-old woman who presents with a new-onset, unilateral right-sided headache, with associated nausea and vomiting. The headache is severe and pulsatile in character and does not radiate anywhere else. Sitting in a dark and quiet room improves her symptoms, whilst light and noise make them worse. She has not had any recent head trauma and has no personal history of headaches or nervous system disorders, but her mother has a history of migraines.

My main differential would be migraine, with differential diagnosis of tension and cluster headache.

I would recommend simple analgesia during acute attacks and possibly prescribe some selective serotonin receptor agonist such as sumatriptan. I'd also advise her to speak to her family care doctor if she would like to consider prophylactic medication such as propranolol, and to avoid triggers

**General Points**

| | | | | | | |
|---|---|---|---|---|---|---|
| Polite to patient | | | | | | |
| Maintains eye contact | | | | | | |
| Appropriate use of open and closed questions | | | | | | |
| No or limited use of medical jargon | | | | | | |

## ? QUESTIONS FROM THE EXAMINER

### What is the difference between a primary and secondary headache?

A primary headache is the most common type of headache. It essentially means the headache is not the result of a specific underlying cause. By contrast, a secondary headache is directly caused by another condition, such as an aneurysm or brain tumour.

### The pathophysiology of aura is thought to be rooted in cortical spreading depression (CSD). What is the definition of CSD?

CSD is a transient and local suppression of spontaneous electrical activity in the cortex which moves slowly across the brain.

### Describe the typical stages of a migraine headache.

Characteristically the individual begins to experience prodrome/premonition, followed by an aura and then a headache. Afterwards, there is usually a postdrome or recovery period.

### Various monoclonal antibodies have been developed to prevent migraine. These monoclonal antibodies act as antagonists to which neuropeptide?

Calcitonin gene-related peptide.

### Give three potential triggers of migraines.

Caffeine, stress, hormonal changes (for example, the menstrual cycle), depression, fatigue, hypoglycaemia and dehydration.

### How long does the aura of a migraine usually last?

Usually under 1 h.

### How is a cluster headache treated?

Acutely, it is treated with high-flow oxygen and triptans. Prophylactically, patients are often given calcium channel blockers, such as verapamil.

### What is the mechanism of action of sumatriptan?

Sumatriptan is a selective serotonin receptor agonist. It is a vasoconstrictor, reducing blood flow in the cerebral vessels.

### Give two common pharmacological treatments for trigeminal neuralgia.

Carbamazepine or pregabalin ± amitriptyline.

### How does a tension headache present?

Usually a dull, aching pain that can be 'band-like', wrapping around the head. It can be a sense of constriction.

## Station 1.13   Collapse

### Doctor Briefing

You are a junior doctor working on the medical assessment unit and have been asked to see Mr Jones, a 65-year-old man, who has been referred from primary care following three episodes of collapse over the last 4 days. Each episode lasted a few minutes with full recovery. He has a history of diabetes and had an MI 5 years ago. Please take a history from Mr Jones, present your findings and formulate an appropriate management plan.

### Patient Briefing

Following a visit to your doctor, due to three previous episodes of collapse, you have been advised to visit the hospital for further assessment. Each episode has occurred shortly after standing up, including two episodes occurring after getting out of bed.

Prior to collapsing, you experience dizziness and changes in your vision. Your wife has been present for all three collapses and describes a complete loss of consciousness for a few minutes, with no tongue biting or abnormal movements. You recover completely but are left with a feeling of nausea and headache.

You take medication for type 2 diabetes and hypertension but have not had a medication review for the past 3 years and admit to only occasionally taking the tablets, and sometimes taking double doses as a 'catch-up'. You currently have no chest pain associated with the collapsing episodes, and episodes do not tend to occur following exertion. You have smoked around 10 cigarettes a day for the last 40 years and drink a few beers at the weekend.

Your father also has type 2 diabetes, but no other medical conditions run in the family.

You are concerned about injuring yourself or your wife due to collapsing when completing activities of daily living.

### Mark Scheme for Examiner

#### Introduction

| | |
|---|---|
| Cleans hands, introduces self, confirms patient identity and gains consent for history taking | |
| Establishes current patient knowledge and concerns | |

#### History of Presenting Complaint

| Question | Justification | Answer | Thoughts | | | | |
|---|---|---|---|---|---|---|---|
| Are the episodes associated with loss of consciousness? | It is important to establish the patient's definition of collapse | 'Yes, unless I sit down' | It is important to take a collateral history to understand any activity while the patient is unconscious | | | | |
| How long do you remain unconscious? | Episodes of unconsciousness due to syncope are usually less than 1 min. Patients experiencing seizures may be unconscious for a longer period of time | 'About 30 s' | Symptoms are more suggestive of syncope than seizures | | | | |
| Has anyone witnessed you collapse? | Assessing for seizure activity | 'My wife' | A collateral history can be taken | | | | |
| Did they observe any jerky movements or tongue biting? Did you experience any urinary or faecal incontinence during the collapses? | It is important to find out whether the patient had any of problems during the collapse as it may point more towards seizure than other causes. | 'No' | No seizure-related symptoms | | | | |

## History of Presenting Complaint

| Question | Justification | Answer | Thoughts | | | | | |
|---|---|---|---|---|---|---|---|---|
| What were you doing before each episode? | Vasovagal syncope may be triggered by severe emotional or orthostatic stress | 'Two episodes were after I got out of bed' | Standing rapidly may trigger orthostatic stress | | | | | |
| Do you experience any symptoms before you collapse, such as light-headedness or vision changes? | Seizures may be associated with aura. Vasovagal syncope may be preceded by light-headedness and visual disturbances. There are often no preceding symptoms with cardiovascular syncope | 'I feel dizzy, sweaty and get a ringing in my ears' | Symptoms may suggest vasovagal collapse | | | | | |
| Does anything prevent you collapsing? | Sitting or lying down may prevent collapse in orthostatic hypotension | 'Lying down stops me collapsing' | Indicative of orthostatic hypotension | | | | | |
| Do you have any chest pain or palpitations? | Chest pain may be associated with cardiovascular syncope | 'No' | Less indicative of a cardiovascular collapse | | | | | |
| Do you experience any symptoms after collapsing, including confusion or drowsiness? | A postictal period may be associated with seizures | 'I felt sick for about 30 min but was not drowsy or confused' | Symptoms are more suggestive of syncope than seizures | | | | | |
| Have you hit your head during any of the episodes? | It is important to assess for head trauma that may need further investigation | 'No' | No additional concerns | | | | | |
| Did you vomit while unconscious? | Vomit may be aspirated during a collapse, which may cause further symptoms, such as acute inflammatory respiratory reactions | 'No' | No additional concerns | | | | | |

## Past Medical and Surgical History

| Question | Justification | Answer | Thoughts | | | | | |
|---|---|---|---|---|---|---|---|---|
| Have you experienced these symptoms before? | Episodes of collapse may have been investigated and treated previously | 'No' | No additional concerns | | | | | |
| Do you have any other medical problems? | Cardiovascular causes of collapse may be associated with a known murmur, or previous cardiac disorders. Medication such as antihypertensives and diuretics may contribute to orthostatic hypotension | 'Type 2 diabetes and I had a heart attack 3 years ago' | Diabetic control should be assessed, and a medication review conducted | | | | | |
| How well controlled is your diabetes? | Hypoglycaemia may be associated with loss of consciousness | 'I haven't been to the doctor to check in 2 years' | Important to assess HbA1c and review medication(s) | | | | | |

## Drug History

| Question | Justification | Answer | Thoughts | | | |
|---|---|---|---|---|---|---|
| Are you currently taking any medication, or have any allergies? | Antihypertensives, prescribed following the MI, may be contributing to orthostatic hypertension | 'Atenolol and metformin, no allergies' | Need to address the patient's medication compliance | | | |
| How often do you take your medication? Do you ever forget to take a dose? | Assessing medication compliance | 'Sometimes I forget and take two doses when I remember' | The patient may be hypotensive following taking multiple doses of atenolol | | | |
| When was the last time your doctor assessed your medication? | Important to understand if a medication review has recently been undertaken | 'A few years ago' | The patient is due for a more up to date review of his medications. | | | |

## Family History

| Question | Justification | Answer | Thoughts | | | |
|---|---|---|---|---|---|---|
| Are there any diseases that run in the family, including any cancers? | Always check for relevant heritable conditions | 'My dad has type 2 diabetes' | The patient is presenting with high cardiovascular risk factors | | | |

## Social and Travel History

| Question | Justification | Answer | Thoughts | | | |
|---|---|---|---|---|---|---|
| Who is currently at home? Are you working? | Explore possible social concerns or if wider support is needed | 'I live with my wife and am a retired train driver' | No social concerns; able to educate the patient's wife regarding the episodes of collapse | | | |
| Do you smoke? | Explore wider risk factors | 'Around 10 a day for the last 40 years' | 20 pack-years. The patient has increased cardiovascular risk | | | |
| What is your average weekly alcohol consumption? | | 'A few beers at the weekend' | No additional concerns | | | |

## Systems Review

| Question | Justification | Answer | Thoughts | | | |
|---|---|---|---|---|---|---|
| Have you had any bowel changes or vomiting? | Diarrhoea and vomiting may contribute to hypotension | 'No' | No additional concerns | | | |
| Have you experienced any headaches or motor or sensory changes? | These symptoms may indicate a neurological cause of symptoms such as a stroke or brain tumour | 'No' | No additional concerns | | | |
| Have you had any recent night sweats, fever, weight loss or fatigue? | It is essential to ask about B symptoms to rule out certain causes, such as infection | 'No' | No additional concerns | | | |

## Finishing the Consultation

| Question | Justification | Answer | Thoughts | | | | |
|---|---|---|---|---|---|---|---|
| Is there anything that I've missed that you would like to tell me about? | May identify useful information that has been missed. Will also help to build rapport with the patient | 'I hope it's nothing serious' | Take the time to explain what will happen from here | | | | |
| Do you have any questions? | Allows any final concerns to be addressed | | | | | | |

## Present Your Findings

Mr Jones, a 65-year-old man with a past medical history of a previous MI (2 years ago) and type 2 diabetes, presented with a series of collapsing episodes. Episodes are associated with loss of consciousness, preceded by dizziness, tinnitus and sweats, with full recovery after about 30 s. Episodes appear to be triggered by standing from lying. No symptom indicative of seizure activity has been described. Mr Jones takes atenolol and metformin and describes poor compliance, forgetting doses and taking double catch-up doses. Mr Jones has not had a medication review in 2 years.

My main differential is orthostatic hypotension, secondary to antihypertensive medication usage or autonomic dysfunction due to diabetes.

I will complete an ECG to exclude cardiac causes, routine blood tests including FBC, and HbA$_{1c}$. I will also conduct a medication review, measure standing and sitting blood pressure and perform the tilt table test

## General Points

Polite to patient

Maintains good eye contact

Appropriate use of open and closed questions

No or limited use of medical jargon

## ❓ QUESTIONS FROM THE EXAMINER

### Describe the baroreceptor reflex.

Baroreceptors are stretch receptors that aim to maintain blood pressure, and if pressure decreases, tonic baroreceptor firing decreases. Afferent activity travels to the nucleus tractus solitarius, with efferent activity increasing sympathetic activity and decreasing parasympathetic activity. The pressure therefore increases as cardiac output increases and total peripheral resistance increases.

### Where are baroreceptors located?

The aortic arch and carotid sinuses.

### Why is orthostatic hypotension more prevalent in older patients?

Elderly patients have a blunted baroreflex. They may also be taking medication that reduces their blood pressure (antihypertensives) or decreases their circulating volume (diuretics).

### How may orthostatic hypertension be managed conservatively?

Advise patients to take care and time when moving from lying to standing to reduce the risk of collapse, and to increase water and salt ingestion. Consider use of compression stockings and abdominal binders to reduce venous pooling. Inform the patient of manoeuvres to reduce venous pooling (such as leg crossing) and review the patient's medications.

### What pharmacological management may be used for orthostatic hypertension?

Fludrocortisone, which is a mineralocorticoid that can used for neuropathic orthostatic hypotension. Midodrine is a vasopressor which may be used in orthostatic hypotension due to autonomic dysfunction.

### Why are patients taking long-term steroids advised against stopping the medication suddenly?

Adrenal atrophy can occur, as exogenous steroids are present. Therefore, acute adrenal insufficiency may occur upon abruptly stopping medication, as the adrenal glands are unable to produce the quantity of steroids required.

### What is a Stokes–Adams attack?

A sudden collapse without prodrome due to transient arrhythmias which result in decreased cardiac output and therefore loss of consciousness.

### Describe the mechanism of a vasovagal collapse.

Blood pressure suddenly decreases due to reflex bradycardia and decreased peripheral vasodilation in response to a stressor. Stressors may include extreme emotions such as fear, pain or orthostatic stress caused by prolonged standing.

### What symptoms may indicate a seizure as opposed to a collapse?

Signs suggestive of a seizure include tongue biting, urinary or faecal incontinence, involuntary movements and a long recovery period.

### State two cardiac causes of collapse.

Aortic stenosis and arrhythmias including ventricular fibrillation (due to being associated with a significant decrease in blood pressure).

## Station 1.14 Weakness

### Doctor Briefing

You are a junior doctor in primary care and have been asked to see James Harper, a 67-year-old man, who has presented with right-leg weakness. His past medical history includes hypertension and hypercholesterolaemia. Please take a history from Mr Harper, present your findings and formulate an appropriate management plan

### Patient Briefing

You are visiting your doctor, as you experienced an episode of weakness and numbness in your right leg yesterday. The episode lasted around 4 h, during which you found it hard to balance and to coordinate your actions. On questioning, you found yourself walking into doorframes and furniture numerous times during the period.

You further recall feeling confused, which is out of character, and unable to communicate as normal, as you 'could not get the words out'. You recall having a previous episode of similar weakness about 4 months ago, but as the symptoms only lasted around 1 h, you did not seek any medical assistance.

You have hypertension and hypercholesterolaemia, for which you are taking amlodipine. You are allergic to penicillin. Your brother had a heart attack at 60 years old, but no other conditions run in the family.

You are retired and live alone. You quit smoking around 10 years ago, after smoking about 20 cigarettes a day for 20 years, and do not drink alcohol.

Although the weakness has now completely resolved, you are still very concerned the symptoms may return and affect your ability to walk and communicate.

### Mark Scheme for Examiner

#### Introduction

| | | | |
|---|---|---|---|
| Cleans hands, introduces self, confirms patient identity and gains consent for history taking | | | |
| Establishes current patient knowledge and concerns | | | |

#### History of Presenting Complaint

| Question | Justification | Answer | Thoughts | | | |
|---|---|---|---|---|---|---|
| Please can you describe what you mean by weakness | It is important to understand the patient's definition of weakness | 'I was struggling to stand, walk or move my leg' | The patient appears to be describing a Muscle Power Scale score of 3 | | | |
| When did you first notice the weakness? | This helps to determine if this is acute or chronic | 'About 24 h ago' | Acute causes should be ruled out | | | |
| How long did the weakness last? | Symptoms associated with a stroke or progressive neurological disorders such as Guillain–Barré syndrome may persist. In transient ischaemic attacks (TIAs), patients display symptoms for less than 24 h | 'About 4 h' | More indicative of a reversible cause or relapsing and remitting disease progression | | | |
| Have all of your symptoms completely resolved? | In TIAs symptoms resolve fully within 24h. In a stroke, symptoms may persist | 'Yes, after around 4 h' | Symptoms are more indicative of a TIA | | | |

## History of Presenting Complaint

| Question | Justification | Answer | Thoughts | | | | | | |
|---|---|---|---|---|---|---|---|---|---|
| Where was the weakness? | This enquires whether weakness is bilateral or unilateral. The location of weakness may provide information regarding the site of a lesion | 'My right leg only.' | Unilateral weakness in the lower extremity suggests focal neurology | | | | | | |
| How quickly did the weakness start? | Onset of progressive diseases may be more gradual. Strokes and TIAs often present acutely | 'Very suddenly' | More indicative of a vascular cause | | | | | | |
| Did you experience any changes in sensation, such as numbness or tingling? | It is important to assess associated symptoms | 'Numbness' | Need to exclude acute causes of nerve compression | | | | | | |
| Have you experienced any back pain? | Assessing for spinal cord compression | 'No' | No additional concerns | | | | | | |
| Have you experienced any changes in sensation when passing urine, or urinary incontinence? | | 'No' | | | | | | | |
| Did anything make the weakness worse or better? | Symptoms worsening on exertion may be associated with myasthenia gravis | 'No' | The weakness is not influenced by fatigue | | | | | | |
| How did the weakness affect your walking? | Assesses for changes in coordination and gait | 'I felt off balance and walked into furniture' | Co-ordination may be impaired. It is important to assess for associated visual changes | | | | | | |
| Did you experience any changes in your vision? | Visual changes may help to identify the site of a lesion | 'My vision was blurry' | This suggests the visual pathway has been affected | | | | | | |
| Did you experience any headaches? | Subarachnoid haemorrhages may be associated with a thunderclap headache. Hemiplegic migraines may be associated with limb weakness | 'No' | No additional concerns | | | | | | |
| Did you experience any changes in your speech? | Dysarthria and aphasia may be associated with TIAs or a stroke | 'I was unable to get words out' | Suggestive of expressive aphasia | | | | | | |

**Past Medical and Surgical History**

| Question | Justification | Answer | Thoughts | | | | |
|---|---|---|---|---|---|---|---|
| Have you ever experienced similar symptoms before? | Checking symptoms are not recurring to explore past medical history | 'Yes, about 4 months ago' | Relapsing and remitting conditions (such as multiple sclerosis) should be considered. TIAs may occur repeatedly in patients with high cardiovascular risk | | | | |
| Did you seek medical help, or undergo any medical investigations? | The patient may have already undergone investigations or trialled medications | 'No' | Unable to be guided by previous investigations | | | | |
| Do you have a history of seizures or a diagnosis of epilepsy? | Todd's paresis presents in patients with epilepsy following seizures | 'No' | No additional concerns | | | | |
| Do you have any other medical conditions? | Assess the patient's global cardiovascular risk | 'Hypertension and hypercholesterolaemia' | High cardiovascular risk may be associated with ischaemic stroke due to an embolus | | | | |
| Have you ever had a heart attack or previous stroke? | | 'No' | No additional concerns | | | | |

**Drug History**

| Question | Justification | Answer | Thoughts | | | | |
|---|---|---|---|---|---|---|---|
| Are you currently taking any medication, or have any allergies? | Anticoagulants may be associated with increased risk of intracranial haemorrhage. Myopathy is associated with steroid and statin use | 'Amlodipine and allergic to penicillin' | No additional concerns | | | | |

**Family History**

| Question | Justification | Answer | Thoughts | | | | |
|---|---|---|---|---|---|---|---|
| Are there any diseases that run in the family, including any cancers? | Always check for relevant heritable conditions | 'My brother had a heart attack at 60' | This may require further investigation but currently is not a concern | | | | |
| Has anyone in your family previously experienced a stroke or been diagnosed with an aneurysm? | Familial intracranial aneurysms may be heritable | 'No' | No additional concerns | | | | |

## Social and Travel History

| Question | Justification | Answer | Thoughts | | | | | |
|---|---|---|---|---|---|---|---|---|
| Who is currently at home? Are you working? | Explore possible social concerns or if wider support is needed | 'I live alone and am retired' | Wider support may be required | | | | | |
| Do you smoke? | Explore wider risk factors | 'I quit 10 years ago, but smoked 20 a day for 20 years' | 20 pack-years. Smoking increases cardiovascular risk | | | | | |
| What is your average weekly alcohol consumption? | | 'I don't drink alcohol' | No additional concerns | | | | | |

## Systems Review

| | | | | | | | | |
|---|---|---|---|---|---|---|---|---|
| Have you had a fever? | Assess for any infective causes such as bacterial meningitis | 'No' | No additional concerns | | | | | |
| Have you experienced any nausea and vomiting? | These symptoms may be associated with raised intracranial pressure, such as from a haematoma | 'No' | Symptoms are more indicative of an ischaemic rather than haemorrhagic cause of symptoms | | | | | |
| Have you experienced any joint pain or stiffness? | Assess for musculoskeletal symptoms | 'No' | No additional concerns | | | | | |

## Finishing the Consultation

| | | | | | | | | |
|---|---|---|---|---|---|---|---|---|
| Is there anything that I've missed that you would like to tell me about? | May identify useful information that has been missed. Will also help to build rapport with the patient | 'I felt a bit confused and clumsy during the episode, which I am concerned about' | Take the time to explain what will happen from here | | | | | |
| Do you have any questions? | Allows any final concerns to be addressed | | | | | | | |

## Present Your Findings

Mr Harper, a 67-year-old man with known hypertension and hypercholesterolaemia, presented with a single episode of right-leg weakness lasting around 4 h, then fully resolving. Mr Harper also experienced expressive dysphasia, confusion, coordination impairments and numbness, with blurred vision.

My main differential is a TIA, due to an ischaemic cause following an embolus.

I would like to complete a FBC, urea and electrolytes, LFT, serum glucose level, serum lipid levels and a clotting screen. I will also conduct an MRI head and carotid Doppler

| General Points | | | | |
|---|---|---|---|---|
| Polite to patient | | | | |
| Maintains good eye contact | | | | |
| Appropriate use of open and closed questions | | | | |
| No or limited use of medical jargon | | | | |

## ❓ QUESTIONS FROM THE EXAMINER

### Is it necessary to inform the Driver and Vehicle Licensing Agency (DVLA) if a patient has a TIA?

Patients should avoid driving for 1 month following a stroke or TIA, or 3 months if experiencing frequent TIAs. It is only necessary to inform the DVLA if neurological deficits persist longer than 1 month.

### What is the difference between haemorrhagic and ischaemic stroke?

Haemorrhagic strokes are due to a ruptured blood vessel, and are responsible for 15% of strokes. Ischaemic strokes are due to a reduction in blood flow, usually following an occlusion such as an embolus in the cerebral artery. These are responsible for 85% of strokes.

### What is the mechanism of injury in haemorrhagic strokes?

Primary injury is due to increased intracerebral pressure secondary to the haemorrhage. Secondary injury is due to inflammation, leading to overproduction of toxic free radical species. Haem from the red blood cells is toxic to neural tissue.

### What are the three types of haemorrhagic stroke?

Spontaneous intracerebral haemorrhage, burst aneurysm and subarachnoid haemorrhage.

### What is a berry aneurysm?

Berry aneurysms are the most common type of aneurysm, and describe vascular swellings in congenital weak spots in arterial walls. They occur most commonly in the circle of Willis. Rupture of berry aneurysms can lead to subarachnoid haemorrhage.

### Which brain areas are involved in speech and language, and where are they located?

Language tends to be left-lateralised, especially in right-handed individuals. Broca's area is responsible for speech production and is located in the frontal cortex (inferior frontal gyrus). Wernicke's area is responsible for speech comprehension and is located in the temporal parietal junction.

### How may a patient with Broca's aphasia present?

A patient may present with expressive aphasia, with an inability to articulate words. The patient will retain understanding, speech comprehension and intelligence.

### How may a patient with Wernicke's area present?

A patient may present with receptive aphasia, with an inability to form comprehensive sentences. Patients will able to talk freely, and be able to read clearly; however, they will be unable to understand language; meaning is impaired.

### What is meant by spatial neglect?

Neglect is an attentional deficit which may develop following a stroke, most commonly following damage to the right hemisphere. Patients may fail to identify stimuli presented on the opposite side to their brain lesion. For example, patients may only eat food on the right side of their plate following a right-hemisphere stroke.

### How may a patient present with bilateral hemianopia, and where is the likely location of a lesion?

A patient may describe a loss of the outer half of the vision in both eyes (loss of temporal vision bilaterally). A lesion is likely to be present in the optic chiasm.

## Station 1.15    Hypothyroidism

### Doctor Briefing

You are a junior doctor in primary care and have been asked to see Mr Long, a 45-year-old man, who noticed a lump in his neck 2 weeks ago. He thinks this has got bigger and is worried about what is causing it. He is a smoker with a 20-pack-year history and drinks around 30 units of alcohol each week. He has no other medical history. Please take a history from Mr Long, present your findings and formulate an appropriate management plan.

### Patient Briefing

You are a 45-year-old man presenting to your primary care doctor for the first time in several years. Please behave in a restless way throughout the consultation, including tapping your foot repeatedly. Only wear a t-shirt during the consultation.

You have noticed a swelling in your neck that you think has grown in size over the last few weeks. The swelling is not painful or sensitive to touch. You think you first noticed the swelling 3 weeks ago, but it may have been there for longer.

On specific questioning, over the last month you have noticed some unintentional weight loss of about 4 kg. You have also had difficulty sleeping. Furthermore, you feel very warm even when it is cold outside and have felt some 'fluttering in your chest'. Your partner has noticed that you have been more irritable than normal as well.

Otherwise, you are well and have not had any fevers. You are smoker, roughly 1 pack per day for the past 20 years. You drink approximately 30 units of alcohol, but do not take recreational drugs. You live at home with your partner and have not travelled recently. There is no significant family history of cancer or thyroid disease.

You have never had this problem previously but are worried that this neck lump is a sign of cancer.

### Mark Scheme for Examiner

#### Introduction

| | |
|---|---|
| Cleans hands, introduces self, confirms patient identity and gains consent for history taking | |
| Establishes current patient knowledge and concerns | |

#### History of Presenting Complaint

| Question | Justification | Answer | Thoughts | |
|---|---|---|---|---|
| When did you first notice the lump in your neck? | Establishing onset of the lump is important. Some lumps may be transient, with an acute onset; others may have more insidious onset | 'About 3 weeks ago' | Three weeks renders an infectious cause less likely. However, further exploration is required | |
| Have you noticed any changes in the size of the lump? | A rapidly growing lump may be a sign of an aggressive thyroid cancer | 'I think it's slowly getting bigger' | This suggests the lump is growing in size, but not rapidly. This suggests an aggressive cancer is less likely | |
| Is the lump painful to touch? | A painful, tender neck lump may suggest an inflammatory or infective cause. Cervical lymphadenopathy may present with a tender, mobile lump, whilst a thyroglossal cyst tends to be painless | 'No' | This suggests an infective cause is less likely | |
| Have you noticed anything makes the lump better or worse? | Establishing exacerbating and relieving factors for any pain or swelling is important | 'No' | A thyroid problem is becoming the more likely differential diagnosis | |

## History of Presenting Complaint

| Question | Justification | Answer | Thoughts | | | | | |
|---|---|---|---|---|---|---|---|---|
| Have you noticed any recent unintentional weight changes? | Unintentional weight loss can be a feature of hyperthyroidism | 'I've lost about 4 kg without trying' | Unintentional weight loss can be a sign of thyroid disease and is also seen in malignancy | | | | | |
| Have you noticed any changes in appetite? | In hyperthyroidism, appetite can be increased, whilst the opposite occurs in hypothyroidism | 'Not really' | No additional concerns | | | | | |
| Do you have a fever, or have you recently been unwell? | Neck lumps can be enlarged lymph nodes as a result of infections. It is important to ask about any signs of existing or recent infection | 'No' | Suggests an infectious cause is less likely | | | | | |
| Have you noticed any changes to your sleep? | In hyperthyroidism, people may suffer from restlessness and difficulty sleeping | 'I'm finding it hard to get to bed' | Consider hyperthyroidism as a top differential diagnosis | | | | | |
| Have you been feeling particularly warm or cold when others have been feeling or comfortable? | In hyperthyroidism, people can have heat intolerance. Conversely, in hypothyroidism, people may complain of feeling unusually cold | 'I've been feeling hot more than usual' | This is in keeping with hyperthyroidism being the top differential diagnosis at present | | | | | |
| Have you noticed any chest pain or unusual feelings in your chest? | Enquire about palpitations, which can occur in hyperthyroidism | 'I've had some fluttering in my chest' | Presence of palpitations is in keeping with hyperthyroidism | | | | | |
| Have you noticed any changes to your mood? | Mood changes can be a feature of thyroid disease. Typically, in hyperthyroidism patients can have irritability, whilst in hypothyroidism, patients can have mood swings or low mood | 'My wife has said that I've been a bit more irritable lately' | Irritability may be a sign of hyperthyroidism | | | | | |
| Have you noticed any changes to your hair, such as thinning? | Hair changes on both the scalp and thinning of the eyebrows can be a sign of thyroid disease | 'No' | No additional concerns | | | | | |
| Have you noticed any changes to your bowel habits? | In hyperthyroidism, patients can complain of diarrhoea. In hypothyroidism, patients can complain of constipation | 'No' | No additional concerns | | | | | |

## Past Medical History

| Question | Justification | Answer | Thoughts | | | | | |
|---|---|---|---|---|---|---|---|---|
| Do you have any chronic medical conditions? | Comorbidities have implications for both diagnosis and management of thyroid disease | 'No' | No additional concerns | | | | | |
| Do you have any history of thyroid disease? | An existing or previous diagnosis of thyroid disease would help inform this diagnosis | 'No' | No additional concerns | | | | | |

**Past Medical History**

| Question | Justification | Answer | Thoughts | | | | | |
|---|---|---|---|---|---|---|---|---|
| Do you have any history of cancer? | Malignancy may result in enlarged lymph nodes and cervical lymphadenopathy. A metastatic spread of an existing cancer could present in this way, as could a primary haematological malignancy | 'No' | Less likely to be a metastatic spread of an existing cancer, but could be a new-onset malignancy | | | | | |

**Drug History**

| Question | Justification | Answer | Thoughts | | | | | |
|---|---|---|---|---|---|---|---|---|
| Are you on any regular medications? | Important to check for contraindications in potential management plan, or to check if certain medications may be causing iatrogenic effects explaining the symptoms, such as lithium or phenytoin | 'No' | No additional concerns | | | | | |
| Do you have any allergies? | Always ask. Important for potential management plans | 'No' | No additional concerns | | | | | |

**Family History**

| Question | Justification | Answer | Thoughts | | | | | |
|---|---|---|---|---|---|---|---|---|
| Has anyone in your family had a diagnosis of cancer? | Family history of malignancy may render malignancy or metastatic spread a higher differential diagnosis, especially if it is a particularly heritable cancer | 'No' | No additional concerns | | | | | |
| Do you have any family history of other medical conditions? | Other hereditary medical conditions may impact management plans or reveal other possible risk factors for thyroid disease | 'No' | No additional concerns | | | | | |

**Social and Travel History**

| Question | Justification | Answer | Thoughts | | | | | |
|---|---|---|---|---|---|---|---|---|
| Do you drink alcohol? | Always important to take an alcohol history. It may have important implications for the management plan | 'Yes, I like a drink every night so around 30 units a week' | Should remind the patient that the weekly recommended alcohol limit per week is 14 units. | | | | | |
| Do you smoke? | Smoking is a risk factor for malignancy, which is an important differential diagnosis | 'Yes, I've been smoking around 1 pack a day for 20 years' | A significant smoking history is a cause for concern for cancer. | | | | | |
| How is your diet? | Poor diet and raised BMI can be a risk factor for certain malignancies | 'I'm pretty healthy' | No additional concerns | | | | | |
| Do you take any recreational drugs? | Important to document any illicit drug use, as it may have an impact on management plan | 'No' | No additional concerns | | | | | |

## Systems Review

| Question | Justification | Answer | Thoughts | | | | |
|---|---|---|---|---|---|---|---|
| Have you had any difficulty swallowing? | If the neck swelling is large or located particularly close to the oesophagus, compression could cause swallowing difficulties | 'No' | No additional concerns | | | | |
| Have you noticed any breathlessness? | If the neck swelling is large or located particularly close to the trachea, it could compress it, causing breathing difficulties | 'No' | No additional concerns | | | | |

## Finishing the Consultation

| | | | | | | | |
|---|---|---|---|---|---|---|---|
| Is there anything that I've missed, or anything that you are particularly concerned about? | May identify useful information that has been missed. Will also help when framing communication with the patient | 'I think that's all'. | Take the time to explain what will happen from here | | | | |
| Do you have any questions for me at the moment? | | | | | | | |

## Present Your Findings

Mr Long is a 45-year-old man who has presented with unintentional weight loss, insomnia, heat intolerance and palpitations. He also has a progressively growing, non-tender swelling in his neck. These symptoms have all been persistent for the last month. He has no further systemic symptoms of fever and has not recently been travelling.

My main differential for Mr Long is hyperthyroidism. I would also consider cardiac causes, including arrhythmias, as well as malignancy.

I would like to do a full thyroid examination on Mr Long. I would then like to do thyroid function tests and an ECG and organise an ultrasound of the neck lump

## General Points

| | | | | |
|---|---|---|---|---|
| Polite to patient | | | | |
| Maintains good eye contact | | | | |
| Appropriate use of open and closed questions | | | | |
| No or limited use of medical jargon | | | | |

## ❓ QUESTIONS FROM THE EXAMINER

### What are the hormones involved in the hypothalamic–pituitary–thyroid axis?

Thyroid-releasing hormone is released from the hypothalamus and signals to the pituitary gland. The pituitary gland releases thyroid-stimulating hormone (TSH) that signals to the thyroid. Finally, the thyroid releases triiodothyronine and thyroxine.

### What are the autoantibodies involved in Graves' disease?

Anti-TSH-receptor (anti-TSHR) autoantibodies.

### What are the five main types of thyroid cancer and their relative incidences?

Papillary thyroid cancer is the most common, followed by follicular thyroid cancer, medullary thyroid cancer and Hurthle cell thyroid cancer, and anaplastic thyroid cancer in descending order.

### What is the proportion of patients still alive at **5 years with a diagnosis of anaplastic thyroid carcinoma?**

One in 10 patients.

### What are the potential ocular problems that occur in Graves' ophthalmopathy?

Sensitivity to light, watering, red eyes, blurred or double vision and exophthalmos (bulging eyes).

### What pregnancy difficulties can patients with hyperthyroidism have?

Pre-eclampsia, premature labour and birth, miscarriage and low birth weight.

### What can trigger thyrotoxicosis?

Poorly managed hyperthyroidism, infection, pregnancy and trauma to the thyroid.

### Vitamin D deficiency presents as different clinical entities in children compared with adults. What are they respectively?

In children it presents as rickets whereas in adults, it presents as osteomalacia.

### What is the difference between primary, secondary and tertiary hyperparathyroidism?

In primary hyperparathyroidism, the parathyroid glands simply release excessive parathyroid hormone due to a functional issue with the glands, such as adenoma, carcinoma or hyperplasia. In secondary hyperparathyroidism, the parathyroid glands release excess parathyroid hormone in response to a separate pathology, such as hypocalcaemia or vitamin D deficiency. In tertiary hyperparathyroidism, the parathyroid glands autonomously secrete parathyroid hormone following chronic secondary hyperparathyroidism.

### What is the phrase to help remember the signs of hypercalcaemia and what symptoms does it refer to?

Bones, stones, (abdominal) moans and (psychic) groans. This refers to bony pain, renal stones, constipation or abdominal pain, and psychiatric conditions, such as depression.

## Station 1.16   Intermittent Claudication

### Doctor Briefing

You are a junior doctor in primary care and have been asked to see Mr Brown, a 63-year-old man who presents with worsening leg pain on exertion. He is a long-term cigarette smoker and has type 2 diabetes, with a recent HbA$_{1c}$ of 9%. Please take a history from Mr Brown, present your findings and formulate an appropriate management plan.

### Patient Briefing

You are visiting your doctor due to burning pain in both legs for the past 8 days. The pain initially started in your feet and is now present in both legs until halfway up your calves. Although present most of the time, the pain is worse when you move and at night. The pain is not relieved by ibuprofen, and nothing can reduce the pain at night. It can also present as a sharp stabbing, and you have noticed a tingling sensation in your legs.

You currently have an ulcer on your right foot, which you have attributed to your poorly controlled type 2 diabetes. You further have recently been diagnosed with diabetic nephropathy and retinopathy.

On questioning, you are a long-term smoker, having smoked around 20 cigarettes a day for the past 30 years, and have no intention of quitting. You drink around 5 units of alcohol each week. You live with your son and are a retired gardener. Your mother had a stroke at the age of 60.

You are concerned you may need your legs amputated, as one of your friends has recently required an amputation due to uncontrolled diabetes.

### Mark Scheme for Examiner

#### Introduction

| | | | | |
|---|---|---|---|---|
| Cleans hands, introduces self, confirms patient identity and gains consent for history taking | | | | |
| Establishes current patient knowledge and concerns | | | | |

#### History of Presenting Complaint

| Question | Justification | Answer | Thoughts | | | |
|---|---|---|---|---|---|---|
| When did the pain start? | This helps to determine if symptoms are acute or chronic | 'About 8 days ago' | An acute onset may suggest a neurovascular cause | | | |
| Where is the pain? Is it in both legs? | The region of pain may correlate with an ischaemic territory | 'The pain started under my feet and is now in both my legs until about halfway up my calf' | Bilateral leg pain is unlikely to have an infective cause | | | |
| Is the pain consistent or intermittent? | Infective causes and mechanical injuries may present with constant pain. Vascular pain may be intermittent and exertion-dependent | 'There is constant background pain, but the pain increases at night and when I am walking' | Exacerbating factors should be explored | | | |
| Does anything reduce the pain at night? | Intermittent claudication pain can often be relieved by the patient hanging his legs off the bed | 'No' | Symptoms are not typical of intermittent claudication | | | |

**History of Presenting Complaint**

| Question | Justification | Answer | Thoughts | | | | | |
|---|---|---|---|---|---|---|---|---|
| Does the pain increase on movement? | Pain on exertion may indicate a vascular cause, or irritation of underlying structures due to movement. | 'Yes' | Claudication distance should be assessed | | | | | |
| How far are you able to walk before the pain starts? | Assessing claudication distance is important if a vascular cause is being considered | 'The pain increases as soon as I start walking' | Suggestive of neurogenic pain, which increases on pressure | | | | | |
| Does the pain resolve upon rest? | Intermittent claudication and osteoarthritic pain often resolve on rest | 'Slightly, when I raise my feet' | This is not typical in intermittent claudication | | | | | |
| Did any trauma or injury precede the pain? | Assess for previous trauma | 'No' | No previous trauma | | | | | |
| Have you experienced any weakness or tingling? | Neuropathic pain may present with weakness or tingling | 'Yes, tingling' | Indicative of neuropathic pain | | | | | |
| Does anything make the pain better, including painkillers? | NSAIDs may reduce pain due to swelling such as in arthritis | 'No, ibuprofen does not reduce the pain' | The pain is unlikely to be inflammatory | | | | | |
| Please describe the pain | The type of pain may be indicative of the cause; for example, a sharp pain may be associated with neurological pain | 'Sharp, burning pain' | Both neuropathy and vascular pain may present with a burning sensation | | | | | |
| Have you experienced changes in sensation, including increased sensitivity to touch? | Diabetic neuropathy may be associated with increased sensitivity to touch | 'I have pain on light touch' | The patient is describing allodynia | | | | | |
| Do you have any ulcers, redness or swelling? | Peripheral vascular disease may lead to ulcers. It is important to exclude infective causes | 'I have an ulcer on my right foot' | Ulcers may indicate reduced blood flow | | | | | |
| How severe is the pain? | It is important to assess pain severity | '5/10 at rest. 8/10 when I stand or touch my legs' | The patient is describing severe pain | | | | | |
| Have your legs changed in temperature? | Cold feet may be associated with reduced vascular supply. Increased temperature is observed with inflammation or infection | 'No' | No additional concerns regarding acute limb ischaemia | | | | | |
| Do you experience cramping in your calf or thigh? | Such symptoms are typical in intermittent claudication | 'No' | Symptoms are less indicative of intermittent claudication | | | | | |

## Past Medical and Surgical History

| Question | Justification | Answer | Thoughts | | | | | |
|---|---|---|---|---|---|---|---|---|
| Do you have any medical conditions, including heart problems, stroke, high blood pressure or diabetes? | It is important to assess the patient's vascular risk | 'I have hypertension and type 2 diabetes, with nephropathy and retinopathy' | The patient has an increased vascular risk | | | | | |
| How well controlled is your diabetes? What is your blood glucose, and do you have any complications? | Symptoms described may be related to diabetic neuropathy. Uncontrolled diabetes is more likely to present with complications | 'I have diabetic nephropathy, eye problems, and an ulcer on my right foot. My HbA$_{1c}$ is 9%' | Uncontrolled diabetes may contribute to the symptoms described | | | | | |

## Drug History

| Question | Justification | Answer | Thoughts | | | | | |
|---|---|---|---|---|---|---|---|---|
| Are you on any medication currently, or have any allergies? | People may not disclose their whole medical history. You must always check for allergies | 'Metformin, losartan and no allergies' | The patient's blood pressure is controlled on only one antihypertensive agent | | | | | |

## Family History

| Question | Justification | Answer | Thoughts | | | | | |
|---|---|---|---|---|---|---|---|---|
| Are there any diseases that run in the family, including cancers, strokes or ischaemic heart disease? | Important to check for relevant heritable conditions | 'My mother had a stroke at 60' | A family history of hypercoagulability may be relevant | | | | | |

## Social and Travel History

| Question | Justification | Answer | Thoughts | | | | | |
|---|---|---|---|---|---|---|---|---|
| Who is currently at home? Are you working? | Explore social concerns | 'I live with my son and am a retired gardener' | No social concerns at present | | | | | |
| Do you smoke? | Smoking is associated with peripheral vascular disease and diabetes | '30 a day for 30 years' | The patient has increased risk due to smoking status of 30 pack years | | | | | |
| What is your average weekly alcohol consumption? | Explore wider risk factors | 'Around 5 units a week' | No additional concerns | | | | | |

## Systems Review

| Question | Justification | Answer | Thoughts | | | | | |
|---|---|---|---|---|---|---|---|---|
| Have you a cough or chest pain? | Haemoptysis and pleuritic chest pain may be associated with PE and DVT | 'No' | No additional concerns | | | | | |

**Systems Review**

| Question | Justification | Answer | Thoughts | | | | |
|---|---|---|---|---|---|---|---|
| Just to check, have you had any problems with bladder or bowel function? | Find out if there are any wider concerns that have not arisen yet | 'No, they have been normal' | No additional concerns | | | | |
| Have you had any recent night sweats, fever, weight loss or fatigue? | It is essential to ask about B symptoms to rule out certain causes, such as infection | 'No' | No additional concerns | | | | |

**Finishing the Consultation**

| Question | Justification | Answer | Thoughts | | | | |
|---|---|---|---|---|---|---|---|
| Is there anything that I've missed that you would like to tell me about? | May identify useful information that has been missed. Will also help to build rapport with the patient | 'I am concerned I will require an amputation' | Take the time to explain what will happen from here | | | | |
| Do you have any questions? | Allows any final concerns to be addressed | | | | | | |

**Present Your Findings**

Mr Brown, a 63-year-old man, with uncontrolled type 2 diabetes and hypertension and 30 pack-years, presented with an 8-day history of bilateral leg and foot pain. The pain is worse on touch or standing, associated with a tingling sensation, and is described as a burning pain. The patient has further presented with an ulcer on his right foot.

My main differential is diabetic neuropathy; however, I would also like to investigate for intermittent claudication.

I am going to examine Mr Brown, including examination of pulses and reflexes. I will take blood tests including $HbA_{1c}$, FBC, urea and electrolytes. I will also measure for an ankle brachial pressure index (ABPI) and conduct a duplex ultrasound and nerve conduction tests if indicated

**General Points**

| | | | | |
|---|---|---|---|---|
| Polite to patient | | | | |
| Maintains good eye contact | | | | |
| Appropriate use of open and closed questions | | | | |
| No or limited use of medical jargon | | | | |

## ? QUESTIONS FROM THE EXAMINER

**What scoring system may be used to assess a patient's cardiovascular risk?**

QRISK can be calculated. This includes age, sex, ethnicity, smoking status, diabetes status, family history of angina or MI, CKD and atrial fibrillation, amongst other risk factors.

**Describe how an ABPI may be calculated. What is a normal ABPI ratio?**

ABPI compares the blood pressure in the upper limbs to that in the lower limbs. The blood pressure at the ankle is divided by the brachial blood pressure. A normal ABPI is between 1.0 and 1.4.

## What does a high ABPI ratio indicate?

High ABPI may be indicative of subclinical atherosclerosis and suggests arterial stiffness in the peripheral arteries.

## What clinical test may be conducted to assess for limb ischaemia?

Buerger's test, which involves raising both of the patient's legs to 45° while supine, can be used to assess arterial insufficiency.

## What Buerger's angle is indicative of severe limb ischaemia?

Less than 20°.

## Describe why reactive hyperaemia may occur.

During ischaemia, anaerobic respiration occurs, leading to an accumulation of metabolic waste. Local vasodilation will therefore occur, causing redness.

## What pattern of neurological pain may be expected in diabetic neuropathy?

A glove-and-stocking distribution, describing a loss of sensation initially in the hands and feet.

## Describe what is meant by gangrene. Describe the difference between wet and dry gangrene.

Gangrene describes tissue death due to insufficient vascular supply which may present in peripheral vascular disease. Dry gangrene describes tissue death in the absence of infection whereas wet gangrene describes tissue death with associated infection which may present with discharge.

## What is the management of gangrene?

Patients may be treated with broad-spectrum antibiotics such as ceftriaxone (cephalosporin) intravenously, and surgical debridement. In severe cases, amputation may be required.

## What pulses can be palpated in the foot and where are they located?

Dorsalis pedis is located dorsally on the foot, lateral to the extensor hallucis longus tendon. Posterior tibial is inferior and posterior to the medial malleolus.

## Station 1.17    Swollen Calf

### Doctor Briefing

You are a junior doctor in primary care and have been asked to see Mrs Maynard, a 70-year-old woman, who presented with a 3-week history of leg swelling. The swelling has got progressively worse and is affecting her mobility. She has a history of angina, hypertension, recurrent urinary tract infections (UTIs) and COPD. Please take a history from Mrs Maynard, present your findings and formulate an appropriate management plan.

### Patient Briefing

You are visiting your doctor as you noticed swelling in both of your legs around 3 weeks ago. You are struggling to fit into your shoes and the swelling has increased, impairing your walking. You have not noticed any other specific symptoms and are not experiencing any pain. However, you feel generally fatigued and nauseous. You have experienced some breathlessness on exertion but have attributed this to your COPD and have not experienced a new-onset cough.

On questioning, you are passing less urine than usual, and it is a darker colour. You have not noticed any blood in your urine, and have no other urinary problems, including no pain or burning sensation, despite previously experiencing recurrent waterwork infections.

You are known to have angina, hypertension and COPD, for which you are taking GTN spray, amlodipine, furosemide, atorvastatin and steroid inhalers. You are aware that high blood pressure runs in your family. You are a retired nurse, have never smoked and drink alcohol infrequently.

You are concerned that the leg swelling is due to the medications you take and are keen to not add any more medication if possible.

### Mark Scheme for Examiner

#### Introduction

| | | | |
|---|---|---|---|
| Cleans hands, introduces self, confirms patient identity and gains consent for history taking | | | |
| Establishes current patient knowledge and concerns | | | |

#### History of Presenting Complaint

| Question | Justification | Answer | Thoughts | | | | |
|---|---|---|---|---|---|---|---|
| When did you notice the swelling? | Helps determine if this is acute or chronic | '3 weeks ago' | Chronic causes need to be ruled out | | | | |
| Is the swelling in both legs? | Unilateral swelling may be associated with cellulitis or DVT. Bilateral swelling may be more indicative of congestive heart failure | 'Both' | The cause is less likely to be infective | | | | |
| Are there overlying skin changes? | Skin changes may be observed with infective causes such cellulitis | 'No' | No dermatological manifestation of any underlying condition | | | | |
| Do you have calf pain? | Exclude symptoms of DVT | 'No' | Symptoms not indicative of DVT | | | | |
| Does the swelling stay the same throughout the day? | Allows assessment of whether oedema is dependent | 'It increases when I stand' | The patient has described dependent oedema | | | | |
| Do you have chest pain or palpitations? | Cardiac causes of oedema, including congestive heart failure, may be associated with chest pain and palpitations | 'No' | The patient is not experiencing symptoms associated with cardiac conditions | | | | |

## History of Presenting Complaint

| Question | Justification | Answer | Thoughts | | | | |
|---|---|---|---|---|---|---|---|
| Do you have a cough? Is it productive? Is it worse at night? | Patients with congestive cardiac failure may have a cough with white or pink (blood-tinged) frothy sputum, that is worse at night. Patients with severe CKD may experience haemoptysis | 'No new cough' | No additional concerns | | | | |
| Are you experiencing shortness of breath? | Patients may experience shortness of breath in cardiac or renal failure. Anaemia due to CKD may also contribute to breathlessness | 'Yes, on walking' | Indicative of cardiac or renal failure | | | | |
| Is the shortness of breath worse when lying down? | Orthopnoea is associated with congestive cardiac failure | 'No' | No additional concerns | | | | |
| Does anything reduce the swelling? | The patient may be taking medication to relieve the symptoms | 'Raising my legs' | The patient has described dependent oedema | | | | |
| If you press into your leg, does a pit remain when you stop pressing? | Assess for pitting oedema. Lymphoedema presents with non-pitting oedema | 'Yes' | Symptoms not indicative of lymphoedema | | | | |
| Have you experienced any recent episodes of collapse or dizziness? | Congestive cardiac failure may be associated with syncope | 'No' | No additional concerns | | | | |
| Have you experienced nausea, vomiting or lethargy? | Such symptoms may be associated with congestive heart failure or CKD | 'I'm very tired and feel nauseous' | Although symptoms are broad, they may be indicative of congestive heart failure or CKD | | | | |
| Have you noticed changes in your urine? | CKD may present with changes in urine, including oliguria | 'I am passing less urine and it is very dark' | This may indicate a renal cause | | | | |
| Do you have increased urgency, or pain when urinating? | Exclude acute infective causes of urinary symptoms, including UTIs | 'No' | No additional concerns | | | | |
| Do you have any blood in your urine? | Haematuria may be present in CKD | 'No' | No additional concerns | | | | |

## Past Medical/Surgical History

| | | | | | | | |
|---|---|---|---|---|---|---|---|
| Do you have any other medical conditions? | Assesses risk factors for heart failure and renal failure | 'Angina, hypertension and COPD' | The patient has risk factors for heart failure and renal failure | | | | |
| Do you have a previous history of DVT or varicose veins? | Such conditions may be associated with venous insufficiency | 'I have varicose veins on my legs' | The patient may have venous insufficiency leading to oedema | | | | |

**Past Medical/Surgical History**

| Question | Justification | Answer | Thoughts | | | | |
|---|---|---|---|---|---|---|---|
| Have you ever been diagnosed with diabetes, renal stones or a kidney disorder? | Such conditions are associated with CKD | 'I have recurrent UTI's' | Recurrent UTIs may be associated with CKD | | | | |
| Have you previously been diagnosed with cancer? | Lymphoedema may occur secondary to cancer | 'No' | No additional concerns | | | | |

**Drug History**

| Question | Justification | Answer | Thoughts | | | | |
|---|---|---|---|---|---|---|---|
| Are you currently taking any medication, or have any allergies? | Numerous medications are cardio- or nephrotoxic, including ACE inhibitors and gentamicin. Calcium channel blockers can increase fluid retention. Diuretics may mask symptoms of oedema | 'GTN spray, amlodipine, furosemide, atorvastatin, steroid inhalers' | The patient is frequently taking nephrotoxic medications | | | | |
| Do you take any NSAIDs? | Long-term NSAID usage is associated with CKD. | 'Every day' | Possible that long term NSAID use has cause damage to the kidneys. | | | | |

**Family History**

| Question | Justification | Answer | Thoughts | | | | |
|---|---|---|---|---|---|---|---|
| Are there any diseases that run in the family, including any cancers? | Always check for relevant heritable conditions | 'High blood pressure runs in the family' | Hypertension is a risk factor for congestive cardiac failure and CKD | | | | |

**Social and Travel History**

| Question | Justification | Answer | Thoughts | | | | |
|---|---|---|---|---|---|---|---|
| Who is currently at home? Are you working? | Explore possible social concerns or if wider support is needed | 'I live with my husband and am a retired nurse' | No social concerns at present | | | | |
| Do you smoke? | Explore wider risk factors | 'Never' | No additional concerns | | | | |
| What is your average weekly alcohol consumption? | | 'I drink alcohol infrequently' | No additional concerns | | | | |
| Is the leg swelling affecting your mobility? | Assess the impact on activities of daily living | 'I am struggling walking' | The patient's activities of daily living are affected | | | | |

## Systems Review

| Question | Justification | Answer | Thoughts | | | | |
|---|---|---|---|---|---|---|---|
| Have you had any bowel changes? | Malabsorption may contribute to hypoalbuminaemia | 'No' | No additional concerns | | | | |
| Have you experienced any swelling in your neck, dry skin and dry hair? | Assess for symptoms of hypothyroidism which may present with pretibial myxoedema | 'No' | No additional concerns | | | | |
| Have you experienced any unintentional weight loss, fever or malaise? | It is important to assess associated symptoms | 'No' | No additional concerns | | | | |

## Finishing the Consultation

| Question | Justification | Answer | Thoughts | | | | |
|---|---|---|---|---|---|---|---|
| Is there anything that I've missed that you would like to tell me about? | May identify useful information that has been missed. Will also help to build rapport with the patient | 'I'm concerned this is because of all the medication I need to take' | Take the time to explain what will happen from here | | | | |
| Do you have any questions? | Allows any final concerns to be addressed | | | | | | |

## Present Your Findings

Mrs Maynard, a 70-year-old woman, with a past medial history of angina, hypertension, recurrent UTIs and COPD, presented with a 3-week history of progressive bilateral pitting oedema with no calf pain or overlying skin changes. Mrs Maynard is experiencing exertional shortness of breath, with no new cough, chest pain or palpitations. She is experiencing general fatigue and nausea with oliguria without gross haematuria or symptoms indicative of an infective cause.

My main differential is CKD, secondary to hypertension and nephrotoxic medication. I will also investigate for hypoalbuminaemia and congestive cardiac failure.

I will complete a urine dip and blood tests including urea and electrolytes, FBC and kidney function tests, including creatinine, creatinine:albumin ratio and estimated glomerular filtration rate. I would also examine brain natriuretic peptide (BNP) and conduct a chest X-ray and echocardiogram to exclude congestive cardiac failure

## General Points

| | | | | |
|---|---|---|---|---|
| Polite to patient | | | | |
| Maintains good eye contact | | | | |
| Appropriate use of open and closed questions | | | | |
| No or limited use of medical jargon | | | | |

## ❓ QUESTIONS FROM THE EXAMINER

### What clinical signs may be present in a patient with congestive cardiac failure?

Raised fluid status, including a raised jugular venous pressure, bilateral crackles in the lung bases, ascites and peripheral oedema. Patients may also present with a displaced apex beat due to left ventricular dilation, and a right ventricular heave due to pulmonary hypertension.

## Providing examples, what may cause low-output cardiac failure?

Excessive preload from increased central venous pressure (for example, due to fluid overload in renal failure), pump failure (for example, systolic or diastolic failure) and chronic increased afterload (for example, in hypertension).

## Describe high-output cardiac failure, and provide examples of possible causes.

High-output cardiac failure describes a normal output but increased demand, meaning the output is not sufficient. This may occur in anaemia, pregnancy or hyperthyroidism.

## Why is BNP a marker of congestive cardiac failure?

BNP is released by the ventricles in response to stretch due to increased ventricular blood volume, which causes dilation of the ventricles. Raised BNP therefore indicates myocytes are strained due to increased volume.

## What is the action of BNP?

BNP acts to decrease blood pressure by decreasing systemic and central vascular resistance. BNP also increases the glomerular filtration rate in the kidneys and decreases sodium reabsorption in the tubules to reduce fluid load. Consequently, both preload and afterload are reduced.

## Using Starling's law, describe preload.

Preload describes the initial stretching force on the ventricular myocytes. Starling's law describes the relationship between the stretch of the myocytes and the force of the contraction, with the contraction force increasing as the stretch increases. Preload is therefore determined by the end diastolic volume which is influenced by heart rate, arterial contraction and central venous pressure.

## What is the most common causative agent of cellulitis?

Typically, cellulitis is caused by beta-haemolytic streptococci, where group A streptococcus is the most common causative agent.

## What are the risk factors for lymphoedema?

Lymphadenectomy (for example, axillary node clearance in patients with breast cancer), elderly patients, obesity, rheumatoid or psoriatic arthritis, radiotherapy (such as during cancer treatment) and cellulitis.

## What are the possible complications associated with chronic lymphoedema?

Delayed wound healing (as blood flow to the wound may be disrupted), infection, including cellulitis due to decreased immune surveillance, pain (due to compression or stretching or nerves) and an increased risk of cancer (due to decreased immune surveillance).

## Describe the appearance of leg ulcers that arise due to venous insufficiency.

Venous ulcers are often located in the gaiter area (below the knee but above the ankle). Unlike the deep, punched-out appearance of arterial ulcers, venous ulcers are often shallow, with irregular edges, and are mildly painful.

## Station 1.18   Back Pain

### Doctor Briefing

You are a junior doctor in primary care and have been asked to see Mrs Fletcher, a 60-year-old woman who presented with back pain. She has also become incontinent and is feeling unsteady on her feet. Please take a history from Mrs Fletcher, present your findings and formulate an appropriate management plan.

### Patient Briefing

You are visiting the doctor as you have had lower-back pain for the last 2 months. You have visited your doctor previously for the same pain; however, it has not subsided with the suggested treatment of ibuprofen, and is worsening.

You have also been experiencing incontinence over the past 3 days. You recall feeling sudden strong urges to urinate even after you have just been, and have been unable to reach the bathroom in time.

On questioning you recall feeling thirstier than usual recently and have been experiencing headaches and dizziness, which you have attributed to being dehydrated. You also feel more tired than usual but again have dismissed this as 'getting old'.

You currently have no long-term medical conditions and do not take any regular medications. You are a retired dentist who lives alone independently and are a non-smoker who doesn't drink alcohol. You are aware that your mother died of blood cancer at 72 years old.

You are very concerned as the pain is preventing you from leaving the house and visiting your grandchildren, so you are feeling isolated at home.

### Mark Scheme for Examiner

#### Introduction

| | | | | |
|---|---|---|---|---|
| Cleans hands, introduces self, confirms patient identity and gains consent for history taking | | | | |
| Establishes current patient knowledge and concerns | | | | |

#### History of Presenting Complaint

| Question | Justification | Answer | Thoughts | | | |
|---|---|---|---|---|---|---|
| Whereabouts is your back pain? | Allows consideration of structures around the specific site of pain | 'My lower back' (around T11 on examination) | Need to assess neurology of the patient | | | |
| When did you first notice your back pain? | This helps to determine if this is acute or chronic | 'About 2 months ago' | Need to investigate previous treatment options the patient has tried | | | |
| Did the pain come on suddenly or more gradually? | Assess if there was a precipitating factor | 'Gradually' | There appears to be no event directly attributable to the pain onset. Less likely to be mechanical back pain | | | |
| Do you remember what you were doing when the pain started? | | 'No' | | | | |
| How would you describe the pain? | Neuropathic pain may present as a sharp, stabbing pain. Bone pain is more frequently dull | 'A dull ache that is always present' | Consider bone aetiology | | | |

## History of Presenting Complaint

| Question | Justification | Answer | Thoughts | | | | |
|---|---|---|---|---|---|---|---|
| Does the pain spread anywhere else? | Assess for radiation | 'No' | No signs of radiation | | | | |
| Have you experienced any numbness, tingling or weakness? | Nerve compression may be associated with the aforementioned symptoms | 'I have had pins and needles in my legs a lot over the past 2 days' | Concerned about nerve compression | | | | |
| What treatment have you tried to relieve the pain? | Response to treatment options may give an indication of the source and severity of the pain | 'Ibuprofen, and heat and ice packs' | Consider escalation through the National Institute for Health and Care Excellence (NICE) pain ladder. More concerned as NSAIDs are not relieving the pain | | | | |
| Does anything make the pain worse? | Mechanical pain may be worse on movement | 'Movement, but the pain is still there at night and when I rest' | More concerned, as the pain does not appear to be mechanical | | | | |
| How severe is the pain? | More severe, sudden-onset pain may need treating more urgently | 'About 5/10 for the past 3 months, but much more severe for the last few days' | Concerned about the recent increase in severity | | | | |
| Have you experienced any night sweats, fever or unintentional weight loss? | Assesses malignancy red-flag symptoms | 'I have had a fever, and lost 5 kg in the last 4 months' | Increased concern due to red-flag symptoms | | | | |
| Have you experienced a change in sensation in your perineum? | Assessing neurological complications | 'No' | No additional concerns | | | | |
| Have you experienced any urinary or faecal incontinence? | | 'I have needed to run to the bathroom to urinate recently and have sometimes been unable to make it in time' | Concerned regarding urge incontinence | | | | |

## Past Medical and Surgical History

| Question | Justification | Answer | Thoughts | | | | |
|---|---|---|---|---|---|---|---|
| Do you have any other medical conditions, including arthritis or osteoporosis? | Previous joint pain may be associated with future pain in different joints | 'No' | Pain is less likely to be of rheumatological origin | | | | |

## Past Medical and Surgical History

| Question | Justification | Answer | Thoughts | | | | | |
|---|---|---|---|---|---|---|---|---|
| Have you had any previous spinal problems or spinal surgery? | Spinal surgery may be associated with future weakness. A previous medical problem may be recurring | 'No' | No additional concerns | | | | | |
| Have you ever received treatment for kidney stones? | Kidney stones may be associated with hypercalcaemia | 'No' | No additional concerns | | | | | |

## Drug History

| Question | Justification | Answer | Thoughts | | | | | |
|---|---|---|---|---|---|---|---|---|
| Are you currently on any medication, or have any allergies? | People may not disclose their whole medical history. You must always check for allergies | 'Ibuprofen for pain and no allergies' | Pain not resolved by NSAIDs | | | | | |
| Have you ever taken steroids? | Assess risk of osteoporosis | 'No' | No additional concerns | | | | | |

## Family History

| Question | Justification | Answer | Thoughts | | | | | |
|---|---|---|---|---|---|---|---|---|
| Are there any diseases that run in the family, including cancers? | Important always to check for relevant heritable conditions | 'My mum died of blood cancer at 72 years old' | Family history of haematological malignancies | | | | | |

## Social and Travel History

| Question | Justification | Answer | Thoughts | | | | | |
|---|---|---|---|---|---|---|---|---|
| Who is currently at home? Are you working? | Find out if there are any social concerns or if wider support is needed | 'I live alone and am a retired dentist' | Support at home needs to be considered | | | | | |
| Do you smoke? | Assess wider risk factors | 'Never' | No additional concerns | | | | | |
| What is your average weekly alcohol consumption? | | 'I don't drink alcohol' | No additional concerns | | | | | |

## Systems Review

| Question | Justification | Answer | Thoughts | | | | | |
|---|---|---|---|---|---|---|---|---|
| Have you noticed any light-headedness, breathlessness or palpitations? | May potentially be a result of anaemia and malignancy. These symptoms can also suggest a cardiovascular issue | 'Yes, I'm short of breath when climbing the stairs, and feel a bit dizzy' | Potential signs of anaemia | | | | | |
| Have you noticed any abnormal bleeding or bruising? | Bleeding disorders are common in malignancy | 'I've been having heavy nose bleeds recently' | Concerns regarding reduced platelet production | | | | | |

**Systems Review**

| Question | Justification | Answer | Thoughts | | | | | |
|---|---|---|---|---|---|---|---|---|
| Have you come across any new noticeable lumps? | This is checking for enlarged lymph nodes | 'No' | No additional symptoms indicating lymphoma | | | | | |
| Just to check, have you had any problems with bladder or bowel function? | Find out if there are any wider concerns that have not arisen yet | 'No, they have been normal' | No additional concerns | | | | | |
| Have you had any recent night sweats, fever, weight loss or fatigue? | It is essential to ask about B symptoms to rule out certain causes, such as infection | 'No' | No additional concerns | | | | | |
| Have you noticed any other new symptoms? Is there anything else that is concerning you? | This allows for assessment of more systemic symptoms | 'I am feeling very thirsty at the moment and having frequent headaches' | The patient may be describing symptoms of hypercalcaemia | | | | | |

**Finishing the Consultation**

| Question | Justification | Answer | Thoughts | | | | | |
|---|---|---|---|---|---|---|---|---|
| Is there anything that I've missed that you would like to tell me about? | May identify useful information that has been missed. Will also help to build rapport with the patient | 'I'm concerned I have cancer like my mum' | Take the time to explain what will happen from here | | | | | |
| Do you have any questions? | Allows any final concerns to be addressed | | | | | | | |

**Present Your Findings**

Mrs Fletcher, a 60-year-old woman, with no significant past medical history, presented with chronic dull, achy lower-back pain persistent on rest. The pain is recently associated with leg paraesthesia, urge incontinence and systemic symptoms of dizziness, shortness of breath, recurrent nose bleeds and polydipsia. Mrs Fletcher further describes red flags of fever and unintentional weight loss and has a first-degree relative with a haematological malignancy.

My main differential would be spinal cord compression secondary to multiple myeloma.

I would like to undertake an FBC and urine electrophoresis and conduct a bone marrow biopsy. I will further treat spinal cord compression as an oncological emergency

**General Points**

| | | | | | |
|---|---|---|---|---|---|
| Polite to patient | | | | | |
| Maintains good eye contact | | | | | |
| Appropriate use of open and closed questions | | | | | |
| No or limited use of medical jargon | | | | | |

## ❓ QUESTIONS FROM THE EXAMINER

### What are the clinical features of myeloma?

Clinical features of myeloma often include osteolytic bone lesions present on radiological imaging. Blood tests may further demonstrate hypercalcaemia, anaemia, neutropenia and thrombocytopenia as well as impaired renal function. Neutropenia patients may therefore present with recurrent bacterial infections.

### What complications may be associated with multiple myeloma?

Spinal cord compression, peripheral neuropathy and hyperviscosity. The latter may present with neurological symptoms due to decreased blood flow to the brain, such as confusion, symptoms of stroke and dizziness.

### Why is myeloma associated with renal disease?

Myeloma can cause tubular obstruction due to deposits of light-chain immunoglobulin G (IgG) in the glomerulus. The IgG chains have a toxic and inflammatory effect on the proximal tubule. Most damage is due to light chains in the distal loop of Henle.

### What protein may be present in the urine in a patient with suspected myeloma?

Bence Jones proteins, which are free immunoglobulin light chains that are filtered by the kidneys. These are commonly kappa or lambda types of light chains.

### What are the diagnostic criteria for myeloma?

Myeloma is defined by the presence of monoclonal protein bands either in the blood or present on urine electrophoresis. Radiological findings of bone lesions and a high proportion of plasma cells present in a bone marrow biopsy are also required for diagnosis. End-organ damage is the final diagnostic criterion that may present as hypercalcaemia, renal insufficiency or anaemia.

### How would spinal cord compression be treated?

An urgent MRI is required if spinal cord compression is suspected. Dexamethasone should be started, and assessment for neurosurgery or local radiotherapy should be made. It is important to assess the patient's neurological status repeatedly prior to surgical or radiological interventions, and record any changes.

### What urinary symptoms might be present in a spinal cord compression above T12 and why?

Afferent signals from the bladder wall providing information regarding the fullness of the bladder are unable to reach the pontine micturition centre. Therefore, patients will have no conscious awareness of their bladder being full, and their bladder will empty automatically with the bladder stretch reflex.

### What urinary symptoms might be present in a spinal cord compression below T12 and why?

The parasympathetic neurons responsible for contracting the detrusor muscle and prompting micturition in response to afferent stretch receptors will be paralysed as they exit around the T12 vertebral body. The bladder stretch reflex is therefore unable to function, and this may result in overflow incontinence due to urinary retention.

### At what vertebral level does the spinal cord commonly end in adults?

L1/2.

### What group of conditions might be associated with early-morning stiffness that reduces throughout the day?

Inflammatory conditions such as rheumatoid arthritis or ankylosing spondylitis.

## Station 1.19    Inherited Disease

### Doctor Briefing

You are a doctor in cardiology clinic and have been asked to see Mr Jones, a 42-year-old man, who has been referred to outpatient clinic by his primary care doctor who recently diagnosed a heart murmur. His primary care doctor has noted that Mr Jones is very tall with long extremities and hyperextendable joints. He has a family history of cardiac problems and wonders whether this may be genetic. Please take a history from Mr Jones, present your findings and formulate an appropriate management plan.

### Patient Briefing

You recently visited your doctor, as you have been experiencing fatigue and breathlessness for about 1 month. You have also occasionally experienced dizziness and palpitations; however, you do not have a cough or any chest pain. Following your appointment, you have been referred to cardiology clinic.

On questioning, you are short-sighted and have joint hyperextensibility but no other medical problems. You are not currently taking any regular medications.

You note that both your father and grandfather were also very tall and wore glasses. There is no consanguinity in your immediate family, and you have only one brother who is 38 years old and does not have any symptoms that you are aware of.

You are an engineer who lives with your wife and children (14-year-old son and 10-year-old daughter), who are all doing well. You are not currently trying for any more children. You drink around one bottle of wine over the weekend with your wife and do not smoke.

As your father and grandfather both required medication for cardiac problems, you are most concerned your symptoms are due to a genetic disease, and therefore your children may also experience similar problems.

### Mark Scheme for Examiner

#### Introduction

| | | | | |
|---|---|---|---|---|
| Cleans hands, introduces self, confirms patient identity and gains consent for history taking | | | | |
| Establishes current patient knowledge and concerns | | | | |

#### History of Presenting Complaint

| Question | Justification | Answer | Thoughts | | | | |
|---|---|---|---|---|---|---|---|
| Why did you initially visit your GP? | Assess if the patient is symptomatic | 'I was feeling fatigued and breathless' | The patient is symptomatic | | | | |
| When did you first notice you were experiencing breathlessness? | This helps to assess if breathlessness is related to the newly diagnosed murmur | 'About 1 month ago' | Chronic breathlessness may indicate a cardiac origin | | | | |
| Do you have a cough? | A cough may be associated with chronic respiratory diseases, infection or pulmonary oedema | 'No' | No additional concerns | | | | |
| Do you have any chest pain? | Breathlessness may be associated with cardiac or respiratory causes which may present with chest pain | 'No' | No additional concerns | | | | |
| Do you ever experience palpitations? | Palpitations would prompt towards a cardiac cause of symptoms | 'Yes' | Suggests a cardiac cause | | | | |

## History of Presenting Complaint

| Question | Justification | Answer | Thoughts | | | | | | | |
|---|---|---|---|---|---|---|---|---|---|---|
| Do you have episodes of dizziness or have you fainted? | Important to assess as the patient has a recently diagnosed murmur | 'Yes, I get dizzy frequently' | May be associated with the murmur | | | | | | | |
| Do you have increased flexibility in your joints? | Associated with Marfan's syndrome, which the GP has highlighted as a concern | 'Yes, at my elbows, knees and thumbs' | Cardinal symptoms of Marfan's | | | | | | | |
| How tall are you? (Measure on examination for accuracy) | Marfan's syndrome is associated with being tall and having long limbs | '6 ft 4' (1.93 m) | Tall height is a possible sign of Marfan's syndrome. | | | | | | | |

## Past Medical and Surgical History

| Question | Justification | Answer | Thoughts | | | | | | | |
|---|---|---|---|---|---|---|---|---|---|---|
| Do you have any other medical conditions? | Assess wider concerns | 'No' | No additional concerns | | | | | | | |
| Have you ever been diagnosed with scoliosis or suffered with joint pain? | Associated with Marfan's syndrome | 'Yes, I had an operation as a child for scoliosis' | Marfan's may be associated with scoliosis | | | | | | | |
| Do you have any vision problems? | Marfan's syndrome has been linked to a variety of visual problems such as, cataracts, glaucoma and high myopia | 'I have been short-sighted since early childhood' | Marfan's may be associated with lens dislocation | | | | | | | |
| Have you ever been diagnosed with hypertension? | Associated with coarctation of the aorta | 'No, I normally have low blood pressure' | Consider if prescribing beta-blockers to slow aortic root dilatation | | | | | | | |

## Drug History

| Question | Justification | Answer | Thoughts | | | | | | | |
|---|---|---|---|---|---|---|---|---|---|---|
| Are you currently taking any medication, or have any allergies? | Medication may identify conditions the patient has not yet disclosed | 'No medications or allergies' | No additional concerns | | | | | | | |

## Family History

| Question | Justification | Answer | Thoughts | | | | | | | |
|---|---|---|---|---|---|---|---|---|---|---|
| Are there any diseases that run in the family? | Always check for relevant heritable conditions | 'My dad and grandad both had heart problems' | Supportive of current thinking regarding Marfan's syndrome | | | | | | | |
| Has anyone in the family been diagnosed with Marfan's syndrome? | If there is a specific disease you are considering, ask separately | 'I'm not sure' | The patient may not be aware of Marfan's syndrome, so symptoms experienced by family members should be assessed | | | | | | | |

**Family History**

| Question | Justification | Answer | Thoughts | | | | | |
|---|---|---|---|---|---|---|---|---|
| Does your mother or father experience any of the symptoms you have described? | Assess if the patient's parents are symptomatic as Marfan's is an autosomal-dominant syndrome. Allows creation of a family tree | 'My dad also has heart problems, is very tall and wears glasses My mum has no symptoms' | Father displays symptoms of Marfan's. Patient has a 50% chance of inheriting an autosomal-dominant condition if one parent displays symptoms | | | | | |
| How old was your father when he first experienced symptoms? | Genetic conditions may present at an earlier age | 'Early 20s' | Young age of symptom onset suggests potential genetic cause | | | | | |
| Is there any consanguinity in the family? | Increases chances of inheriting an autosomal-recessive disease, like Ehlers–Danlos syndrome, which can present similarly | 'No' | No additional concerns | | | | | |
| Do you have any siblings, how old are they and do they experience similar symptoms? | Allows creation of a family tree to assess inheritance patterns | 'One brother, who is 38 and without any symptoms' | No additional concerns | | | | | |
| Did any of your grandparents experience similar symptoms? If so, what side of the family are they on? | | 'My grandad on my dad's side' | Suggests autosomal-dominant condition from the patient's father's side | | | | | |
| Do you have any children, how old are they and do they have symptoms? | Assess who might be at risk in the future or require screening | '14-year-old son and 10-year-old daughter, neither with symptoms, but I am concerned they may develop them in the future' | Consider referral for genetic counselling | | | | | |
| Is anyone in the family pregnant or trying to get pregnant? | | 'No' | No additional concerns | | | | | |

**Social and Travel History**

| | | | | | | | | |
|---|---|---|---|---|---|---|---|---|
| Who is currently at home? Are you working? | Explore possible social concerns or if wider support is needed | 'I live with my wife and children and am an engineer' | No social concerns | | | | | |

## Social and Travel History

| Question | Justification | Answer | Thoughts | | | | |
|---|---|---|---|---|---|---|---|
| Do you smoke? | Explore wider risk factors | 'No' | No additional concerns | | | | |
| What is your average weekly alcohol consumption? | | 'A bottle of wine at the weekend' | No additional concerns | | | | |

## Systems Review

| | | | | | | | |
|---|---|---|---|---|---|---|---|
| Just to check, have you had any problems with bladder or bowel function? | Find out if there are any wider concerns that have not arisen yet | 'No, they have been normal' | No additional concerns | | | | |
| Have you had any recent night sweats, fever, weight loss or fatigue? | It is essential to ask about B symptoms to rule out certain causes, such as infection | 'No' | No additional concerns | | | | |

## Finishing the Consultation

| | | | | | | | |
|---|---|---|---|---|---|---|---|
| Is there anything that I've missed that you would like to tell me about? | May identify useful information that has been missed. Will also help to build rapport with the patient | 'I'm concerned my children will also have the same symptoms when they are older' | Take the time to explain what will happen from here | | | | |
| Do you have any questions? | Allows any final concerns to be addressed | | | | | | |

## Present Your Findings

Mr Jones, a 42-year-old man, recently diagnosed with a new murmur, presented with a 1-month history of fatigue, palpitations and breathlessness without an associated cough or chest pain. Mr Jones is 6 ft 4 in (1.93 m), experiences dizziness, describes hyperextensibility in his joints and has been myopic since childhood. He has had scoliosis-corrective surgery.

Mr Jones is unsure if there is a family history of Marfan's syndrome, but both his father and grandfather on his father's side experienced similar cardiac symptoms, suggesting an autosomal-dominant pattern of inheritance.

I would also like to investigate for Marfan's syndrome using the Ghent criteria for diagnosis. This would include fundoscopy and an echocardiogram. I would further refer Mr Jones for genetic counselling if a diagnosis is made

## General Points

| | | | | | |
|---|---|---|---|---|---|
| Polite to patient | | | | | |
| Maintains good eye contact | | | | | |
| Appropriate use of open and closed questions | | | | | |
| No or limited use of medical jargon | | | | | |

## ❓ QUESTIONS FROM THE EXAMINER

### Describe the different prenatal genetic screening options available in the UK.

Ultrasound scanning to detect structural abnormalities at 12 and 20 weeks in low-risk pregnancies. Chorionic villous sampling for chromosome and DNA analysis after 11 weeks of gestation. Amniocentesis for sampling the amniotic fluid to allow chromosome and DNA analysis after 15 weeks of gestation. Non-invasive genetic testing, as free fetal DNA circulates in the maternal blood after 8–9 weeks; a maternal blood test can be used to diagnose genetic conditions in the fetus.

### What are the rates of miscarriage with chorionic villous sampling and amniocentesis?

Chorionic villous sampling is 1–2%, amniocentesis is 0.5–1%.

### What is meant by 'anticipation'?

Genetic conditions may present at an earlier age or in a more severe form in younger generations. For example, the age of symptom onset for Huntington's disease usually gets younger through the generations, with an increased severity of symptoms experienced.

### Describe the patterns of inheritance of haemophilia.

Haemophilia demonstrates an X-linked recessive pattern.

### Why are males more commonly affected by X-linked disorders?

X-linked disorders are influenced by chromosomes present only on the X chromosome. As males only have one X chromosome, they will display signs of the condition if the single copy they inherit is mutated. As females have two X chromosomes, they may not display symptoms or display less severe symptoms if one copy of the gene is functional and able to compensate for the mutated copy.

### What do you expect to see on a family tree if there is an autosomal-dominant pattern of inheritance?

Affected family members in each generation, the condition to be present in both males and females and both males and females have affected children.

### Describe robertsonian (centric fusion) and reciprocal translocations.

Robertsonian translocations describe when acrocentric chromosomes break close to their centromeres, and fusion of their long arms, with loss of short arms, occurs. Reciprocal translocations describe exchange of fragments from two non-homologous chromosomes.

### What are acrocentric chromosomes?

Acrocentric chromosomes are those with centromeres located near the end of the chromosome, meaning such chromosomes have a long and short arm. They include chromosomes 13, 14, 15, 21 and 22.

### What do you expect to see on a family tree in conditions caused by translocations?

A family tree may contain multiple miscarriages. Many individuals will have various congenital abnormalities affecting multiple organ systems. Individuals without symptoms are likely to be balanced carriers.

### With an example, explain what is meant by aneuploidy.

Humans normally have 23 pairs of chromosomes. Aneuploidy describes when there is an incorrect number of chromosomes, such as in trisomy, where 47 chromosomes are present. An example includes trisomy 21, where three 21 chromosomes are present, leading to Down syndrome.

## Station 1.20 Joint Pain

### Doctor Briefing

You are a junior doctor in the ED and have been asked to see Jack Hassall, a 30-year-old man, who presented with a 2-day history of pain and swelling in his right knee. He is fit and well with no significant medical history. Please take a history from Jack, present your findings and formulate an appropriate management plan.

### Patient Briefing

You are visiting the doctor due to a pain in your knee that is preventing you from going to work. The pain, which feels like a tight band, started 5 days ago and came on suddenly. On questioning you have noticed that the area behind your knee is red and swollen, with a palpable lump.

You have experienced aching in your joints for a few years, particularly in your hands and wrists, but have attributed this to over-use from work. You work as a builder, which involves significant amounts of manual labour, and play rugby in your spare time. You are otherwise healthy and don't frequently visit the doctor.

You have a previous injury in your right knee from a rugby accident 7 years ago, when you damaged your ligaments, but completed a course of physiotherapy as treatment. You have no other medical conditions and do not take any regular medications.

Your father suffers from type 2 diabetes and gout.

You live an active lifestyle, playing rugby often. You currently live with your two children, do not smoke, but drink around 3 pints of beer an evening.

You are most concerned about requiring time off work, as you are the only source of income in the household.

### Mark Scheme for Examiner

#### Introduction

| | | | |
|---|---|---|---|
| Cleans hands, introduces self, confirms patient identity and gains consent for history taking | | | |
| Establishes current patient knowledge and concerns | | | |

#### History of Presenting Complaint

| Question | Justification | Answer | Thoughts | | | | |
|---|---|---|---|---|---|---|---|
| Where is the pain? | The site of pain may indicate the underlying structures affected | 'Behind my knee' | Structures in the popliteal fossa may be affected | | | | |
| Did the pain start suddenly or gradually worsen? | Degenerative disorders progress gradually. Trauma, septic arthritis and gout may present acutely | 'Suddenly' | Acute causes should be excluded | | | | |
| Did any activity precede the pain? | Allows trauma to be excluded | 'I hurt my knee playing rugby recently' | The patient may have an injury from mechanical trauma | | | | |
| Please describe the pain | Arthritis usually presents as stiffness | 'A tightness and fullness behind my knee' | This suggests the pain may not be arthritic. Cysts may create a feeling of fullness | | | | |
| Are you experiencing joint stiffness? | | 'Stiffness and difficulty extending' | | | | | |

**History of Presenting Complaint**

| Question | Justification | Answer | Thoughts | | | | | |
|---|---|---|---|---|---|---|---|---|
| Does the pain radiate? | Assesses if other structures are affected | 'No' | No additional concerns | | | | | |
| Do you have a rash or fever? | Rheumatoid arthritis may present alongside a rash. Septic arthritis is associated with a fever | 'No' | No additional concerns | | | | | |
| Does anything make the pain better or worse? | NSAIDs may reduce pain due to inflammation | 'Ibuprofen has partially helped to reduce the pain' | There may be an inflammatory cause | | | | | |
| Are the symptoms worse in the morning? | Rheumatoid arthritis is often worse in the morning. Osteoarthritis is often worse in the evening | 'No, pain is worse on movement' | Symptoms are not indicative of rheumatoid arthritis | | | | | |
| How severe is the pain? | This allows assessment of severity | 'Around 7/10' | Analgesia should be prescribed | | | | | |
| Is there any redness, swelling or lumps? | This allows identification of cysts or inflammation | 'Swelling and a painful lump' | This suggests a collection of fluid is present | | | | | |
| Are any other joints painful or swollen? | Trauma is less likely to affect multiple joints. Degenerative and rheumatological conditions often affect multiple joints | 'Sometimes my hands and wrist ache and swell, but I think this is due to overuse at work' | The patient may be describing degenerative damage, which may indicate an underlying more chronic condition. This should be assessed and investigated separately | | | | | |
| Do you have calf pain or swelling? | Allows assessment of a ruptured Baker's cyst and exclusion of DVT symptoms | 'No' | No additional concerns | | | | | |
| Do you feel generally well? | It is vital to exclude septic arthritis in sudden-onset pain in a single joint | 'Yes' | No additional concerns | | | | | |
| Has the pain limited your function? | This provides an indication of the impact of the pain on activities of daily living | 'I am unable to work' | The patient may need financial support and assistance returning to work | | | | | |
| Have you experienced these symptoms before? | Checking symptoms are not recurring to explore past medical history | 'Never' | No additional concerns | | | | | |

## Past Medical and Surgical History

| Question | Justification | Answer | Thoughts | | | | | |
|---|---|---|---|---|---|---|---|---|
| Do you have any known joint problems, including arthritis? | Symptoms may be caused by an acute episode of a chronic joint condition. A Baker's cyst may be associated with underlying joint problems, such as rheumatoid arthritis | 'I injured my right-knee ligaments playing rugby 7 years ago' | No additional concerns | | | | | |
| Do you have any dermatological conditions, including psoriasis? | Psoriatic arthritis should be excluded | 'No' | No additional concerns | | | | | |
| Have you had any previous fractures or orthopaedic surgery? | Previously injured joints may be more prone to degenerative disorders, including osteoarthritis | 'No' | No additional concerns | | | | | |

## Drug History

| Question | Justification | Answer | Thoughts | | | | | |
|---|---|---|---|---|---|---|---|---|
| Are you currently taking any medication, or have any allergies? | Steroids and disease-modifying antirheumatic drugs cause immunosuppression, which may make patients more susceptible to septic arthritis. Diuretics are associated with an increased risk of gout | 'No medications or allergies' | No additional concerns | | | | | |

## Family History

| Question | Justification | Answer | Thoughts | | | | | |
|---|---|---|---|---|---|---|---|---|
| Are there any diseases that run in the family, including any cancers? | Always check for relevant heritable conditions | 'My father has type 2 diabetes and gout' | A family history of gout may suggest hereditary hyperuricaemia | | | | | |

## Social and Travel History

| Question | Justification | Answer | Thoughts | | | | | |
|---|---|---|---|---|---|---|---|---|
| Who is currently at home? Are you working? | Explores social concerns | 'I live with my two children and am a full-time builder' | Concerned about the impact on the patient's work. The patient describes strenuous activity at work. Excessive kneeling may cause prepatellar bursitis | | | | | |
| Do you smoke? | Explore wider risk factors | 'No' | No additional concerns | | | | | |
| What is your weekly alcohol consumption? | Excessive alcohol consumption is associated with gout | '2/3 pints a night' | The patient may have increased risk factors for gout | | | | | |

## Social and Travel History

| Question | Justification | Answer | Thoughts | | | | |
|---|---|---|---|---|---|---|---|
| Have you recently undertaken strenuous exercise? | Mechanical trauma may cause pain, such as through as a meniscal tear | 'I play rugby weekly' | Pain may be due to mechanical trauma | | | | |
| Have you engaged in unprotected sexual activity with any new partners, or any partners who may be carrying a sexually transmitted disease? | Sexually transmitted diseases may be associated with reactive arthritis | 'No' | No additional concerns | | | | |

## Systems Review

| Question | Justification | Answer | Thoughts | | | | |
|---|---|---|---|---|---|---|---|
| Have you had any bowel changes, or recently been diagnosed with gastroenteritis? | Gastroenteritis is associated with reactive arthritis | 'No' | No additional concerns | | | | |
| Have you had vision changes, or painful, itchy eyes? | Reiter's syndrome is associated with conjunctivitis or urethritis | 'No.' | No additional concerns | | | | |
| Have you had any changes with your urinary system? | | 'No' | No additional concerns | | | | |
| Have you noticed any changes in your nails? | Rheumatological conditions may be associated with nail changes, including onycholysis | 'No' | No additional concerns | | | | |

## Finishing the Consultation

| Question | Justification | Answer | Thoughts | | | | |
|---|---|---|---|---|---|---|---|
| Is there anything that I've missed that you would like to tell me about? | May identify useful information that has been missed. Will also help to build rapport with the patient | 'I am really concerned as I need to return to work quickly' | Take the time to explain what will happen from here | | | | |
| Do you have any questions? | Allows any final concerns to be addressed | | | | | | |

## Present Your Findings

Mr Hassall, a 30-year-old man, with no significant past medical history, presented with a 5-day history of 7/10 pain, swelling and mass in the popliteal fossa. The pain is reduced by NSAIDs and worsened on movement. The patient has a family history of type 2 diabetes and gout. Mr Hassall has a previous ligament injury to his right knee and undertakes frequent strenuous manual labour and activity.

My main differential is a Baker's cyst following previous trauma. However, I would also like to investigate for early-onset osteoarthritis, as the patient describes a separate chronic aching pain and inflammation in his hands and wrists.

I will complete knee examination, with an examination of the joint above and below. I will also complete an ultrasound scan to confirm the diagnosis and evaluate any complications

| General Points | | | |
|---|---|---|---|
| Polite to patient | | | |
| Maintains good eye contact | | | |
| Appropriate use of open and closed questions | | | |
| No or limited use of medical jargon | | | |

## ❓ QUESTIONS FROM THE EXAMINER

### What complications are associated with a Baker's cyst?

Most Baker's cysts are uncomplicated; however, they may be associated with chronic pain, rupture, haemorrhage (especially in patients taking anticoagulants) or compression of nearby structures leading to a DVT or compartment syndrome.

### What differential needs to be excluded in the case of a ruptured Baker's cyst?

A ruptured Baker's cyst may present very similar clinically to a DVT. Presentation may include swelling and redness in the calf.

### How long is spontaneous recovery of a Baker's cyst expected to take?

Around 10–20 months.

### How may compartment syndrome present?

Patients may present with a pain disproportionate to the injury. Symptoms may include the 5 Ps, consisting of pain, pallor, paraesthesia, pulselessness and paralysis.

### What are the main signs of osteoarthritis on plain-film X-ray?

Loss of joint space, osteophytes, subchondral cysts and subchondral sclerosis. This can be remembered with the mnemonic LOSS.

### What are the main findings of rheumatoid arthritis on plain-film X-ray?

Loss of joint space, erosions, soft-tissue swelling, soft bones (osteopenia). This can be remembered with the mnemonic LESS.

### List five extra-articular manifestations of rheumatoid arthritis.

Vasculitis, interstitial fibrosis, pericarditis, carpal tunnel syndrome and scleritis.

### What are the three types of joints in humans?

Synovial (such as the shoulder), fibrous and cartilaginous joints.

### Describe the main features of a synovial joint.

Synovial joints contain an articular capsule, with both a fibrous and synovial layer, articular cartilage and synovial fluid (contained in bursae).

### What is a sesamoid bone? Please provide an example.

A sesamoid bone describes a small bone that is embedded within a tendon. An example includes the patella.

## Station 1.21    Breast Lump

### Doctor Briefing

You are a junior doctor in primary care and have been asked to see Mrs Patterson, a 45-year-old woman, who has noticed a lump in her left breast. Please take a history, present your findings and formulate an appropriate plan.

### Patient Briefing

You are visiting the doctor as you have had pain in the top right of your left breast for about 2 days. A small, movable lump around 4 cm underlies the site of the pain, and your overlying skin is red, hot and swollen. You have flu-like symptoms as well as a high temperature, and don't feel very well. You have not noticed any nipple discharge or changes.

On questioning, you are perimenopausal with your last menstrual period 3 weeks ago, and first menstrual period at 12 years old. You have been experiencing hot flushes and breast tenderness for the last 6 months. You breastfed both your children, who are now of secondary-school age.

You have no significant past medical history and are not taking any regular medications, including no hormone replacement or contraceptive pills.

You currently live with your husband and work full-time as a teacher. You have never smoked and drink around 8 units of alcohol a week.

You are concerned, as your mother was diagnosed with breast cancer recently (at 72 years old).

### Mark Scheme for Examiner

#### Introduction

| | | | | |
|---|---|---|---|---|
| Cleans hands, introduces self, confirms patient identity and gains consent for history taking | | | | |
| Establishes current patient knowledge and concerns | | | | |

#### History of Presenting Complaint

| Question | Justification | Answer | Thoughts | | | | |
|---|---|---|---|---|---|---|---|
| When did you notice the lump in your breast? | This helps to determine if this is acute or chronic. If malignancy is suspected, a triple assessment is required urgently | 'About 2 days ago' | Suggests acute onset. I would like to consider if there is a precipitating event | | | | |
| Where is the lump? | Helps to guide the breast examination | 'In the top right corner of my left breast' | Need to question further about the shape and size of the lump to allow accurate assessment | | | | |
| What is the size and shape of the lump? | To assess the lump shape and consistency | 'About 4 cm and round' | Smooth round edges are less likely to be associated with malignancy. Need to assess the lump and lymph nodes upon assessment | | | | |
| Have you noticed a lump in your breast before? | Benign breast changes may present with a lump which changes with the menstrual cycle. Previous personal history of breast cancer is associated with increased future risk of breast cancer | 'No' | No previous breast lump to compare the current presentation with | | | | |

## History of Presenting Complaint

| Question | Justification | Answer | Thoughts | | | | |
|---|---|---|---|---|---|---|---|
| When was your last menstrual period? | Assess if the patient is postmenopausal. Assess if changes are related to the menstrual cycle | '3 weeks ago' | Need to confirm the patient is not perimenopausal | | | | |
| Are you experiencing any symptoms of menopause? | Assess if the patient is postmenopausal. Assessing malignancy risk due to oestrogen exposure | 'I have been experiencing hot flushes and breast tenderness for the last 6 months' | Patient is perimenopausal | | | | |
| What age did you have your first menstrual period? | Assessing malignancy risk due to oestrogen exposure | '12 years old' | No evidence of precocious puberty and increased oestrogen exposure | | | | |
| Do you have any children and how old are they? | Assessing malignancy risk due to oestrogen exposure. Allows questioning regarding recent breastfeeding | 'I have two children, aged 12 and 14' | Not currently breastfeeding | | | | |
| Do you have any pain in your breast? | Fibroadenomas and malignancies may present with painless lumps | 'Yes' | May suggest an infective cause | | | | |
| Have you noticed any skin changes? | Skin changes may be associated with malignancy, or infection and inflammation | 'My skin is hot and red' | Suggestive of an infective cause | | | | |
| Have you noticed any nipple changes or discharge? | Blood-stained nipple discharge and nipple inversion may be associated with malignancy. Milky discharge may be associated with galactocele or mastitis | 'No' | No additional concerns | | | | |
| Have you experienced any chest trauma recently? | Fat necrosis usually presents following a history of trauma | 'No' | No additional concerns | | | | |
| Do you have any other symptoms? | Assess for systemic signs of infection | 'I feel like I have the flu and have a high temperature' | Indicative of systemic infection | | | | |

## Drug History

| Question | Justification | Answer | Thoughts | | | | |
|---|---|---|---|---|---|---|---|
| Are you on any medication at the moment, or have any allergies? | You must always check for allergies | 'No medications and no allergies' | No additional concerns | | | | |

### Drug History

| Question | Justification | Answer | Thoughts | | | | | |
|---|---|---|---|---|---|---|---|---|
| Have you ever taken the oral contraceptive pill? | If there is a specific drug you need to consider, always ask. The patient may have recently stopped taking it. These drugs increase exposure to oestrogen and may be associated with a small increased risk of breast cancer | 'No. I have never taken those medications' | No additional concerns | | | | | |
| Have you ever taken hormone replacement therapy (HRT)? | HRT is associated with increased risk of breast cancer | 'No' | No additional concerns | | | | | |

### Family History

| Question | Justification | Answer | Thoughts | | | | | |
|---|---|---|---|---|---|---|---|---|
| Are there any diseases that run in the family, including any cancers? | Important always to check for relevant heritable conditions | 'My mother was diagnosed with breast cancer a few months ago' | Possible concern. The patient may have hereditary *BRCA1/2* and *TP53* mutations; however, this is unlikely due to the age her mother was diagnosed | | | | | |
| How old was your mother when she was diagnosed? | Important to check the age at diagnosis | '72' | | | | | | |

### Social and Travel History

| Question | Justification | Answer | Thoughts | | | | | |
|---|---|---|---|---|---|---|---|---|
| Who is currently at home? Are you working? | Find out if there are any social concerns or if wider support is needed | 'I live with my husband and work full-time in a school' | No social concerns at present | | | | | |
| Do you smoke? | Find out a patient's wider risk factors | 'No, I have never smoked' | No additional concerns | | | | | |
| What is your average weekly alcohol consumption? | Find out a patient's wider risk factors as well as exploring causes for symptom changes | 'I drink around 8 units a week' | Patient not disclosing any further concerns at present | | | | | |
| Have you recently travelled abroad? | Ensure no tropical infections as a cause of the patient's symptoms | 'No, not for several years' | No travel concerns at present | | | | | |

### Systems Review

| Question | Justification | Answer | Thoughts | | | | | |
|---|---|---|---|---|---|---|---|---|
| Do you have any chest pain or trouble breathing? | Find out if there are any wider concerns that have not arisen yet | 'No' | No additional concerns | | | | | |
| Just to check, have you had any problems with bladder or bowel function? | Find out if there are any wider concerns that have not arisen yet | 'No, they have been normal' | No additional concerns | | | | | |

**Systems Review**

| Question | Justification | Answer | Thoughts | | | | |
|---|---|---|---|---|---|---|---|
| Have you had any recent night sweats, fever, weight loss or fatigue? | It is essential to ask about B symptoms to rule out certain causes, such as infection | 'No' | No additional concerns | | | | |

**Finishing the Consultation**

| Question | Justification | Answer | Thoughts | | | | |
|---|---|---|---|---|---|---|---|
| Is there anything that I've missed that you would like to tell me about? | May identify useful information that has been missed. Will also help to build rapport with the patient | 'I'm concerned I have cancer like my mum' | Take the time to explain what will happen from here | | | | |
| Do you have any questions? | Allows any final concerns to be addressed | | | | | | |

**Present Your Findings**

Mrs Patterson, a 45-year-old woman, has noticed a painful 2-cm round lump in her left breast, with hot, red skin over the lump. Mrs Patterson described no nipple changes or discharge. She feels unwell with a temperature and flu-like symptoms.

My main differential would be breast cyst or mastitis, but I will also investigate for a fibroadenoma.

I will refer Mrs Patterson to a one-stop clinic for a triple assessment which will include a breast examination, mammography and fine-needle aspiration biopsy

**General Points**

Polite to patient

Maintains good eye contact

Appropriate use of open and closed questions

No or limited use of medical jargon

## ❓ QUESTIONS FROM THE EXAMINER

### What imaging is gold standard to investigate breast tissue in women <35 years old and why?

Ultrasound is used for women <35 years old, as the breast tissue is denser and hence lumps may not be detected from mammography.

### Name three risk factors of breast malignancy.

First-degree family history, nulliparity, early menarche or late menopause, HRT/oral contraceptive pill and *BRCA1/2* gene mutations.

### What tumour marker may indicate breast cancer?

CA 15-3.

### What screening programme is in place for breast cancer and what type of prevention is this?

Mammography is offered every 3 years to women aged 50–71 years old. Screening is a type of secondary prevention, aiming for early detection of disease and prevention of complications.

## What are the two types of non-invasive breast cancers, and how are they defined?

In situ malignancies are described as having not yet invaded the basement membrane. In the breast, in situ cancers may arise from either the epithelial cells lining the ducts (ductal carcinoma in situ), or the epithelial cells of the lobules (lobular carcinoma in situ).

## What receptors are assessed on breast cancer cells and why?

Progesterone receptors, oestrogen receptors and HER2 receptors. Targeted hormone treatment can be utilised in receptor-positive malignancies. Therefore, triple-negative cancers have the poorest prognosis.

## What targeted treatment may be used in pre- and postmenopausal women with oestrogen receptor-positive breast cancer?

Treatment for premenopausal women may include selective oestrogen modulators such as tamoxifen. Treatment for postmenopausal women may include aromatase inhibitors.

## Why does treatment differ based on if a patient is pre- or postmenopausal?

The majority of oestrogen production in premenopausal women occurs in the ovaries. However, in postmenopausal women, the majority of oestrogen is produced in the form of androgens from the adrenal glands. Aromatase inhibitors prevent the conversion of androgens to oestrogen.

## What are the common sites of metastasis of breast cancer?

Bone, lungs, liver and brain. The sentinel lymph nodes, which are usually the axillary lymph nodes, should be assessed as breast cancer metastasis most commonly occurs via the lymph.

## What agents may be used to prevent skeletal-related events from bone metastasis and what is the mechanism of action?

Denosumab, a RANK ligand that inhibits osteoclast action, decreasing bone resorption.

## Station 1.22   Urinary Incontinence

### Doctor Briefing

You are a junior doctor in primary care and have been asked to see Mrs Sanchez, a 54-year-old woman, who has presented with a 3-month history of urinary incontinence. She is afraid to leave the house in case she needs the toilet, and this is starting to have a significant affect on her quality of life. Please take a history from Mrs Sanchez, present your findings and formulate an appropriate management plan.

### Patient Briefing

You are visiting the doctor because for the last 3 months you have been experiencing leaking of urine, especially during the night, which you feel unable to control. You are only passing small amounts of urine, despite experiencing feelings of increased urgency and frequency. You have no signs of infection currently and are not experiencing any pain; however, you have had three UTIs in the past 6 months.

On questioning you have type 2 diabetes, for which you take metformin, and your blood glucose has not been very tightly controlled. As such, you have also recently visited the doctor for foot ulcers. You are not aware of any medical conditions that run in the family.

You live with your husband and work in an office; however, you haven't been able to attend work recently due to your symptoms. You have never smoked and drink around 6 units of alcohol each week. You have two children, both delivered by caesarean section.

You have been experiencing a lack of motivation, feeling down, and you are having difficulty sleeping as you are concerned about these symptoms and the impact they are having on your life. You are further feeling embarrassed to discuss this with the doctor.

### Mark Scheme for Examiner

#### Introduction

| | | | | |
|---|---|---|---|---|
| Cleans hands, introduces self, confirms patient identity and gains consent for history taking | | | | |
| Establishes current patient knowledge and concerns | | | | |

#### History of Presenting Complaint

| Question | Justification | Answer | Thoughts | | |
|---|---|---|---|---|---|
| When did you first notice you were leaking urine? | This helps to determine if this is acute or chronic. An acute cause may suggest acute neurological deficits that need urgent treatment | 'About 3 months' | Less concerned as this has been ongoing | | |
| How frequently are you urinating? | Many conditions associated with urinary incontinence are associated with increased frequency, including UTIs | 'About 10 times during the day, six times each night' | Increased frequency should be explored | | |
| Is urinating this frequently normal for you? Are you waking more frequently during the night to urinate? | Assesses the impact on the patient's quality of life | 'I am urinating much more frequently' | | | |
| Are you experiencing a sense of urgency to urinate? | Urgency may be associated with urge incontinence, often due to a UTI or intake of large amounts of fluids | 'Yes' | Fluid intake and symptoms of infection should be assessed | | |

## History of Presenting Complaint

| Question | Justification | Answer | Thoughts | | | | | |
|---|---|---|---|---|---|---|---|---|
| Approximately what volume of urine are you passing each day? | This allows assessment of whether a patient is producing appropriate amounts of urine | 'About 1 L' | Appropriate urine volume produced | | | | | |
| What is your approximate daily fluid intake? How much of this intake is from caffeinated drinks? | Assess if incontinence is due to increased fluid intake (perhaps due to osmotic symptoms) | 'About 2 L, with about 1 cup of coffee' | No concerns regarding fluid intake or diuretic effect of caffeine | | | | | |
| Do you have any difficulties accessing toilets currently? | Assesses the patient's physical ability and mobility | 'No' | No additional concerns | | | | | |
| Does anything trigger the leakage of urine, such as coughing or sneezing? | Assesses symptoms of stress incontinence | 'No' | Symptoms are not indicative of stress incontinence | | | | | |
| Are you experiencing any burning on urination? | Assess if there is an infectious cause; for example, a UTI | 'No' | No indication of an infective agent | | | | | |
| Have you experienced any dragging sensation, or the sensation of a lump? | Assesses symptoms of prolapse | 'No' | No concern regarding prolapse | | | | | |
| Have you experienced any changes in your bowel habits? | Constipation may increase abdominal pressure, increasing frequency of urination | 'No' | No indication of increased abdominal pressure due to constipation | | | | | |
| Have you experienced any change of sensation in your perineum? | This allows assessment of neurological damage leading to incontinence, including the pudendal nerve | 'No' | No concern regarding neurological damage | | | | | |
| Are you able to feel when you need to urinate? | If afferent neurones are damaged, patients may be unable to feel when their bladder is full | 'Sometimes I'm not aware I need to go' | Symptoms may indicate afferent nerve neurological damage | | | | | |
| Do you have a normal stream when urinating? | This allows assessment of the urinary outflow | 'I pass very little urine, very slowly' | This may indicate detrusor muscle dysfunction or urinary outflow obstruction | | | | | |
| Have you noticed any blood in your urine? | Urological malignancies may present with haematuria | 'No' | No additional concerns | | | | | |

## Past Medical History

| | | | | | | | | |
|---|---|---|---|---|---|---|---|---|
| Have you experienced these symptoms before? | Checking these are not recurring symptoms and exploring the past medical history | 'Never' | No additional concerns | | | | | |

**Past Medical History**

| Question | Justification | Answer | Thoughts | | | | | |
|---|---|---|---|---|---|---|---|---|
| Do you have any other medical conditions, including chronic respiratory conditions? | Chronic respiratory conditions may be associated with stress incontinence | 'No' | No additional concerns | | | | | |
| Have you undergone any previous pelvic surgery, including a hysterectomy? | Weakened pelvic floor muscles, which may contribute to stress incontinence | 'No' | No additional stress incontinence risk factors identified | | | | | |
| Do you have any biological children? Were they delivered via vaginal delivery? | | 'Two children, both delivered by caesarean section' | | | | | | |
| Do you have any other medical conditions? | Assesses wider risk factors | 'Type 2 diabetes' | Poorly controlled diabetes | | | | | |
| How well controlled is your blood glucose? | | 'My capillary glucose is around 12 mmol currently' | | | | | | |
| Have you had any recent UTIs? | Urinary retention leading to overflow incontinence may be associated with UTIs | 'Yes, three in the last 6 months' | May suggest urinary stasis in the bladder | | | | | |
| Have you ever been diagnosed with bladder stones? | Bladder stones may form due to urine stasis | 'No' | Bladder stones investigations should be considered | | | | | |

**Drug History**

| Question | Justification | Answer | Thoughts | | | | | |
|---|---|---|---|---|---|---|---|---|
| Are you on any medication at the moment, or have any allergies? | People may not disclose their whole medical history. You must always check for allergies | '1 g metformin a day and no allergies' | No additional concerns | | | | | |

**Family History**

| Question | Justification | Answer | Thoughts | | | | | |
|---|---|---|---|---|---|---|---|---|
| Are there any diseases that run in the family, including any cancers? | Important to check for relevant heritable conditions, including urological malignancies | 'No' | No additional concerns | | | | | |

**Social and Travel History**

| Question | Justification | Answer | Thoughts | | | | | |
|---|---|---|---|---|---|---|---|---|
| Who is currently at home? Are you working? | Explore social concerns | 'I live with my husband and work in an office but haven't been able to work recently' | Address concerns about returning to the workplace | | | | | |

**Social and Travel History**

| Question | Justification | Answer | Thoughts | | | | |
|---|---|---|---|---|---|---|---|
| Do you smoke? | Explore wider risk factors | 'No, never' | No additional concerns | | | | |
| What is your average weekly alcohol consumption? | Explore wider risk factors | 'Around 6 units a week' | No additional concerns | | | | |

**Systems Review**

| Question | Justification | Answer | Thoughts | | | | |
|---|---|---|---|---|---|---|---|
| Have you experienced any back pain or leg weakness recently? | Assesses cauda equina syndrome symptoms | 'No' | No additional concerns | | | | |
| Have you had any recent night sweats, fever, weight loss or fatigue? | It is essential to ask about B symptoms to rule out certain causes, such as infection | 'No' | No additional concerns | | | | |

**Finishing the Consultation**

| Question | Justification | Answer | Thoughts | | | | |
|---|---|---|---|---|---|---|---|
| Is there anything that I've missed that you would like to tell me about? | May identify useful information that has been missed. Will also help to build rapport with the patient | 'I am really embarrassed, so hope this is sorted quickly' | Take the time to explain what will happen from here | | | | |
| Do you have any questions? | Allows any final concerns to be addressed | | | | | | |

**Present Your Findings**

Mrs Sanchez, a 54-year-old woman with poorly controlled type 2 diabetes on metformin, presented with a 3-month history of incontinence, with urgency and frequency. Mrs Sanchez describes a loss of sensation of bladder fullness and a poor stream, with frequent and recurrent UTIs.

My main differential would be neurogenic bladder due to poorly controlled diabetes.

I am going to complete a urine dipstick, midstream urine sample, as well as $HbA_{1c}$ blood test. I would further conduct a cystoscopy and urodynamic studies

**General Points**

| | | | | |
|---|---|---|---|---|
| Polite to patient | | | | |
| Maintains good eye contact | | | | |
| Appropriate use of open and closed questions | | | | |
| No or limited use of medical jargon | | | | |

# ? QUESTIONS FROM THE EXAMINER

## What are the different types of urinary incontinence?

Stress incontinence is often due to weakness in pelvic floor muscles and urine may leak during exertion. Urge incontinence is when a patient experiences a sudden urge to urinate. Mixed incontinence is due to a combination of both stress and urge incontinence. Overflow incontinence occurs if the bladder is unable to be completely emptied and residual urine remains in the bladder, which gradually fills it.

## Where is the sacral micturition centre located and what is its role?

The sacral micturition centre is located in the intermediolateral grey horn of the spinal cord S2–S4 and is responsible for the micturition bladder stretch reflex.

## Describe the bladder stretch reflex.

The afferent pelvic splanchnic nerves (S2–S4) provide information regarding the fullness of the bladder, from the stretch of the detrusor muscle. A feeling of fullness activates the parasympathetic pelvic nerve (S2–S4), which stimulates micturition through detrusor muscle contraction.

## What may cause urinary retention, and what complications may arise following chronic retention?

Urinary retention may be caused from obstruction below the neck of the bladder, most commonly due to benign prostatic hyperplasia in males, or renal stones. Chronic retention may lead to accumulation of urine in the bladder, causing distension. Such retention may lead to the formation of bladder stones due to urine stasis. Urinary stasis may also cause infections.

## What is the normal volume of urine held by the bladder?

1–1.5 L.

## What is diabetes insipidus and how may it present?

Increased production of antidiuretic hormone (ADH), leading to increased amount of urination. Patients may present with increased thirst (polydipsia) and polyuria. Diabetes insipidus may be from a central cause, from the pituitary producing too much ADH or due to the aquaporin receptors on the collecting ducts of the nephrons not responding to ADH (nephrogenic diabetes insipidus).

## How do male and female urinary tracts differ?

Males have both an internal and external sphincter, with the prostate situated between the two. Females only have an external sphincter, with no prostate or internal sphincter. Males also have a longer urethra of around 20 cm compared to a female urethra of around 3–4 cm.

## What is the role of parasympathetic nerve innervation to the bladder?

Parasympathetic innervation arises from the sacral micturition centre (S2–S4), forming the pelvic nerve. It is responsible for facilitating voiding through contraction of the detrusor muscle (through acting on the muscarinic 3 receptors with acetylcholine).

## What is the role of sympathetic nerve innervation to the bladder?

The hypogastric sympathetic nerve arises from T12–L3, and is responsible for relaxation of the detrusor muscle through noradrenergic action on $B_3$ receptors. The hypogastric nerve further promotes internal sphincter muscle contraction in males, through releasing noradrenaline at alpha 1 receptors.

## Which somatic nerves are involved in micturition, where do they act and what is their role?

The pudendal nerve, arising from S2–S4, acts on nicotinic receptors with acetylcholine to cause contraction of the external urethral sphincter, allowing somatic control of micturition by preventing micturition.

## Station 1.23    Haematuria

### Doctor Briefing

You are a junior doctor in the ED and have been asked to see Brian Stevens, a 55-year-old man, who presented with a 24-h history of frank, painless haematuria. He is otherwise fit and well with no significant medical history. Please take a history from Mr Stevens, present your findings and formulate an appropriate management plan.

### Patient Briefing

You are visiting the ED, as your urine has been a pinkish colour and cloudy, with a funny smell for the past 24 h. You are experiencing severe pain in your right lower back, which is now also in your right groin. The pain came on suddenly and comes and goes in waves. You are unable to find a comfortable position. You are passing less urine than usual and have experienced increased frequency but no pain or burning sensation upon passing urine.

On questioning you are experiencing nausea but have not vomited and have a high temperature. You have never experienced these symptoms before, have no other significant medical problems and are not taking any regular medications.

You are not aware of any other medical conditions that run in the family.

You live with your wife and are currently a full-time teacher. You have smoked around 20 cigarettes a day for the last 25 years and drink around 8 units a week.

You are concerned because your brother required renal stones to be removed a few years ago and you are wondering if you are experiencing the same problem.

### Mark Scheme for Examiner

#### Introduction

| | | | | |
|---|---|---|---|---|
| Cleans hands, introduces self, confirms patient identity and gains consent for history taking | | | | |
| Establishes current patient knowledge and concerns | | | | |

#### History of Presenting Complaint

| Question | Justification | Answer | Thoughts | | | | |
|---|---|---|---|---|---|---|---|
| When did you first notice blood in your urine? | Helps determine if this is an acute or chronic presentation | 'About 24 h ago' | 24 h ago implies a sudden onset, therefore we should rule out acute causes | | | | |
| Have you passed any blood clots in your urine? | Blood clots in urine suggest significant bleeding, usually from the urinary tract. Clots may cause urethral blockage | 'No' | No additional concerns | | | | |
| What colour is your urine? Is there any frothing? | This allows assessment of proteinuria and indicates possible location of bleeding | 'Pinkish and cloudy, not frothy' | Macroscopic haematuria commonly suggests a lower urinary tract cause, e.g. UTI. If the urine is not frothy, it is unlikely to be proteinuria. Cloudy urine suggests an infective cause | | | | |
| Does your urine have an unpleasant smell? | Further assesses potential infective cause | 'Yes' | Consider infection | | | | |

## History of Presenting Complaint

| Question | Justification | Answer | Thoughts | | | | |
|---|---|---|---|---|---|---|---|
| Is there any pain or burning sensation when you pass urine? | Screening for UTI symptoms | 'No' | No additional concerns | | | | |
| Do you feel the need to pass urine more frequently? | Associated with benign prostatic hyperplasia UTI, renal stones and systemic conditions, including diabetes mellitus | 'No, I have been passing less urine' | Consider obstructive cause | | | | |
| Are you currently in pain? If so, point to the origin of the pain. | Flank pain is typically associated with kidney origin | 'In my right lower back, coming around to my groin' | Potential kidney origin. Loin to groin suggests potential renal stones | | | | |
| Is the pain constant? | Renal stones classically present with colicky pain | 'It comes and goes' | Colicky pain is associated with obstruction of peristaltic structures | | | | |
| How severe is the pain? | This allows assessment of severity | 'Very severe: 9/10' | Analgesia should be prescribed | | | | |
| How suddenly did the pain start? | Assesses if pain is due to a chronic or acute obstruction | 'Very quickly' | Reduced concern of malignant obstruction. Consider renal stones | | | | |
| Have you experienced any nausea or vomiting? | Pyelonephritis and renal stones are classically associated with nausea and vomiting | 'I feel sick' | Consider pyelonephritis and renal stones as differentials | | | | |
| Have you noticed any unintentional weight loss? | Screening for red flags for urological malignancy | 'No' | No red flags | | | | |

## Past Medical and Surgical History

| Question | Justification | Answer | Thoughts | | | | |
|---|---|---|---|---|---|---|---|
| Have you recently been hospitalised and required a catheter? | Assesses recent urological trauma | 'No' | No additional concerns | | | | |
| Have you ever been treated for renal stones? | Patients frequently experience renal stones repeatedly | 'No' | No additional concerns | | | | |

## Drug History

| Question | Justification | Answer | Thoughts | | | | |
|---|---|---|---|---|---|---|---|
| Are you currently taking any medication, or have any allergies? | Numerous common medications are associated with haematuria, including over-the-counter medications such as NSAIDs | 'No medications or allergies' | No additional concerns | | | | |

**Drug History**

| Question | Justification | Answer | Thoughts | | | | | |
|---|---|---|---|---|---|---|---|---|
| Have you ever taken a drug that could affect your bleeding, including aspirin or warfarin? | If there is a specific drug you need to consider, always ask about it. These drugs can increase bleeding risk | 'Never' | No additional concerns | | | | | |
| Have you taken the antibiotics gentamicin or rifampicin recently? | Gentamicin is nephrotoxic. Rifampicin can discolour urine | 'No' | No additional concerns | | | | | |
| Have you had all your immunisations? | Very important to check. Hepatitis B virus associated with CKD | 'Yes' | No additional concerns | | | | | |

**Family History**

| Question | Justification | Answer | Thoughts | | | | | |
|---|---|---|---|---|---|---|---|---|
| Are there any diseases that run in the family, including any cancers? | Always check for relevant heritable conditions | 'My brother had renal stones removed a few years ago' | Cystine stones may be hereditary | | | | | |

**Social and Travel History**

| Question | Justification | Answer | Thoughts | | | | | |
|---|---|---|---|---|---|---|---|---|
| Who is currently at home? Are you working? | Explore possible social concerns or if wider support is needed | 'I live with my wife and am a full-time teacher' | No social concerns. No suggestion of risk factors for bladder cancer such as work in the dye, rubber and textile industries. | | | | | |
| Do you smoke? | Explore wider risk factors | 'Around 20 a day for the last 25 years' | 25 pack-years. Smoking increases the risk of malignancy and renal stones | | | | | |
| What is your average weekly alcohol consumption? | | 'Around 8 units a week' | No additional concerns | | | | | |
| Have you recently travelled abroad? | Assess for tropical infections. Fresh-water swimming increases urinary schistosomiasis risk | 'Visited family in Spain 6 months ago' | No travel concerns | | | | | |
| Have you altered your diet recently? | Certain foods, e.g. beetroot, may discolour urine | 'No' | Exclude discoloration due to diet | | | | | |
| Have you recently undertaken strenuous exercise? | May cause haematuria | 'No' | Exclude exercise-induced haematuria | | | | | |

## Social and Travel History

| Question | Justification | Answer | Thoughts | | | | |
|---|---|---|---|---|---|---|---|
| Have you engaged in unprotected sexual activity with any new partners, or any partners who may be carrying a sexually transmitted disease? | Chlamydia and gonorrhoea may cause haematuria | 'No' | No additional concerns | | | | |

## Systems Review

| Question | Justification | Answer | Thoughts | | | | |
|---|---|---|---|---|---|---|---|
| Just to check, have you had any problems with bladder or bowel function? | Find out if there are any wider concerns that have not arisen yet | 'No, they have been normal' | No additional concerns | | | | |
| Have you had any recent night sweats, fever, weight loss or fatigue? | It is essential to ask about B symptoms to rule out certain causes, such as infection | 'No' | No additional concerns | | | | |
| Have you developed a rash? | Assess for Henoch–Schönlein purpura | 'No' | No additional concerns | | | | |
| Have you had any recent illnesses or infections? | Recent infection may cause glomerulonephritis. Frequent recent infections may suggest the patient is immunocompromised – HIV is associated with CKD | 'No' | No additional concerns | | | | |

## Finishing the Consultation

| Question | Justification | Answer | Thoughts | | | | |
|---|---|---|---|---|---|---|---|
| Is there anything that I've missed that you would like to tell me about? | May identify useful information that has been missed. Will also help to build rapport with the patient | 'I hope it's nothing serious' | Take the time to explain what will happen from here | | | | |
| Do you have any questions? | Allows any final concerns to be addressed | | | | | | |

## Present Your Findings

Mr Stevens, a 55-year-old man, presented with a 24-h history of frank haematuria and oliguria. Urine is pink and cloudy with an unpleasant odour. No pain or burning on micturition. He describes severe, sudden-onset, colicky loin-to-groin pain, with nausea. No red flags for malignancy or sexually transmitted disease. There is a family history of renal stones.

My main differential is renal stones, with potential associated UTI. I would also like to investigate for benign prostatic disease and ruptured abdominal aortic aneurysm, and refer under the 2-week wait system due to age for urological malignancy if no clear cause is determined.

I will complete a urine dip, urine microscopy, culture and sensitivity and blood tests. I would like to arrange a CT kidneys, ureters and bladder

| General Points | | | | |
|---|---|---|---|---|
| Polite to patient | | | | |
| Maintains good eye contact | | | | |
| Appropriate use of open and closed questions | | | | |
| No or limited use of medical jargon | | | | |

## ❓ QUESTIONS FROM THE EXAMINER

### What would you expect to find when examining a patient with renal stones?

Usually no tenderness on palpation. Percussion tenderness at the renal angle may indicate retroperitoneal inflammation.

### How would you manage and treat a patient with renal stones?

Analgesia, antibiotics and antiemetics. Most stones < 5 mm pass spontaneously. For stones >5 mm or those <5 mm where pain is not resolving, treat with medical expulsive therapy with nifedipine or alpha blockers. If the stone has not passed within 48 h, consider extracorporeal shock-wave lithotripsy or percutaneous nephrolithotomy.

### Where are renal stones anatomically most likely to cause obstruction and why?

Renal stones are most likely to cause an obstruction at anatomical narrowings in the urinary tract, including the pelviureteric junction, pelvic brim and vesicoureteric junction.

### What is a staghorn calculus, and what is a possible complication if it is not appropriately treated?

A large calculus in the renal pelvis, which extends over at least two calyces. A possible complication includes urinary sepsis.

### What does EPO play a role in?

The kidneys produce EPO, which stimulates red blood cell production. Patients with CKD may therefore experience symptoms of anaemia.

### Why are patients with CKD at increased risk of cardiovascular disease?

The kidneys have a role in producing renin, which acts as part of the renin–angiotensin–aldosterone system (RAAS) to regulate blood pressure. Patients with CKD may therefore be at risk of cardiovascular disease, due to increased proinflammatory cytokines caused by overstimulation of the RAAS.

### Describe haemodialysis.

Haemodialysis is when an atrioventricular fistula is accessed to pass the patient's blood through a machine containing a semipermeable membrane and dialysis fluid with the correct concentration of solutes, before being returned into the patient's body.

### Describe peritoneal dialysis.

Peritoneal dialysis is when a catheter is inserted into the peritoneal cavity and fluid with the correct concentration of solutes is infused. The peritoneum is utilised as a semipermeable membrane.

### Why might a patient opt for peritoneal dialysis as opposed to haemodialysis?

Patients may choose peritoneal dialysis as it provides more flexibility, which may be more amenable for a patient's lifestyle. As peritoneal dialysis is conducted at home, patients aren't required to make multiple trips to hospital each week. Furthermore, there are fewer dietary restrictions for peritoneal dialysis.

### What is the first choice of pharmacological treatment following acute rejection of a renal transplant, its mechanism of action and a key side effect?

Glucocorticoids, which decrease the transcription of inflammatory cytokines. Side effects include hyperlipidaemia, diabetes mellitus, impaired wound healing, cataracts, osteoporosis and fragile skin.

# Clinical Examination

2

## Outline

## Station 2.1   Cardiovascular

### Doctor Briefing

You are a junior doctor in the Emergency Department (ED) and have been asked to see Mrs Smith, a 60-year-old woman who has presented with shortness of breath and a new murmur. Please perform a relevant cardiovascular examination on Mrs Smith and present your findings.

### Patient Briefing

Your general practitioner (GP) has referred you to the ED with shortness of breath and generalised fatigue which have been getting worse over the past week. You have also been coughing persistently, waking up with bad night sweats, and you have started to notice swelling in your legs.

You recently had an emergency dentist appointment. The dentist diagnosed you with a dental abscess and prescribed oral antibiotics. He commented on your poor dental hygiene and advised that you should stop smoking. Aside from the recent course of antibiotics, you take a statin, calcium channel blocker and beta-blocker. You have no allergies, and your past medical history includes hypercholesterolaemia, hypertension, recurrent dental abscesses and previous prosthetic valve replacement surgery. You have smoked 20 cigarettes a day for 40 years.

You are concerned that you have got a more serious infection following your dental abscess.

### Mark Scheme for Examiner

| Introduction | | | | | |
|---|---|---|---|---|---|
| Washes hands, introduces self, confirms patient identity and gains consent for examination | | | | | |
| Offers a chaperone | | | | | |
| Appropriately exposes the patient whilst keeping dignity at all times, and repositions into a suitable position for the examination | | | | | |
| Asks if the patient has any pain currently | | | | | |

## General Inspection

| What are you looking for or examining? | Justification | Findings and evolving thought process | | | |
|---|---|---|---|---|---|
| Assess general well-being | On initial glance, does the patient look well, unwell or in pain? | The patient looks pale and sweaty | | | |
| Obvious clues | Gives an indication of the patient's baseline health | The patient has a low body mass index (BMI) and has a bag of regular medications with her | | | |
| Check surroundings | Checks for obvious clues to aid diagnosis or equipment/observations to aid assessment | The patient has had observations which confirm a fever and tachycardia. A 20G cannula is present in the patient's hand and she is on 2 L oxygen via nasal cannula | | | |

## Examination of the Hands and Arms

| | | | | | |
|---|---|---|---|---|---|
| Check hands for signs of infective endocarditis | Checks for clubbing, splinter haemorrhages and Janeway lesions and feels for Osler's nodes | Splinter haemorrhages can be seen in the patient's nailbeds | | | |
| Check the capillary refill time (CRT) and peripheral temperature simultaneously | Assesses peripheral perfusion | CRT is normal at 2 s. Hands appear warm and well perfused | | | |
| Palpate radial pulses | Assesses rate and regularity. Also feel bilateral pulses simultaneously to assess for any radio-radio delay | The pulse rate is tachycardic at 115 bpm and regular in rhythm | | | |
| Check for collapsing pulse | Asks patient if she has any pain before lifting arm. If a collapsing pulse is present, this is suggestive of aortic regurgitation | No collapsing pulse present | | | |
| Palpate brachial or carotid pulse | Assesses volume and character of the pulse. A slow rising pulse is a feature of aortic stenosis | Volume is full-bodied with normal character | | | |
| Check blood pressure | Assesses for a narrow pulse pressure (aortic stenosis) and wide pulse pressure (aortic regurgitation) | Blood pressure is 136/70 mmHg. Pulse pressure is normal | | | |

## Examination of the Face

| | | | | | |
|---|---|---|---|---|---|
| Look for xanthelasma and corneal arcus | These signs are suggestive of hypercholesterolaemia | Xanthelasma present bilaterally on lower eyelids | | | |
| Check for conjunctival pallor | Suggestive of anaemia | Pale conjunctiva present | | | |
| Look in the mouth | Assesses for central cyanosis and hydration status | Tongue looks moist and well perfused | | | |
| (Offer to) perform fundoscopy | Looks for features of hypertensive and/or diabetic retinopathy and Roth spots, which suggest infective endocarditis | Roth spots present on fundoscopy | | | |

## Chest Examination – Inspection

| What are you looking for or examining? | Justification | Findings and evolving thought process | | | | |
|---|---|---|---|---|---|---|
| Look for devices in situ | Looks for evidence of previous cardiac intervention for example, pacemaker, implantable cardioverter defibrillator | No devices present | | | | |
| Look for scars | Looks for evidence of previous cardiac surgery such as median sternotomy, lateral thoracotomy, pacemaker, mitral valvotomy, chest drains | A midline sternotomy scar can be seen, indicating possible previous cardiac surgery | | | | |
| Look for chest wall deformities | Deformities such as pectus excavatum and pectus carinatum can affect the function of the heart | No chest wall deformities | | | | |
| Look for visible pulsation | In a normal heart you should see a single outward pulse over the fifth intercostal space in the midclavicular line | Unremarkable pulsation | | | | |
| Check jugular venous pressure (JVP) | Provides an indirect indicator of central venous pressure. If raised, could indicate right heart failure | The JVP is not raised | | | | |

## Chest Examination – Palpation

| | | | | | | |
|---|---|---|---|---|---|---|
| Feel for apex beat | Usually located in the midclavicular line fifth intercostal space. If displaced, could indicate cardiomegaly | Apex beat felt and located in correct position | | | | |
| Feel for parasternal heaves and precordial impulses | Suggestive of ventricular hypertrophy | No heaves or impulses palpated | | | | |
| Feel for thrills | Suggestive of a severe heart murmur | No thrills palpated | | | | |

## Chest Examination – Auscultation

| | | | | | | |
|---|---|---|---|---|---|---|
| Auscultate all four areas of the precordium | Listens to aortic, pulmonary, tricuspid and mitral valve areas to assess for heart murmurs | An early diastolic murmur can be heard, suggestive of aortic regurgitation | | | | |
| Check for radiation to both carotids and axillae | Radiation to the carotids could indicate severe aortic stenosis, with radiation to the axillae indicating mitral regurgitation | There is no radiation of the murmur | | | | |
| Auscultate mitral area with patient rolled on to the left side | Accentuates mid-late diastolic murmur for mitral stenosis | Murmur is not accentuated | | | | |
| Auscultate lower left sternal edge with patient sat up and breath held on exhalation | Accentuates early diastolic murmur for aortic regurgitation | The murmur heard previously is accentuated with this manoeuvre | | | | |
| Auscultate both lung bases | Listens for bi-basal crackles, which could suggest pulmonary oedema | Fine bi-basal crackles can be heard at both lung bases | | | | |

## Examination of the Abdomen and Legs

| What are you looking for or examining? | Justification | Findings and evolving thought process | | | | |
|---|---|---|---|---|---|---|
| Look for blood vessel grafts, such as saphenous vein | This could indicate previous coronary artery bypass graft surgery | No signs of previous grafts | | | | |
| Assess for hepato-megaly, ascites and peripheral oedema | These signs, if present, could suggest right heart failure | Bilateral pitting peripheral oedema to mid-shins is present | | | | |

## Finishing

| | | | | | | |
|---|---|---|---|---|---|---|
| Check patient is comfortable, offer to help reposition her and give the privacy to change | Keeps the patient's dignity | Treating the patient with respect is important | | | | |
| Remove your gloves and wash hands | Complying with hand hygiene is vital | No additional concerns | | | | |

## Present Your Findings

Mrs Smith is a 60-year-old woman who has presented with shortness of breath and a heart murmur. On examination she is pyrexic, tachycardic and looks pale. On inspection, she has peripheral stigmata of infective endocarditis, with splinter haemor-rhages present on both hands. On auscultation, she has an early diastolic murmur in the aortic area which does not radiate. She has a midline sternotomy scar, due to previous prosthetic valve replacement, and evidence of pulmonary and peripheral oedema.

I feel the most likely diagnosis is infective endocarditis, with the differentials being acute heart failure, pneumonia and mitral stenosis.

I would like to perform a respiratory examination and review bedside electrocardiogram (ECG) monitoring. I will also take bloods (including full blood count (FBCs), urea and electrolyte (U&Es), C-reactive protein (CRP), liver function tests (LFTs)) and blood cultures, request a chest X-ray (CXR), and order a transthoracic echocardiogram and 12-lead ECG. I would also like to ascer-tain whether her heart murmur is new or long-standing

## General Points

| | | | | |
|---|---|---|---|---|
| Polite to patient | | | | |
| Maintains good eye contact | | | | |
| Clear instruction and explanation to patient | | | | |

## ❓ QUESTIONS FROM THE EXAMINER

### What are the main risk factors for infective endocarditis?

Valvular heart disease (including degenerative, aortic stenosis or rheumatic heart disease), prosthetic heart valves, non-sterile ve-nous injections (such as in intravenous (IV) drug use) and immunocompromised states all increase the risk of infective endocarditis.

### What constitutes the main treatment for infective endocarditis?

In unstable patients, empirical antibiotic therapy should be administered. Antibiotics should be given according to culture sensitiv-ities if available, but this should not delay commencement.

## What are the key differences between prosthetic and mechanical heart valves?

Mechanical heart valves are known to last longer than prosthetic valves. Mechanical heart valves require the patient to take lifelong anticoagulation medication.

## What is the first-line modality of imaging used to examine any new heart murmur?

An echocardiogram, preferably transthoracic.

## What is the difference between endocarditis and pericarditis?

Endocarditis is inflammation of the inner lining of the heart's chambers and valves whereas pericarditis is inflammation of the pericardial sac surrounding the heart.

## What symptoms and signs could occur in a patient with aortic stenosis?

A patient with aortic stenosis may initially be asymptomatic. Symptoms may include dyspnoea, angina and dizziness or syncope.

## Classically, how do you describe the murmur associated with aortic stenosis?

Classically it is described as a harsh crescendo–decrescendo late systolic ejection murmur that radiates to the carotids.

## What are the potential reasons for a midline sternotomy scar?

A midline sternotomy scar is performed in many open cardiac procedures, such as heart valve surgery, coronary artery bypass grafting or heart transplantation.

## How might you accentuate the JVP if you are struggling to visualise it?

Elecit the hepatojugular reflex, where applying pressure over the liver causes the JVP to rise.

## How might you describe a murmur?

When describing a heart murmur, it is useful to mention timing of the murmur during the cardiac cycle, intensity, location of maximum intensity, radiation, influence of expiration and inspiration, changes with manoeuvres and any specific characteristics.

## Station 2.2    Respiratory

### Doctor Briefing

You are a junior doctor in general medicine and have been asked to see Mrs Fredrickson, a 76-year-old woman who has presented with severe difficulty in breathing and a cough. Please perform a relevant respiratory examination on Mrs Fredrickson and present your findings.

### Patient Briefing

You have aortic stenosis and have undergone an elective transcatheter aortic valve replacement, and over the last 24 h you have developed difficulty with your breathing, a fever and a productive cough. You are coughing up offensive green/brown-coloured sputum and are finding it difficult to breathe without supplementary oxygen. You are not coughing up any blood and do not have any chest pain.

You have spent very little time in hospital previously and are greatly concerned about hospital-acquired infections.

### Mark Scheme for Examiner

#### Introduction

| | | | | | |
|---|---|---|---|---|---|
| Washes hands, introduces self, confirms patient identity and gains consent for examination | | | | | |
| Offers a chaperone | | | | | |
| Appropriately exposes the patient whilst keeping dignity at all times, and repositions into a suitable position for the examination | | | | | |
| Asks if the patient has any pain currently | | | | | |

#### General Inspection

| What are you looking for or examining? | Justification | Findings and evolving thought process | | | |
|---|---|---|---|---|---|
| Assess general well-being | On initial glance, does the patient look well, unwell or in pain? | The patient looks unwell and is of slim build | | | |
| Obvious clues | Gives an indication of the patient's baseline health | The patient is currently on 15 L oxygen via a non-rebreathe mask, saturating at 93% | | | |
| Take respiratory rate and assess rate and depth of breathing | Hyperventilation could indicate anxiety and predisposes to metabolic acidosis. Hypoventilation could indicate ventilatory failure | The patient is breathing fast and shallow, with a respiration rate of 28 breaths/min | | | |
| Look for nasal flaring, tracheal tug, intercostal recession, lip pursing, use of accessory muscles | Checks for signs of respiratory distress and assesses work of breathing | Patient is seen to be using accessory muscles for breathing | | | |

#### Examination of the Hands

| | | | | | |
|---|---|---|---|---|---|
| Check for clubbing and peripheral cyanosis | May indicate chronic lung pathology | No clubbing or peripheral cyanosis | | | |
| Look for tar staining | May indicate current or previous cigarette smoking | No tar staining present | | | |
| Check for resting tremor | May suggest excessive use of beta-agonists or theophylline bronchodilators | No resting tremor present | | | |

## Examination of the Hands

| What are you looking for or examining? | Justification | Findings and evolving thought process | | | | | |
|---|---|---|---|---|---|---|---|
| Feel the radial pulse | Checks pulse rate, rhythm and volume. Chronic $CO_2$ retainers have warm peripheries and large-volume bounding pulses | The radial pulse is regular and tachycardic at 105 bpm. Volume appears normal. Warm peripheries | | | | | |
| Test for a $CO_2$ retention flap or flapping tremor | This can be performed by asking the patient to lift the arms in front of her, cock the wrists back and hold for 30 s. It is positive if there are signs of tremor. $CO_2$ retention/type 2 respiratory failure can cause a flapping tremor | No tremor noted | | | | | |

## Examination of the Eyes

| | | | | | | | |
|---|---|---|---|---|---|---|---|
| Look for conjunctival pallor | May be suggestive of anaemia | No conjunctival pallor noted | | | | | |
| Look for Horner's syndrome | Horner's syndrome is characterised by ptosis, miosis, anhidrosis, enophthalmos. An apical lung cancer or superior vena cava (SVC) obstruction may invade the sympathetic chain, causing Horner's syndrome | No evidence of Horner's syndrome | | | | | |

## Examination of the Mouth

| | | | | | | | |
|---|---|---|---|---|---|---|---|
| Inspect the mouth | Checks for central cyanosis, hypoxia and oral thrush (which could be secondary to oral steroid use) | No additional concerns | | | | | |

## Examination of the Neck

| | | | | | | | |
|---|---|---|---|---|---|---|---|
| Check JVP | If raised, causes include cor pulmonale, elevated intrathoracic pressures (for example, severe asthma or tension pneumothorax) and SVC obstruction | The JVP is normal | | | | | |
| Check for tracheal deviation | Tracheal deviation may indicate lobar collapse, pneumonectomy, pleural effusion or tension pneumothorax | The trachea is located centrally with no deviation | | | | | |
| Feel and assess lymph nodes in the neck and axilla | Checks for swelling, inflammation or signs of malignancy | The submandibular lymph nodes appear slightly swollen and tender | | | | | |

## Chest Examination – Inspection

| What are you looking for or examining? | Justification | Findings and evolving thought process | | | | | | |
|---|---|---|---|---|---|---|---|---|
| Look for chest wall deformities or asymmetry | Barrel chest, pectus excavatum, thoracic kyphoscoliosis, pectus carinatum are some chest wall deformities that may indicate underlying lung pathology or functional disease | There are no chest wall deformities | | | | | | |
| Look for chest wall lesions, scars and dilated superficial veins | Metastatic tumour nodules and neurofibromas may be present as well as evidence of thoracic surgery. Dilated superficial veins may indicate SVC obstruction | No chest wall lesions or scars present | | | | | | |

## Chest Examination – Palpation

| | | | | | | | | |
|---|---|---|---|---|---|---|---|---|
| Palpate the apex beat | If impalpable, consider diagnosis such as emphysema, obesity, dextrocardia and a large pleural effusion. Tension pneumothoraces can cause a displaced apex beat | Strong and regular apex beat found in the fifth intercostal space, midclavicular line | | | | | | |
| Feel for equal chest expansion | Assesses upper, middle and lower zones. Unilateral reduced expansion may indicate pneumothorax, pleural effusion, pneumonia and collapse | Bilateral equal chest expansion | | | | | | |

## Chest Examination – Percussion

| | | | | | | | | |
|---|---|---|---|---|---|---|---|---|
| Percuss chest wall in a systematic approach, comparing the notes at equivalent positions on both sides | Assesses for resonance and dullness which may indicate lung pathology. Important to compare and contrast to isolate potential disease | Right lower zone is dull to percussion. The left lung is resonant in contrast | | | | | | |

## Chest Examination – Auscultation

| | | | | | | | | |
|---|---|---|---|---|---|---|---|---|
| Auscultate all lung areas in a systematic approach | Listens for quality and volume of breath sounds, bilateral air entry and any added sounds such as crackles, wheeze and plural rub | There is reduced air entry and coarse crackles at the right lung base, with some mild wheeze throughout the lung on expiration | | | | | | |
| Check for whispering pectoriloquy | Can be performed by asking the patient to whisper whilst auscultating the chest. Can help differentiate between pleural effusion and consolidation | Whispered sounds cannot be heard on auscultation (normal finding) | | | | | | |

## Examination of the Back

| | | | | | | | | |
|---|---|---|---|---|---|---|---|---|
| Repeat inspection, palpation, percussion and auscultation on the back, ensuring the patient's arms are folded across the chest | Important to do this so as not to miss any examination findings. The bases of the lung can be best heard from the back | Findings on the anterior wall are also noted posteriorly | | | | | | |

**Additional Tests**

| What are you looking for or examining? | Justification | Findings and evolving thought process | | | | |
|---|---|---|---|---|---|---|
| Offer to check peak flow | Important to assess in any patient with a history of asthma | Peak flow reduced from baseline | | | | |
| Offer to take and examine a sputum sample | Important to test for microorganisms in any suspected respiratory infection. Can help to isolate atypical infection and guide antibiotic therapy | Awaiting results | | | | |

**Finishing**

| | | | | | | |
|---|---|---|---|---|---|---|
| Check patient is comfortable, offer to help reposition them and give the privacy to change | Keeps the patient's dignity | Treating the patient with respect is important | | | | |
| Remove your gloves and wash hands | Complying with hand hygiene is vital | No additional concerns | | | | |

**Present Your Findings**

Mrs Fredrickson is a 76-year-old woman who has presented with a 24-h history of increasing difficulty in breathing, fever and a cough productive of brown/green sputum. On examination she is pyrexial with an oxygen saturation of 93% on 15 L oxygen via a non-rebreathe mask and a raised respiratory rate of 28 breaths/min. There is reduced right air entry and coarse crackle at the right lung base, which is dull to percussion. Chest expansion is normal.

I feel the most likely diagnosis is hospital-acquired pneumonia, with the differentials being a pleural effusion, exacerbation of asthma, heart failure and lung fibrosis.

I would like to request a CXR and take bloods (including FBCs, U&Es, CRP, procalcitonin), as well as an arterial blood gas. My initial management would include IV fluids and antibiotics according to local trust guidelines

**General Points**

| | | | |
|---|---|---|---|
| Polite to patient | | | |
| Maintains good eye contact | | | |
| Clear instruction and explanation to patient | | | |

## ❓ QUESTIONS FROM THE EXAMINER

### What are the most common causative organisms in hospital-acquired pneumonia?

Aerobic Gram-negative bacilli such as *Pseudomonas aeruginosa*, *Escherichia coli*, *Klebsiella pneumoniae*.

### Name a respiratory disease that clubbing could indicate.

Respiratory causes for finger clubbing include lung cancer, interstitial lung disease, cystic fibrosis and bronchiectasis.

### What is the CURB65 score and what parameters does it assess?

CURB65 is a score of pneumonia severity. A point is given for each parameter of confusion, urea greater than 7 mmol/L, respiratory rate ≥ 30 breaths/min, systolic blood pressure < 90 mmHg or diastolic blood pressure ≤ 60 mmHg and age >65 years old.

## What is procalcitonin?

Serum procalcitonin is a biomarker of inflammation, and it is particularly raised in respiratory infections.

## Why is a normal $CO_2$ level concerning in an asthmatic who is having a severe exacerbation of asthma?

As a patient suffering a severe asthma attack struggles to maintain oxygen saturations, their respiratory rate will increase. This will lead to more $CO_2$ being lost. If a patient in these circumstances has a normal $CO_2$, this suggests they are tiring and are unable to maintain this respiratory rate, and the patient will continue to deteriorate without further intervention.

## What is the difference between CPAP and BIPAP?

Continuous positive airway pressure (CPAP) provides a single positive pressure, whereas bilevel positive airway pressure (BIPAP) provides both an exhale and an inhale pressure.

## How would you differentiate between a moderate and severe exacerbation of asthma?

Features of a severe asthma attack include the patient being unable to complete a sentence without taking a breath, respiratory rate >25/min breaths/min, pulse rate > 110 bpm and peak flow 33–50% of predicted.

## Which factors would make you think that someone has life-threatening asthma?

Features of life-threatening asthma are silent chest, cyanosis, exhaustion, altered consciousness, peak expiratory flow <33% of predicted, oxygen saturation <92%.

## Which four drugs are the mainstay of tuberculosis treatment?

Rifampin, isoniazid, pyrazinamide and ethambutol hydrochloride.

## Which opportunistic respiratory infection is seen in immunocompromised individuals (for example, acquired immunodeficiency syndrome (AIDS))?

*Pneumocystis* pneumonia.

## Station 2.3  Abdominal

### Doctor Briefing

You are a junior doctor in general surgery and have been asked to see Miss Payne, a 45-year-old woman, who has presented with severe abdominal pain and vomiting. Please perform a relevant abdominal examination on Miss Payne and present your findings.

### Patient Briefing

Over the past 6 h you have felt unwell with severe abdominal pain and have been vomiting fresh red blood. You feel dizzy and you fainted before being brought into hospital.

On questioning, the stomach pain started suddenly 6 h ago and is now very severe at a 10/10 intensity. It feels like someone is stabbing a knife into your stomach. Nothing makes the pain feel better and eating or drinking makes it worse. You have a history of peptic ulcer disease and have low compliance with taking your omeprazole. You have recently injured your leg running, so have been taking some of your partner's naproxen and ibuprofen to try and help with the pain. You drink 20 units of alcohol a week, and last night drank a particularly large amount at a birthday celebration. The pain and vomiting started later in the night, but you initially put this down to food poisoning.

You are extremely concerned at the appearance of blood in your vomit and are worried that something serious is wrong.

### Mark Scheme for Examiner

#### Introduction

| | | | | |
|---|---|---|---|---|
| Washes hands, introduces self, confirms patient identity and gains consent for examination | | | | |
| Offers a chaperone | | | | |
| Appropriately exposes the patient whilst keeping dignity at all times, and repositions into a suitable position for the examination | | | | |
| Asks if the patient has any pain currently | | | | |

#### General Inspection

| What are you looking for or examining? | Justification | Findings and evolving thought process | | | | |
|---|---|---|---|---|---|---|
| Assess general well-being | On initial glance, does the patient look well, unwell or in pain? | The patient looks unwell and very pale. She is complaining of severe pain in her stomach and appears agitated | | | | |
| Obvious clues | Gives an indication of the patient's baseline health | The patient has an 18G cannula in situ with saline running. There are two vomit bowls by the patient which contain coffee-ground vomit, as well as bright-red haematemesis | | | | |
| Check surroundings | Checks for obvious clues to aid diagnosis or equipment/observations to aid assessment | | | | | |

#### Examination of the Hands

| | | | | | | |
|---|---|---|---|---|---|---|
| Look at the nails | Leukonychia suggests low albumin. Koilonychia suggests iron deficiency. Clubbing suggests underlying chronic disease | There are no abnormalities regarding the nails | | | | |
| Look at the palms | Palmar erythema and Dupuytren's contracture may suggest chronic liver disease | No peripheral stigmata of liver disease | | | | |

## Examination of the Hands

| What are you looking for or examining? | Justification | Findings and evolving thought process | | | | | | |
|---|---|---|---|---|---|---|---|---|
| Check for a liver flap | This can be performed by asking the patient to lift her arms in front of her, cock the wrists back and hold for 30 s. It is positive if there are signs of tremor, which could suggest possible hepatic encephalopathy | No liver flap seen | | | | | | |
| Feel for a radial/brachial pulse | Assesses pulse rate, regularity, volume and character | The pulse is regular but noticeably tachycardic. You note the pulse is thin and thready | | | | | | |
| Offer to measure the blood pressure and check CRT | Important if you suspect gastrointestinal (GI) bleed | The blood pressure is low at 83/53 mmHg and the CRT is prolonged at 4 s | | | | | | |

## Examination of the Face and Neck

| | | | | | | | | |
|---|---|---|---|---|---|---|---|---|
| Look at the eyes | Inspect for jaundice, anaemia (conjunctival pallor), Kayser–Fleischer rings and xanthelasma. Kayser–Fleischer rings occur in Wilson's disease and xanthelasmata are a feature of hypercholesterolaemia | Conjunctival pallor is noted | | | | | | |
| Look at the mouth | Gingivitis may suggest malnutrition. Ulcers are a feature of inflammatory bowel disease (IBD). Perioral pigmentation may suggest Peutz–Jeghers syndrome | The patient's mouth looks dry. There are no other signs to visualise | | | | | | |
| Feel and assess neck lymph nodes | Checks for swelling or inflammation. Troissier's sign (palpable Virchow's node in left supraclavicular fossa) is associated with GI malignancy | The lymph nodes are of normal size and consistency and non-tender | | | | | | |

## Examination of Chest and Back

| | | | | | | | | |
|---|---|---|---|---|---|---|---|---|
| Look at the chest | Hair loss, gynaecomastia and spider naevi can feature in chronic liver disease. Spider naevi can also feature in pregnancy. It is abnormal for men and women to have more than six and four spider naevi, respectively | There are no visual signs to elicit | | | | | | |

## Abdominal Examination – Inspection

| | | | | | | | | |
|---|---|---|---|---|---|---|---|---|
| Look at the abdomen and comment on shape and scars | Observes for generalised distention, obvious masses/organomegaly and cachexia (chronic disease, cancer, malnutrition). May be evidence of laparoscopic and drain scars | There is a McBurney's scar in the right iliac fossa indicating previous open appendectomy | | | | | | |

**Abdominal Examination – Inspection**

| What are you looking for or examining? | Justification | Findings and evolving thought process | | | | | |
|---|---|---|---|---|---|---|---|
| Look at the skin | Bruising, such as Grey Turner's and/or Cullen's sign, may be associated with pancreatitis and/or ruptured abdominal aortic aneurysm (AAA). Jaundice and dilated veins (caput medusae) may suggest chronic liver disease | There is no evidence of bruising, dilated veins or jaundice | | | | | |
| Ask the patient to blow out her abdomen and cough | If pain is elicited, this may suggest peritoneal irritation and it may be possible to visualise herniation | The patient struggles with this due to pain, but no herniation can be seen on active coughing | | | | | |

**Abdominal Examination – Palpation**

| | | | | | | | |
|---|---|---|---|---|---|---|---|
| Ask the patient if she has any pain and start palpation away from the pain. Observe the reaction on the patient's face at all times | Allows accurate assessment of pain and minimises discomfort/shock | Commence palpation away from the site of pain | | | | | |
| Superficial palpation with one hand: assess all nine quadrants of the abdomen in a systematic approach | Checks for tenderness and voluntary/involuntary guarding. Checks for Murphy's sign (palpate over the site of the gallbladder and ask the patient to inhale) and Rovsing's sign (palpates left iliac fossa and enquires about pain in right iliac fossa), which could suggest cholecystitis and appendicitis respectively | There is epigastric tenderness and involuntary guarding. Murphy and Rovsing's sign absent | | | | | |
| Deep palpation with both hands: palpate liver | Measures the liver edge in fingerbreadths from the ribcage. Comments on surface, tenderness, pulsatility and any masses. Checks for hepatomegaly | No hepatomegaly or masses palpated. The surface is smooth, non-nodular, non-pulsatile and non-tender | | | | | |
| Deep palpation with both hands: palpate spleen | Check for splenomegaly. The spleen should not be palpable unless it is at least three times its normal size | The spleen cannot be palpated | | | | | |
| Deep palpation with both hands: palpate kidneys | Checks for tenderness and any masses. Renal angle tenderness suggests pyelonephritis | Kidneys cannot be palpated and there is no renal angle tenderness | | | | | |
| Deep palpation with both hands: palpate bladder | Checks for distended bladder, tenderness and any masses. May indicate urinary retention | Bladder cannot be palpated | | | | | |
| Deep palpation with both hands: palpate abdominal aorta | Feels for expansile and pulsatile masses which would suggest AAA | No expansile or pulsatile masses can be palpated | | | | | |

## Abdominal Examination – Percussion

| What are you looking for or examining? | Justification | Findings and evolving thought process | | | | | | |
|---|---|---|---|---|---|---|---|---|
| Percuss liver (from above and below) | Dullness helps determine the size of the liver and assesses for hepatomegaly | No additional concerns | | | | | | |
| Percuss spleen | Dullness helps determine the size of the spleen and assesses for splenomegaly | No additional concerns | | | | | | |
| Percuss bladder | Helps determine the urinary volume | No additional concerns | | | | | | |
| Percuss for shifting dullness and check for fluid thrill | Suggestive of ascites | Shifting dullness and fluid thrill are absent | | | | | | |

## Abdominal Examination – Auscultation

| | | | | | | | | |
|---|---|---|---|---|---|---|---|---|
| Auscultate for bowel sounds (over the ileocaecal valve) for 30 s | Assesses whether bowel sounds are present (normal), absent (paralytic ileus) or high-pitched/'tinkling' (obstruction) | Active bowel sounds can be heard | | | | | | |
| Auscultate for bruits:<br>• Aortic bruits just above the umbilicus)<br>• Renal bruits 2 cm either side of the umbilicus<br>• Liver bruits over the liver | Aortic bruits may suggest aortic aneurysms<br><br>Renal bruits may suggest renal artery stenosis<br><br>Liver bruits may suggest hepatoma, acute alcoholic hepatitis, transjugular intrahepatic portosystemic stent shunt | No bruits can be heard | | | | | | |

## Additional Tests

| | | | | | | | | |
|---|---|---|---|---|---|---|---|---|
| Offer to examine the external genitalia and hernia orifices | Helps to identify hernias and any disease affecting the genitalia | No additional concerns | | | | | | |
| Look for peripheral oedema | Suggests liver failure or nephrotic syndrome | No peripheral oedema | | | | | | |
| Offer to perform a digital rectal examination (DRE) | Helps to identify abnormalities in the rectum or stool | The DRE is mostly normal, apart from the presence of black tarry stool on the finger. No masses felt | | | | | | |
| Dipstick the urine | Helps identify presence of microorganisms in the urine, infection markers, blood and glucose/ketones (diabetes/diabetic ketoacidosis) | No additional concerns | | | | | | |

**Finishing**

| What are you looking for or examining? | Justification | Findings and evolving thought process | | | | |
|---|---|---|---|---|---|---|
| Check patient is comfortable, offer to help reposition her and give the privacy to change | Keeps the patient's dignity | Treating the patient with respect is important | | | | |
| Remove your gloves and wash hands | Complying with hand hygiene is vital | No additional concerns | | | | |

**Present Your Findings**

Miss Payne is a 45-year-old woman who has presented with severe abdominal pain and vomiting of fresh red and coffee-ground haematemesis. On examination, she is pale and poorly perfused with cool peripheries, and a CRT of 4 s. She is hypotensive and tachycardic with a thin and thready pulse. There is severe epigastric tenderness and involuntary guarding. Her abdomen is tympanic with no shifting dullness. Bowel sounds are present. She has a scar in the right iliac fossa consistent with previous open appendectomy.

I feel the most likely diagnosis is upper GI bleed, likely secondary to a ruptured peptic ulcer, with the differentials being oesophageal varices and Boehaave's syndrome.

I would like to take bloods (including FBCs, U&Es, LFTs, amylase, coagulation, lactate and CRP). I would also like to take a group and save and cross-match 4 units of red blood cells. Additionally, I would request a urinary beta-human chorionic gonadotrophin (β-hCG), organise an erect CXR and abdominal X-ray, and escalate to a senior requesting urgent endoscopy

**General Points**

| | | | | | |
|---|---|---|---|---|---|
| Polite to patient | | | | | |
| Maintains good eye contact | | | | | |
| Clear instruction and explanation to patient | | | | | |
| Warns the patient about potential pain/discomfort prior to palpation | | | | | |

## ❓ QUESTIONS FROM THE EXAMINER

### What is the Rockall scoring system and why might it be helpful in assessing upper GI bleeds?

The Rockall scoring system can be used to identify patients at risk of adverse outcome following a GI bleed. It can help to identify patients at high risk of rebleeding and requiring future interventions. It can be used pre- or post-endoscopy.

### What is the Glasgow Blatchford bleeding score and why is it helpful in the management of upper GI bleeds?

The Glasgow Blatchford score can be used to identify the likelihood a patient with an upper GI bleed will require acute intervention, such as a blood transfusion or endoscopy. This is helpful to decide which patients require urgent endoscopy.

### What is the first-line modality of imaging used to assess a patient with an upper GI bleed?

Oesophagogastroduodenoscopy (OGD) is used both to visualise GI bleeding, and provide treatment.

### What is the first-line investigation for patients who you suspect may have IBD?

Blood tests, including erythrocyte sedimentation rate (ESR), CRP and FBC to look for anaemia as a consequence of IBD. To make a diagnosis of IBD, an endoscopy or colonoscopy is required to evaluate and biopsy lesions.

### What is the first-line investigation in the suspicion of jaundice?

A set of LFTs, to confirm high levels of bilirubin.

### How might you classify the causes of jaundice?

The most common way is location of the underlying case, which can be prehepatic, intrahepatic or posthepatic.

### Which antibodies might you test for in the suspicion of coeliac disease and what modality of imaging might you request?

A serology for immunoglobulin A (IgA) tissue transglutaminase antibody is suggestive of coeliac disease, and the diagnosis can be confirmed by OGD with small intestinal biopsy.

### In any female patient of child-bearing age who presents with abdominal pain/swelling, what must you always consider and how would you test for this?

In any female of reproductive age, it is important to investigate for an ectopic pregnancy, as this is a medical emergency. This can be done by sending for a serum β-hCG, which if positive should be followed by a pelvis ultrasound.

### Which risk factors increase the likelihood of experiencing an upper GI bleed?

The most common causes of upper GI bleeding are gastric and duodenal ulcers and oesophageal varices. Risk factors for these conditions are gastro-oesophageal reflux disease, hiatus hernia, excess alcohol, severe liver disease and history of non-steroidal anti-inflammatory drug use.

### Which cancers commonly metastasise to the liver?

The most common types of primary cancer to metastasise to the liver are breast, bowel, lung, pancreatic and ovarian cancer.

## Station 2.4   Hernia

### Doctor Briefing

You are a junior doctor in the ED and have been asked to see Mr Jarral, a 91-year-old man, who has presented with abdominal pain and distension. He has also been vomiting and has noticed a lump in the groin. Please perform a relevant hernia examination on Mr Jarral and present your findings.

### Patient Briefing

You were brought to the ED by your carer due to an obvious groin lump on the right-hand side, which has appeared over the last 24 h. Your mobility has been worsening over the past 12 months, and yesterday you attempted to lift yourself out of a chair. You found this strenuous and felt a 'popping' sensation in your groin and haven't felt well since.

On questioning, you have no appetite, feel nauseous and have been vomiting. Your stomach feels swollen and is very sore to touch. The lump is appearing more swollen and darkening in colour, from red to purple since it appeared. You suffer with chronic constipation and have not been able to open your bowels for the last week. You have not passed any wind in the last 24 h.

You have suspicions that this might be a hernia, as you have had an inguinal hernia earlier in life which was repaired, but this feels much more painful and you worry that you cannot 'pop the lump back in'.

### Mark Scheme for Examiner

#### Introduction

| | | | | | |
|---|---|---|---|---|---|
| Washes hands, introduces self, confirms patient identity and gains consent for examination | | | | | |
| Offers a chaperone | | | | | |
| Appropriately exposes the patient whilst keeping dignity at all times, and repositions into a suitable position for the examination | | | | | |
| Asks if the patient has any pain currently | | | | | |

#### General Inspection

| What are you looking for or examining? | Justification | Findings and evolving thought process | | | |
|---|---|---|---|---|---|
| Assess general well-being | On initial glance, does the patient look well, unwell or in pain? | The patient is morbidly obese and looks in obvious pain and discomfort | | | |
| Check surroundings | Checks for obvious clues to aid diagnosis or equipment/ observations to aid assessment | There is bilious vomit in a bowl next to the patient | | | |

#### Hernia Examination – Inspection

| | | | | | |
|---|---|---|---|---|---|
| Inspect the groin areas | Look for masses, scars and skin changes (erythema). Important to compare both sides. Scars could indicate previous surgery, and erythema may indicate infection. Remember to compare both sides | There is an obvious groin lump in the right femoral region. The overlying and surrounding skin is erythematous, and the lump looks dark red and purple. The left groin is normal | | | |
| Ask the patient to cough and look for accentuation at the inguinal, femoral and scrotal regions | Coughing may accentuate any hernia | The groin lump remains the same on coughing. The patient complains of pain when doing this | | | |

## Hernia Examination – Palpation

| What are you looking for or examining? | Justification | Findings and evolving thought process | | | | |
|---|---|---|---|---|---|---|
| Gently feel the hernia, observing the patient's face for discomfort | Assessing for tenderness and pain response | The lump is acutely tender, and the patient is in severe pain | | | | |
| Ask the patient to cough while you are palpating | Feeling over the mass for a palpable cough impulse | There is no palpable cough impulse | | | | |
| Define the local anatomy, highlighting each bony prominence in turn with a finger placement | Assessing where the herniation is aids with diagnosis | The hernia can be seen and felt over the femoral canal region, inferolateral to the pubic tubercle and medial to the femoral pulse | | | | |
| Ask the patent if the hernia ever 'goes back in'. If so, ask him to reduce it on his own | Hernias which are irreducible may be at risk of obstruction or strangulation | The patient cannot reduce the hernia himself | | | | |
| Attempt to reduce the hernia, then ask the patient to cough to see if it reappears | If an inguinal hernia is reducible, this test can help differentiate between an indirect (does not reappear on cough) and direct inguinal hernia (reappears on cough) | You cannot reduce the hernia, as the patient complains of severe pain | | | | |

## Hernia Examination – Auscultation

| | | | | | | |
|---|---|---|---|---|---|---|
| Listen over the hernia for bowel sounds | Particularly in large hernias which are more likely to be loops of bowel | No bowel sounds are present | | | | |

## Additional Tests

| | | | | | | |
|---|---|---|---|---|---|---|
| Offer to examine the contralateral side for hernia, the external genitalia, abdomen and rectum | Allows comparison and examination for other hernias. It is also important to assess for other abdominal pathology | No additional concerns | | | | |

## Finishing

| | | | | | | |
|---|---|---|---|---|---|---|
| Check patient is comfortable, offer to help reposition him and give the privacy to change | Keeps the patient's dignity | Treating the patient with respect is important | | | | |
| Remove your gloves and wash hands | Complying with hand hygiene is vital | No additional concerns | | | | |

## Present Your Findings

Mr Jarral is a 91-year-old man who has presented with abdominal pain and distension. On examination he is comfortable at rest. He has a distended abdomen, with a visible lump over the right femoral region. The overlying and surrounding skin is erythematous and warm to touch. The lump is very tender and not reducible. Bowel sounds are not present over the lump.

I feel the most likely diagnosis is strangulated right-sided femoral hernia, with differential diagnosis of obstructed hernia.

I would like to take bloods (including FBCs, U&Es, LFTs, amylase, coagulation, lactate and CRP) and immediately refer him to the general surgeons for urgent consideration of surgery. In the meantime, I will prescribe analgesia for the patient

| General Points | | | | |
|---|---|---|---|---|
| Polite to patient | | | | |
| Maintains good eye contact | | | | |
| Clear instruction and explanation to patient | | | | |
| Warns the patient about potential pain/discomfort before palpation | | | | |

## ? QUESTIONS FROM THE EXAMINER

### How can you tell the difference between an obstructed and strangulated hernia?

A strangulated hernia will be tender and irreducible, with swelling, redness and warmth of the surrounding skin. The patient may also have systemic symptoms of sepsis or fever. In comparison, an obstructed hernia will be painful and irreducible, without these associated symptoms.

### How long would Mr Jarral have to wait for his surgery if his hernia is strangulated?

In the case of a strangulated hernia, surgical repair must be done within 4–6 h from symptom onset to prevent necrotic bowel.

### Why are femoral hernias more common in females?

Women have a larger pelvis size.

### Why are femoral hernias more likely to strangulate than inguinal hernias?

Femoral hernias are at high risk of strangulation due to the narrow femoral canal and rigid borders.

### What are Hesselbach triangle borders and where are they?

An area of the abdominal wall that often weakens with age and is the site of a direct inguinal hernia. The borders are as follows:
Medially: rectus abdominis muscle
Laterally: inferior epigastric vessels
Inferiorly: inguinal ligament

### What are the advantages in performing laparoscopic surgery over open surgery for hernia repair?

Laparoscopic surgery is associated with a reduced risk of complications such as infection, bleeding and nerve injury.

### In general, why do hernias occur?

A weakness, that can be congenital or acquired with age, in the wall of a body cavity allows structures to protrude through it.

### Which type of hernia is the most common in children and why?

The most common hernia present in birth or childhood is an indirect inguinal hernia, most commonly due to incomplete closure of the processus vaginalis during development.

### Which type of hernia is most common in adults and why?

In adults overall, the most common hernia is a direct inguinal hernia, due to weakening of the transversalis fascia with age and increased abdominal pressure.

### Where are the deep and superficial rings within the inguinal canal located?

The deep ring is found just above the midpoint of the inguinal ligament, and the superficial is superior to the pubic tubercle.

## Station 2.5   Testicular

### Doctor Briefing

You are a junior doctor in general surgery and have been asked to see Mr Smith, a 20-year-old man, who has presented with a swelling of his right testicle. Please perform a relevant testicular examination on Mr Smith and present your findings.

### Patient Briefing

Over the last 24 h you have experienced worsening pain and tenderness in your right testicle. The testicle feels larger than normal, and the pain is making you feel very nauseous, though you have not yet vomited.

On questioning, you feel feverish, and the pain has progressed from a dull ache to a severe sharp pain, now 8/10 intensity. You have 'not felt right' for a week. You have noticed some clear discharge from the tip of your penis, and there is a swelling above your right testicle, which is causing discomfort. You have not experienced any other urinary symptoms and are otherwise fit and well. You have no past medical history and no allergies.

You have never had a sexual health screen and have had unprotected sexual intercourse with multiple female partners in the last few weeks after coming out of a long-term relationship.

You are deeply concerned that you have a sexually transmitted infection.

### Mark Scheme for Examiner

#### Introduction

| | | | | |
|---|---|---|---|---|
| Washes hands, introduces self, confirms patient identity and gains consent for examination | | | | |
| Offers a chaperone | | | | |
| Appropriately exposes the patient whilst keeping dignity at all times, and repositions into a suitable position for the examination | | | | |
| Asks if the patient has any pain currently | | | | |

#### General Inspection

| What are you looking for or examining? | Justification | Findings and evolving thought process | | | |
|---|---|---|---|---|---|
| Assess general well-being | On initial glance, does the patient look well, unwell or in pain? | The patient looks distressed and in obvious pain | | | |
| Check surroundings | Checks for obvious clues to aid diagnosis or equipment/observations to aid assessment | The patient is holding a vomit bowl and says the pain is making him feel very nauseous | | | |

#### Examination of the Penis – Inspection/Examination

| | | | | | |
|---|---|---|---|---|---|
| If the patient is not circumcised, retract the foreskin (or ask the patient to do it himself) | Allows exposure to the glans and assesses for phimosis (narrowing of the foreskin) | Mild phimosis noted, but the foreskin is able to retract fully | | | |
| Inspect the penis | Look for: asymmetry, lumps, ulcers, discharge, position of the urethral meatus. May indicate underlying disease, including sexually transmitted infections or congenital abnormalities (hypospadias) | Clear urethral discharge can be seen on examination. The patient can expel this himself | | | |

**Examination of the Penis – Inspection/Examination**

| What are you looking for or examining? | Justification | Findings and evolving thought process | | | | | |
|---|---|---|---|---|---|---|---|
| Open the urethral meatus | Further assesses for discharge and patency | The urethral meatus is patent | | | | | |
| If retracted, replace the foreskin | Prevents paraphimosis (a condition where retracted foreskin obstructs the blood supply, resulting in pain and swelling) | No additional concerns | | | | | |

**Examination of the Testes – Inspection**

| | | | | | | | |
|---|---|---|---|---|---|---|---|
| Look both anteriorly and posteriorly for the size and shape of each scrotum | Allows a general assessment of the size and shape of each scrotum. Note that the left testicle is often lower than the right in normal men | The right testicle looks significantly swollen and enlarged compared to the left | | | | | |
| Carefully inspect the testicles | Look for asymmetry, lumps, ulcers, swelling, rashes, scrotal oedema, scars, distribution of pubic hair, necrotic tissue (Fournier's gangrene). May help establish diagnosis and identify any relevant pathology | There is marked asymmetry between the testicles, as the right is swollen with overlying scrotal erythema | | | | | |

**Examination of the Testes – Palpation**

| | | | | | | | |
|---|---|---|---|---|---|---|---|
| Ask the patient if he is in any pain | Important to check before examination for patient comfort | The patient complains of severe pain in the right testicle | | | | | |
| Examine the asymptomatic side first; systematically palpate the testicles with good technique (both thumbs and index fingers) | Check that both testicles are present or if one may be undescended. Note the size and symmetry and feel for any swelling or masses | Both testicles are present and descended. It is difficult to perform this examination due to patient discomfort. The right testicle feels firm and significantly swollen compared to the left. There is marked tenderness on palpation | | | | | |
| Assess any scrotal masses | Important to assess any testicular lump accurately. Describe the site, size, shape, consistency, fluctuance, tenderness, ability to get above the lump and cough impulse. If cough impulse present and unable to get above the lump, consider hernia | No isolated masses or lumps can be felt and there is no evidence of a hernia. Swelling is isolated to the entire right testicle | | | | | |
| Palpate the epididymis (head, body and tail) | If swollen and tender, consider epididymitis | The right-sided epididymal head, body and tail feel swollen and tender | | | | | |
| Feel the spermatic cord using two fingers, tracing it from the testes to the inguinal region | Assesses for masses (such as spermatocele) and tenderness | No additional concerns | | | | | |

**Examination of the Testes – Palpation**

| What are you looking for or examining? | Justification | Findings and evolving thought process | | | | |
|---|---|---|---|---|---|---|
| Offer to transilluminate any masses that are present | Assesses whether cystic or non-cystic and solid vs. fluid | The testicular swelling does not transilluminate | | | | |
| Repeat the examination with the patient standing and inspect/palpate the posterior scrotum | Allows reassessment with gravity and greater access to the posterior aspect. This may accentuate hernias or varicoceles | No additional concerns | | | | |

**Additional Tests**

| | | | | | | |
|---|---|---|---|---|---|---|
| Perform Phren's test | This is done by elevating the testes and assessing the impact on testicular pain. Used to differentiate testicular pain caused by acute epididymitis and testicular torsion. A reduction in testicular pain is associated with epididymitis | The pain is somewhat reduced on testicular elevation | | | | |
| Assess for cremasteric reflex | This is performed by stroking the inner-thigh skin, which causes the ipsilateral testicle to rise. Loss of the cremasteric reflex is associated with testicular torsion | The cremasteric reflex is present | | | | |
| Feel the inguinal lymph nodes | May indicate scrotal pathology. However, testicular infection/malignancy tends to spread to para-aortic nodes | The inguinal lymph nodes cannot be palpated | | | | |
| Offer to examine the abdomen and hernia orifices, and do a urine dipstick | Testicular pathology can present with abdominal signs. Hernias can present as testicular lumps, and the urine may indicate urinary infection | No additional concerns | | | | |

**Finishing**

| | | | | | | |
|---|---|---|---|---|---|---|
| Check patient is comfortable, offer to help reposition him and give the privacy to change | Keeps the patient's dignity | Treating the patient with respect is important | | | | |
| Remove your gloves and wash hands | Complying with hand hygiene is vital | No additional concerns | | | | |
| Provide the patient with information on how to perform a self-exam | Enables the patient to identify problems on his own | No additional concerns | | | | |

**Present Your Findings**

Mr Smith is a 20-year-old man who has presented with a right-sided testicular swelling. On examination, the right testicle is significantly swollen and tender when compared to the left, with overlying scrotal erythema. Additionally, the epidydimal head, body and tail are swollen and tender, with clear urethral discharge visualised on examination. Examination of the left testicle and the rest of the external genitalia was otherwise unremarkable.

I feel the most likely diagnosis is epididymo-orchitis with the differential being testicular torsion.

I would like to perform additional tests on the urine sample, specifically nucleic acid amplification test urine testing for chlamydia and gonorrhoea. I would also take bloods (including FBCs, U&Es and CRP), request a testicular ultrasound and urgently refer to urology

| General Points | | | | |
|---|---|---|---|---|
| Polite to patient | | | | |
| Maintains good eye contact | | | | |
| Clear instruction and explanation to patient | | | | |
| Warns the patient about potential pain/discomfort prior to palpation | | | | |

## ? QUESTIONS FROM THE EXAMINER

### What is the first-line modality of imaging for any testicular lump/swelling?

Scrotal ultrasound is the best imaging choice initially.

### What previous surgery may come to mind if you notice scrotal scars on examination?

It may suggest a patient has had a previous testicular torsion and has undergone surgery.

### Which side do varicoceles classically present on and why?

They present on the left testicle in the majority of cases, as the left spermatic vein is longer and inserts into the left renal vein at 90°, putting it at increased hydrostatic pressure and slower drainage.

### Describe the route the testicles travel on descent into the scrotum.

The testes descend through the inguinal canal in the anterior abdominal wall and into the scrotum of the perineum.

### Describe the lymphatic drainage of the testicles and scrotum.

The testicles drain to the para-aortic and lumbar lymph nodes. The scrotum drains to superficial inguinal lymph nodes.

### What sexually transmitted infection require blood testing for detection?

Human immunodeficiency virus (HIV) and syphilis both require a blood sample for testing. Other sexually transmitted infections, such as chlamydia and gonorrhoea, are better tested for with a swab or urine sample.

### Which anatomical layers form part of the scrotum?

From external to internal, these layers are:
- Skin
- Dartos fascia and muscle
- External spermatic fascia
- Cremasteric fascia
- Internal spermatic fascia
- Tunica vaginalis
- Tunica albuginea

### How might you tell the difference between an epididymal cyst and a hydrocele?

Epididymal cysts are lumps caused by a build-up of fluid in the epididymis, whereas a hydrocele is accumulation of fluid in the sac surrounding the testes. A hydrocele will show painless swelling of the testes, whereas an epididymal cyst will show a swelling separate from the testes, located posteriorly and superiorly.

### Which viral infection can lead to orchitis as a complication in males, and what further complication can this lead to?

Mumps can lead to orchitis, inflammation of the testis. In a small number of cases, this can cause testicular atrophy and hypofertility.

### Why is looking for gynaecomastia relevant in a testicular examination?

Gynaecomastia may be a symptom of decreased testosterone, which can be due to testicular disorders such as orchitis or testicular trauma.

## Station 2.6    Stoma

### Doctor Briefing

You are a junior doctor in general surgery and have been asked to see Mrs Pouch, a 40-year-old woman, in clinic for a routine postoperative follow-up. She has a stoma bag in situ. Please perform a relevant stoma examination on Mrs Pouch and present your findings.

### Patient Briefing

You are attending a clinic for a routine postoperative follow-up after a total abdominoperineal resection for the treatment of colorectal cancer.

Since your surgery, you have felt well and have not been feverish. Your stoma output has been regular with semiformed stool, and you have received good support from your husband in adapting to this change. You have mostly had no issues with changing your own colostomy device, but have noticed that in hot weather, the surrounding stoma site can sometimes become slightly itchy.

You have no concerns and are happy with how your recovery is going following the surgery.

### Mark Scheme for Examiner

**Introduction**

| | | | | | | |
|---|---|---|---|---|---|---|
| Washes hands, introduces self, confirms patient identity and gains consent for examination | | | | | | |
| Offers a chaperone | | | | | | |
| Appropriately exposes the patient whilst keeping dignity at all times, and repositions into a suitable position for the examination | | | | | | |
| Asks if the patient has any pain currently or if she has had any recent issues with the stoma (for example, bleeding, change in output) | | | | | | |

**General Inspection**

| What are you looking for or examining? | Justification | Findings and evolving thought process | | | |
|---|---|---|---|---|---|
| Assess general well-being | On initial glance, does the patient look well, unwell or in pain? | The patient looks well, is of average build and looks well nourished | | | |
| Check surroundings | Checks for obvious clues to aid diagnosis or equipment/observations to aid assessment | There is a stoma bag situated in the left lower abdominal quadrant | | | |

**Examination of the Stoma – Inspection**

| | | | | | |
|---|---|---|---|---|---|
| Look for abdominal scars | Can give vital clues as to the operative history | There is a midline laparotomy scar | | | |
| Describe the site of stoma | Colostomies are typically located in the left iliac fossa whereas ileostomies and urostomies are typically located in the right iliac fossa | The stoma is located in the left iliac fossa | | | |
| State the number of lumens | One lumen would indicate an end ileostomy/colostomy or a urostomy. Two lumens close together may indicate a loop ileostomy/colostomy depending on the site | On inspection, one lumen can be identified | | | |

## Examination of the Stoma – Inspection

| What are you looking for or examining? | Justification | Findings and evolving thought process | | | | |
|---|---|---|---|---|---|---|
| Describe the stoma spout | The presence/absence of a spout can help to differentiate between ileostomies/urostomies and colostomies | You cannot visualise a spout, and the stoma appears to be flush with the skin | | | | |
| Describe the contents of the stoma bag (effluent) | The presence of semisolid faecal contents would suggest a colostomy. Liquid faecal contents would suggest an ileostomy, and urine would suggest a urostomy | On inspection, you can see around 50 mL of semisolid faecal contents | | | | |
| Inspect the skin around the stoma | Looks for signs of infection, fistula or skin excoriation | There is a slight skin excoriation to the left of the stoma but no surrounding erythema or pus content | | | | |
| Observe for any obvious complications: parastomal hernia, prolapse, retraction or infarction | These complications could be suspected purely on inspection. Infarction may present with a black, painful stoma | There is no evidence of further complications | | | | |

## Examination of the Stoma – Palpation

| | | | | | | |
|---|---|---|---|---|---|---|
| Enquire about pain, before palpating around the stoma | Checks for surrounding tenderness, which may indicate infection or obstruction | There is no surrounding tenderness | | | | |
| Offer to remove the ostomy bag, being cautious to avoid leakage (or ask the patient to do this herself) | Exposes the stoma to more in-depth examination and allows you to identify the bag contents further | The patient prefers to remove her own ostomy device | | | | |
| With gloves and lubrication, insert an index finger into the stoma opening | Assesses for stenosis (narrowing of opening conduit) and end type (confirms number of openings) | The stoma opening feels healthy with one lumen present and no evidence of stenosis | | | | |
| Offer to replace a new ostomy bag at the site | Patients may prefer to do this themselves. Treating the patient with respect is important | The patient is happy to replace her ostomy device herself | | | | |

## Additional Tests

| | | | | | | |
|---|---|---|---|---|---|---|
| Ask the patient to cough and assess for parastomal and incisional hernias | Potential complications of new stoma creation that can be accentuated by coughing | No parastomal or incisional hernias observed | | | | |
| Offer to perform a full abdominal examination, including assessment for the presence of an anus | Important if there are any suspicions of GI pathology. Assessing the presence of an anus can help distinguish between an end colostomy or loop colostomy | No additional concerns | | | | |

**Finishing**

| What are you looking for or examining? | Justification | Findings and evolving thought process | | | | |
|---|---|---|---|---|---|---|
| Check patient is comfortable, offer to help reposition her and give the privacy to change | Keeps the patient's dignity | Treating the patient with respect is important | | | | |
| Remove your gloves and wash hands | Complying with hand hygiene is vital | No additional concerns | | | | |

**Present Your Findings**

Mrs Pouch is a 40-year-old woman attending a routine outpatient appointment. On examination, she is comfortable at rest and has a stoma located in the lower left quadrant of her abdomen. The stoma appears healthy, with semiformed stool, and a single that which is flush with the skin. In keeping with the history, a minor skin excoriation can be seen to the left of the stoma, which has produced a minimal quantity of blood within the stoma contents. There is a midline laparotomy scar and no evidence of incisional or parastomal hernia.

I feel the most likely diagnosis is a healthy-looking end colostomy following a total abdominoperineal resection.

To complete my examination, I would like to arrange the next routine follow-up appointment and update the stoma care community team

**General Points**

| | | | | |
|---|---|---|---|---|
| Polite to patient | | | | |
| Maintains good eye contact | | | | |
| Clear instruction and explanation to patient | | | | |
| Warns the patient about potential pain/discomfort prior to palpation | | | | |

## ❓ QUESTIONS FROM THE EXAMINER

### What is a Hartmann's procedure?

Hartmann's procedure is a complete surgical resection of the rectosigmoid colon, with the formation of an end colostomy.

### Which stoma-producing procedure results in the closure of the anus?

An end colostomy, with closure of the rectal stump.

### What psychological effects can affect individuals with stomas?

Problems such as depression, anxiety, low self-esteem, body image concerns, sexual dysfunction, fear of stoma leakage and concerns about being away from home which may lead to social isolation.

### Why are ileostomies and urostomies spouted stomas? What is the importance of this?

They must be spouted due to the contents being more acidic and, hence, at risk of irritation and causing skin damage.

### What is the purpose of a temporary end colostomy?

This may be done in emergency bowel surgery, or in inflammation such as diverticulosis. It allows for acute inflammation to settle before the ends of the bowel are reattached and the stoma is removed.

## How do a stoma prolapse and a stoma retraction differ in their clinical presentation?

A stoma prolapse would show more bowel protruding through the stomal opening, whereas a stomal retraction is when the opening appears sunken.

## How would a parastomal hernia be managed?

Small or asymptomatic parastomal hernias can be managed conservatively, with input from stoma care nurses. In large or symptomatic hernias, a mesh repair can be carried out.

## What is wound dehiscence?

A surgical complication where the wound that has been sutured closed reopens spontaneously postoperatively.

## What surgical intervention can be offered to patients with familial adenomatous polyposis?

Due to the very high lifetime risk of developing colon cancer, prophylactic proctocolectomy and ileoanal anastomosis can be offered.

## Which important nerve plexus lies between the sacrum and rectum and what might be the consequence if these parasympathetic fibres are damaged during surgery?

The pelvic splanchnic nerves, arising from sacral spinal nerves S2, S3 and S4. If damaged, this can cause neurogenic bladder dysfunction and faecal incontinence.

## Station 2.7    Rectal

### Doctor Briefing

You are a junior doctor in general surgery and have been asked to perform a DRE on Mr Wilson, a 69-year-old man, who has presented with vomiting, abdominal pain and reduced bowel movements. Treat and address the model as you would a real patient and perform a DRE, stating your positive and negative findings. The patient has already consented to the procedure.

### Patient Briefing

You are in hospital following a surgical procedure. You do not recall opening your bowels over the weekend and have lower abdominal pain. You understand that the doctor must perform a rectal examination to check whether you are constipated and are able to understand and consent to this examination.

On further questioning, you have felt slightly confused today. However, you are able to recall your name and date of birth and recognise the doctors taking care of you. You recall the nurse giving you some 'strong pain medication' this morning which made you feel quite nauseous and dizzy, and you vomited an hour later. You recall being on pain medication throughout your hospital stay. Prior to this hospital admission, you think that you were able to open your bowels normally.

You are concerned as to why you feel dizzy and 'not quite yourself' today.

### Mark Scheme for Examiner

#### Introduction

| | | | | |
|---|---|---|---|---|
| Washes hands, introduces self, confirms patient identity and gains consent for examination | | | | |
| Offers a chaperone | | | | |
| Appropriately exposes the patient whilst keeping dignity at all times, and repositions into a suitable position for the examination. Only removes the underwear when necessary and provides a sheet to cover the patient's lower body. Places an incontinence sheet between the patient's buttocks and the bed | | | | |
| Asks if the patient has any pain currently | | | | |

#### General Inspection

| What are you looking for or examining? | Justification | Findings and evolving thought process | | |
|---|---|---|---|---|
| Assess general well-being | On initial glance, does the patient look well, unwell or in pain? | The patient looks disoriented and slightly confused, repeating the fact that he has stomach pain and has not been able to open his bowels | | |
| Check surroundings | Checks for obvious clues to aid diagnosis or equipment/observations to aid assessment | The patient is holding a vomit bowl, and a nearby prescription chart shows that he has recently been started on oral morphine | | |

#### Rectal Examination – Inspection

| Gently separate the buttocks and inspect the anus and perianal area | Looks for fissures, skin tags, erythema, sinuses/fistulae, pilonidal sinuses, haemorrhoids. Describe anything that you notice | There is evidence of a thrombosed external haemorrhoid at the 3 o'clock position: 1 cm × 1 cm | | |
|---|---|---|---|---|

## Rectal Examination – Procedure

| What are you looking for or examining? | Justification | Findings and evolving thought process | | | | | |
|---|---|---|---|---|---|---|---|
| Lubricate your index finger | Minimises patient discomfort | The patient is aware of what to expect | | | | | |
| Warn the patient prior to finger insertion | Treating the patient with respect is important | | | | | | |
| Apply pressure to the external anal sphincter, before inserting your finger into the anus | This pressure can help the external sphincter to relax, increasing ease of examination and minimising patient discomfort. It may not be possible to insert a finger in the rectum due to potential faecal impaction | The patient complains of pain when your finger applies pressure around the thrombosed haemorrhoid. You are unable to insert your finger fully into the rectum due to the presence of hard stool | | | | | |
| Palpate the anterior, right lateral, posterior and left lateral walls in turn | Attempts to identify any masses, stool or tenderness within the rectum | Due to the reason above, you are unable to palpate the rectal walls or the prostate | | | | | |
| In males, palpate the prostate gland | Assesses size, surface and consistency of both lobes. Palpates the median sulcus. Identifies any swelling or masses | Due to the reason above, you are unable to palpate the rectal walls or the prostate | | | | | |
| Ask the patient to squeeze his buttocks or bear down on your finger | Tests anal tone | The patient is able to bear down on your finger | | | | | |
| Withdraw your finger and inspect for faeces, blood, mucus or melaena | May provide evidence of pathology. Assesses consistency of faeces and presence of blood/mucus | There is evidence of faeces on your finger on withdrawal but no blood, mucus or melaena | | | | | |

## Additional Tests

| | | | | | | | |
|---|---|---|---|---|---|---|---|
| Offer to perform an abdominal examination, inspect a stool sample and dipstick the urine | Important to aid diagnosis | Abdominal examination shows marked lower abdominal tenderness, and you can feel a hard mass in the left lower quadrant. You are unable to get a stool sample, and urinalysis is clear | | | | | |

## Finishing

| | | | | | | | |
|---|---|---|---|---|---|---|---|
| Check patient is comfortable, offer to help reposition him and give the privacy to change | Keeps the patient's dignity | Treating the patient with respect is important | | | | | |
| Remove your gloves and wash hands | Complying with hand hygiene is vital | No additional concerns | | | | | |

**Present Your Findings**

Mr Wilson is a 69-year-old man who has presented with vomiting, abdominal pain and reduced bowel movements. With his consent, I performed a rectal examination on him. On inspection, there was evidence of a thrombosed haemorrhoid in the 3 o'clock position with overlying tenderness. On palpation, there was evidence of very firm stool in the rectum, suggesting severe faecal impaction, which prevented further continuation of the examination. There was no stool, blood or mucus present.

I feel the most likely diagnosis is constipation with faecal impaction, likely secondary to opioid use, with the differentials being irritable bowel disease, hypercalcaemia and colorectal malignancy (in this age group).

To complete my examination, I would like to perform a full abdominal examination, inspect a stool sample and dipstick the urine. I would perform an abdominal X-ray and consider a rectal enema, suppository and/or laxatives. I would also offer to switch the morphine to another reasonable alternative

**General Points**

Polite to patient

Maintains good eye contact

Clear instruction and explanation to patient

Warns the patient about potential pain/discomfort prior to examination

## ❓ QUESTIONS FROM THE EXAMINER

**What would you expect to find on rectal examination in a patient with benign prostatic hyperplasia?**

The prostate will be symmetrically enlarged and smooth, with no nodules.

**What is the difference between an anal fistula and an anal fissure?**

An anal fistula is an abnormal opening between the anal canal and perianal skin, usually caused by a chronic anal abscess. An anal fissure is a longitudinal tear of the perianal skin, and is usually shallow.

**What virus causes anal warts and what can now be done to help protect patients against this?**

Anal warts are caused by the human papillomavirus (HPV types 6 and 11 most commonly), like genital warts. The HPV vaccine is the most effective way to prevent this. Using barrier protection during sexual intercourse also reduces the risk of contracting HPV.

**What would you be concerned about if a patient does not appear to have good anal tone and what investigation would you want to request urgently?**

Loss of anal tone may indicate a spinal cord pathology, such as cauda equina syndrome. An urgent magnetic resonance imaging (MRI) spine is necessary to investigate this.

**What tool can be used to assess the different types of stools and how is this helpful in practice?**

The Bristol stool chart can be used as a standardised method of describing stool samples. This can be useful to monitor any changes in a patient's bowel habits using picture reference.

**What differentiates between external and internal haemorrhoids?**

Internal haemorrhoids are located above the dentate line (the histological transition zone between squamous of the rectum and the columnar epithelium of the anus), and external haemorrhoids are located below the dentate line.

**What is the treatment for patients with faecal impaction?**

This can be managed by enemas, suppositories or, in cases where these fail, manual evacuation.

**Why might a patient with severe constipation and faecal impaction also experience episodic diarrhoea?**

Overflow diarrhoea, where watery stools progress around and past a faecal impaction in the bowel, but firmer stools cannot.

**What is the difference between melaena and fresh red blood, and the diagnostic significance of each?**

Melaena is digested blood, after it has come in contact with stomach acid and suggests an upper GI bleed, whereas fresh red blood suggests a source lower in the bowel/anus.

**What is the scoring system used to grade prostate cancer based on histological appearance?**

The Gleason score.

## Station 2.8    Cranial Nerve

### Doctor Briefing

You are a junior doctor in general medicine and have been asked to see Mr Wade, a 48-year-old man, who has presented with a droopy eyelid. Please perform a relevant cranial nerve examination on Mr Wade and present your findings.

### Patient Briefing

You have been suffering with a troublesome cough and cold for several weeks. This has been mostly self-managed with rest, paracetamol and good hydration. However, you woke up today with left facial drooping, noticeable mainly in your left eye and mouth.

On further questioning, your left eye feels irritated and dry, and you are struggling to blink. You attempted to drink a glass of water but found it difficult to keep the liquid in your mouth, with most of it ending up down your shirt. Your partner says your speech sounds slurred and half of your face looks paralysed. You have no other weakness in any of your limbs. You have no other medical conditions and have never experienced anything like this before.

You are extremely health-anxious and are worried that you are having a stroke.

### Mark Scheme for Examiner

**Introduction**

| | | | | | | |
|---|---|---|---|---|---|---|
| Washes hands, introduces self and confirms patient identity | | | | | | |
| Offers a chaperone | | | | | | |
| Appropriately exposes the patient whilst keeping dignity at all times, and repositions into a suitable position for the examination | | | | | | |
| Asks if the patient has any pain currently | | | | | | |

**General Inspection**

| What are you looking for or examining? | Justification | Findings and evolving thought process | | | |
|---|---|---|---|---|---|
| Assess general well-being | On initial glance, does the patient look well, unwell or in pain? | There is obvious facial asymmetry, with left facial drooping | | | |
| Check surroundings | Checks for obvious clues to aid diagnosis or equipment/observations to aid assessment | There are no surrounding items indicative of underlying disease | | | |

**Examination of the Olfactory Nerve (CN I)**

| | | | | | |
|---|---|---|---|---|---|
| Ask about any recent changes in sense of smell | Tests sensory function of CN I (no motor component) | The patient has no change in sense of smell or taste | | | |

**Examination of the Optic Nerve (CN II)**

| | | | | | |
|---|---|---|---|---|---|
| Ask about glasses or contact lens use | To gauge the patient's baseline vision. Tests sensory function of CN II (no motor component) | The patient does not usually require glasses or contact lens | | | |
| Inspect the pupils | Assess pupil size, symmetry and shape. Tests sensory function of CN II (no motor component) | Pupils are normal in size and equal in symmetry and shape | | | |

## Examination of the Optic Nerve (CN II)

| What are you looking for or examining? | Justification | Findings and evolving thought process | | | | | |
|---|---|---|---|---|---|---|---|
| Check visual acuity | Test one eye at a time with a Snellen chart or get the patient to read something.<br>Tests sensory function of CN II (no motor component) | Visual acuity appears intact and the same in both eyes | | | | | |
| Check visual fields | Sit opposite the patient and ask him to look straight ahead. Test all four quadrants of both eyes separately by moving a finger into the visual field from outside it.<br>Tests sensory function of CN II (no motor component) | Visual fields appear intact and the same in both eyes | | | | | |
| Check blind spots | Test for this using a red hat pin.<br>Tests sensory function of CN II (no motor component) | Blind spots elicited and normal | | | | | |
| Assess colour vision using Ishihara plates | This can be performed using Ishihara plates | Colour vision assessment normal | | | | | |
| Offer to perform fundoscopy | Assess the optic disc for signs of pathology; for example, papilloedema | No additional concerns | | | | | |

## Examination of the Oculomotor, Trochlear, Abducens Nerves (CN III, IV, VI)

| | | | | | | | |
|---|---|---|---|---|---|---|---|
| Inspect the eyelids for evidence of ptosis | Can be associated with oculomotor nerve palsy and Horner's syndrome | There is no evidence of ptosis | | | | | |
| Test eye movements | Ask the patient (while keeping his head still) to follow the movements of your finger in all directions. Ask about double vision and look for nystagmus.<br>Tests motor function of CN III, IV and VI to the extraocular muscles which control eye movement and eyelid function.<br>Assess for oculomotor, trochlear or abducens nerve palsy | Eye movements are normal and intact in both eyes. The patient does not experience double vision and there is no obvious nystagmus | | | | | |
| Test accommodation reflex | Ask the patient to look to a distant point and then something closer. Observe convergence of the eyes and constriction of the pupils | Accommodation reflex is normal | | | | | |
| Test pupillary light reflexes | Test for both direct and consensual light reflexes and look for relative afferent pupillary defect.<br>For both reflexes, the sensory limb is dependent on CN II and the motor limb on CN III | Pupillary light reflexes are normal with pupils equal and reactive to light | | | | | |

## Examination of the Trigeminal Nerve (CN V)

| What are you looking for or examining? | Justification | Findings and evolving thought process | | | | |
|---|---|---|---|---|---|---|
| Feel for contraction of masseter and temporalis muscles under your fingers while the patient clenches his jaw | Tests motor function of CN V to the muscles of mastication | Normal contraction of the masseter and temporalis muscles | | | | |
| Ask the patient to open his jaw against your resistance | | Normal jaw power against resistance | | | | |
| Test sensation to the face<br><br>Offer to assess pain and temperature sensation in all branches | Test sensation first, demonstrating the sensation centrally (sternum). Then test light touch to the corresponding areas for ophthalmic, maxillary and mandibular branches bilaterally whilst patient's eyes are shut. Compare each side. Tests sensory function of CN V to the face.<br>• Ophthalmic (V1) branch – forehead.<br>• Maxillary (V2) branch – cheek.<br>• Mandibular (V3) branch – lower jaw | Sensation to all areas of the face is intact and the same bilaterally<br><br>Not performed (not appropriate in OSCE) | | | | |
| Offer to assess corneal reflex | This can be done using cotton wool. The afferent pathway involves the trigeminal nerve whereas the efferent pathway involves branches of the facial nerve. This reflex should cause the involuntary blinking of both eyes | The left eyelid does not blink in response to the corneal reflex on both eyes | | | | |
| Offer to assess jaw jerk reflex | This can be done by striking the chin with a tendon hammer while the mouth is open. Both afferent/efferent pathways of this reflex involve the trigeminal nerve. The jaw should jerk upwards (slight mouth closure) in response to a downward tap | Jaw jerk reflex is present and normal | | | | |

## Examination of the Facial Nerve (CN VII)

| | | | | | | |
|---|---|---|---|---|---|---|
| Ask about any recent changes in sense of taste | Tests the sensory function of CN VII for taste from the anterior two-thirds of the tongue | No changes in taste | | | | |
| Inspect the patient's face at rest for asymmetry<br><br>Test all related movements for each branch of the facial nerve with relaxation between each movement<br><br>Test each movement against resistance | Tests the motor function of CN VII to the muscles of facial expression.<br>• Temporal: raising eyebrows<br>• Zygomatic: scrunching the eyes<br>• Buccal: blowing out the cheeks<br>• Mandibular: showing the teeth or whistling<br>• Cervical: sticking the chin forward | There is obvious facial asymmetry with left facial drooping at the eye and angle of the mouth<br><br>The patient is unable to perform any of these movements on the left side and against resistance. There is no forehead sparing | | | | |

**Examination of the Vestibulocochlear Nerve (CN VIII)**

| What are you looking for or examining? | Justification | Findings and evolving thought process | | | | | |
|---|---|---|---|---|---|---|---|
| Ask about any recent changes in hearing

Test hearing | Starting with the unaffected side first, obscure the entrance to the contralateral ear canal by pressing the tragus into the canal. Whisper into the ear and ask the patient to repeat what you are saying. Gradually increase your volume and ensure the patient's eyes are shut. Assesses the sensory function of CN VIII in the conveyance of sound (no motor component) | No changes in hearing | | | | | |
| Perform Rinne's and Weber's tests | Assesses for sensorineural and conductive hearing loss | No evidence of sensorineural or conductive hearing loss | | | | | |
| Offer to assess balance | Assesses the sensory function of CN VIII in balance control | No abnormalities in balance | | | | | |

**Examination of the Glossopharyngeal and Vagus Nerves (CN IX and X)**

| | | | | | | | |
|---|---|---|---|---|---|---|---|
| Ask the patient to cough and swallow water | Tests the motor function of CN IX and X to the stylopharyngeus muscle and muscles of the mouth. A bovine cough may indicate a vagus nerve lesion | Swallow and cough are normal | | | | | |
| Ask the patient to open his mouth and say 'ahh' (while you look for palate movement and uvula deviation) | Vagus nerve lesions result in deviation of the uvula and asymmetrical elevation of the palate towards the unaffected side | There is no uvula deviation, and the palate remains symmetrical | | | | | |
| Offer to test the gag reflex | This can be done by sticking a tongue depressor gently into the back of the throat.
Involves both the afferent glossopharyngeal nerve and efferent vagus nerve. Absent gag reflex may indicate CN IX/X lesion | Not performed (not appropriate in OSCE) | | | | | |

**Examination of the Accessory (Spinal Root) Nerve (CN XI)**

| | | | | | | | |
|---|---|---|---|---|---|---|---|
| Ask the patient to shrug his shoulders against resistance

Ask the patient to touch each shoulder with his chin against resistance | Assesses the motor function of CN XI to the sternocleidomastoid and trapezius muscles (no sensory component) | Motor function intact | | | | | |

**Examination of the Hypoglossal Nerve (CN XII)**

| What are you looking for or examining? | Justification | Findings and evolving thought process | | | | |
|---|---|---|---|---|---|---|
| Inspect the patient's tongue with the mouth open | Wasting/fasciculation could indicate an ipsilateral hypoglossal lesion | No wasting or fasciculation | | | | |
| Ask the patient to protrude his tongue and assess for deviation | May indicate hypoglossal lesion with the tongue deviating towards the side of the lesion | No tongue deviation | | | | |
| Ask the patient to push his tongue into his cheek and resist the movement by pushing on to the tongue through the outside of the cheek | Assesses the motor function of CN XII to the extrinsic muscles of the tongue (no sensory component). Weakness would present on the side of the hypoglossal lesion | Motor function of the tongue intact and equal on both sides | | | | |

**Additional Tests**

| | | | | | | |
|---|---|---|---|---|---|---|
| Offer to perform a full neurological examination, including: cerebellar, upper- and lower-limb examination | Assesses for any neurological signs elsewhere which may aid diagnosis or prompt further investigation | Cerebellar, lower- and upper-limb examinations are unremarkable | | | | |
| Offer to assess sweating on both sides of the face | Unilateral anhidrosis may indicate Horner's syndrome | No abnormal sweating evident | | | | |
| Offer to perform a cognitive assessment, including speech | Gross abnormality may indicate brain lesion and prompt further investigation | Cognitive assessment is normal | | | | |

**Finishing**

| | | | | | | |
|---|---|---|---|---|---|---|
| Check patient is comfortable, offer to help reposition him and give the privacy to change | Keeps the patient's dignity | Treating the patient with respect is important | | | | |
| Remove your gloves and wash hands | Complying with hand hygiene is vital | No additional concerns | | | | |

**Present Your Findings**

Mr Wade is a 48-year-old man who has presented with a droopy eyelid. On examination he has left-sided facial paralysis with no forehead sparing. The patient is unable to perform any facial nerve movements against resistance on the left side, including inability to close the left eye fully. Facial movements are all intact on the right side. Pupils are equal and responsive to light with no abnormalities in movement. Corneal reflex is absent on the affected side. All other cranial nerves are intact.

I feel the most likely diagnosis is Bell's palsy, secondary to a recent viral infection, with differentials being an intracranial stroke.

I would like to take bloods (including FBCs, U&Es, LFTs, bone profile and thyroid function tests (TFTs)) and discuss with the neurologists to rule out an intracranial stroke and subsequently make a referral to ear, nose and throat for further assessment

| General Points | | | | |
|---|---|---|---|---|
| Polite to patient | | | | |
| Maintains good eye contact | | | | |
| Clear instruction and explanation to patient | | | | |
| Warns the patient about potential pain/discomfort prior to palpation | | | | |

## ❓ QUESTIONS FROM THE EXAMINER

### What is visual neglect/inattention and what might cause this?

Visual neglect is a neuropsychological disorder in which a person is unable to acknowledge or perceive stimuli in one hemispace of the visual field. This is commonly caused by a right-parietal-lobe injury, for example, cerebrovascular disease, with neglect occurring towards the side of space contralateral (opposite) to their unilateral lesion.

### Describe the afferent and efferent limb functions of the pupillary light reflex.

There is one ipsilateral and one contralateral efferent limb for every afferent limb of the pupillary reflex. The afferent limb functions to receive sensory input (such as light) which is transmitted along the optic nerve to the ipsilateral relevant nucleus of the midbrain. The efferent limbs transmit motor output to the oculomotor nerve which innervates the ciliary sphincter and bilaterally controls pupillary constriction.

### What is the difference between the presentation and causes of bitemporal hemianopia and homonymous hemianopia?

Bitemporal hemianopia describes the bilateral loss of the temporal visual fields resulting in central tunnel vision, usually the result of optic chiasm compression by a tumour; for example, pituitary adenoma. Homonymous hemianopia describes the same-sided loss of visual field in each eye and is mostly caused by strokes and tumours posterior to the optic chiasm.

### What are the innervations of the extraocular muscles?

A useful way to remember extraocular innervation is by remembering $LR_6SO_4O_3$. The lateral rectus is innervated by CN VI, superior oblique is innervated by CN IV, and all of the other extraocular muscles are innervated by CN III.

### How do oculomotor, trochlear and abducens nerve palsies typically present?

With an oculomotor nerve palsy, the affected eye is usually displaced laterally and inferiorly ('down and out'). With a trochlear nerve palsy, the patient will complain of vertical diplopia (double vision) and may develop a head tilt away from the affected eye. With an abducens palsy, the affected eye will appear adducted, and the patient may complain of horizontal diplopia.

### What is strabismus?

Strabismus (or squint) is a condition in which both eyes do not line up in the same direction when focusing on an object. This can be further categorised depending on whether the strabismus is present permanently (manifest) or when binocular vision is interrupted (latent), i.e. by covering one eye.

### How is conductive hearing loss noted in Rinne's and Weber's tests?

The normal interpretation for each ear should be that air conduction is louder than bone conduction (Rinne's positive) with equal sound in both ears. However, in the context of conductive hearing loss, the sound will be heard best in the abnormal ear and bone conduction will transmit sound better than air conduction (Rinne's negative).

### How does a facial nerve palsy differ in presentation from a cerebral stroke?

As the muscles of the forehead have bilateral innervation from the brain (bilateral cortical representation), any upper motor neurone cause (for example, cerebral palsy) will not involve the forehead and the occipitofrontalis muscle. Any lower motor neurone cause (for example, facial nerve palsy) will therefore include the forehead muscles on the ipsilateral side to the lesion.

### How does a vagus nerve lesion typically affect the palate and the uvula?

Vagus nerve lesions typically cause paralysis and ipsilateral lowering of the soft palate. This leads to deviation of the uvula away from the side of the lesion. There may be loss of the gag and cough reflex, leading to a weak bovine cough. Dysfunction of the pharyngeal muscles may lead to dysphagia and recurrent laryngeal nerve involvement may cause dysphonia.

### How does a hypoglossal nerve lesion typically affect the tongue?

A hypoglossal nerve lesion typically causes paralysis, fasciculations and eventual atrophy of the tongue muscles on the affected side. As a result, this causes deviation of the tongue towards the side of the lesion.

## Station 2.9   Peripheral Nerves (Upper Limb)

### Doctor Briefing

You are a junior doctor in the ED and have been asked to see Mr Reilly, a 64-year-old man, who has recently had a fall and fractured his humerus. He is now struggling to perform everyday tasks with his right hand. Please perform a relevant neurological examination on Mr Reilly's upper limbs and present your findings.

### Patient Briefing

Several months ago, you attended ED following a fall where you were told you had fractured the surgical neck of your right humerus. Ever since this injury, you have had difficulty with certain movements involving your right limb.

On further questioning, you are struggling to lift anything with your right arm, as you have problems with most shoulder movements. You have difficulty raising your arm away from your body and have had to use your left side to undertake the majority of tasks. This has been particularly troublesome, as you enjoy writing but are right-handed. Additionally, you have noticed that the sensation in your right shoulder is reduced and feels different against your clothing.

You were never told you would experience these difficulties following this fracture and you worry that you may have damaged a nerve. You would like further assessment.

### Mark Scheme for Examiner

#### Introduction

| | | | | | |
|---|---|---|---|---|---|
| Washes hands, introduces self and confirms patient identity | | | | | |
| Offers a chaperone | | | | | |
| Appropriately exposes the patient whilst keeping dignity at all times, and repositions into a suitable position for the examination | | | | | |
| Asks if the patient has any pain currently | | | | | |

#### General Inspection

| What are you looking for or examining? | Justification | Findings and evolving thought process | | | |
|---|---|---|---|---|---|
| Assess general well-being | On initial glance, does the patient look well, unwell or in pain? | The right shoulder appears slightly adducted and internally rotated | | | |
| Check surroundings | Checks for obvious clues to aid diagnosis or equipment/observations to aid assessment | There are no relevant findings | | | |

#### Examination of the Upper Limbs – Inspection

| | | | | | |
|---|---|---|---|---|---|
| Look for SWIFT: scars, wasting of muscles, involuntary movements, fasciculations and tremor | May be manifestations of upper or lower motor neurone disease | The right shoulder appears to have less deltoid muscle bulk compared to the left | | | |
| Look for pronator drift | Ask the patient to hold out his arms in supination and to close his eyes. If the palm turns involuntarily to face the floor, this indicates a contralateral upper motor neurone lesion | The patient does not have any evidence of pronator drift | | | |

**Examination of the Upper Limbs – Inspection**

| What are you looking for or examining? | Justification | Findings and evolving thought process | | | | |
|---|---|---|---|---|---|---|
| Assess function | Gross assessment for functional deficit and impact on patient's quality of life; for example, asking the patient to do up a button | The patient has problems in doing up his buttons due to movement deficit in the right shoulder | | | | |

**Examination of the Upper Limbs – Tone**

| | | | | | | |
|---|---|---|---|---|---|---|
| Hold the patient's hand in a handshake position, then use your other hand to support his elbow | Ensure that the patient is relaxed and good technique is used | There are no abnormalities in tone | | | | |
| Passively move the muscle groups of the shoulder, elbow and wrist through their full range of movement | Ensures full range of movement through shoulder circumduction, elbow flexion/extension and wrist circumduction | | | | | |
| Feel for any abnormalities of tone | Examples include spasticity, rigidity, cogwheeling, hypotonia, hypertonia, supinator 'catch'. May indicate upper motor neurone disease or pyramidal tract lesions; for example, stroke (rigidity) and extrapyramidal tract lesions such as Parkinson's disease (spasticity) | | | | | |

**Examination of the Upper Limbs – Reflexes**

| | | | | | | |
|---|---|---|---|---|---|---|
| Test for biceps reflex | This is done by striking the bicep tendon in the antecubital fossa. Note flexion of the elbow | Normal biceps reflex elicited bilaterally | | | | |
| Test for brachioradialis reflex | This is done by striking the brachioradialis tendon roughly 5–8 cm above the wrist. Note supination of the wrist | Normal brachioradialis reflex elicited bilaterally | | | | |
| Test for triceps reflex | This is done by taking the weight of the arm and striking the tricep tendon at the elbow just above the olecranon. Note extension of the elbow | Normal triceps reflex elicited bilaterally | | | | |
| Reinforce reflexes as necessary by asking patient to clench teeth | May make reflexes more apparent | No additional concerns | | | | |

**Examination of the Upper Limbs – Power**

| What are you looking for or examining? | Justification | Findings and evolving thought process | | | | | |
|---|---|---|---|---|---|---|---|
| Test for power by performing the actions described, isolating each relevant joint and testing against resistance:<br>• Shoulder abduction/ abduction ('Arms out like a chicken')<br>• Elbow flexion/extension ('Hands up like a boxer')<br>• Wrist flexion/extension ('Arms out, wrists back like you're riding a motorbike')<br>• Grip strength ('Squeeze my fingers')<br>• Finger extension ('Fingers out straight')<br>• Finger abduction ('Splay your fingers outwards')<br>• Thumb abduction ('Thumbs to the ceiling') | Assessment of power in the upper limb is important and it is useful to know the innervation for various muscle groups and actions:<br>• Shoulder abduction: C5 – axillary nerve<br>• Shoulder adduction: C6/7 – thoracodorsal nerve<br>• Elbow flexion: C5/6 – musculocutaneous and radial nerve<br>• Elbow extension: C7 – radial nerve<br>• Wrist extension: C6 – radial nerve<br>• Wrist flexion: C6/7 – median nerve<br>• Finger extension: C7 – radial nerve<br>• Finger abduction: T1 – ulnar nerve<br>• Thumb abduction: T1 – median nerve | The shoulder appears to have a significant deficit on right-sided movements and the patient is unable to lift the right arm without support from the left arm. The patient has 1/5 power on abduction (15–90°), flexion, extension and external rotation of the shoulder.<br>The left upper limb and small muscles of the hand appear intact with 5/5 power of movements | | | | | |
| Rate the power | This is based on the Medical Research Council scale and is as follows:<br>  0 = no movement<br>  1 = flicker of movement<br>  2 = isogravitational movements only<br>  3 = able to move against gravity<br>  4 = able to move against resistance but not fully<br>  5 = full power | | | | | | |
| At each stage of assessment, compare both sides | Allows comparison to distinguish between 'normal' and 'abnormal' and unilateral vs. bilateral signs | The power of movements in the right upper limb is markedly reduced compared to movements in the left | | | | | |

**Examination of the Upper Limbs – Coordination**

See 'Station 2.11 Cerebellar' for more in-depth assessment of coordination, but as a minimum:

| | | | | | | | |
|---|---|---|---|---|---|---|---|
| Gross assessment of coordination | Perform finger–nose testing and assess for dysdiadochokinesia. If impaired, may indicate cerebellar pathology | Coordination fully intact with no deficits | | | | | |

**Examination of the Upper Limbs – Sensation**

| | | | | | | | |
|---|---|---|---|---|---|---|---|
| Provide a reference stimulus by touching the sternum first | Allows comparison for 'normal' dermatome sensation.<br>Ensure the patient's eyes are closed to provide confidence in the results of the assessment | The patient can acknowledge the reference stimulus | | | | | |

## Examination of the Upper Limbs – Sensation

| What are you looking for or examining? | Justification | Findings and evolving thought process | | | | | | |
|---|---|---|---|---|---|---|---|---|
| Test for light touch stimulus | This can be done by using a piece of cotton wool and stroking each dermatome (C5, C6, C7, C8, T1) in sequence, comparing both sides.<br>• C5 – upper, lateral aspect of the arm (axillary nerve)<br>• C6 – outer forearm (lateral cutaneous nerve of forearm)<br>• C7 – middle finger (median nerve)<br>• C8 – little finger (radial nerve)<br>• T1 – medial aspect of antecubital fossa (medial cutaneous nerve of forearm)<br>Assesses sensation involving the dorsal columns and spinothalamic tracts | There is reduced sensation over the C5/C6 dermatome (the 'regimental badge area') on the right side. The patient also complains of paraesthesia in this area | | | | | | |
| Repeat for pain (pinprick) stimulus. | This can be done using a Neurotip. Assesses sensation involving the spinothalamic tracts | Pain sensation is also reduced over the C5/C6 dermatome on the right side | | | | | | |
| Test proprioception | Start with a small demonstration of upwards/downwards movement in the most distal joint. Then ask the patient to close his eyes and to tell you whether the joint is pointing upwards/downwards after a random sequence. Assesses sensation and awareness of movements involving the dorsal columns | Proprioception is normal and the patient is able to recognise peripheral limb movements | | | | | | |
| Test vibration sense | This is done by placing a tuning fork on a bony prominence and asking the patient when he feels the vibration start and stop. Assesses sensation involving the dorsal columns | Vibration sense is intact on all bony prominences of the upper limbs | | | | | | |

## Additional Tests

| | | | | | | | | |
|---|---|---|---|---|---|---|---|---|
| Offer to perform a full neurological examination, including: cerebellar, cranial nerve and lower-limb examination | Assesses for any neurological signs elsewhere which may aid diagnosis or prompt further investigation | Cerebellar, cranial nerve and lower-limb examination are unremarkable | | | | | | |
| Offer to perform a vascular exam of the upper limbs | Vascular pathology may mimic neurological signs; for example, reduced sensation, peripheral neuropathy | Vascular examination is unremarkable | | | | | | |

**Additional Tests**

| What are you looking for or examining? | Justification | Findings and evolving thought process | | | | | |
|---|---|---|---|---|---|---|---|
| Offer to perform fundoscopy | Raised intracranial pressure may indicate brain lesions and prompt further investigation | Fundoscopy is unremarkable | | | | | |
| Perform a cognitive assessment, including speech | Gross abnormality may indicate brain lesion and prompt further investigation | Cognitive assessment is normal | | | | | |
| Perform a DRE if there are any concerns regarding cauda equina syndrome | Assess for anal sphincter tone and perianal sensation. Deficit could indicate cauda equina syndrome | DRE not indicated here | | | | | |

**Finishing**

| | | | | | | | |
|---|---|---|---|---|---|---|---|
| Check patient is comfortable, offer to help reposition him and give the privacy to change | Keeps the patient's dignity | Treating the patient with respect is important | | | | | |
| Remove your gloves and wash hands | Complying with hand hygiene is vital | No additional concerns | | | | | |

**Present Your Findings**

Mr Reilly is a 64-year-old man who has presented with difficulty performing everyday tasks with his right upper limb following a right-sided surgical fracture of the neck of the humerus. On examination he is comfortable at rest with the right shoulder appearing adducted and internally rotated at rest. Assessment of the upper limbs revealed normal tone and coordination. The patient has 1/5 power on abduction (15–90°), flexion, extension and external rotation of the shoulder. There is reduced sensation and pain response over the C5/C6 dermatome (the 'regimental badge area') on the right side with reports of paraesthesia. Reflexes are normal and intact bilaterally. There are no other abnormalities.

I feel the most likely diagnosis is a right-sided axillary nerve palsy secondary to a surgical fracture of neck of the humerus.

I would like to examine for fractures elsewhere, refer to physiotherapy and optimise analgesia

**General Points**

Polite to patient

Maintains good eye contact

Clear instruction and explanation to patient

Warns the patient about potential pain/discomfort prior to palpation

## ❓ QUESTIONS FROM THE EXAMINER

### What is the difference between the location of an upper or lower motor neurone?

The upper motor neurones originate in the cerebral cortex and travel down to the brainstem or spinal cord, terminating in the brainstem or the anterior horn of the spinal cord, whereas lower motor neurones begin in the spinal cord and terminate on the muscle fibre they provide innervation to.

### When assessing power, which pattern of weakness do upper motor neurone lesions commonly cause?

Upper motor neurone lesions show weakness in muscles groups, whereas lower motor neurone lesions show weakness in single muscle fibres.

### What is the difference between the clinical presentation of spasticity and rigidity?

Spasticity is velocity-dependent increased muscle tone, which presents as stiffness/tightness of muscles against resistance, with increased tendon reflexes. Rigidity shows increased tone at rest, with normal tendon reflexes.

### What is the difference between the causes of spasticity and rigidity?

Spasticity is caused by lesions in the pyramidal tracts (upper motor neurone lesions). Rigidity is caused by extrapyramidal lesions.

### Where does the axillary nerve originate and what is its innervation?

It is derived from the posterior cord of the brachial plexus, spinal roots C5 and C6. It provides sensory innervation to the skin over the lower deltoid (known as the 'regimental badge area'), and provides motor function to the teres minor and deltoid muscles.

### What is Erb's palsy and which nerve roots are affected?

It is a form of brachial plexus palsy, classically associated with birth trauma, with excessive lateral traction on the neck and shoulder dystocia. Usually, it involves injury to the upper trunk of the brachial plexus (C5–C6).

### What causes wrist drop and which nerve injury causes this palsy?

Damage to the radial nerve or its branches, which causes weakness in the extensor muscles of the forearm and impairs wrist extension.

### What nerve injury causes the hand of Benedict sign?

This sign describes when, while attempting to make a fist, a patient can only flex the ring finger and the little finger, with the middle, index and thumb remaining extended. This is caused by proximal median nerve injury (where the injury is above the anterior interosseous nerve origin).

### Which nerve is affected in carpal tunnel syndrome, and which clinical tests can be used to evoke symptoms?

It is caused by compression of the median nerve at the wrist. Both the Phalen test of holding the patient's wrist in full flexion (90°) for 1 min or Tinel's test with percussing or tapping over the carpal tunnel can elicit pain and tingling in the region innervated by the median nerve.

### What is the best modality of imaging for assessing brachial plexus nerve injury?

MRI, as it allows visualisation of soft tissues.

## Station 2.10 Peripheral Nerves (Lower Limb)

### Doctor Briefing

You are a junior doctor in a neurology clinic and have been asked to see Mr Romberg, a 64-year-old man, who has long-standing diabetes mellitus. He is continually injuring his feet without realising it. Please perform a relevant neurological examination on Mr Romberg's lower limbs and present your findings.

### Patient Briefing

You were diagnosed with diabetes 25 years ago and your blood glucose is regularly high with difficult control.

On further questioning, your wife has recently spotted wounds to your feet, which you have not noticed as they have not been painful. There is also numbness in your feet and legs, noted mainly when putting on your socks, with the sensory loss getting worse over the years. You now struggle to feel hot temperatures when standing in a bath and frequently trip over your feet when you walk. You use a walking stick to help your mobility.

Your GP advised you attend a neurology clinic to investigate these changes further. You are worried that you are going to need an amputation.

### Mark Scheme for Examiner

#### Introduction

| | | | |
|---|---|---|---|
| Washes hands, introduces self and confirms patient identity | | | |
| Offers a chaperone | | | |
| Appropriately exposes the patient whilst keeping dignity at all times, and repositions into a suitable position for the examination | | | |
| Asks if the patient has any pain currently | | | |

#### General Inspection

| What are you looking for or examining? | Justification | Findings and evolving thought process | | | |
|---|---|---|---|---|---|
| Assess general well-being | On initial glance, does the patient look well, unwell or in pain? | The patient has a raised BMI | | | |
| Check surroundings | Checks for obvious clues to aid diagnosis or equipment/observations to aid assessment | The patient is using a walking stick to aid mobility | | | |

#### Examination of the Lower Limbs – Inspection

| | | | | | |
|---|---|---|---|---|---|
| Assess gait | Ask the patient to walk from one end of the room to another. Look for signs suggestive of an underlying neurological deficit. For example, a festinant gait suggests Parkinson's disease, an antalgic gait suggests osteoarthritis, a scissoring gait suggests cerebral palsy, an ataxic gait suggests cerebellar dysfunction, marche à petits pas suggests diffuse cerebrovascular disease, foot slapping suggests sensory polyneuropathy, and high stepping suggests weakness of ankle dorsiflexion | The patient appears to have difficulty walking and appears unsteady on his feet. Both feet regularly slap together with toes catching on the floor. The patient walks better when looking downwards | | | |
| Look for SWIFT | May be manifestations of upper or lower motor neurone disease | There are no obvious neurological signs in the lower limbs | | | |

## Examination of the Lower Limbs – Tone

| What are you looking for or examining? | Justification | Findings and evolving thought process | | | | | |
|---|---|---|---|---|---|---|---|
| Ask the patient to lie flat and ensure the lower limbs are relaxed | Ensures good technique for testing tone | There are no abnormalities in tone | | | | | |
| Roll the patient's legs from side to side, looking at the feet for resistance. Abruptly lift the knee and note the movement of the lower leg | Assesses tone in hip, knee and ankle muscle groups. In hypertonia, the ankle will come off the examination couch, even if the patient is relaxed | | | | | | |
| Passively flex and extend the knee joint | Ensures full range of movement through knee flexion and extension | | | | | | |
| Feel for any abnormalities of tone | Spasticity, rigidity, hypotonia and hypertonia may indicate upper motor neurone disease | | | | | | |

## Examination of the Upper Limbs – Power

| | | | | | | | |
|---|---|---|---|---|---|---|---|
| Test for power by performing the actions described, isolating each relevant joint and testing against resistance:<br>• Hip flexion/extension<br>• Hip adduction/abduction<br>• Knee flexion/extension<br>• Ankle plantar flexion/extension<br>• Ankle dorsiflexion<br>• Hallux/toe extension | Assessment of power in the lower limb is important, and it is useful to know the innervation for various muscle groups and actions:<br>• Hip flexion: L1/2 – iliofemoral nerve<br>• Hip extension: L5/S1/S2 – inferior gluteal nerve<br>• Knee flexion: S1 – sciatic nerve<br>• Knee extension: L3/4 – femoral nerve<br>• Ankle plantarflexion/extension: S1/2 – tibial nerve<br>• Ankle dorsiflexion: L4/5 – deep peroneal nerve<br>• Hallux/toe extension: L5 – deep peroneal nerve | No apparent deficits in movement. 5/5 power in all movements, performed against resistance | | | | | |
| Rate the power | This is based on the Medical Research Council scale and is as follows:<br>0 = no movement<br>1 = flicker of movement<br>2 = isogravitational movements only<br>3 = able to move against gravity<br>4 = able to move against resistance but not fully<br>5 = full power | 5/5 power bilaterally | | | | | |
| At each stage of assessment, compare both sides | Allows comparison to distinguish between 'normal' and 'abnormal' and unilateral vs. bilateral signs | | | | | | |

**Examination of the Upper Limbs – Reflexes**

| What are you looking for or examining? | Justification | Findings and evolving thought process | | | | | |
|---|---|---|---|---|---|---|---|
| Test for knee tendon reflex | This is done by striking the ligamentum patellae. Note contraction of the quadriceps muscle | Normal knee tendon reflex elicited bilaterally | | | | | |
| Test for ankle tendon reflex | This is done by pulling the foot up with one hand into dorsiflexion, before striking the Achilles. Note contraction in the gastrocnemius muscle and plantarflexion of the foot | Normal ankle tendon reflex elicited bilaterally | | | | | |
| Test for plantar reflex | This is done by using the reverse end of the tendon hammer, running the sharp edge up the lateral aspect of the sole of an unsocked foot.<br>A normal response is for the big toe to flex downward. In an abnormal response, the big toe extends and the other toes splay out (implies upper motor neurone disease) | The big toes flex downwards bilaterally | | | | | |
| Test for ankle clonus | This is done by rapidly flexing the foot into dorsiflexion. Observe for clonus – when the foot subsequently beats, rapidly moving from flexion to extension.<br>Clonus is a series of rhythmic muscle contractions/relaxations which are involuntary. More than five beats is abnormal and may signify upper motor neurone lesions | There are only two clonus beats. No additional concern | | | | | |
| Reinforce reflexes as necessary by asking patient to clench teeth | May make reflexes more apparent | Not required | | | | | |

**Examination of the Upper Limbs – Coordination**

See 'Station 2.11 Cerebellar' for more in-depth assessent of co-ordination, but as a minimum:

| Gross assessment of coordination | Ask the patient to run his left heel from the right knee down along the shin of the right leg. Ask him then to make an arc in the air with the heel and repeat the previous movement. Repeat on both sides.<br>An abnormal response is if this cannot be completed smoothly | Coordination fully intact with no deficits | | | | | |
|---|---|---|---|---|---|---|---|

**Examination of the Upper Limbs – Sensation**

| Provide a reference stimulus by touching the sternum first | Allows comparison for 'normal' dermatome sensation<br>Ensure the patient's eyes are closed to provide confidence in the results of the assessment | The patient can acknowledge the reference stimulus | | | | | |
|---|---|---|---|---|---|---|---|

**Examination of the Upper Limbs – Sensation**

| What are you looking for or examining? | Justification | Findings and evolving thought process | | | | |
|---|---|---|---|---|---|---|
| Test for light touch stimulus | This can be done using a piece of cotton wool and stroking each dermatome (L1, L2, L3, L4, L5, S1, S2) in sequence, comparing both sides.<br>• L1 – inguinal region/top of medial thigh (ilioinguinal nerve)<br>• L2 – upper outer thigh (lateral cutaneous nerve of thigh)<br>• L3 – inner aspect of the thigh (femoral nerve)<br>• L4 – medial lower leg (saphenous nerve)<br>• L5 – upper outer aspect of lower leg (common peroneal nerve), dorsal surface, medial aspect of big toes (superficial peroneal nerve)<br>• S1 – heel of foot (tibial nerve)<br>• S2 – posterior aspect of knee (sciatic nerve)<br>Assesses sensation involving the dorsal columns and spinothalamic tracts | Absent light touch sensation up to the level of the mid-knee in a stocking-like distribution | | | | |
| Repeat for pain (pin-prick) stimulus using a Neurotip | Assesses sensation involving the spinothalamic tracts | Reduced pain sensation up to the level of the mid-knee in a stocking-like distribution | | | | |
| Test proprioception | Start with a small demonstration of upwards/downwards movement in the most distal joint. Ask the patient to close his eyes and to tell you whether the joint is pointing upwards/downwards after a random sequence.<br>Assesses sensation and awareness of movements involving the dorsal columns | Proprioception is normal and the patient can recognise peripheral limb movements | | | | |
| Test vibration sense | This is done by placing a tuning fork on a bony prominence and asking the patient when they feel the vibration start and stop.<br>Assesses sensation involving the dorsal columns | Vibration sense is intact on all bony prominences of the lower limb | | | | |
| **Additional Tests** | | | | | | |
| Perform Romberg's test | Remain within arm's reach, ask the patient to keep his feet together and arms by side. Ask the patient to close his eyes and observe for falling without correction.<br>Assesses for sensory ataxia with gross assessment of proprioception, vision and vestibular function. If there is a deficit, the patient will struggle to remain standing when his eyes are closed (positive Romberg's sign) | Romberg's sign is positive | | | | |

**Additional Tests**

| What are you looking for or examining? | Justification | Findings and evolving thought process | | | | | |
|---|---|---|---|---|---|---|---|
| Offer to perform a full neurological examination, including: cerebellar, cranial nerve and lower-limb examination | Assesses for any neurological signs elsewhere which may aid diagnosis or prompt further investigation | Cerebellar, cranial nerve and upper-limb examination are unremarkable | | | | | |
| Offer to perform a vascular exam of the lower limbs | Vascular pathology may mimic neurological signs; for example, reduced sensation, peripheral neuropathy | Vascular examination is unremarkable | | | | | |
| Offer to perform fundoscopy | Raised intracranial pressure may indicate brain lesions and prompt further investigation | Fundoscopy is unremarkable | | | | | |
| Perform a cognitive assessment, including speech | Gross abnormality may indicate brain lesion and prompt further investigation | Cognitive assessment is normal | | | | | |
| Perform a DRE if there are any concerns regarding cauda equina syndrome | Assess for anal sphincter tone and perianal sensation. Deficit could indicate cauda equina syndrome | DRE not indicated here | | | | | |

**Finishing**

| | | | | | | | |
|---|---|---|---|---|---|---|---|
| Check patient is comfortable, offer to help reposition him and give the privacy to change | Keeps the patient's dignity | Treating the patient with respect is important | | | | | |
| Remove your gloves and wash hands | Complying with hand hygiene is vital | No additional concerns | | | | | |

**Present Your Findings**

Mr Romberg is a 64-year-old man who has presented with increasing foot injuries and reduced sensation. On examination he is overweight and walks with the aid of one stick. He has a foot-slapping gait and a positive Romberg's test. He has decreased sensation to light touch and pain up to his mid-shin, in a stocking distribution. Motor examination is unremarkable.

I feel the most likely diagnosis is diabetic polyneuropathy with differential being peripheral vascular disease.

I would like to dipstick the urine, perform blood tests and check the other organ systems for complications for diabetes

**General Points**

Polite to patient

Maintains good eye contact

Clear instruction and explanation to patient

Warns the patient about potential pain/discomfort prior to palpation

# ❓ QUESTIONS FROM THE EXAMINER

## How does diabetes lead to diabetic neuropathy?

Uncontrolled high blood sugar is thought to damage nerves and interfere with their ability to send signals. This is mainly due to the weakening of the capillaries, which supply the nerves with nutrients and oxygen, leading to diabetic neuropathy.

## What constitutes the main route of treatment for diabetic neuropathy?

As diabetic neuropathy is mostly irreversible, the mainstay of treatment is preventive, aiming for good glycaemic control with healthy diet and exercise. Frequent checking of the feet can help acknowledge any ulcers and prompt early recognition. There are also medications that can help reduce the pain associated with peripheral neuropathy, such as amitriptyline.

## How does sciatica present and what causes it?

Sciatica describes nerve pain in the leg, which is caused by irritation or compression of the sciatic nerve. Often tingling, numbness or weakness may also be associated in the buttocks, posterior aspect of the affected leg, the feet and toes.

## What vitamin deficiencies can lead to neurological disease?

A deficiency in vitamin $B_{12}$ can lead to neurological problems such as visual changes, memory loss, paraesthesia, ataxia, limb weakness and peripheral neuropathy.

## At what level of the lower spinal cord are lumbar punctures performed, and why?

The lumbar puncture is usually performed between L3/4 or L4/5. This is because the conus medullaris (bottom of the spinal cord and beginning of the cauda equina) terminates at the level of L1/2 in adults, meaning an insertion site below this point minimises the risk of spinal cord trauma.

## Which lower-limb neurological signs tend to occur with Parkinson's disease?

Parkinson's disease usually presents with a triad of tremor, rigidity and bradykinesia (slowness of movement). In addition to impaired balance and coordination of the lower limbs, Parkinson's' disease often causes a slow shuffling gait, which may appear rushed or get stuck at times.

## What is cauda equina syndrome and what complication does it lead to if left untreated?

The cauda equina is a bundle of nerve roots at the lumbar end of the spinal cord, mostly providing motor and sensory function to the legs and pelvic organs. Cauda equina syndrome occurs when the cauda equina is compressed. If left untreated, it can lead to permanent paralysis and impaired bladder/bowel control.

## What is a positive Trendelenburg sign, and which lower motor nerve does it involve?

A positive Trendelenburg sign describes a pelvic drop on the contralateral side during a single-leg stand on the affected side. This usually indicates weakness in the hip abductor muscles, commonly caused by damage to the superior gluteal nerve.

## Which nerve roots are anaesthetised in a femoral nerve block and when might this be performed?

The femoral nerve originates from L2, L3 and L4. A femoral nerve block (in combination with a sciatic nerve block) may be indicated in patients requiring lower-limb surgery. It may also be indicated as analgesia in patients with a fractured neck of femur.

## Which nerve palsy leads to foot drop, and which muscle groups are affected?

Foot drop occurs due to damage or compression of the common peroneal nerve, a derivative nerve from the terminal branch of the sciatic nerve. With damage to this nerve, there will be weakness of tibialis anterior and other key dorsiflexors of the foot, leading to a loss of active dorsiflexion of the ankle.

## Station 2.11   Cerebellar

### Doctor Briefing

You are a junior doctor in general medicine, and have been asked to see Mr Gordon, a 75-year-old man, who has presented with persistent falling. He also finds that when reaching for objects, he keeps missing them. Please perform a relevant cerebellar examination on Mr Gordon and then present your findings.

### Patient Briefing

You have had long-standing kidney disease, for which you receive haemodialysis three times a week. Over the past few months, you have been feeling increasingly unwell, and have not been eating regularly. Recently you have been feeling confused and have been experiencing falls and difficulty walking. Your family also mentioned some strange eye movements, but you haven't noticed this yourself.

You have a background of alcohol abuse but have not been drinking recently.

You are concerned as you do not feel safe at home with your increased falls.

### Mark Scheme for Examiner

#### Introduction

Washes hands, introduces self, confirms patient identity and gains consent for examination

Offers a chaperone

Appropriately exposes the patient whilst keeping dignity at all times, and repositions into a suitable position for the examination

Asks if the patient has any pain currently

#### General Inspection

| What are you looking for or examining? | Justification | Findings and evolving thought process | | | | | |
|---|---|---|---|---|---|---|---|
| General well-being | On initial glance, does the patient look well, unwell or in pain? | Patient appears comfortable | | | | | |
| Obvious clues | Gives an indication of the patient's baseline health | Patient looks generally well | | | | | |
| Surroundings | Checks for obvious clues to aid diagnosis or equipment/observations to aid assessment | Patient mobilises with a walking stick | | | | | |

#### Cerebellar Examination – Gait

| | | | | | | | |
|---|---|---|---|---|---|---|---|
| Assess gait | Ask the patient to walk up and down the room. Look for a broad-based gait with irregular stride rhythm or length and instability. To pick up more subtle ataxic gait, ask the patient to tandem walk, i.e. walk by placing one foot in front of the other as if on a tightrope | Patient shows a wide-based, small-stepped gait. Unable to carry out tandem walk due to unsteadiness | | | | | |

**Cerebellar Examination – Eyes**

| What are you looking for or examining? | Justification | Findings and evolving thought process | | | | |
|---|---|---|---|---|---|---|
| Assess for slow-pursuit movements | Hold up a pen and ask the patient to follow its movement with his eyes, keeping the head still. Move the pen horizontally and vertically, as for ocular muscle examination, in all directions. Hold the patient's gaze at lateral and vertical positions to try and elicit nystagmus | Lateral gaze induced. Vertical nystagmus elicited. Loss of smooth pursuit | | | | |
| Assess for rapid eye movements | Make a fist with one hand and an open palm with the other. Rapidly shout 'fist' and 'palm', while asking the patient to look at the respective hand in response. Look for square-wave jerks and saccadic intrusions. A saccade is a fast eye movement<br>SWJ are inappropriate saccades that take the eye away from its focus. There is then a pause, followed by a corrective saccade back to the original target.<br>Saccadic intrusions are similar but not necessarily followed by a return movement. They may be associated with cerebellar disease | Patient's eyes overshoot before correcting (saccadic intrusions), consistent with cerebellar pathology | | | | |

**Cerebellar Examination – Speech**

| | | | | | | |
|---|---|---|---|---|---|---|
| Assess speech | Assess for slurring of speech by asking the patient to say 'British constitution', 'West Register Street' and 'baby hippopotamus'.<br>Assess for staccato speech by asking the patient how to make a cup of tea | Slurred, scanning speech consistent with cerebellar pathology | | | | |

**Cerebellar Examination – Upper Limb**

| | | | | | | |
|---|---|---|---|---|---|---|
| Assess for cerebellar rebound | With the patient's arms held out in front of him, press his arm downwards and let go, with the patient resisting. When you let go, he should try to restore the arms to the original position. Look for overshoot. A small distance of overshooting before correction is normal.<br>An exaggerated rebound is suggestive of spasticity, such as in stroke. A complete absence is suggestive of cerebellar disease | No rebound phenomena, suggestive of cerebellar disease | | | | |
| Perform the finger–nose test | Ask the patient to bring his index finger out to touch your finger, which should be positioned at roughly arm's length away from him. Then ask him to touch his nose and repeat from your finger to his nose as quickly and accurately as he can. Look for intention tremor and poor coordination | Patient exhibits poor coordination | | | | |
| Assess for dysdiadochokinesis | Ask the patient to slap his hand with the palm of his other hand, then to slap it with the other side of his hand (dorsal) and repeat, lifting his hand up in between, as fast as he can. Look for poor coordination | Patient shows poor coordination, consistent with cerebellar pathology | | | | |

**Finishing**

| What are you looking for or examining? | Justification | Findings and evolving thought process | | | |
|---|---|---|---|---|---|
| Check patient is comfortable, offer to help reposition him and give the privacy to change | Keeps the patient's dignity | Treating the patient with respect is important | | | |
| Remove your gloves and wash hands | Complying with hand hygiene is vital | No additional concerns | | | |

**Present Your Findings**

Mr Gordon is a 75-year-old man who has presented with persistent falling. On examination, Mr Gordon has a wide-based, short-stepped gait. On testing ocular pursuit movements, lateral nystagmus was elicited, with fast saccadic eye movements. He has slurred scanning speech, poor coordination and past pointing. I also noted that he has stigmata of chronic liver disease.

I feel the most likely diagnosis is cerebellar dysfunction, potentially Wernicke's syndrome due to long-standing dialysis.

I would like to do a full neurological examination, including cerebellar, peripheral and cranial nerve examination, and perform fundoscopy and a cognitive assessment, including speech. I would also consider commencing Mr Gordon on medication after speaking to his renal team

**General Points**

Polite to patient

Maintains good eye contact

Clear instruction and explanation to patient

## ❓ QUESTIONS FROM THE EXAMINER

**Mr Gordon asks whether his condition will get better if he has Wernicke's encephalopathy.**

Yes, Wernicke's encephalopathy is considered reversible if treated, though it can take days to weeks.

**What name is given to the syndrome when the symptoms of Wernicke's become irreversible?**

Korsakoff syndrome.

**How would a patient presenting with both hypoglycaemia and Wernicke's encephalopathy be managed?**

IV thiamine must be administered before IV glucose, as glucose without thiamine can worsen encephalopathy and confusion.

**What is confabulation?**

Confabulation, a symptom of Korsakoff syndrome, is when a patient produces fabricated memories to fill in lapses of memory.

**How would an ischaemic stroke of the cerebellum present clinically?**

Classically there would be sudden-onset headache, nausea, vomiting, vertigo and poor balance whilst standing or walking.

**Why can Romberg's test not be carried out in a patient with cerebellar pathology?**

A patient with cerebellar pathology would likely be unable to complete the first step, standing upright, with the feet together and eyes open without losing balance.

### What would a positive Romberg's test suggest in a patient presenting with ataxia?

Romberg's test assesses proprioception and vestibular function (known as sensory ataxia). A positive test suggests a sensory ataxia, or a non-cerebellar cause of balance issues.

### What are the causes of thiamine deficiency?

Chronic heavy alcohol use is the most common cause. Others include malnutrition (such as in anorexia), malabsorption (as with IBD), increased demand states (pregnancy, hyperthyroidism and malignancy) and increased loss (diarrhoea or dialysis).

### What direction nystagmus would you expect to see in a right-sided cerebellar lesion?

Fast phase of the movement towards the side of the lesion, therefore right-sided nystagmus in a right-sided cerebellar lesion.

### What is Charcot's neurologic triad?

The triad of nystagmus, intention tremor and scanning or staccato speech, which is associated with multiple sclerosis.

## Station 2.12   Parkinson's Disease

### Doctor Briefing

You are a junior doctor in neurology outpatients and have been asked to see Mr Smith, a 62-year-old man, who has been referred by his primary care physician with signs of parkinsonism. Please perform a relevant examination on Mr Smith and present your findings.

### Patient Briefing

You have been increasingly confused over the past year and have been feeling depressed. You have been experiencing visual hallucinations, anxiety and sleep disturbance over the past 6 months, and during this time you have been having difficulty walking and getting dressed. You have been more prone to falling and experiencing tremors.

You are concerned as your primary care physician mentioned this could be Parkinson's disease and you've heard that this is serious.

### Mark Scheme for Examiner

| Introduction | | | | | | | |
|---|---|---|---|---|---|---|---|
| Washes hands, introduces self, confirms patient identity and gains consent for examination | | | | | | | |
| Offers a chaperone | | | | | | | |
| Appropriately exposes the patient whilst keeping dignity at all times, and repositions into a suitable position for the examination | | | | | | | |
| Asks if the patient has any pain currently | | | | | | | |

| General Inspection | | | | | | | |
|---|---|---|---|---|---|---|---|
| **What are you looking for or examining?** | **Justification** | | **Findings and evolving thought process** | | | | |
| General well-being | On initial glance, does the patient look well, unwell or in pain? | | Patient appears agitated | | | | |
| Obvious clues | Gives an indication of the patient's baseline health | | Patient looks generally well. Unilateral resting tremor of his right hand. Appearance is slightly dishevelled | | | | |
| Surroundings | Checks for obvious clues to aid diagnosis or equipment/ observations to aid assessment | | Patient mobilises with a walking stick | | | | |

| Parkinson's Examination – Movement | | | | | | | |
|---|---|---|---|---|---|---|---|
| Assess for tremor | Ask the patient to hold his arms straight out with the palms facing the floor (postural). Ask the patient to close his eyes and slowly count backwards from 20 (this should elicit and accentuate any tremor). Perform the finger–nose test to look for intention tremor due to cerebellar disease. Note that the finger–nose test should dampen a Parkinson's disease tremor but accentuate a benign essential tremor. A Parkinson's disease tremor is normally markedly asymmetrical. Classic tremor of Parkinson's disease is a 'pill-rolling' tremor of the index finger and thumb | | Resting tremor of the right hand. Tremor dampened by finger–nose test. Appearance of pill-rolling tremor consistent with Parkinson's disease | | | | |

**Parkinson's Examination – Movement**

| What are you looking for or examining? | Justification | Findings and evolving thought process | | | | |
|---|---|---|---|---|---|---|
| Assess for bradykinesia | Ask the patient to perform the following rapid alternating movements:<br>Using one hand first, ask the patient to move his fingers towards his thumbs as though closing a duck's beak, then opening it and closing it. Ask him to repeat this as quickly and accurately as he can.<br>Ask him to mimic playing the piano with both hands as fast as possible in mid-air.<br>Look for slow initiation, asymmetry and reduction of speed and amplitude | Reduction of movement speed and amplitude after 5 s | | | | |
| Assess for micrographia | Ask the patient to write a phrase; for example, 'Little red riding hood'.<br>Ask him to repeat it about five times.<br>Look for abnormally small writing | Progressively smaller handwriting | | | | |
| Assess for rigidity | Passively circumduct a wrist and then flex and/or extend at the elbow.<br>Repeat on the other side.<br>Feel for lead-pipe rigidity (rigidity throughout movement) and cogwheeling (ratchety stiffness of limb through passive movement) | Rigidity and cogwheeling present in both arms | | | | |

**Parkinson's Examination – Gait**

| | | | | | | |
|---|---|---|---|---|---|---|
| Assess gait | Ask the patient to walk normally from one side of the room to the other, and then to turn around and come back, whilst ensuring he is supported.<br>Look for gait ignition failure, festinance, reduced arm swing, stooped posture and en bloc turning.<br>Parkinsonian gait is described as a slow shuffling gait with difficulty initiating movement | Slow, short-stepped gait, with difficulty turning, consistent with Parkinson's disease | | | | |
| Perform the pull test | This assesses for postural instability. With the patient still standing, warn him that you need to test his tendency to fall backwards (retropulsion) and will need to pull him back, but you will be behind to support him.<br>Then, with both hands on each of the patient's shoulders, pull him back sharply.<br>In idiopathic Parkinson's disease, postural instability is a late sign to develop. Therefore, if this was present early or at onset, an alternative diagnosis should be sought | Patient unable to correct balance | | | | |

**Parkinson's Examination – Parkinson-Plus Syndrome**

| | | | | | | |
|---|---|---|---|---|---|---|
| Examine eye movements | Vertical gaze palsy and slow saccadic eye movements are associated with progressive supranuclear palsy | No gaze palsy observed | | | | |
| Assess speech | Nasal or staccato quality is a feature of multiple-system atrophy | Quiet speech | | | | |
| Measure the erect and supine blood pressure | Orthostatic hypotension is a feature of multiple-system atrophy | No drop in standing blood pressure | | | | |

**Finishing**

| What are you looking for or examining? | Justification | Findings and evolving thought process | | | | |
|---|---|---|---|---|---|---|
| Check patient is comfortable, offer to help reposition him and give the privacy to change | Keeps the patient's dignity | Treating the patient with respect is important | | | | |
| Remove your gloves and wash hands | Complying with hand hygiene is vital | No additional concerns | | | | |

**Present Your Findings**

Mr Smith is a 62-year-old man who has presented with signs of parkinsonism. He has a unilateral, pill-rolling, resting tremor of his right hand, dampened by movement. He has bradykinesia of his right side and marked micrographia. He has bilateral rigidity with noticeable cogwheel rigidity at the right wrist. He walks with the aid of one stick and has a stooped, festinant gait.

I feel the most likely diagnosis is Lewy body dementia, due to the features of Parkinson's with confusion and agitation.

I would like to do a full neurological examination, including cerebellar, peripheral and cranial nerve examination, perform fundoscopy and do a cognitive assessment, including speech. I would consider commencing Mr Smith on medication; for example, levodopa

**General Points**

Polite to patient

Maintains good eye contact

Clear instruction and explanation to patient

## ❓ QUESTIONS FROM THE EXAMINER

**What triad of signs classifies parkinsonism?**

Bradykinesia, resting tremor and rigidity.

**Why would anticholinergics be avoided or used with caution in a patient with Lewy body dementia?**

They can worsen psychiatric symptoms, such as dementia and confusion.

**Why do patients with Parkinson's disease display hypomimia?**

Bradykinesia of the facial movements leads to less produced and slow facial expressions.

**What pathology is the cause of Parkinson's disease?**

Progressive dopaminergic neuron degeneration in the substantia nigra, leading to a deficiency of dopamine.

**How would a diagnosis of Parkinson's disease be made?**

Parkinson's disease is based on the presence of typical parkinsonian features and excluding any other potential causes. Imaging is not required unless it is an atypical presentation.

### How would a presentation of vascular Parkinson's differ?

Vascular Parkinson's classically affects the lower limbs and is symmetrical.

### Name the risk factors for the development of idiopathic Parkinson's disease.

Age, family history and previous traumatic brain injury.

### Why is levodopa not the first-line treatment in younger Parkinson's patients?

Levodopa's efficacy decreases and its side-effect profile increases with time. Patients with limited comorbidity or those under the age of 65 are usually given dopamine agonists initially, to delay these effects.

### What role do COMT inhibitors play in Parkinson's treatment?

COMT inhibitors do not treat Parkinson's symptoms themselves, but they can improve the efficacy of levodopa by inhibiting its metabolism.

### What surgical treatments for Parkinson's disease are available?

Deep-brain stimulation can be conducted in specialist centres for some patients.

## Station 2.13    Peripheral Vascular

### Doctor Briefing

You are a junior doctor in vascular surgery and have been asked to see Mr O'Neil, a 60-year-old man, who has developed pain in his right leg on walking and at rest. Please perform a relevant vascular examination on Mr O'Neil and present your findings.

### Patient Briefing

You have a history of critical-limb ischaemia for which you are on secondary preventive medications. However, in the early hours of the morning, you experienced severe and persistent pain in your right leg which prompted your urgent transfer to hospital. You were unable to walk on the leg and lost all power, sensation and movement, requiring ambulatory transfer.

On questioning, your leg is extremely cold and pale, and this came on very suddenly. You have a history of cardiovascular disease, with previous heart attacks and transient ischaemic attacks. You have poorly controlled hypertension and diabetes and have a 60-pack-year smoking history.

You are concerned that your vascular disease has worsened, and you might require an amputation.

### Mark Scheme for Examiner

#### Introduction

| | | | | | |
|---|---|---|---|---|---|
| Washes hands, introduces self, confirms patient identity and gains consent for examination | | | | | |
| Offers a chaperone | | | | | |
| Appropriately exposes the patient whilst keeping dignity at all times, and repositions into a suitable position for the examination | | | | | |
| Asks if the patient has any pain currently | | | | | |

#### General Inspection

| What are you looking for or examining? | Justification | Findings and evolving thought process | | | |
|---|---|---|---|---|---|
| General well-being | On initial glance, does the patient look well, unwell or in pain? | The patient is in severe pain and extremely agitated. The patient is morbidly obese and has xanthelasmata and fingernail tar stains | | | |
| Surroundings | Checks for obvious clues to aid diagnosis or equipment/observations to aid assessment | The patient has a crutch which he uses as a walking aid | | | |

#### Examination of the Legs – Inspection

| | | | | | |
|---|---|---|---|---|---|
| Inspect and compare the lower limbs for any obvious changes | Specifically inspect for muscle bulk, asymmetry, swelling, nail changes and gangrene | The right leg is white compared to the left with noticeable hair loss. Several toes appear gangrenous | | | |
| Inspect the skin | Comment on colour (pale, blue, dusky red or black, brown), scars, hair loss, skin thickening and dry skin | | | | |
| Look for ulcers | Comment on site, shape, depth and edges. Look in between the toes, heels and under any dressings | There are two painful, necrotic-looking ulcers on the big toe. They are regularly shaped and 0.5 cm deep with the punched-out appearance of an arterial ulcer | | | |

**Examination of the Legs – Inspection**

| What are you looking for or examining? | Justification | Findings and evolving thought process | | | | | |
|---|---|---|---|---|---|---|---|
| Look for varicose veins, lipoderma-tosclerosis, venous eczema, skin pigmentation and oedema | May suggest chronic venous disease | There is no evidence of varicose veins or signs of chronic venous disease | | | | | |
| Assess functional ability in a corridor walking test | Important to establish limitations of vascular disease and function of limbs | The patient is unable to walk due to pain and has no movement in the affected limb | | | | | |

**Examination of the Legs – Palpation**

| | | | | | | | |
|---|---|---|---|---|---|---|---|
| Feel for the temper-ature of both lower limbs | If the vascular supply is compromised, the lower limbs will be cool to touch | The right lower limb is severely cold to touch in contrast to the left lower limb, which feels warm | | | | | |
| Check the CRT | Quickly assesses peripheral perfusion | You cannot elicit a CRT from the right lower limb, but the left CRT is elon-gated at 4 s | | | | | |
| Check for peripheral oedema | May be suggestive of underlying heart failure or chronic venous disease | There is no peripheral oedema | | | | | |
| Squeeze the calves gently and assess for tenderness | The lower limbs will be tender in acute limb ischaemia | The right limb is acutely painful and tender | | | | | |
| Check sensation in both legs | Progressive peripheral neuropathy is common in patients with significant peripheral vascular disease | There is no sensation in the right limb and reduced sensation in the left | | | | | |

**Examination of the Legs – Pulses**

| | | | | | | | |
|---|---|---|---|---|---|---|---|
| Feel for the pres-ence of femoral pulses bilaterally | Weakening or absence of the pulses suggests severe arterial disease or occlusion | All pulses are absent on the right at and below the femoral artery. Pulses are weakly present on the left | | | | | |
| Assess for radi-ofemoral delay (feel for radial and femoral pulse simultaneously) | | | | | | | |
| Feel for the pres-ence of popliteal pulses, posterior tibial pulses and dorsalis pedis pulses bilaterally | | | | | | | |
| Auscultate the femo-ral arteries | Listens for bruits which may suggest arterial disease | You cannot hear any femoral bruits or a pulse | | | | | |

## Examination of the Abdomen

| What are you looking for or examining? | Justification | Findings and evolving thought process | | | | |
|---|---|---|---|---|---|---|
| Inspect the abdomen looking for any obvious pulsation | May indicate an AAA | No evidence of an AAA | | | | |
| Palpate the aorta for pulsating masses | | | | | | |
| Auscultate the aorta and renal arteries for vascular bruits | Suggestive of turbulent blood flow which may indicate arterial disease (partial occlusion) | No bruits can be auscultated | | | | |

## Additional Tests

| | | | | | | |
|---|---|---|---|---|---|---|
| Perform Buerger's test | This is done by raising both legs and noting at which degree a limb develops pallor. Assesses adequacy of the arterial supply to the leg. In a healthy individual, the entire leg should remain pink, even at 90°. A Buerger's angle of >20° indicates severe limb ischaemia | The right leg is pale and lacking arterial perfusion at rest | | | | |
| Offer to measure ankle brachial pressure index (ABPI) | Assesses the severity of arterial disease | The ABPI cannot be calculated due to the acute severity of this presentation. Previous readings indicate values <0.5, indicating severe arterial disease and critical limb ischaemia | | | | |
| Offer to perform a full cardiovascular examination, fundoscopy and dipstick the urine | Findings may indicate underlying cardiovascular disease, hypertensive/diabetic retinopathy or glucose in the urine (suggestive of diabetes) | Cardiovascular examination is unremarkable. There are high quantities of glucose in the urine | | | | |

## Finishing

| | | | | | | |
|---|---|---|---|---|---|---|
| Check patient is comfortable, offer to help reposition him and give the privacy to change | Keeps the patient's dignity | Treating the patient with respect is important | | | | |
| Remove your gloves and wash hands | Complying with hand hygiene is vital | No additional concerns | | | | |

## Present Your Findings

Mr O'Neil is a 60-year-old man who has presented with right-leg pain on walking and at rest. On examination he has tar-stained fingers and xanthalasmata. His entire right limb is thin, white and perishingly cold up to the hip. There is evidence of hair loss and no reperfusion on CRT. There are no pulses palpable in the right limb and no power or sensation elicited. There are several painful, necrotic-looking ulcers on the dorsal aspects of the right foot, with several gangrenous toes. Examination of the left leg and upper limbs was unremarkable with all pulses palpable.

I feel the most likely diagnosis is acute limb ischaemia with embolic occlusion likely at the right femoral artery.

I would like to perform an A–E assessment and seek emergency senior input, with the aim of revascularising the affected limb immediately as quickly as possible, with either medical or surgical intervention. Initial management would include high-flow oxygen, gaining IV access, performing an ECG and starting anticoagulation and antiplatelet therapy according to local trust guidelines

| General Points | | | |
|---|---|---|---|
| Polite to patient | | | |
| Maintains good eye contact | | | |
| Clear instruction and explanation to patient | | | |
| Warns the patient about potential pain/discomfort prior to palpation | | | |

## ❓ QUESTIONS FROM THE EXAMINER

### What are the relevance and purpose of measuring ABPI?

The ABPI is a non-invasive test used in the diagnosis of peripheral arterial disease and in the assessment of peripheral arterial perfusion in the lower limbs. An ABPI of <1.0 indicates some degree of peripheral arterial disease, with <0.5 commonly alerting you to critical limb ischaemia.

### Which AAAs are typically managed by surgery?

Surveillance is offered to all people with an asymptomatic AAA depending on its size. Aneurysm repair is considered for all symptomatic AAAs, large (>5.5 cm) asymptomatic AAAs or large (>4.0 cm) asymptomatic AAAs that have grown by 1 cm in a year. Surgical intervention is also offered for any AAAs that may have ruptured.

### What is the first initial investigation when suspecting peripheral vascular compromise?

Often basic observations are performed initially as a reflection of cardiovascular health; for example, heart rate, blood pressure, CRT. The ABPI is a good first-line non-invasive test to assess for peripheral arterial disease.

### What is the difference in clinical presentation between a venous and arterial ulcer?

Venous ulcers are often shallow with a granulated base, sloping edges with surrounding changes of venous insufficiency. Arterial ulcers are often found at distal sites with well-defined punched-out borders with surrounding changes of arterial insufficiency and limb ischaemia.

### Why does diabetes increase your risk of peripheral vascular disease?

Diabetes increases your risk as it leads to vascular inflammation and blood vessel changes which promote atherosclerosis and blood vessel damage. Diabetes also increases your risk of clotting and insulin resistance may play a role in peripheral vascular disease.

### What is the difference between critical limb ischaemia and acute limb ischaemia?

Critical limb ischaemia describes the chronic ischaemia that occurs with severe peripheral vascular disease. Acute limb ischaemia is defined as the sudden decrease in arterial blood flow to a limb which threatens its viability. This is a vascular emergency due to its risk of tissue necrosis and potential for limb amputation and death.

### How does lower-limb vascular pain usually present clinically?

Vascular pain is usually described as claudication, which is pain that arises with continuous movement of the limbs. This is caused by restricted blood flow to the upper or lower limbs secondary to blood vessel narrowing and atherosclerosis. Often this occurs intermittently and improves on cessation of movement as the limb reperfuses.

### What is radio-radial delay and what might this indicate?

Radio-radial delay describes a delay between the radial pulses on both sides and may indicate a subclavian artery stenosis or aortic dissection.

### What findings might you visualise on fundoscopy of a patient with diabetic or hypertensive retinopathy?

Diabetic retinopathy may reveal microaneurysms, dot-and-blot haemorrhages or pre-proliferative changes. Hypertensive retinopathy may cause arteriolar narrowing, arteriovenous nipping, retinal haemorrhages, cotton-wool spots and hard exudates.

### Give examples of medications that are commonly used in peripheral vascular disease.

Examples include medications to prevent the progression of peripheral vascular disease, such as antiplatelet or anticlotting agents, statins (to lower circulating cholesterol), antihypertensives and vasodilators for problematic and painful intermitted claudication.

## Station 2.14   Varicose Vein

### Doctor Briefing

You are a junior doctor in vascular clinic and have been asked to see Mr Wilson, a 45-year-old man, who is known to suffer from varicose veins. Please perform a relevant vascular examination on Mr Wilson and present your findings.

### Patient Briefing

You are attending clinic after being referred from your primary care doctor due to a collection of bothersome veins in your left leg.

On questioning, you work as a fitness instructor, but refuse to wear shorts as you are very conscious of how these veins look to clients. Additionally, you have to purchase trousers a size larger for comfort due to the swollen veins in your leg. You also frequently experience leg pain and a heavy sensation in areas where the veins are, with nighttime itching and aching proving particularly bothersome. You have no other relevant medical history and no allergies.

You have privately managed this problem for a long time but are open to discussing treatment options to try and improve the troublesome symptoms and build your self-esteem.

### Mark Scheme for Examiner

#### Introduction

| | | | | | | |
|---|---|---|---|---|---|---|
| Washes hands, introduces self and confirms patient identity | | | | | | |
| Offers a chaperone | | | | | | |
| Appropriately exposes the patient whilst keeping dignity at all times, and repositions into a suitable position for the examination | | | | | | |
| Asks if the patient has any pain currently | | | | | | |

#### General Inspection

| What are you looking for or examining? | Justification | Findings and evolving thought process | | | | |
|---|---|---|---|---|---|---|
| General well-being | On initial glance, does the patient look well, unwell or in pain? | The patient looks well, though appears anxious | | | | |
| Surroundings | Checks for obvious clues to aid diagnosis or equipment/observations to aid assessment | There are no surrounding items of relevance | | | | |

#### Examination of the Legs – Inspection

| | | | | | | |
|---|---|---|---|---|---|---|
| Inspect the patient's legs whilst he is standing | Standing makes the varicose veins more prominent if present (due to the effect of gravity on venous pooling) | Varicose veins can be seen on standing | | | | |
| Look for varicose veins along the paths of long and short saphenous veins | These are where varicose veins are usually located | Large, engorged superficial varicose veins can be seen on both the medial and lateral aspects of the left leg, along the courses of the long and short saphenous veins | | | | |
| Assess both legs for signs of chronic venous disease | Look for lipodermatosclerosis, venous eczema, skin pigmentation, oedema and atrophie blanche. Varicose veins are a common cause of chronic venous insufficiency | There are mild signs of venous eczema and lipodermatosclerosis on the left leg | | | | |

**Examination of the Legs – Inspection**

| What are you looking for or examining? | Justification | Findings and evolving thought process | | | | | |
|---|---|---|---|---|---|---|---|
| Look for venous ulcers and scars | Thought to be caused by the malfunction of venous valves and sustained by chronic venous disease | There are no venous ulcers present on examination | | | | | |
| Look for a saphena varix (dilation of saphenous vein at its junction) | Common manifestation of venous valve malfunction and may be mistaken for an inguinal hernia | There is a saphena varix present on the left side, 2 cm inferior and lateral to the pubic tubercle | | | | | |

**Examination of the Legs – Palpation**

| | | | | | | | |
|---|---|---|---|---|---|---|---|
| Palpate any visible varicose veins and assess for temperature, tenderness and phlebitis | Increased warmth and tenderness suggest superficial thrombophlebitis | There is no sign of thrombophlebitis | | | | | |
| Feel for lipodermatosclerosis and compare the consistency of the subcutaneous fat of both legs | May only be appreciated by gentle palpation | Mild lipodermatosclerosis on the left side can be palpated | | | | | |
| Check for pitting oedema | Can impact the skin and the management of venous disease | There is no pitting oedema | | | | | |
| Ask the patient to cough and palpate over the saphenofemoral junction (SFJ) and at the saphenopopliteal junction | Allows for detection of any valvular incompetence | An impulse can be felt over the SFJ | | | | | |
| Palpate the pulses in the lower limbs bilaterally | Palpate for femoral, popliteal, posterior tibial and dorsalis pedis pulses. Assesses the arterial blood supply of each leg | All pulses are regular and present on both sides | | | | | |

**Examination of the Legs – Percussion**

| | | | | | | | |
|---|---|---|---|---|---|---|---|
| Perform the tap test | This is done by placing one finger over the SFJ to detect any thrills and tapping the varicose vein. Allows assessment of valvular incompetence. The presence of a thrill suggests incompetent valves where there is continuity of the vein | A palpable thrill can be felt over the SFJ | | | | | |

**Examination of the Legs – Auscultation**

| | | | | | | | |
|---|---|---|---|---|---|---|---|
| Auscultate any visible varicose veins for bruits | Auscultate with the bell. If present, bruits may suggest underlying arteriovenous malformation | No bruits can be heard on auscultation | | | | | |

**Additional Tests**

| What are you looking for or examining? | Justification | Findings and evolving thought process | | | | |
|---|---|---|---|---|---|---|
| Perform the Trendelenburg test | This is done by emptying the varicose veins and placing a tourniquet or pressure over the SFJ, asking the patient to stand and observing for filling. If the veins fill up again, repeatedly place the tourniquet at lower intervals (to assess at which point the veins stop filling). Used to locate the site of incompetent venous valves. The point at which the tourniquet prevents the veins from refilling indicates the location of the valve incompetence | The veins stop filling when the tourniquet is at the level of the SFJ | | | | |
| Perform Perthes test | This is done by applying a tourniquet at proximal midthigh and asking the patient to walk around the room. If the varicose veins become less distended, this suggests that there is no deep venous valvular insufficiency. If the varicose veins remain or become more distended, this suggests there is a problem with the deep venous system | The varicose veins become more distended | | | | |
| Offer to perform venous duplex ultrasound | Assesses site of venous incompetence and patency of deep veins | This has been requested | | | | |
| Offer to perform full lower-limb peripheral (arterial) vascular examination | Further assesses for coexisting arterial disease, which is important when thinking about varicose vein management | There is no evidence of arterial disease on examination | | | | |

**Finishing**

| | | | | | | |
|---|---|---|---|---|---|---|
| Check patient is comfortable, offer to help reposition him and give the privacy to change | Keeps the patient's dignity | Treating the patient with respect is important | | | | |
| Remove your gloves and wash hands | Complying with hand hygiene is vital | No additional concerns | | | | |

**Present Your Findings**

Mr Wilson is a 45-year-old man who has presented with extensive varicose veins. On examination he has dilated superficial veins on the lateral and medial side of the left leg. There are no ulcers present, but there is evidence of venous eczema and lipodermatosclerosis. There is no temperature difference, tenderness or oedema evident. A cough impulse is palpable at the SFJ on the left side. Trendelenburg's and Perthes test suggest valve incompetence at the SFJ and additional incompetence within the deep venous system.

I feel the most likely diagnosis is long and short saphenous varicose veins, with likely involvement of the deep venous system, and initial signs of chronic venous disease.

I would like to perform an abdominal examination to identify any masses and await the results from the venous duplex ultrasound scan. I would then explore the impact of the varicose veins on Mr Wilson in more depth and discuss conservative and operative management options with him

**General Points**

| | | | | | | |
|---|---|---|---|---|---|---|
| Polite to patient | | | | | | |
| Maintains good eye contact | | | | | | |

| General Points | | | | |
|---|---|---|---|---|
| Clear instruction and explanation to patient | | | | |
| Warns the patient about potential pain/discomfort prior to palpation | | | | |

## ❓ QUESTIONS FROM THE EXAMINER

### What causes a saphena varix?

A saphena varix is a dilatation at the superior aspect of the long saphenous vein as it joins the femoral vein, known as the SFJ, located within the groin. This is due to valvular incompetence.

### How might you distinguish between a saphena varix and inguinal hernia on examination?

These often present similarly due to the presence of a cough impulse in both. However, a saphena varix often has a bluish tinge and will vanish when the patient lies down and a venous 'hum' may be heard on auscultation. The only true way to distinguish between the two definitively is to perform a duplex ultrasound scan.

### Why is it important to assess for arterial disease in a patient with varicose veins?

One of the main treatment options for varicose veins is compression therapy. However, this can be detrimental to patients with severe arterial disease as compression therapy may lead to secondary limb ischaemia.

### Why might chronic alcohol consumption increase the risk of varicose veins?

Chronic alcohol consumption leads to vasodilation and increased blood viscosity. Alcohol also stimulates blood flow while the veins attempt to work as they normally would. This means faulty valves are more likely to generate backflow, as venous blood accumulates in the veins.

### Why is an abdominal examination relevant in the presence of varicose veins?

Although a less common cause, it is important to palpate for abdominal masses as increased pressure in the abdomen/pelvis, such as a large tumour, could occlude venous return from the legs, presenting with varicose veins.

### Varicose veins increase your risk of developing what complication? Why is this?

Varicose veins increase your risk of developing a deep-vein thrombosis (DVT) as blood pools in the venous system and has more time to clot. Therefore, this is one of the criteria in the DVT Well's score criteria when assessing likelihood of DVT in a patient.

### What is the difference between a DVT and superficial thrombophlebitis?

DVT describes a clot that occurs within one of the large deep veins within your leg, whereas superficial thrombophlebitis describes a blood clot that occurs in the superficial veins of the leg. While not usually life-threatening, superficial clots can cause significant discomfort, tenderness and pain.

### What is the difference between telangiectasias and varicose veins?

Telangiectasias are very small thread-like veins that are less than 1 mm in diameter, otherwise known as spider veins. They are superficial and dilated under the surface of the skin. Varicose veins are commonly bigger, raised and clearly swollen. Varicose veins are caused by venous insufficiency, whereas telangiectasias are linked to ageing and sun exposure.

### How might varicose veins be managed conservatively without further surgical intervention?

Varicose veins can be managed with lifestyle changes such as exercising, reducing alcohol intake, elevating the legs, weight loss and graduated compression stocking therapy. Topical gel and anti-inflammatory medication can also decrease associated discomfort.

### What is the difference between sclerotherapy and ablation for the treatment of troublesome varicose veins?

Sclerotherapy is when medicine is injected into the affected veins to make them shrink. Endothermal ablation involves using energy from high-frequency radio waves or lasers to seal the affected veins. Both treat varicose veins, though there is still risk of recurrence.

## Station 2.15   Ulcer

### Doctor Briefing

You are a junior doctor in vascular surgery and have been asked to see Mr Simpson, a 67-year-old man with diabetes, whose wife has noticed an ulcer under his foot. Please examine Mr Simpson's foot ulcer and present your findings.

### Patient Briefing

Over the past 2 weeks, you have noticed increasing pain in the heel of your right foot when you are walking and at night. You do not remember a trigger for this, but on inspection your wife says it looks like you have a hole in your foot and advised medical attention.

On questioning, you have noticed that your legs feel cold often and sometimes look quite pale. You take over-the-counter pain-killers for a regular cramping sensation in your legs on walking, which has been ongoing for several years. A recent check-up indicated that you were newly diabetic and have high blood pressure and cholesterol, but you decided against medication as you do not like taking it. You smoke a cigar often and have done since you were a teenager.

You are concerned as the pain is worsening.

### Mark Scheme for Examiner

#### Introduction

| | | | | | | |
|---|---|---|---|---|---|---|
| Washes hands, introduces self, confirms patient identity and gains consent for examination | | | | | | |
| Offers a chaperone | | | | | | |
| Appropriately exposes the patient whilst keeping dignity at all times, and repositions into a suitable position for the examination | | | | | | |
| Asks if the patient has any pain currently | | | | | | |

#### General Inspection

| What are you looking for or examining? | Justification | Findings and evolving thought process | | | |
|---|---|---|---|---|---|
| General well-being | On initial glance, does the patient look well, unwell or in pain? | The patient has xanthelasma around his eyes and has a strong odour of cigarette smoke. There is tar staining on the nails | | | |
| Surroundings | Checks for obvious clues to aid diagnosis or equipment/observations to aid assessment | The patient is limping and complains of pain in his right foot. There is a loose bandage wrapped around the right foot base | | | |

#### Examination of the Ulcer – Inspection

| | | | | | |
|---|---|---|---|---|---|
| Look at the limb for surrounding scars, skin grafts or other surgery | May indicate previous ulcers or vascular surgery | There are no signs of previous surgery | | | |
| Look for ulcers | Comment on the site, shape, base, colour, depth and size of any ulcers. Helps to distinguish between different types of ulcers, such as venous, arterial, neuropathic | The ulcer is round, with punched-out edges, measuring 2 cm × 2 cm on the heel of the right foot. The base of the ulcer is sloughed with no red granulation tissue visible | | | |
| Look at the surrounding skin | Comment on colour, hair loss, signs of chronic venous disease (haemosiderin deposits, eczema, lipodermatosclerosis) and signs of infection | The surrounding skin is cold to touch with significant hair loss. There are no signs of infection or chronic venous disease | | | |

## Examination of the Ulcer – Palpation

| What are you looking for or examining? | Justification | Findings and evolving thought process | | | | |
|---|---|---|---|---|---|---|
| Palpate the ulcer and comment on tenderness | Arterial ulcers tend to be painful whereas venous/neuropathic ulcers tend to be painless. Tenderness may also indicate infection | The patient complains of pain on palpation | | | | |
| Feel the surrounding skin with the back of your hand | Assesses temperature of the limb which may indicate arterial disease if cold, or infection if warm | The surrounding skin is cold to touch | | | | |
| Palpate local lymph nodes | Lymphadenopathy may suggest underlying infection | There is no surrounding lymphadenopathy | | | | |
| Assess the neurovascular status of the limb | Important in distinguishing any underlying disease, for example, arterial disease or peripheral neuropathy | The limb is mostly neurovascularly intact with some reduced sensation in the right foot and absent distal pulses | | | | |

## Additional Tests

| | | | | | | |
|---|---|---|---|---|---|---|
| Offer to measure APBI | Assesses the presence and severity of arterial disease | ABPI readings are 0.6, indicating arterial disease | | | | |
| Offer to check blood glucose and urine dipstick | Screens for diabetes, if not already known | A recent blood glucose is visible on the patient's record, indicating new uncontrolled diabetes | | | | |
| Offer to perform a full vascular examination | Assess the pulses and look for signs of chronic venous insufficiency. Findings may help to distinguish between different ulcer causes and associated underlying disease | Vascular examination finds signs of chronic undiagnosed arterial disease | | | · | |

## Finishing

| | | | | | | |
|---|---|---|---|---|---|---|
| Check patient is comfortable, offer to help reposition him and give the privacy to change | Keeps the patient's dignity | Treating the patient with respect is important | | | | |
| Remove your gloves and wash hands | Complying with hand hygiene is vital | No additional concerns | | | | |

## Present Your Findings

Mr Simpson is a 67-year-old man who has presented with a foot ulcer. On examination the ulcer is round, with punched-out edges, measuring 2 cm × 2 cm on the heel of the right foot. The base of the ulcer is sloughed with no red granulation tissue visible and painful to palpation. The affected leg is pale with significant hair loss and thin skin which is cold to touch. Distal pulses are not present.

I feel the most likely diagnosis is arterial ulceration, with differential diagnosis of neuropathic ulcer secondary to diabetes.

I would like to perform a Doppler ultrasound and peripheral nerve examination, check glycated haemoglobin (HbA1c) levels and dipstick the urine. I would then like to discuss both conservative and surgical management of the arterial disease with the patient

| General Points | | | |
|---|---|---|---|
| Polite to patient | | | |
| Maintains good eye contact | | | |
| Clear instruction and explanation to patient | | | |
| Warns the patient about potential pain/discomfort prior to palpation | | | |

## ❓ QUESTIONS FROM THE EXAMINER

### What is the difference between wet and dry gangrene?

Wet gangrene usually occurs from venous obstruction associated with infections. Bacteria invade the tissue, causing swelling and blistering, with a rotten, wet and dark appearance. Dry gangrene occurs if the arterial blood supply to the tissue is cut off, causing the area to become dry, shrink and turn black as the tissue necroses.

### What is the difference in sites between arterial and venous ulcers?

Venous ulcers are commonly found in the area between the ankle and calf, often on the medial aspect of the leg. In contrast, arterial ulcers are commonly found lower on the outside of the ankle, feet, heels or toes towards the distal periphery of joints.

### How do arterial and venous ulcers differ in depth, base and edges?

Arterial ulcers tend to have punched-out edges with no red granulation base, but the base can be sloughed or infective. Venous ulcers more commonly have sloping edges with a red/white granulation base. Arterial ulcers are more commonly deeper than venous ulcers, which are usually wider and cover a greater area.

### Where do neuropathic ulcers tend to occur?

Neuropathic ulcers are commonly found at pressure points on the plantar (bottom) surface of the foot, such as the heel, metatarsophalangeal joint or the hallux.

### How would you manage an arterial ulcer?

The main treatment for arterial ulcers usually involves good wound care using appropriate wound dressings and physical/chemical debridement. This includes treating any potential infection with appropriate antibiotics. Surgical interventions can include skin grafting or surgical revascularisation (bypassing or angioplasty of narrowed vessels).

### How would you manage a venous ulcer?

The main treatment for venous ulcers is similar to that of arterial ulcers with good wound care and physical/chemical debridement. However, compression therapy of the limb is more effective here and leg elevation to aid venous return to the heart. Surgical management may be considered for larger, more troublesome ulcers.

### What is lipodermatosclerosis?

Lipodermatosclerosis describes a type of chronic inflammation of the layer of fat underneath the skin (panniculitis). This is mainly caused by underlying venous insufficiency.

### Why do arterial ulcers tend to be more painful at night?

The pain from arterial ulcers can be worse at night because when the legs are elevated, the arterial supply to the feet is reduced. The pain often improves when the legs are lowered; for example, by hanging them over the side of the bed.

### How do arterial and venous leg ulcers form?

A leg ulcer is a break in the skin, usually caused by local minor trauma. Arterial ulcers form due to poor perfusion of nutrient-rich blood to the lower extremities due to damaged arteries. Venous ulcers form due to insufficient return of blood to the heart due to damaged veins.

### Which is the most common type of leg ulcer and why?

A venous leg ulcer is the most common type as venous disease is much more common than arterial disease. Venous disease causes skin damage due to persistently high pressure in the veins of the legs, easily leading to ulceration.

## Station 2.16    Neck Lump

### Doctor Briefing

You are a primary care physician and have been asked to see Mr Gardner, a 60-year-old man, whose has presented with a neck lump. Please perform a relevant examination on Mr Gardner and present your findings.

### Patient Briefing

You have noticed a lump in your neck that is becoming more noticeable and larger in the last few months, to the point where your partner has commented on its presence. It is painless, firm, rubbery and around the size of a grape.

On questioning, you have been feeling increasingly tired and have unintentionally lost 8 kg in the past month. You have also experienced severe night sweats and have been recovering from a presumed viral infection. You have lost your appetite and have noticed a persistent cough and pressure in your chest, which have troubled you for several weeks. You were recently started on omeprazole for gastro-oesophageal reflux disease and have no allergies. You have had a previous thyroidectomy and take levothyroxine.

Your partner asked you to check this neck lump with a doctor and you are worried that it may be cancerous.

### Mark Scheme for Examiner

#### Introduction

| | |
|---|---|
| Washes hands, introduces self, confirms patient identity and gains consent for examination | |
| Offers a chaperone | |
| Appropriately exposes the patient whilst keeping dignity at all times, and repositions into a suitable position for the examination | |
| Asks if the patient has any pain currently | |

#### General Inspection

| What are you looking for or examining? | Justification | Findings and evolving thought process | |
|---|---|---|---|
| General well-being | On initial glance, does the patient look well, unwell or in pain? | The patient looks cachexic and pale, though not in any obvious pain | |

#### Examination of the Neck – Inspection

| | | | |
|---|---|---|---|
| Ask the patient to point out the neck lump location if relevant | Alerts you to where the patient thinks the neck lump is | The patient points to the right side of the neck in the cervical region | |
| Inspect the neck at eye level from the front, sides and back of the neck | Looks for obvious masses or scars which may indicate previous surgery. If so, then describe the neck lump by commenting on site, size, shape, colour, edge (smooth or irregular) | The patient has a previous thyroidectomy scar, and you can see a small bulge in the right side of the neck. There is no overlying erythema, and the lump appears to be roughly the size of a grape. It appears to be smooth and located in the cervical region | |
| Ask the patient to open his mouth and protrude his tongue | Looks for thyroglossal cyst, which would move upwards with this action | The lump does not appear to move on tongue protrusion | |

## Examination of the Neck – Inspection

| What are you looking for or examining? | Justification | Findings and evolving thought process | | | | | |
|---|---|---|---|---|---|---|---|
| Ask the patient to take a mouthful of water and swallow as you are inspecting | You may identify movement, which suggest a thyroid mass | The lump does not appear to move on swallowing | | | | | |

## Examination of the Neck – Palpation

| | | | | | | | |
|---|---|---|---|---|---|---|---|
| Repeat the above (tongue protrusion and swallow) while gently palpating from behind | May be difficult to identify mass and acknowledge movement on inspection alone | The lump does not appear to move during palpation | | | | | |
| Palpate the local lymph nodes | Palpate for submental, submandibular, tonsillar, parotid, pre/postauricular, superficial/deep/posterior cervical, occipital and supraclavicular nodes. Assesses for lymphadenopathy, which may indicate underlying pathology. If a lump is found, comment on site, size, shape, tenderness, temperature, consistency, mobility and pulsatility | The lump appears to be an enlarged anterior cervical lymph node. The lump is located in the cervical lymph node region and is roughly 3 cm × 2 cm. It is non-tender, smooth, firm and rubbery in consistency. The lump appears tethered to the underlying tissue | | | | | |
| Offer to perform a full examination of the thyroid gland if relevant | Thyroid masses and pathology can present as neck lumps | Not relevant due to previous thyroidectomy | | | | | |

## Additional Tests

| | | | | | | | |
|---|---|---|---|---|---|---|---|
| If a lump is found, test for transillumination | Allows you to distinguish between a cystic and solid mass | The mass does not transilluminate | | | | | |
| If a lump is found, auscultate to listen for bruit | May be suggestive of vascular aetiology; for example a carotid artery aneurysm | No bruits can be heard | | | | | |
| Offer to look in the mouth, as well as palpate (bimanually) the floor of the mouth | This allows assessment of the submandibular gland. Salivary gland masses may also be seen within the mouth. There may be infection within the mouth or tonsils, which could cause surrounding lymphadenopathy | No masses present | | | | | |
| Offer to examine the nose and ears | Checks for infection which may cause surrounding lymphadenopathy | Ear and nose examination appear normal | | | | | |
| If a parotid mass is obvious, offer to examine the face and scalp, including the facial nerve | Parotid masses can compress the facial nerve, leading to facial muscle paralysis | There is no parotid mass present | | | | | |

**Finishing**

| What are you looking for or examining? | Justification | Findings and evolving thought process | | | |
|---|---|---|---|---|---|
| Check patient is comfortable, offer to help reposition him and give the privacy to change | Keeps the patient's dignity | Treating the patient with respect is important | | | |
| Remove your gloves and wash hands | Complying with hand hygiene is vital | No additional concerns | | | |

**Present Your Findings**

Mr Gardner is a 60-year-old man who has presented with a neck lump. On examination there is a single enlarged cervical lymph node in the right anterior triangle, which measures 3 cm × 2 cm. It is firm and rubbery, has a smooth surface, is well circumscribed, non-tender to palpation and is non-mobile over the deep tissue. There is no pulsation, transillumination or surrounding lymphadenopathy of any other nodes.

I feel the most likely diagnosis is non-Hodgkin's lymphoma, with the differentials being other types of lymphoma, reactive lymphadenopathy or lymphadenitis.

I would like to refer this patient urgently to haematology under the 2-week suspected cancer referral pathway for a lymph node biopsy. I would also like to request a CXR and an ECG and take bloods (including FBCs, U&Es, CRP and LFTs)

**General Points**

| | | | |
|---|---|---|---|
| Polite to patient | | | |
| Maintains good eye contact | | | |
| Clear instruction and explanation to patient | | | |
| Warns the patient about potential pain/discomfort prior to palpation | | | |

## ❓ QUESTIONS FROM THE EXAMINER

**What is the difference between a branchial cyst and a cystic hygroma?**

A branchial cyst is a painless, firm neck mass presenting in the anterior triangle of the neck, whereas a cystic hygroma is a softer painless mass in the posterior triangle.

**What are the borders of the anterior and posterior anatomical triangle?**

The anterior triangle is bordered by the inferior border of the mandible superiorly, the anterior border of the sternocleidomastoid laterally and the midline of the neck medially. The posterior triangle is bordered by the posterior border of the sternocleidomastoid anteriorly, the anterior border of the trapezius muscle posteriorly and the middle one-third of the clavicle inferiorly.

**Where can the submandibular gland be palpated?**

The best way to palpate the submandibular gland is to perform bimanual palpation, with one hand on the lateral floor inside the mouth, and the other at the inferior border of the mandible.

**On clinical examination, how does a benign neck lump typically differ from a malignant neck lump?**

Benign neck lumps are classically soft and mobile, often less than 1 cm and are smooth and painless. A malignant neck lump is more commonly hard, firm, irregular and tethered to underlying structures.

## Which clinical characteristics of a lymph node may alert you to a haematological malignancy as opposed to metastatic cancer?

Haematological malignancy often leads to a widespread group of rubbery or boggy lymph nodes, whereas metastatic cancer will affect lymph nodes draining from the affected organ, and appear firm, irregular and non-mobile.

## What obstructive symptoms suggest a neck mass is causing airway compromise?

Shortness of breath, particularly on exertion and eventually stridor or wheeze are concerning features that can indicate airway compromise.

## What are the autoimmune causes of a thyroid goitre?

Hashimoto thyroiditis and Graves' disease can both cause a thyroid goitre.

## What are the most common neck lumps in children?

Lymphadenopathy is the most common cause of neck lumps in children and is most commonly reactive due to infections, such as an upper respiratory infection.

## What is the first-line investigation for a suspicious neck lump?

An ultrasound scan.

## What is the most common head and neck cancer in adults?

Squamous cell carcinoma.

## Station 2.17    Thyroid

### Doctor Briefing

You are a junior doctor in general medicine and have been asked to see Mr Hashimoto, a 50-year-old man, who has presented with weight loss and profound diarrhoea. He has also developed a lump in his neck. Please perform a relevant thyroid examination on Mr Hashimoto and present your findings.

### Patient Briefing

Over the last few days, you have had frequent diarrhoea and noticed that your trousers are looser than normal. You have also noticed increasing pain and tenderness in your neck, which your partner says looks swollen. The pain extends to the jaw and ears. You feel hot and sweaty during the consultation and that your heart is racing.

On questioning, you have not felt well in the week prior to these new symptoms starting. Your partner checked your temperature twice and confirmed a fever. You have not been sleeping well recently and have found it hard to concentrate on simple tasks. You do not take any regular medications and do not have any known past medical history. You are allergic to penicillin.

You are concerned as you have never experienced anything like this before and worry that you have an infection or cancer in your neck.

### Mark Scheme for Examiner

#### Introduction

| | | | |
|---|---|---|---|
| Cleans hands, introduces self, confirms patient identity and gains consent for examination | | | |
| Offers a chaperone | | | |
| Appropriately exposes the patient whilst keeping dignity at all times, and repositions into a suitable position for the examination | | | |
| Asks if the patient has any pain currently | | | |

#### General Inspection

| What are you looking for or examining? | Justification | Findings and evolving thought process | | | |
|---|---|---|---|---|---|
| General well-being | On initial glance, does the patient look well, unwell or in pain? | The patient looks sweaty and unwell, appearing restless | | | |
| Obvious clues | Gives an indication of the patient's baseline health | The patient has a low BMI and his clothes appear loose-fitting, implying recent weight loss | | | |
| Surroundings | Checks for obvious clues to aid diagnosis or equipment/observations to aid assessment | The patient has had observations which confirm a fever and tachycardia but has not been cannulated yet | | | |

#### Examination of the Hands

| | | | | | |
|---|---|---|---|---|---|
| Look at the hands | Checking for thyroid acropachy, onycholysis, sweatiness, palmar erythema, fine tremor | The patient has a resting fine tremor and appears sweaty and warm | | | |
| Feel for pulse | Assessing the rate and rhythm of the patient's radial pulse | The patient's pulse is irregular and tachycardic at 110 bpm | | | |

## Examination of the Eyes

| What are you looking for or examining? | Justification | Findings and evolving thought process | | | | |
|---|---|---|---|---|---|---|
| Look at the eyes from the side and above | Checking for chemosis, periorbital oedema, erythema, lid retraction, exophthalmos | Visual manifestation of thyroid disease in the eyes not present | | | | |
| Assess for ophthalmoplegia and pain on ocular movements | Assessing cranial nerves III, IV, VI | Ophthalmoplegia and pain not present | | | | |
| Assess for lid lag | Checking for ocular manifestations of hyperthyroid states | Lid lag not present | | | | |

## Neck Examination – Inspection

| | | | | | | |
|---|---|---|---|---|---|---|
| Look at the neck from the front and side | Checking for scars, hyperaemia, swelling and distended neck veins | The neck looks diffusely swollen with no other obvious signs | | | | |
| Inspect while the patient is swallowing water | Checking for evidence of thyroid gland masses and thyroglossal cysts | The patient struggles to sip water due to his sore throat, but you can see that the swelling rises when he swallows | | | | |
| Inspect while the patient protrudes the tongue | Checking for thyroglossal cysts | The swelling does not move on tongue protrusion | | | | |

## Neck Examination – Palpation

| | | | | | | |
|---|---|---|---|---|---|---|
| Assess any swelling | Checking site, size, shape, consistency, edge, mobility, fluctuance, transillumination, relationship to skin and deep structures for thyroid mass | You can feel a smooth, diffuse bilateral neck swelling. It has a circumscribed border and is firm in consistency, though you struggle to press too hard as the thyroid is tender | | | | |
| Assess temperature | Checking whether patient is warm or cold to touch, and reviewing recent temperature recordings | The patient feels warm to touch and recent observations display a temperature of 37.9°C | | | | |
| Palpate while swallowing | Checking whether the mass rises with swallowing | You can feel the swelling rise on swallowing | | | | |
| Palpate while protruding the tongue | Checking whether the mass rises with tongue protrusion | You can feel the swelling does not move on tongue protrusion | | | | |
| Assess lymph nodes | Checking submental, submandibular, anterior chain, supraclavicular, posterior chain, parotid nodes, mastoid nodes, occipital nodes | The patient appears to have slightly enlarged and tender submental and submandibular lymph nodes | | | | |
| Feel for the trachea | Checking for evidence of tracheal deviation, which can be caused by a large goitre | The trachea is not deviated | | | | |

## Neck/Chest Examination – Percussion

| What are you looking for or examining? | Justification | Findings and evolving thought process | | | | | |
|---|---|---|---|---|---|---|---|
| Percuss from the thyroid down the sternum | Checking for extension of retrosternal goitre | The swelling does not extend to the chest | | | | | |

## Neck Examination – Auscultation

| | | | | | | | |
|---|---|---|---|---|---|---|---|
| Auscultate each lobe using the bell of the stethoscope | Checking to see if any bruits are present | No bruit can be heard | | | | | |

## Additional Tests

| | | | | | | | |
|---|---|---|---|---|---|---|---|
| Assess tendon reflexes | Checking for hypo/hyperreflexia by checking biceps or knee jerk reflex | Reflexes are elicited and normal | | | | | |
| Look for lower-limb skin changes | Checking for pretibial myxoedema, which is typically seen in Graves' disease, but can also be associated with hypothyroidism or Hashimoto's thyroiditis | No evidence of pretibial myxoedema | | | | | |
| Ask the patient to stand from sitting position with his arms crossed | Checking for proximal myopathy which, if present, may suggest an underlying hyperthyroidism | No evidence of proximal myopathy | | | | | |

## Finishing

| | | | | | | | |
|---|---|---|---|---|---|---|---|
| Check patient is comfortable, offer to help reposition him and give the privacy to change | Keeps the patient's dignity | Treating the patient with respect is important | | | | | |
| Remove your gloves and wash hands | Complying with hand hygiene is vital | No additional concerns | | | | | |

## Present Your Findings

Mr Hashimoto is a 50-year-old man who has presented with a painful swollen neck, profound diarrhoea and weight loss on a background of recent sore throat and flu-like symptoms. On examination he appears anxious and sweaty with a fine bilateral hand tremor, irregular tachycardic pulse and fever. He has a smooth, diffuse neck swelling which elevates on swallowing but not on tongue protrusion. His thyroid is tender on palpation, has a well-circumscribed border and is firm in consistency. Surrounding lymph nodes appear slightly swollen and tender.

I feel the most likely diagnosis is hyperthyroidism secondary to De Quervain's (subacute) thyroiditis, with the differentials being thyroid cancer and Graves' disease.

I would like to measure the blood pressure, dipstick the urine, take bloods (including TFTs, FBCs, U&Es, LFTs, bone profile, CRP, ESR and blood glucose) and perform an ECG. I would then like to arrange an ultrasound of the neck to assess any thyroid masses further and seek a senior review

| General Points | | | |
|---|---|---|---|
| Polite to patient | | | |
| Maintains good eye contact | | | |
| Clear instruction and explanation to patient | | | |
| Warns the patient about potential pain/discomfort prior to neck palpation | | | |

## ❓ QUESTIONS FROM THE EXAMINER

### What is an important initial bedside investigation to perform in a patient showing signs of thyrotoxicosis?

In a patient with clinical signs of hyperthyroidism it is important to get a baseline ECG to check for arrhythmias, notably atrial fibrillation, which can co-present with thyrotoxicosis.

### What blood test is important when investigating suspected hyperthyroidism?

It is important to check TFTs in anyone presenting with signs and symptoms of thyroid disease to aid in diagnosis and distinguish between primary and secondary causes. Other tests to include are FBC, U&Es, LFTs, bone profile, CRP, ESR and blood glucose.

### Describe the differences in TFTs between primary and secondary hyperthyroidism.

In most cases of hyperthyroidism, the TFTs will reflect a primary cause with increased production of thyroid hormone in the thyroid gland and decreased production of thyroid-stimulating hormone (TSH) due to negative feedback of the hypothalamic–pituitary–thyroid axis. Secondary hyperthyroidism suggests a fault within the pituitary gland and not the thyroid, which causes increased production of TSH, leading to excess thyroid hormone production.

### What is the most common cause of hyperthyroidism and how would you test for this specifically?

The most common cause of hyperthyroidism is Graves' disease. After initial confirmation of a primary hyperthyroidism with TFTs, Graves' disease can be specifically tested for by checking levels for TSH receptor-stimulating antibodies. Additionally, antithyroid peroxidase antibodies are found in 70% of patients, but these are less specific.

### Which clinical features are specific to Graves' disease?

Thyroid eye disease (such as exophthalmos and ophthalmoplegia), thyroid acropachy (triad of digital clubbing, soft-tissue swelling of the hands/feet and periosteal new bone formation) and pretibial myxoedema.

### What is the first-line modality of imaging used to examine any thyroid masses?

Ultrasound scan would be first line.

### What is de Quervain's (subacute) thyroiditis?

De Quervain's (subacute) thyroiditis is an inflammatory response within the thyroid thought to be triggered by a viral infection, such as mumps or flu. Patients commonly present following flu-like symptoms with a tender thyroid swelling and fever. Initially, there is a transient thyrotoxicosis which can later progress to a hypothyroid state, which can last weeks to months.

### What is Hashimoto's thyroiditis?

Hashimoto's thyroiditis is an autoimmune condition where antibodies attack the thyroid gland, causing damage where the thyroid is unable to produce enough thyroid hormone. Patients usually present with a non-tender goitre and signs/symptoms of hypothyroidism, such as tiredness, weight gain and dry skin.

### Which medications can cause hyperthyroidism?

Any medications used to treat hypothyroidism, such as levothyroxine and iodine, or any medication with a high iodine content, such as amiodarone, can induce a hyperthyroid state.

### Give three complications of thyrotoxicosis.

Thyrotoxic crisis (thyrotoxic storm), atrial fibrillation, heart failure, angina, osteoporosis and gynaecomastia.

## Station 2.18    Cushing's Syndrome

### Doctor Briefing

You are a junior doctor in general medicine and have been asked to see Mrs Kain, a 30-year-old woman, who has presented with feelings of low mood, weight gain and amenorrhoea for 3 months. Please perform a relevant examination on Mrs Kain's endocrine system and present your findings.

### Patient Briefing

You have not been feeling yourself for a few months, struggling with low mood and weight gain. You cannot think of any reason why you should feel down. You have also noted that your periods have become less frequent, and it has been over 10 weeks since your last menstrual cycle.

On further questioning, you note that the weight gain appears worse around your face and abdomen. You have not been eating more than usual and exercise regularly. You are not sexually active or pregnant. You suffer with lupus erythematosus and therefore take long-term oral steroids. You have no known drug allergies.

You are confused as to why you are experiencing these symptoms and would like further investigations to work out the cause.

### Mark Scheme for Examiner

| Introduction | | | | | | |
|---|---|---|---|---|---|---|
| Washes hands, introduces self, confirms patient identity and gains consent for examination | | | | | | |
| Offers a chaperone | | | | | | |
| Appropriately exposes the patient whilst keeping dignity at all times, and repositions into a suitable position for the examination | | | | | | |
| Asks if the patient has any pain currently | | | | | | |

| General Inspection | | | | | | |
|---|---|---|---|---|---|---|
| **What are you looking for or examining?** | **Justification** | **Findings and evolving thought process** | | | | |
| General well-being | On initial glance, does the patient look well, unwell or in pain? | You note obvious truncal obesity and a significant dorsocervical fat pad | | | | |
| Surroundings | Checks for obvious clues to aid diagnosis or equipment/observations to aid assessment | The patient has her regular glucocorticoid medication by her bedside | | | | |

| Examination of the Upper Limbs | | | | | | |
|---|---|---|---|---|---|---|
| Assess the skin | Look for skin changes, including thin skin, bruising and wounds. Minor injuries more likely to persist due to poor healing. Bruises can be common in the back of the hands/forearm | You note some minor bruising on the forearms | | | | |
| Check for proximal myopathy | This is done by asking the patient to raise both arms out and assessing power. Proximal myopathy is a common feature of Cushing's due to glucocorticoid-induced muscle atrophy | The patient has reduced power in the proximal upper limbs | | | | |
| Check blood pressure | May be elevated in Cushing's syndrome due to excess cortisol | The blood pressure is elevated, at 160/90 mmHg | | | | |

**Examination of the Upper Limbs**

| What are you looking for or examining? | Justification | Findings and evolving thought process | | | | |
|---|---|---|---|---|---|---|
| Comment on trunk-to-limb ratio | Centripetal adiposity associated with Cushing's syndrome results in thin arms/legs with a large trunk | You notice a significantly large trunk-to-limb ratio | | | | |

**Examination of the Face**

| | | | | | | |
|---|---|---|---|---|---|---|
| Look for facial features associated with Cushing's syndrome | This includes facial 'mooning', acne, plethoric cheeks, hirsutism, hair thinning, cataracts | The patient has characteristic moon-like facies and thinning of the front of the hairline. There is hair growth above the upper limb and plethoric cheeks | | | | |

**Examination of the Neck**

| | | | | | | |
|---|---|---|---|---|---|---|
| Inspect and palpate the supraclavicular fossae | 'Fat pads' are associated with Cushing's syndrome | You can palpate significant supraclavicular fat pads | | | | |

**Examination of the Back**

| | | | | | | |
|---|---|---|---|---|---|---|
| Inspect and palpate the back | Interscapular fat pads ('buffalo hump') and thoracic kyphosis are associated with Cushing's syndrome | You can palpate significant interscapular fat pads | | | | |
| Comment on stature and any clinical evidence of osteoporosis and scoliosis | Long-term steroid use may predispose patients to osteoporosis and bone demineralisation | There is no evidence of osteoporosis and scoliosis | | | | |

**Examination of the Chest**

| | | | | | | |
|---|---|---|---|---|---|---|
| Inspect for breathlessness and auscultate for wheeze | May indicate underlying respiratory illness, for which long-term oral steroids may cause a cushingoid appearance | There are no signs implying an underlying respiratory diagnosis | | | | |
| In males, examine for gynaecomastia | Associated with Cushing's syndrome | Not applicable in this patient | | | | |

**Examination of the Abdomen**

| | | | | | | |
|---|---|---|---|---|---|---|
| Inspect the abdomen | Specifically look for centripetal adiposity, scars of adrenalectomy and purple striae | You note significant centripetal adiposity and purple striae on the abdomen | | | | |

## Examination of the Lower Limbs

| What are you looking for or examining? | Justification | Findings and evolving thought process | | | | | |
|---|---|---|---|---|---|---|---|
| Inspect the lower limbs | Look for skin changes, including thin skin, bruising, leg ulcers and peripheral oedema | There is minor bruising on the shins and mild pitting oedema to mid-shin | | | | | |
| Check for proximal myopathy | Ask the patient to cross her arms and stand from sitting. Proximal myopathy is a common feature of Cushing's due to glucocorticoid-induced muscle atrophy | The patient has reduced power in the proximal lower limbs | | | | | |

## Additional Tests

| | | | | | | | |
|---|---|---|---|---|---|---|---|
| Offer to perform a cardiovascular examination and dipstick the urine | Cardiovascular disease (stroke, myocardial infarction, peripheral vascular disease) can occur as complications from Cushing's | Cardiovascular disease and urinalysis are unremarkable | | | | | |

## Finishing

| | | | | | | | |
|---|---|---|---|---|---|---|---|
| Check patient is comfortable, offer to help reposition her and give the privacy to change | Keeps the patient's dignity | Treating the patient with respect is important | | | | | |
| Remove your gloves and wash hands | Complying with hand hygiene is vital | No additional concerns | | | | | |

## Present Your Findings

Mrs Kain is a 30-year-old woman who has presented with low mood, weight gain and amenorrhoea. On examination she has centripetal obesity, dorsal fat pads, multiple bruising to the forearms and shins and thin skin. Her face is plethoric with hirsutism. She has a proximal myopathy with reduced power for hip flexion and shoulder abduction.

I feel the most likely diagnosis is Cushing's syndrome, secondary to long-term oral steroid use.

I would like to check a random cortisol level while taking other blood tests (including FBCs, U&Es, LFTs, bone profile and blood glucose) and review her steroid use

## General Points

| | | | | | | |
|---|---|---|---|---|---|---|
| Polite to patient | | | | | | |
| Maintains good eye contact | | | | | | |
| Clear instruction and explanation to patient | | | | | | |
| Warns the patient about potential pain/discomfort prior to palpation | | | | | | |

# ❓ QUESTIONS FROM THE EXAMINER

### What is the difference between Cushing's disease and Cushing's syndrome?

Cushing's disease refers to hypercortisolism that is specifically caused by an adrenocorticotrophic hormone (ACTH)-producing pituitary adenoma. Cushing's syndrome refers to any cause of hypercortisolism.

### What imaging tests might be requested to further investigate a person with Cushing's syndrome, and which glands might these look specifically at?

Computed tomography (CT) or MRI of the abdomen and head, to look for adrenal tumours or pituitary adenomas respectively.

### What is the difference between ACTH-dependent and ACTH-independent causes of Cushing's syndrome?

ACTH-independent or primary hypercortisolism is caused by increased cortisol production by the adrenal glands and shows low levels of ACTH. ATCH-dependent or secondary hypercortisolism is when cortisol overproduction is driven by high levels of ACTH, from pituitary adenomas or paraneoplastic syndromes.

### How is Cushing's syndrome definitively diagnosed?

An overnight dexamethasone suppression test is the most sensitive way to diagnose Cushing's syndrome. However further testing is needed to determine the cause.

### What comorbidities are commonly associated with Cushing's syndrome?

Diabetes, hypertension, osteoporosis and cardiovascular disease are all commonly seen in patients with Cushing's syndrome.

### How do Conn's syndrome and Cushing's syndrome differ?

Conn's syndrome refers to primary hyperaldosteronism by an adrenal tumour (aldosteronoma), whereas Cushing's syndrome is caused by hypercortisolism, one cause of which is an adrenal tumour.

### Why would you not suddenly stop long-term steroids in someone you suspect may have Cushing's syndrome for exogenous steroid use?

Patients taking steroids on a long-term basis cannot be suddenly stopped, as exogenous steroids will cause suppression of endogenous steroid production by the adrenal glands. Stopping steroids without tapering will lead to symptoms such as weakness, fatigue, dizziness, nausea and vomiting. The most serious consequence is adrenal crisis.

### How do the low- and high-dose dexamethasone suppression tests feature in the diagnosis of a patient with Cushing's syndrome?

A low dose of dexamethasone will normally suppress cortisol levels, but they will remain raised in an individual with Cushing's syndrome. A high-dose dexamethasone test can help differentiate between Cushing's disease and other cause of hypercortisolism; in pituitary adenomas this will suppress cortisol production, but it will not in ectopic ACTH production or adrenal adenomas.

### What is Nelson's syndrome?

Also known as postadrenalectomy syndrome, this refers to rapid enlargement of a pituitary adenoma following bilateral adrenalectomy for Cushing's syndrome. It is rare as bilateral adrenalectomy is no longer commonly carried out.

### Which cancer is the most common cause of ectopic ACTH production?

Small-cell lung cancer, which can cause Cushing's syndrome through the paraneoplastic production of ACTH.

## Station 2.19    Acromegaly

### Doctor Briefing

You are a junior doctor in general medicine and have been asked to see Mr Black, a 34-year-old man, who has noticed that his hands and feet have swollen up over the last few months. His wedding ring no longer fits his finger and his shoe size has increased. He also reports increased sweating. Please perform a relevant examination on Mr Black's endocrine system and present your findings.

### Patient Briefing

You attend the doctors concerned as you have noticed that your hands and feet have swollen up over the last few months, along with the fact that your wedding ring no longer fits on your finger. You have also become aware that you can no longer fit into your work shoes and have had to buy a bigger size.

On further questioning, you are sweating more and when you have looked at old photos of yourself, you note that your facial features look significantly different – with your brow and lower jaw appearing more prominent and the bridge of your nose slightly larger. Alongside these appearance changes, you have experienced frequent headaches and joint aches. You have recently been told that you are 'borderline' diabetic.

You do not know what might cause these symptoms but are concerned that your appearance is changing and would like to find out why.

### Mark Scheme for Examiner

#### Introduction

| | | | | |
|---|---|---|---|---|
| Washes hands, introduces self, confirms patient identity and gains consent for examination | | | | |
| Offers a chaperone | | | | |
| Appropriately exposes the patient whilst keeping dignity at all times, and repositions into a suitable position for the examination | | | | |
| Asks if the patient has any pain currently | | | | |

#### General Inspection

| What are you looking for or examining? | Justification | Findings and evolving thought process | | | |
|---|---|---|---|---|---|
| General well-being | On initial glance, does the patient look well, unwell or in pain? | The patient is of large, broad build with long limbs and digits. The patient speaks with a deep and slow voice | | | |
| Surroundings | Checks for obvious clues to aid diagnosis or equipment/observations to aid assessment | The patient has a 12-lead ECG attached due to a recent episode of racing heart | | | |

#### Examination of the Hands

| | | | | | |
|---|---|---|---|---|---|
| Inspect the hands | Comment on size and shape. 'Spade-like', enlarged hands are common in acromegaly. Wasting of thenar eminence may indicate carpal tunnel syndrome | The patient's hands are visibly enlarged with wasting of the thenar eminence | | | |
| Palpate the texture of the hands | Boggy palms and moisture are signs of active disease, due to increased sweating and oiliness | The skin is moist and rubber-like with boggy palms evident | | | |

## Examination of the Hands

| What are you looking for or examining? | Justification | Findings and evolving thought process | | | | |
|---|---|---|---|---|---|---|
| Check skin fold thickness | This is done by gently pinching the skin on the back of the hands. The skin may appear thickened and 'doughy' in acromegaly | The skin is notably thickened and 'doughy' | | | | |
| Check sensation in the median nerve distribution | Median nerve supplies the lateral palm. Compression of the median nerve from local oedema may cause carpal tunnel syndrome | Sensation is reduced | | | | |
| Perform Phalen's test | Ask the patient to flex the wrists and hold them together for 60 s. Positive test (paraesthesia in the median nerve distribution) would indicate carpal tunnel syndrome | Phalen's test is positive with paraesthesia occurring on wrist flexion | | | | |
| Perform Tinel's test | Percuss over the carpal tunnel region. Positive test (paraesthesia in the median nerve distribution) would indicate carpal tunnel syndrome | Tinel's test is positive with paraesthesia occurring on percussion | | | | |
| Feel for radial pulse | Tachycardia is associated with a high-output cardiac state | The pulse is tachycardic at 102 bpm | | | | |

## Examination of the Arms

| | | | | | | |
|---|---|---|---|---|---|---|
| Check for axillary hair loss | Hypopituitarism may be associated with acromegaly | There is some evidence of axillary hair loss | | | | |
| Check for proximal myopathy | Ask the patient to raise his arms and check individual power. Proximal myopathy can occur due to excess growth hormone (GH) | The patient has weakened power in both upper limbs, 3/5 bilaterally | | | | |
| Offer to check the blood pressure | Often increased in acromegaly | The blood pressure is raised at 160/95 mmHg | | | | |

## Examination of the Face

| | | | | | | |
|---|---|---|---|---|---|---|
| Inspect the face | Comment on prominent supraorbital ridges, protrusion of the lower jaw (prognathism), large nose/ears/lips and coarse facial appearance, which are all associated with acromegaly | The patient has prominent supraorbital ridges, prognathism, large facial features and a coarse appearance | | | | |
| Ask the patent to stick out his tongue and inspect it | The tongue is often enlarged in acromegaly | The tongue appears to be enlarged | | | | |
| Ask the patient to open his mouth and inspect the gums | Diastema (increased space between the teeth) is common in acromegaly | Diastema is evident on examination | | | | |

## Examination of the Face

| What are you looking for or examining? | Justification | Findings and evolving thought process | | | | | | |
|---|---|---|---|---|---|---|---|---|
| Ask the patient to repeat a simple phrase | The patient may have a husky, deep and slow voice in acromegaly | The patient's voice is deep and slow | | | | | | |
| Assess visual fields | Optic chiasm compression may lead to bitemporal hemianopia | The visual fields test reflects a bitemporal hemianopia | | | | | | |

## Examination of the Neck

| | | | | | | | | |
|---|---|---|---|---|---|---|---|---|
| Check the JVP | Raised JVP may indicate heart failure secondary to hypertension, cardiomyopathy or both | The JVP is raised, at 6 cm | | | | | | |
| Feel for goitre | Approximately 10% of patients with acromegaly have a goitre | There is no goitre present | | | | | | |

## Examination of the Chest

| | | | | | | | | |
|---|---|---|---|---|---|---|---|---|
| Feel for apex beat | A displaced apex beat may indicate cardiomegaly | The apex beat is slightly displaced to the left | | | | | | |
| Auscultate the precordium | A third heart sound may be present, indicating underlying heart failure | Heart sounds are normal | | | | | | |
| Auscultate the lung bases | Left heart failure may lead to pulmonary oedema | There is no sign of pulmonary oedema | | | | | | |

## Examination of the Abdomen

| | | | | | | | | |
|---|---|---|---|---|---|---|---|---|
| Assess for hepatomegaly | May indicate right heart failure | There is no hepatomegaly on examination | | | | | | |

## Examination of the Lower Limbs

| | | | | | | | | |
|---|---|---|---|---|---|---|---|---|
| Assess for proximal myopathy | Ask the patient to cross his arms and stand from sitting. Proximal myopathy can occur due to excess GH | The patient is unable to stand from sitting without use of the arms | | | | | | |
| Look for enlarged feet | Enlarged width and length of the feet are common findings in acromegaly | Both feet are enlarged | | | | | | |
| Check the heel pad thickness | Heel pad thickness can be enlarged in acromegaly | Heel pad thickness is increased | | | | | | |
| Assess for peripheral oedema | Left heart failure may lead to peripheral oedema | There is no sign of peripheral pitting oedema | | | | | | |

**Additional Tests**

| What are you looking for or examining? | Justification | Findings and evolving thought process | | | | | | |
|---|---|---|---|---|---|---|---|---|
| Offer to perform a cardiovascular examination and dipstick the urine | It is important to check the heart as those with acromegaly can suffer from heart complications due to the excess GH, namely cardiomegaly and heart failure. The urine may reflect hyperglycaemia | Cardiovascular examination reveals no further findings. The urine tests positive (+++) for glucose | | | | | | |
| Offer to review old photos | Old photos can be used to compare new features | Old photos confirm the changes in facial features | | | | | | |

**Finishing**

| | | | | | | | | |
|---|---|---|---|---|---|---|---|---|
| Check patient is comfortable, offer to help reposition him and give the privacy to change | Keeps the patient's dignity | Treating the patient with respect is important | | | | | | |
| Remove your gloves and wash hands | Complying with hand hygiene is vital | No additional concerns | | | | | | |

**Present Your Findings**

Mr Black is a 34-year-old man who has presented with hand and foot swelling. On examination he has thick, moist skin, with 'bogginess' in both palms. He has prominent supraorbital ridges with relatively large nose, lips and tongue. Proximal myopathy is evident in both the upper and lower limbs. There was evidence of reduced sensation in the distribution of the median nerve bilaterally, with paraesthesia elicited during Tinel's and Phalen's test. Assessment of the visual fields revealed a bitemporal hemianopia.

I feel the most likely diagnosis is acromegaly associated with carpal tunnel syndrome, likely secondary to a pituitary tumour.

To complete my examination, I would like to take bloods (including FBCs, U&Es, LFTs, bone profile, blood glucose) and check GH/insulin-like growth factor 1 levels

**General Points**

| | | | | |
|---|---|---|---|---|
| Polite to patient | | | | |
| Maintains good eye contact | | | | |
| Clear instruction and explanation to patient | | | | |
| Warns the patient about potential pain/discomfort prior to palpation | | | | |

## ❓ QUESTIONS FROM THE EXAMINER

### What is the most common cause of acromegaly?

Pituitary adenoma, a benign tumour of the pituitary gland. The tumour produces excessive amounts of GH, leading to the signs and symptoms associated with acromegaly.

## What is the difference between acromegaly and gigantism?

Overproduction of GH causes excessive growth and can be labelled as acromegaly or gigantism. The disease process is the same; however, gigantism begins in infancy, prior to bone growth and fusion of the long bone epiphysis. Acromegaly occurs later in life, when the disease process occurs postpuberty and plate fusion.

## How does an oral glucose tolerance test check for acromegaly?

Circulating GH levels tend to fluctuate during the day but are usually suppressed after oral glucose intake. However, with acromegaly, sugar consumption will not reduce the GH levels. If GH levels remain high at serial intervals after high glucose intake, this supports a diagnosis of GH hypersecretion.

## What is the first-line modality of imaging if blood tests confirm excess GH?

As acromegaly is most commonly caused by a benign pituitary adenoma, initial imaging usually takes the form of a contrast-enhanced pituitary MRI scan to look for this probable cause.

## Why might you examine visual fields and what findings might you observe?

Larger tumours can compress the optic chiasm and typically lead to a bitemporal hemianopia, a type of visual loss where the outer half of both the right and left visual field is lost.

## Which type of cancer most commonly secretes GH or GH-releasing hormone (GHRH)?

Pancreatic cancers, small-cell lung cancers, adrenal adenomas and phaeochromocytomas have all been reported to secrete GHRH, leading to the subsequent release of GH.

## What is the clinical consequence of excess GH in childhood compared to in adulthood?

In children this usually results in the child being abnormally tall due to excessive growth of long bones. This is unlikely to occur in adults, as the long bones have typically formed at a set length prior to plate fusion.

## How is GH released?

GHRH is released from the hypothalamus, stimulating GH secretion from the anterior pituitary into the blood. Circulating GH then acts on all tissues in the body, promoting metabolism and growth.

## What treatment is available for acromegaly?

The treatment depends on the cause of increased GH production. For pituitary adenomas, surgery usually forms the main treatment option. Medical injections can also work to slow down the release of GH, shrink tumours and block the effects of GH.

## What is the main complication of acromegaly and what is the significance of this?

The main complications associated with acromegaly are due to the effects of GH on the cardiovascular system, worsening prognosis if left untreated. Hypersecretion of GH can lead to an increase in the risk of cardiomegaly and other cardiac disorders, such as arrhythmias, valve disease and hypertension.

## Station 2.20   Breast

### Doctor Briefing

You are a junior doctor in breast surgery and have been asked to see Mrs Dodd, a 25-year-old woman, who has noticed a breast lump. Please perform a relevant breast examination on Mrs Dodd and present your findings.

### Patient Briefing

You have noticed increased pain and the formation of a hard lump in your breast over the past 2 weeks. The pain has been worsening and you now have a fever of 38°C. You have been breastfeeding for several months but have recently started to reduce the number of feeds following advice from your midwife to introduce soft food slowly.On further questioning, you have noticed that your right breast feels warm and swollen. The pain can be described as a burning sensation and is worse when you breastfeed. You have not noticed any nipple discharge. You do not have any other medical conditions and have no known drug allergies.

You are concerned as you have been unable to continue with your current weaning plan and worry that this could mean that your child does not take to food as well as you would like.

### Mark Scheme for Examiner

#### Introduction

| | | | | |
|---|---|---|---|---|
| Washes hands, introduces self, confirms patient identity and gains consent for examination | | | | |
| Ensures that a chaperone is present and wears gloves | | | | |
| Appropriately exposes the patient whilst keeping dignity at all times, and repositions into a suitable position for the examination | | | | |
| Asks if the patient has any pain currently | | | | |

#### General Inspection

| What are you looking for or examining? | Justification | Findings and evolving thought process | | | |
|---|---|---|---|---|---|
| General well-being | On initial glance, does the patient look well, unwell or in pain? | The patient looks slightly sweaty and warm, but otherwise well | | | |

#### Examination of the Breasts – Inspection

| | | | | | |
|---|---|---|---|---|---|
| With the following positions (below), observe for: asymmetry, swelling or masses, scars, skin changes, nipple changes | These clinical features help to aid diagnosis | The right breast looks erythematous, more swollen and 'fuller' compared to the left. There are no scars or obvious nipple changes | | | |
| Inspect the breasts at rest | To see any obvious masses or skin changes | | | | |
| Inspect the breasts with both arms raised above the head and leaning forwards | This will expose the entire breast and exaggerate any asymmetrical changes | | | | |

## Examination of the Breasts – Inspection

| What are you looking for or examining? | Justification | Findings and evolving thought process | | | | | |
|---|---|---|---|---|---|---|---|
| Inspect the breasts while the patient is sitting and pushing her body up off the bed with both hands | These manoeuvres may accentuate any puckering, asymmetry or changes if any mass is tethered to deep musculature | There are no additional observations or changes with these manoeuvres. There does not appear to be any muscle tethering | | | | | |
| Inspect the breasts with the patient putting her hands on her hips and pushing inwards | | | | | | | |
| Inspect the breasts with the patient leaning forward and observe for muscle tethering of any breast lump | | | | | | | |

## Examination of the Breasts – Palpation

| | | | | | | | |
|---|---|---|---|---|---|---|---|
| Ask the patient to lie back to 45° and relax her head on the pillow, while placing the arm, on the same side of the breast to be examined, behind her head | This lifts the arm out of the way, exposes the breast tissue for examination and spreads the breast flat for examination | The patient appears slightly in pain while doing this | | | | | |
| If it is a unilateral presenting complaint, examine the asymptomatic breast first. Palpate the four quadrants of the breast in turn (with flat fingers, not the palm) | Allows comparison to a 'normal' breast. A systematic approach is important in ensuring all the breast tissues is assessed. For any lump describe size, location, shape, colour, tenderness, temperature, consistency, surface, borders, tethering/mobility, overlying skin changes | No abnormalities detected in the left breast. The right breast is tender to palpation. A fluctuant 'wedge-like' mass can be felt lateral to the areola at the 3 o'clock position. The rough area measures 4 cm × 4 cm. The mass feels hot to touch. There is no overlying skin necrosis | | | | | |
| Palpate the area underneath the nipple and areola | Feel for any masses and observe for any discharge | There are no nipple changes or discharge | | | | | |
| Palpate the axillary breast tail tissue | A large proportion of breast cancers develop in the upper outer quadrant | There are no masses or changes in the axillary breast tissue | | | | | |
| Palpate in the axilla while supporting the arm | Checks for masses and lymphadenopathy | There is some mild axillary lymphadenopathy | | | | | |

## Additional Tests

| | | | | | | | |
|---|---|---|---|---|---|---|---|
| Ask the patient to attempt to produce discharge, if present, by squeezing the nipple between the index finger and thumb | If discharge is present, comment on colour, consistency and volume | Not applicable as no history of nipple discharge | | | | | |
| Elevate the breast with your hand to inspect any pathology not visible during main examination | Lifting the breast may accentuate any changes | No additional concerns | | | | | |

**Additional Tests**

| What are you looking for or examining? | Justification | Findings and evolving thought process | | | |
|---|---|---|---|---|---|
| Offer to palpate the supraclavicular lymph nodes, check for hepatomegaly and lymphoedema, palpate for bony tenderness and auscultate the lung bases | May support diagnosis and provide useful information on metastases in suspect breast carcinoma | No additional concerns | | | |

**Finishing**

| | | | | | |
|---|---|---|---|---|---|
| Check patient is comfortable, offer to help reposition her and give the privacy to change | Keeps the patient's dignity | Treating the patient with respect is important | | | |
| Remove your gloves and wash hands | Complying with hand hygiene is vital | No additional concerns | | | |

**Present Your Findings**

Mrs Dodd is a 25-year-old woman who has presented with a new breast lump. On examination the right breast looks erythematous and more swollen compared to the left. The right breast is tender to palpation with a fluctuant 'wedge-like' mass palpated laterally in relation to the areola at the 3 o'clock position, measuring roughly 4 cm × 4 cm. The mass feels hot to touch, though there is no overlying skin necrosis. Breast examination on the left was unremarkable, with no scars or obvious nipple changes bilaterally. Mild axillary lymphadenopathy was noted.

I feel the most likely diagnosis is acute mastitis secondary to breastfeeding, with the differentials being a breast abscess or inflammatory breast pathology.

I would like to auscultate the lung bases, examine for hepatomegaly and lymphadenopathy and palpate for bony tenderness. I would take a full set of observations, encourage breastfeeding and consider antibiotic therapy. I would then like to refer Mrs Dodd to a one-stop breast clinic for triple assessment ±+/- potential incision and drainage of a breast abscess depending on imaging

**General Points**

| | | | |
|---|---|---|---|
| Polite to patient | | | |
| Maintains good eye contact | | | |
| Clear instruction and explanation to patient | | | |
| Warns the patient about potential pain/discomfort prior to palpation | | | |

## ❓ QUESTIONS FROM THE EXAMINER

### What is the most common cancer in women and what are the main risk factors?

Breast cancer, with the main risk factors of age, family history (breast/ovarian), previous breast cancer/lump, exposure to oestrogen, hormone replacement therapy, alcohol, smoking and radiation exposure to the breast.

### What is the difference between adjuvant and neoadjuvant therapy in the relevance of breast malignancy?

Neoadjuvant therapies are delivered before the main treatment to destroy spread cancer cells or reduce the size of the tumour. Adjuvant therapies are delivered after the primary treatment to destroy any remaining cancer cells. Both may include chemotherapy, hormone therapy, radiation therapy or immunotherapy.

### When would you refer a patient under the 2-week criteria for assessment of a potential malignancy?

All women 30+ years should be referred under the suspected cancer pathway if they have an unexplained breast lump. Women over 50 should also be referred with any nipple changes (discharge, retraction, other changes of concerns). Referral should be considered in those with skin changes suggestive of breast cancer or an unexplained lump in the axilla.

### What is peau d'orange and which pathology is this associated with?

Peau d'orange describes the appearance of an oedematous breast where the follicles get buried, often resembling the look of an orange peel. This can be a sign of inflammatory breast cancer.

### How might you distinguish between mastitis and a breast abscess?

Mastitis is a painful inflammatory condition of the breast. A breast abscess is a severe complication of mastitis and is caused when there is a localised collection of pus within the breast tissue. Breast abscess should be suspected with a fever and an acutely painful and swollen breast, with redness, heat and overlying swelling.

### What advice should be given to a patient with mastitis with regard to breastfeeding?

The patient should continue to breastfeed during an episode of mastitis as although it may be painful, sudden cessation of breastfeeding may cause a blockage to get worse. Breastfeeding will help clear the breast from any milk build-up and even with an infection, breastfeeding will not harm the baby.

### How might the characteristic of nipple discharge change your differential diagnosis?

Yellow/green discharge is more likely to indicate infection. Blood-stained discharge is more likely to be cancerous. White, creamy discharge is more likely to be a side effect to medication, indicate pregnancy or normal physiological milk production (postpregnancy).

### What is the difference between a ductal papilloma and duct ectasia?

A ductal papilloma is a benign wart-like lump that develops in one or more milk ducts in the breast, often presenting with clear or blood-stained nipple discharge. A duct ectasia is a benign thickening within a milk duct, which can become blocked and lead to fluid build-up. This can also cause nipple discharge with surrounding tenderness.

### What are the most common benign breast lumps and how do they present?

Breast cysts and fibroadenomas. Fibroadenomas are solid, smooth and rubbery rounded lumps that are easy to move. Breast cysts present similarly but are fluid-filled, whereas fibroadenomas contain connective tissue. Breast cysts can sometimes be painful and tend to occur later in life (usually in perimenopausal women over the age of 40).

### When are women invited for the National Health Service (NHS) breast-screening programme and what does this entail?

Anyone registered with a GP as female will be invited for NHS breast screening in the form of a mammogram every 3 years between the ages of 50 and 70 years.

## Station 2.21   Dermatological

### Doctor Briefing

You are a junior doctor in primary care and have been asked to see Mrs Barton, a 45-year-old woman, who has presented with a rash on her scalp and elbows. Please perform a relevant dermatological examination on Mrs Barton and present your findings.

### Patient Briefing

You have developed an intensely itchy rash over your elbows and scalp over the past few weeks. You have not changed your washing power or soap, and you cannot think of anything that could be irritating your skin. You have never had any problems with your skin before.

You have a past medical history of coeliac disease, which is normally well controlled, but you have been struggling with avoiding gluten in your diet recently, and so you have been experiencing some tummy pain and diarrhoea.

You are concerned because the itching is particularly bad at night and is disturbing your sleep.

### Mark Scheme for Examiner

#### Introduction

Washes hands, introduces self, confirms patient identity and gains consent for examination

Offers a chaperone

Appropriately exposes the patient whilst keeping dignity at all times, and repositions into a suitable position for the examination

Asks if the patient has any pain currently

#### General Inspection

| What are you looking for or examining? | Justification | Findings and evolving thought process |
|---|---|---|
| General well-being | On initial glance, does the patient look well, unwell or in pain? | Patient looks comfortable at rest |
| Obvious clues | Gives an indication of the patient's baseline health | Patient looks generally well, normal body habitus |

#### Dermatology Examination – Look

| | | |
|---|---|---|
| Determine the number and location of skin lesions | The site and distribution pattern of a lesion can indicate a diagnosis.<br>• Psoriasis is most commonly seen at the knees, elbows, scalp and lower back<br>• Eczema is found on the flexor surfaces of the body<br>• Acne is mostly located on the face and upper trunk<br>• Basal cell carcinoma is usually seen on the head or neck<br>• Herpes zoster infection (shingles) follows a dermatomal distribution<br>It is important to examine all lesions | Patient has a rash over the back of her neck at the hair line and bilaterally on each elbow.<br>The distribution is symmetrical |

**Dermatology Examination – Look**

| What are you looking for or examining? | Justification | Findings and evolving thought process | | | | | |
|---|---|---|---|---|---|---|---|
| Closer inspection of individual lesions | For each lesion, describe the headings listed below | Both her neck and elbows have groups of raised red skin lesions. Clusters of papules and vesicles can be observed as well | | | | | |
| Comment on appearance | It is important to use specific terminology in describing a skin lesion:<br>• Pustule: lesion containing pus<br>• Erosion: loss of epidermis<br>• Ulcer: loss of epidermis and dermis<br>• Weal: circumscribed, elevated area of dermal oedema<br>• Macule: flat, circumscribed area of skin discoloration<br>• Papule: circumscribed raised lesion < 5 mm in diameter at the widest point<br>• Nodule: circumscribed raised lesion > 10 mm in diameter at the widest point<br>• Plaque: circumscribed, disc-shaped, elevated lesion<br> • Small < 2 cm<br> • Large > 2 cm<br>• Vesicle: lesion < 5 mm in diameter at the widest point, containing fluid<br>• Bulla: lesion greater than 10 mm in diameter at the widest point, containing fluid | | | | | | |
| Comment on morphology | Measure the diameter at widest point. Increasing size and lesions > 6 mm raise suspicion of malignancy.<br>Describe the shape of the lesion (round, oval, annular, linear, irregular) and the border (regular/well-demarcated or irregular/ill-defined). Asymmetrical lesions with ill-defined borders are associated with malignancy.<br>Assess whether the lesions are discrete (clearly separated) or confluent | Small discrete lesions, all approximately 5 mm in size, with regular borders | | | | | |
| Comment on surface | Describe whether the surface of the lesion appears rough or smooth.<br>• Excoriation: break in the epidermis, often due to trauma<br>• Crust: coating formed by dried blood and debris<br>• Scales: fragments of the outermost epidermis shedding, commonly seen in psoriasis<br>• Lichenification: thickening of the epidermis associated with chronic scratching (such as eczema) | Excoriations over skin lesions, consistent with an itchy rash | | | | | |

## Dermatology Examination – Look

| What are you looking for or examining? | Justification | Findings and evolving thought process | | | | | |
|---|---|---|---|---|---|---|---|
| Comment on colour | • Erythematous: redness due to increased blood supply.<br>• Erythematous lesions will blanch with pressure<br>• Purpuric lesions: non-blanching reddish/purple discoloration caused by the bursting of small blood vessels into the skin<br>• Pigmented: commonly due to excess melanin; lesions can be benign or malignant<br>• Hypopigmented: loss or absence of melanin, such as conditions including vitiligo<br>The presence of colour variation within a skin lesion is suggestive of malignancy. | Erythematous lesions that blanch with pressure | | | | | |

## Dermatology Examination – Special Techniques

| | | | | | | | |
|---|---|---|---|---|---|---|---|
| Scraping a plaque | If the plaque is psoriatic, it will cause capillary bleeding | No bleeding observed | | | | | |
| Look for Nikolsky's sign | Positive Nikolsky's sign if rubbing of the skin results in exfoliation of the epidermis in blistering diseases, such as toxic epidermal necrolysis or pemphigus vulgaris | No exfoliation observed | | | | | |
| Offer to perform further examination depending on your differential diagnosis | Examine the nails and scalp in psoriasis. Examine the fingers and wrists in scabies. Examine the toe webs in fungal infection. Examine the mouth in lichen planus. Examine regional lymph nodes if suspicion of malignancy | No additional concerns | | | | | |

## Finishing

| | | | | | | | |
|---|---|---|---|---|---|---|---|
| Check patient is comfortable, offer to help reposition her and give the privacy to change | Keeps the patient's dignity | Treating the patient with respect is important | | | | | |
| Remove your gloves and wash hands | Complying with hand hygiene is vital | No additional concerns | | | | | |

### Present Your Findings

Mrs Barton, a 45-year-old woman, has presented with a rash on her scalp and elbows. On examination she looked comfortable at rest. There were small raised red skin lesions on the extensor surfaces of her elbows, and the back of her scalp. There was evidence of excoriations over these areas, consistent with a pruritic rash.

Based on these findings, and her history of coeliac disease which has been poorly controlled of late, I feel the most likely diagnosis is dermatitis herpetiformis, with a differential diagnosis of psoriasis.

To complete my examination, I would like to examine Mrs Barton fully for further skin lesions. For treatment, I would recommend Mrs Barton closely follow a gluten-free diet and, in the meantime, I will prescribe some dapsone for symptomatic relief of pruritus

### General Points

Polite to patient

Maintains good eye contact

Clear instruction and explanation to patient

## ? QUESTIONS FROM THE EXAMINER

**What genes are associated with both dermatitis herpetiformis and coeliac disease?**

HLA-DQ2 or HLA-DQ8.

**What is the single best investigation to confirm a diagnosis of dermatitis herpetiformis?**

Skin biopsy showing deposits of IgA at tips of dermal papillae.

**What are two other forms of autoimmune blistering diseases?**

Bullous pemphigoid and pemphigus vulgaris.

**What further treatment could be considered for Mrs Barton if an improved gluten-free diet did not control her symptoms?**

Dapsone, an antifolate antibiotic, is known to help control itching and rash development.

**What malignancy is thought to be more common in patients with dermatitis herpetiformis and coeliac disease?**

Both dermatitis herpetiformis and coeliac disease are associated with an increased incidence of small-bowel lymphoma.

**What is the precursor lesion to squamous cell carcinoma?**

Actinic keratosis is a premalignant lesion that has the potential to develop into malignant squamous cell carcinoma.

**What type of skin cancer has the highest morality rate?**

Melanoma is considered the most dangerous type of skin cancer, with the highest morality rate and most likely to metastasise.

**What virus is responsible for a shingles rash?**

Human herpesvirus-3, which is also known as herpes zoster.

**What are most common causative organisms for cellulitis?**

*Streptococcus pyogenes* (group A beta-haemolytic streptococci) and *Staphylococcus aureus.*

**What is the mainstay management of necrotising faucitis?**

Urgent surgical debridement of all affected tissue.

## Station 2.22   Haematological

### Doctor Briefing

You are a junior doctor in haematology and have been asked to see, Mrs Hodgkins, a 44-year-old woman, who has been feeling 'under the weather' for the last few weeks. She has lost a considerable amount of weight, bruises more easily than before and has recently been sweating profusely. Please perform a relevant haematological examination on Mrs Hodgkins and present your findings.

### Patient Briefing

You have been feeling increasingly unwell over the past few weeks. Your clothes don't fit as you have lost a lot of weight, and you have trouble sleeping as you feel hot and sweaty. You feel tired all the time. You have also been experiencing back pain and have noticed that your urine looks quite bubbly when you go to the toilet.

You are worried this could be something serious, as you know cancer can cause weight loss.

### Mark Scheme for Examiner

#### Introduction

| | | | |
|---|---|---|---|
| Washes hands, introduces self, confirms patient identity and gains consent for examination | | | |
| Offers a chaperone | | | |
| Appropriately exposes the patient whilst keeping dignity at all times, and repositions into a suitable position for the examination | | | |
| Asks if the patient has any pain currently | | | |

#### General Inspection

| What are you looking for or examining? | Justification | Findings and evolving thought process | | | |
|---|---|---|---|---|---|
| General well-being | On initial glance, does the patient look well, unwell or in pain? | Patient looks in comfortable | | | |
| Obvious clues | Gives an indication of the patient's baseline health | Low BMI. Loose clothing suggestive of weight loss | | | |
| Surroundings | Checks for obvious clues to aid diagnosis or equipment/observations to aid assessment | Patient usually mobilises with stick | | | |

#### Haematological Examination – Inspection

| | | | | | |
|---|---|---|---|---|---|
| Inspect closely for muscle wasting, spider naevi, gynae-comastia, bruising, petechial bleeding, peripheral oedema and general colour | Muscle wasting is seen in chronic diseases or long-standing immobility. Spider naevi or gynaecomastia may indicate liver disease. Bruising or petechial bleeding may indicate clotting disorders, thrombocytopenia or malignancy. Peripheral oedema is a sign of possible liver disease. Colour of the patient could be pallor (anaemia), plethora (polycythaemia) or jaundice (liver disease) | Bruising visible on patients' lower legs and forearms | | | |

**Haematology Examination – Hands**

| What are you looking for or examining? | Justification | Findings and evolving thought process | | | | | |
|---|---|---|---|---|---|---|---|
| Inspect the hands | Pallor of the palm skin creases is seen in anaemia. Telangiectasia suggests hepatic dysfunction. Koilonychia (spoon nails) is seen in iron-deficiency anaemia | Palmar creases appear pale, consistent with anaemia | | | | | |
| Palpate the pulse and CRT | Comment on the rate, rhythm and volume of the radial pulse. There may be sinus tachycardia with anaemia. CRT should be <2 s | Heart rate regular, pulse of 84 bpm, CRT <2 s | | | | | |

**Haematology Examination – Face**

| | | | | | | | |
|---|---|---|---|---|---|---|---|
| Inspect the tongue | Comment on colour and smoothness. Atrophic glossitis or a fissured appearance is associated with vitamin $B_{12}$ deficiency | Tongue appears normal | | | | | |
| Inspect the mouth | Look at the lips for angular stomatitis and telangiectasia. Look at the gum for hypertrophy (associated with leukaemia) or bleeding. Note any petechiae at the buccal mucosa | Bleeding gums noted | | | | | |
| Inspect the tonsils | Enlarged tonsils could imply infection or a palatal or pharyngeal lymphoma | Tonsils appear normal | | | | | |
| Examine the eyes | Inspect the conjunctiva for pallor or jaundice. On fundoscopy, look for haemorrhage, signs of hyperviscosity; for example, engorged veins, papilloedema (secondary to polycythaemia) | No abnormalities noted on fundi examination and inspection of the eye | | | | | |

**Haematology Examination – Lymph Nodes**

| | | | | | | | |
|---|---|---|---|---|---|---|---|
| Palpate lymph nodes | Palpate the neck in sequence: submental, submandibular, deep cervical, preauricular, postauricular, occipital, supraclavicular, infraclavicular nodes. Other lymph nodes to consider include the epitrochlear, axillary, inguinal and femoral nodes. Assess the size and consistency. If it is hard, like pressing your forehead, consider malignancy (lymphoma less likely). If the lymph node feels rubbery, like pressing the end of your nose, consider malignancy (especially lymphoma). If it is soft, like pressing your lips, most likely associated with infection. Note any tenderness | No palpable or tender lymph nodes | | | | | |

## Haematology Examination – Abdominal Exam

| What are you looking for or examining? | Justification | Findings and evolving thought process | | | |
|---|---|---|---|---|---|
| Examine the abdomen | Palpate the abdomen for tenderness. Look for abdominal distension, which can suggest ascites or liver pathology. Check for shifting dullness, which suggests ascites | No tenderness or distension | | | |
| Percuss and palpate for the spleen and liver | Hepatosplenomegaly suggests lymphoproliferative or myeloproliferative disease. Hepatomegaly is smooth and/or non-tender in haematological disease and common causes include lymphoma and leukaemia | No evidence of hepatomegaly or splenomegaly | | | |

## Haematology Examination – Legs

| | | | | | |
|---|---|---|---|---|---|
| Inspect the legs | Check the peripheral circulation and note any associated gangrene (toes). Also examine for pitting oedema, from lymphatic obstruction | No additional concerns | | | |

## Finishing

| | | | | | |
|---|---|---|---|---|---|
| Check patient is comfortable, offer to help reposition her and give the privacy to change | Keeps the patient's dignity | Treating the patient with respect is important | | | |
| Remove your gloves and wash hands | Complying with hand hygiene is vital | No additional concerns | | | |

## Present Your Findings

Mrs Hodgkins is a 44-year-old woman presenting with lethargy, weight loss, bruising and sweating. On examination, she is comfortable at rest, and is underweight. There is bruising on her lower legs and forearms. She has pallor of the palmar creases, and bleeding gums. There was no evidence of palpable or tender lymph nodes, or hepatosplenomegaly.

I feel the most likely diagnosis is multiple myeloma, with differentials being another form of malignancy or anaemia.

To complete my examination, I would like to take bloods (including FBCs, creatinine, albumin, bone profile). I would also examine the joints, dipstick the urine and request a CXR

## General Points

| | | | | |
|---|---|---|---|---|
| Polite to patient | | | | |
| Maintains good eye contact | | | | |
| Clear instruction and explanation to patient | | | | |

## ❓ QUESTIONS FROM THE EXAMINER

### What is the definition of thrombocytopenia?

Low platelet count ($< 150 \times 10^9$/L).

## Why would a patient with multiple myeloma have 'foamy' urine?

Foamy or bubbly urine in these patients is caused by Bence Jones proteinuria.

## What is the main diagnostic criteria for multiple myeloma?

≥ 10% clonal plasma cells on bone marrow biopsy.

## Would you expect this patient to have proteinuria on dipstick?

No, as a urine dipstick test will only detect raised levels of albumin. In multiple myeloma, it is paraproteins produced by malignancy cells that lead to increased levels of protein.

## What type of leukaemia most commonly affects young children?

Acute lymphoblastic leukaemia.

## What bleeding disorder is a result of clotting factor IX deficiency?

Deficiency of clotting factor IX is known as haemophilia B, or Christmas disease.

## How is sickle cell anaemia inherited?

Sickle cell anaemia is an autosomal-recessive condition, which means an affected individual must inherit a mutated copy of the gene from each parent.

## What genetic abnormality is found in most cases of chronic myeloid leukaemia?

The translocation of sections of chromosome 9 and 22, known as the Philadelphia chromosome.

## What is the most common cause of megaloblastic anaemia?

Vitamin $B_{12}$ and/or folate deficiency.

## What are the symptoms of hypercalcaemia?

Patients with hypercalcaemia may experience bone pain, abdominal pain, polyuria, muscle weakness, cardiac dysrhythmias and anxiety.

## Station 2.23  Ear

### Doctor Briefing

You are a junior doctor in primary care and have been asked to see, Mrs Mason, an 82-year-old woman, who has presented with worsening hearing. Please perform a relevant hearing examination on Mrs Mason and present your findings.

### Patient Briefing

You have noticed that your hearing has been worse over the past few weeks. You feel it is worse in your right ear, compared to your left. You recently were unable to hear a high-pitched fire alarm, which was very concerning for you. You have also noticed a faint ringing in your right ear when it is otherwise quiet.

You were recently admitted to hospital with an infection that required you to stay in and have antibiotics and get bloods taken every day, but you are now feeling better. You have no other health problems.

You are concerned about whether you will need a hearing aid.

### Mark Scheme for Examiner

#### Introduction

| | | | | |
|---|---|---|---|---|
| Washes hands, introduces self, confirms patient identity and gains consent for examination | | | | |
| Offers a chaperone | | | | |
| Appropriately exposes the patient whilst keeping dignity at all times, and repositions into a suitable position for the examination | | | | |
| Asks if the patient has any pain currently | | | | |

#### General Inspection

| What are you looking for or examining? | Justification | Findings and evolving thought process | | | |
|---|---|---|---|---|---|
| General well-being | On initial glance, does the patient look well, unwell or in pain? | Patient looks conformable at rest | | | |
| Obvious clues | Gives an indication of the patient's baseline health | Patient looks generally well, normal body habitus | | | |
| Surroundings | Checks for obvious clues to aid diagnosis or equipment/observations to aid assessment | Patient uses a stick to mobilise. No hearing aids visible | | | |

#### Ear Examination – External Ear

| | | | | | |
|---|---|---|---|---|---|
| Inspect the preauricular area and pinna | Look for an endaural incision scar (suggests previous ear surgery). Comment on any lesions seen | No lesions or scars indicative of surgery | | | |
| Inspect the postauricular area | Look for postauricular incision scar suggesting previous surgery, such as mastoid surgery | No scars noted | | | |
| Palpate the postauricular area | Feel for a cochlear implant (Bone Anchored Hearing Aids (BAHA) abutment may be palpable here). Assess the mastoid area for tenderness (mastoiditis). Lymphadenopathy may be associated with an ear infection; for example, otitis media, otitis externa | No tenderness or hearing devices | | | |

## Ear Examination – Auditory Meatus and Tympanic Membrane

| What are you looking for or examining? | Justification | Findings and evolving thought process | | | | | |
|---|---|---|---|---|---|---|---|
| Select the appropriately sized speculum | 4-mm: safer (less likelihood of damaging the ear canal and drum) and greater visibility. 3-mm: paediatrics or for a small ear canal | 4-mm speculum for adults | | | | | |
| Correctly hold and position the otoscope | Grip the otoscope like a pencil. For the right ear use the right hand and for the left ear use the left hand. Hold the otoscope by placing your little finger on the patient's zygoma. This acts as an anchor, preventing damage if sudden head movements occur. Elevate the pinna upwards and backwards with your free hand. You may also ask the patient to tilt her head away from you. Put the speculum on the back of the tragus, under direct vision and then slowly insert the speculum whilst looking through the earpiece | Correct technique applied when using the otoscope | | | | | |
| Comment on the ear canal and tympanic membrane | In the ear canal, look for wax (impaction can cause hearing loss), dry skin and foreign objects such as cotton buds that may be causing irritation. Redness and discharge may suggest an infection (otitis externa or otitis media with eardrum perforation). A healthy tympanic membrane should appear translucent and pink-grey. If there an abnormality, describe whether it involves the pars flaccida or pars tensa. Describe what quadrant it is in. In general, the tympanic membrane is about 1 cm diameter. Describe the size of any perforation | A small amount of earwax is visible in both ears. No redness or discharge. Translucent and pale tympanic membrane bilaterally, with no sign of infection or perforation | | | | | |

## Ear Examination – Hearing

| | | | | | | | |
|---|---|---|---|---|---|---|---|
| Perform the whisper test | This is a crude bedside method of establishing hearing levels. Remember to start with the 'better' side first. With one hand, obscure the entrance to the contralateral ear canal by rubbing the tragus gently. This will muffle this ear and ensure that you are only testing one ear at a time. Cover the patient's eyes so that she cannot lip read. Ensure that you are at full arm's length. Whisper a combination of a number and a letter; for example, 'N4', and ask the patient to repeat what you are saying. Get increasingly louder until they can hear you | Patient able to hear voice at whisper level bilaterally | | | | | |

## Ear Examination – Hearing

| What are you looking for or examining? | Justification | Findings and evolving thought process | | | | | |
|---|---|---|---|---|---|---|---|
| Perform Rinne's tuning fork test | Tap a 512-Hertz (Hz) tuning fork on your elbow (not on a hard surface). Check that you have made the tuning fork ring by placing it next to your own ear first. Place it in the following two positions and ask where the patient hears it loudest: • Position 1: on the mastoid process • Position 2: in front of the ear canal Rinne's positive is when air conduction is greater than bone conduction (louder in front of ear than on mastoid process). This may suggest normal hearing or sensorineural deafness. Rinne's negative is when bone conduction is greater than air conduction (louder on mastoid process than in front of ear). This may suggest conductive deafness | Rinne's positive (right ear), air conduction is greater than bone conduction | | | | | |
| Perform Weber's tuning fork test | Tap the tuning fork as before and place the base on the vertex of the head or forehead. Support the patient's head with your other hand. Ask the patient where they hear the sound loudest: In normal hearing or symmetrical loss, sound is heard in the midline, equally in both ears. In sensorineural deafness, sound is loudest in the less-affected ear. In conductive deafness, sound is loudest in affected ear | Sound heard loudest in left ear, consistent with sensorineural hearing loss | | | | | |

## Finishing

| | | | | | | | |
|---|---|---|---|---|---|---|---|
| Check patient is comfortable, offer to help reposition her and give the privacy to change | Keeps the patient's dignity | Treating the patient with respect is important | | | | | |
| Remove your gloves and wash hands | Complying with hand hygiene is vital | No additional concerns | | | | | |

## Present Your Findings

Mrs Mason is an 85-year-old woman presenting with worsening hearing, and tinnitus in her right ear. On examination of the external ear, there are no pinnal lesions or scars. She wears no hearing aids or implant devices. On examination of the external auditory meatus and tympanic membrane, she has bilateral dry ears with no mastoid cavities. Her tympanic membranes look healthy bilaterally. Whispering test was normal in both ears. There was lateralisation to the left ear on Weber's test and Rinne's test was positive, suggesting sensorineural hearing loss.

Based on the history and examination, I feel the most likely diagnosis is sensorineural hearing loss secondary to ototoxic medications, with alternative differentials being other causes of sensorineural hearing loss, such as presbyacusis.

To complete my examination, I would like to perform a pure-tone audiogram and a tympanogram and examine the facial nerve.

| General Points | | | |
|---|---|---|---|
| Polite to patient | | | |
| Maintains good eye contact | | | |
| Clear instruction and explanation to patient | | | |

## ❓ QUESTIONS FROM THE EXAMINER

### What is presbycusis?

Presbycusis is sensorineural hearing loss that occurs due to progressive irreversible damage to hair cells of the organ of Corti, due to age.

### Why are children with Down syndrome at increased risk of otitis media with effusion?

Eustachian tube dysfunction is more common in these patients.

### How would a case of acute mastoiditis be managed?

Immediate empirical antibiotics (such as levofloxacin or ceftriaxone) and consider surgical debridement or myringotomy. Severe or refractory cases may require mastoidectomy.

### Ototoxicity is a well-known side effect of which type of antibiotic?

Systemic aminoglycosides, the most common of which is gentamicin, are associated with ototoxicity.

### What are the names of the middle-ear ossicles?

The malleus, incus and stapes.

### Which muscles attach to the ossicles of the middle ear?

The tensor tympani and the stapedius.

### Where do you expect to find the cone of light on otoscopy?

In a healthy tympanic membrane, the cone-shaped reflection of light will be seen in the anterior inferior quadrant.

### What pattern of hearing loss would you expect in a patient with acoustic neuroma at the left cerebellopontine angle?

This would present clinically as unilateral sensorineural hearing loss of the left ear, Rinne's positive (right ear) and Weber's positive (left ear).

### Which cranial nerve is responsible for hearing and balance?

Cranial nerve VIII, the vestibulocochlear nerve.

### What is the most common causative organism for necrotising otitis externa?

*Pseudomonas*.

# Orthopaedic Examinations

**3**

## Outline

## Station 3.1 Cervical Spine

### Doctor Briefing

You are a junior doctor working in orthopaedics and have been asked to see Leanne Jamieson, a 68-year-old woman, who has been referred by her primary care physician with a stiff and painful neck. She is also complaining of headaches in the back of her head. Please examine Mrs Jamieson's cervical spine and then present your findings.

### Patient Briefing

You have a stiff and painful neck that has been getting worse for several weeks, with pain that goes to your shoulders and the back of your head. The stiffness in your neck is worse when waking up, but it improves in less than an hour. However, it gets worse when you are out and about during the day, and you need to take breaks when reading or cooking to rest your neck, and this helps relieve the pain slightly.

You normally get around fine, apart from occasional pain in your knees the past few years, which you assume is down to getting older, as it is mostly when you have had an active day. You haven't had any numbness, tingling or weakness in your legs.

You saw a doctor who said you had symptoms that warranted further investigation. You are concerned because you don't know why you are experiencing neck pain as you don't remember injuring or straining it, and the pain hasn't improved.

### Mark Scheme for Examiner

| Introduction | | |
|---|---|---|
| Washes hands, introduces self, confirms patient identity and gains consent for examination | | |
| Ensures a chaperone is present | | |
| Appropriately exposes the patient's spine whilst keeping dignity at all times, and repositions into a suitable position for the examination | | |
| Asks if the patient has any pain currently | | |

| General Inspection | | | |
|---|---|---|---|
| **What are you looking for or examining?** | **Justification** | **Findings and evolving thought process** | |
| General well-being | On initial glance, does the patient look well/unwell/in pain? | The patient looks comfortable at rest | |

| General Inspection | | | | | | | |
|---|---|---|---|---|---|---|---|
| **What are you looking for or examining?** | **Justification** | **Findings and evolving thought process** | | | | | |
| Obvious clues | Gives an indication of the patient's baseline health | Patient looks generally well, normal body habitus | | | | | |
| Surroundings | Look to see if the patient uses any mobility aids or supportive equipment | No mobility aids | | | | | |

| Orthopaedic Examination – Look | | | | | | | |
|---|---|---|---|---|---|---|---|
| Inspects from the front, side and back<br><br>Closer inspection of the neck | Look for scars. Longitudinal midline posterior scars or transverse scars adjacent to the midline anteriorly are indicative of previous surgery.<br>Assess for muscle wasting, as seen in nerve injury or chronic inactivity.<br>Check for normal cervical lordosis, lumbar kyphosis and thoracic kyphosis. Loss of cervical lordosis (best seen from the side) is commonly due to muscle spasm.<br>Assess for skin changes, including any lumps or swellings, such as enlarged posterior cervical lymph nodes, which may indicate infection or malignancy | Loss of cervical lordosis, which would be consistent with muscle spasm associated with pain | | | | | |

| Orthopaedic Examination – Feel | | | | | | | |
|---|---|---|---|---|---|---|---|
| Ask the patient if she has any pain and start palpation away from the pain. Observe the reactions on the patient's face at all times | Allows accurate assessment of pain and minimises discomfort/shock | Patient complains of diffuse pain around her lower neck, radiating to her shoulders. Commence palpation away from the site of pain | | | | | |
| Palpate the spine with the patient standing | Palpate along the midline starting from the occiput and moving downwards, looking for alignment and tenderness. The cervical spine from C2 downwards is palpable.<br>Palpate 2.5 cm lateral to the spinous processes to assess for facet joint tenderness. The joints between C5 and C6 are those most often affected by osteoarthritis.<br>Palpate the paraspinal and trapezius muscles for tension, spasm or tenderness.<br>Palpate above the clavicle for a cervical rib.<br>Feel for crepitus on flexion and extension, seen in osteoarthritis | Tenderness elicited at the facet joints at C5 and C6. Crepitus on flexion and extension of the neck at this level is consistent with cervical osteoarthritis | | | | | |

## Orthopaedic Examination – Move

| What are you looking for or examining? | Justification | Findings and evolving thought process | | | | | |
|---|---|---|---|---|---|---|---|
| Assess the cervical spine movement with the patient sitting | Do not move if cervical spine injury is suspected.<br>• Flexion: the patient should be able to touch her chin to her chest. Normal is 80°. Chin–chest distance can be measured<br>• Extension: ask the patient to tilt her head back. Normal is 50°, and the plane of the nose and forehead should be almost horizontal<br>• Rotation: ask the patient to turn her head to the side. The chin normally falls just short of the plane of the shoulders. Normal is 80°<br>• Lateral flexion: the patient should nearly be able to touch the ear on to her shoulder. Normal is 45°.<br>Note any reduced movements. If there is pain on active movement, examine passive movement further | No indication of cervical spine injury, so you can proceed with examination.<br>Patient describes pain at the back of the lower neck that radiates to her shoulder at extremes of movement. Restricted range of movement both actively and passively. Consistent with osteoarthritis | | | | | |

## Orthopaedic Examination – Special Tests

| | | | | | | | |
|---|---|---|---|---|---|---|---|
| Perform Lhermitte's test | Positive result if patient experiences electric shock-like sensations in the spine or limbs on neck flexion.<br>Can be caused by multiple sclerosis, myelopathy from cervical spondylosis, vitamin $B_{12}$ deficiency or whiplash injury | Negative Lhermitte's test | | | | | |
| Gait assessment | Gait disturbance and ataxia can be seen in patients with cervical myelopathy | Patient's gait is unremarkable | | | | | |
| Neurovascular assessment | Perform a neurological examination of the limbs, looking for any lower or upper motor neurone signs | No reduction in sensation or weakness noted | | | | | |
| Offers to perform rectal examination and to palpate and percuss the bladder | Assessment of anal tone.<br>Determine whether loss of sharp/crude sensation restricted in perianal region.<br>Assessment of urinary retention.<br>If absent/reduced anal tone, or features of urinary retention, consider cord compression | Anal tone present, and perianal sensation intact. Non-palpable bladder. No evidence of spinal cord compression | | | | | |

## Finishing

| | | | | | | | |
|---|---|---|---|---|---|---|---|
| Check patient is comfortable, offer to help reposition her and give privacy to change | Keeps the patient's dignity | Treating the patient with respect is important | | | | | |
| Remove your gloves and wash hands | Complying with hand hygiene is vital | No additional concerns | | | | | |

**Present Your Findings**

Mrs Jamieson is a 68-year-old woman who presented with a stiff and painful neck.

On examination she looks comfortable at rest. She has tenderness and crepitus on palpation of the C5–6 facet joints. Both active and passive movements were limited. Her neurovascular examination was unremarkable, as was her gait. Lhermitte's test was negative. There was no indication of cauda equina or a cervical rib.

I feel the most likely diagnosis is cervical osteoarthritis, with differential diagnosis being chronic disc degeneration.

To complete my examination, I would like to examine Mrs Jamieson's shoulders, hips and knees, as she complained of similar knee pain. I would perform X-rays of the cervical spine and other affected joints to assess for osteoarthritis. Initial management for Mrs Jamieson would involve analgesia and physiotherapy. If pain continues for a further 3 months, referral to pain clinic would be advised

**General Points**

Polite to patient

Maintains good eye contact

Clear instruction and explanation to patient

# ❓ QUESTIONS FROM THE EXAMINER

### What is the recommended modality of imaging used to assess spinal cord compression?

Magnetic resonance imaging (MRI). Plain X-rays and computed tomography (CT) are suitable alternatives in acute traumatic spinal cord injury.

### What is the approach taken in trauma situations with a possible cervical spine injury?

In any patient with suspected cervical spine injury, use a prioritising approach (such as ABCDE), and keep the patient's spine immobilised. This includes keeping the patient's cervical spine in line whilst assessing the airway, and log rolling the patient to expose her fully.

### What airway manoeuvres can be performed in a patient with suspected cervical spine injury and why?

If you are concerned about a patient's airway, perform a jaw thrust instead of a head tilt, chin lift, as this involves less movement of the cervical vertebrae.

### What are the common differential diagnoses for neck pain associated with a history of trauma or strain?

Vertebral fracture, whiplash and acute intervertebral prolapse should all be considered when a patient presents with neck pain postinjury.

### How can cervical rib contribute to cold hands and weak pulse?

Overdevelopment of the seventh cervical vertebra can affect the subclavian artery, causing thoracic outlet syndrome. This is tested directly by palpating the radial pulse and then applying traction on the arm for several seconds. Reduction of radial pulsation after this manoeuvre suggests the presence of cervical rib.

### How would you confirm whether a patient with suspected spinal cord compression was in urinary retention?

Feel for a palpable bladder and perform a bladder scan pre- and postvoiding to assess for bladder emptying.

### What is the management of chronic disc degeneration?

Encourage the patient to perform exercises to ease symptoms. Consider muscle relaxants or other medication if the patient is experiencing chronic pain. Surgery may be considered in patients who present with cervical radiculopathy or cervical myelopathy to prevent worsening of symptoms.

## What is the management of cauda equina syndrome?

Cauda equina syndrome is a medical emergency and, if proven, needs emergency surgical decompression by the neurosurgical team

## If you thought the patient's gait was abnormal, what would you do?

Perform a full neurological examination (upper limb, lower limb, cranial nerves) as well as completing gait, arms, legs and spine (GALS) assessment.

## What are the different upper and lower motor neurone signs to cover when assessing patients?

Lower motor neurone signs include hypotonia, muscle wasting, fasciculations and hyporeflexia. Upper motor neurone signs include hypertonia, muscle weakness, upgoing plantar reflex and hyperreflexia.

## Station 3.2    Thoracolumbar Spine

### Doctor Briefing

You are a junior doctor working in orthopaedics and have been asked to see Simon MacPherson, an 85-year-old man, who has recently developed back pain. He is known to have prostate cancer. Please examine his thoracolumbar spine and present your findings.

### Patient Briefing

For the past 3 weeks, you have been experiencing sudden back pain when standing up from a chair or on bending forward. The pain is central and radiates to the sides. It is worse after a long day on your feet and has stopped you from doing daily activities that you enjoy, such as gardening and cooking, where you now need help due to the pain. The pain is not improving on rest and has not been relieved by any massages or compression. There is no reduced range of movement. You saw the general practitioner (GP) who said you had symptoms that warranted further investigation due to your prostate cancer.

You are concerned because you don't know why you are experiencing back pain as you have not injured yourself and are worried that this is a sign of cancer progression.

### Mark Scheme for Examiner

#### Introduction

| | | |
|---|---|---|
| Washes hands, introduces self, confirms patient identity and gains consent for examination | | |
| Ensures a chaperone is present | | |
| Appropriately exposes the patient's hands, wrists and elbows whilst keeping dignity at all times, and repositions into a suitable position for the examination | | |
| Asks if the patient has any pain currently | | |

#### General Inspection

| What are you looking for or examining? | Justification | Findings and evolving thought process | | | |
|---|---|---|---|---|---|
| General well-being | On initial glance, does the patient look well/unwell/in pain? Does the patient appear frail? | The patient looks unwell and in pain whilst sitting at rest. He is pale, and his clothes are loose. You are clinically concerned | | | |
| Any obvious signs | Look for symmetrical or asymmetrical changes, suggested by shoulder asymmetry or pelvic tilt. Any other signs, such as bruising or swelling, muscle wasting and any lumps that may indicate trauma or irregularity, should be considered | No other apparent signs or asymmetry noted on inspection | | | |
| Surroundings | Look to see if the patient uses any walking aids. Does the patient have a cannula and fluids or medication running? Is he attached to an observation monitor? | The patient uses a walking stick | | | |

## Orthopaedic Examination – Look

| What are you looking for or examining? | Justification | Findings and evolving thought process | | | | | |
|---|---|---|---|---|---|---|---|
| Inspect from the front, side and back | Observe the posture or position of the back. Check whether the shoulders, hips, knees and ankles are parallel. Note any obvious asymmetrical changes, such as winged scapula, suggestive of long thoracic nerve injury | No indication of abnormal posture or position. Comment on normal lordosis (or loss) | | | | | |
| Inspect the back | Notes any scars (location, size) from previous surgery, skin changes (such as café-au-lait spots, suggestive of neurofibromatosis and fat pad or hairy patches, suggestive of spina bifida), muscle spasm or wasting. Assess patient's thoracic, lumbar and lateral curvatures. Increased thoracic kyphosis is suggestive of osteoporosis. Lateral curvature is a sign of scoliosis | Currently, no evidence that the patient has had previous surgery or any visible pathology. The patient has mild thoracic kyphosis and flattening of lumbar lordosis. No sign of abnormal lateral curvature | | | | | |
| Repeat inspection with the patient standing with his back against the wall | Check that the heels, pelvis, shoulders and occiput can lean against the wall simultaneously. This is difficult in patients with increased thoracic kyphosis | The patient has difficulty standing up from the seat and walking to the wall, due to pain | | | | | |

## Orthopaedic Examination – Feel

| | | | | | | | |
|---|---|---|---|---|---|---|---|
| Ask the patient if he has any pain and start palpation away from the pain. Observe the reaction on the patient's face at all times | Allows accurate assessment of pain and minimises discomfort/shock | The patient locates the pain to the centre of his lower back, the L4 vertebra, and complains of diffuse pain around this area and to the sides of his back. Commence palpation away from the site of pain | | | | | |
| Feel for spinous processes | Palpate along midline for tenderness from T1 to the sacrum | No indication of tenderness | | | | | |
| Feel for sacroiliac joints | Palpate lateral to spinous process for tenderness | No indication of tenderness | | | | | |
| Feel for muscles | Palpate paraspinal muscles for tenderness | The patient complains of generalised pain in paraspinal muscles in the region of L3–L5 vertebrae | | | | | |

**Orthopaedic Examination – Percussion**

| What are you looking for or examining? | Justification | Findings and evolving thought process | | | | | |
|---|---|---|---|---|---|---|---|
| Percuss the spine | Percuss the spine lightly starting from the top of the neck towards the sacrum. Significant pain is associated with infection, malignancy and fractures | No indication of significant pain on percussion of the spine | | | | | |

**Orthopaedic Examination – Move**

| | | | | | | | |
|---|---|---|---|---|---|---|---|
| Instruct the patient to flex, extend, rotate and laterally flex his back | Note any reduced active movements or pain on movement, which is suggestive of spinal pathology | No reduced active movements. The patient complains of sudden pain with every movement, particularly on extension and rotation | | | | | |

**Orthopaedic Examination – Special Tests**

| | | | | | | | |
|---|---|---|---|---|---|---|---|
| Perform straight-leg raise | Elicit whether a positive test is present by noting pain in the entire lower limb while keeping patient's legs straight flexed at the hip as he lies back. A positive test suggests pathology in L4, L5, S1 nerve roots (sciatic nerve) and therefore, L4/5, L5/S1 and S1/S2 intervertebral spaces, suggestive of lumbar disc prolapse | Pain is reported in thigh and leg on the assessment of both legs | | | | | |
| Perform tibial stretch test | With the patient lying on his back, flexing knee and hip, then extending the knee, press over both hamstring tendons and then the middle of the popliteal fossa. A positive finding is with pain in popliteal fossa but not when hamstring tendons are pressed, suggesting tibial nerve involvement in L4–S3 nerve roots | No reported pain on pressing hamstring tendons or popliteal fossa | | | | | |
| Perform femoral stretch test | With the patient lying on his front, flex his knee and maximally extend the hip. A positive finding is noted with pain in the back or pain radiating down the anterior thigh | No reported pain on maximal extension of the hip | | | | | |
| Perform a gait assessment by asking the patient to walk to the door and back | Note any gait disturbance or ataxia. Difficulty with tiptoe and heel walking suggests S1 and L5 weakness, respectively | Gait is unremarkable | | | | | |

## Orthopaedic Examination – Neurovascular Assessment

| What are you looking for or examining? | Justification | Findings and evolving thought process | | | | |
|---|---|---|---|---|---|---|
| Neurovascular assessment | Note reduced sensation and weakness of the lower limbs, reflexes and pain on myotome assessment | The patient complains of pain on movement of lower limbs during the assessment of hip flexion. No reported reduced sensations and reflexes present | | | | |
| Offer to perform rectal examination | Assessment of anal tone and for saddle anaesthesia is important to rule out cord compression | No evidence of reduced anal tone or evidence of saddle anaesthesia | | | | |

## Finishing

| | | | | | | |
|---|---|---|---|---|---|---|
| Check patient is comfortable, offer to help reposition him and give the privacy to change | Keeps the patient's dignity | Treating the patient with respect is important | | | | |
| Wash hands | Complying with hand hygiene is vital | No additional concerns | | | | |

## Present Your Findings

Mr Simon MacPherson is an 85-year-old man who presented with back pain. On examination, he looks uncomfortable at rest with sudden pain on standing in his lower back, at approximately T4/T5 level. On neurovascular examination, pain on myotome assessment was noted with no reduced sensation or absence of reflexes. Positive findings during the straight-leg raise test of both legs. There was pain on passive and active movement of the back. No concern for cord compression.

My main diagnosis is pathological fracture due to the patient's medical history, with the differential diagnosis being degenerative disc disease, such as osteoarthritis, and I would like to rule out cord compression in view of his risks.

I would like to examine Mr MacPherson's hip, shoulders and cervical spine. I would also perform X-rays of the thoracolumbar spine to assess for disc degeneration and fracture. Initial management would involve analgesia and occupational therapy support, with discussion with an oncologist to rule out pathological fracture due to metastasis

## General Points

| | | | | |
|---|---|---|---|---|
| Polite to patient | | | | |
| Maintains good eye contact | | | | |
| Clear instruction and explanation to the patient | | | | |

##  QUESTIONS FROM THE EXAMINER

### What is the typical presentation of a patient with cauda equina syndrome?

The patient would be complaining of severe back pain, associated with lower motor neurone weakness, flaccid tone and loss of reflexes bilaterally. There may be absent plantar reflexes, with perianal or saddle anaesthesia. The patient may present with bladder, bowel or sexual dysfunction.

### How many phases of gait are there and what are they?

There are six phases: heel strike, foot flat, mid-stance, heel-off, toe-off and swing.

### What are some extra-articular symptoms of ankylosing spondylarthritis?

Anterior uveitis, psoriasis and inflammatory bowel disease.

### What are likely examination findings for metastatic spinal cord compression?

You may find upper motor neurone weakness, upgoing plantar, brisk reflexes bilaterally in lower limbs and increased tone in lower limbs.

### What is a pathological fracture?

A break in the bone that was not caused by injury or trauma, commonly caused by bone weakening due to disease.

### What are some causes of a pathological fracture?

This includes osteoporosis, osteomalacia, benign bone tumours and cysts and primary or secondary malignant bone tumour.

### What is the management for spinal fractures?

The majority of fractures will heal with analgesia, rest and a back brace to limit motion. X-rays are taken regularly to monitor the progress of healing.

### What are the important questions to elicit in a patient presenting with back pain?

Ask the patient to describe the back pain using SOCRATES (site, onset, character, radiation, associated symptoms, time, exacerbating and/or alleviating symptoms and severity) and if it's associated with stiffness or sciatica. Neurological symptoms such as pain, numbness and weakness in the lower limbs should be explored.

### What are the red flags for back pain?

These include urinary or faecal retention or incontinence, bilateral leg pain, decreased anal tone, saddle anaesthesia, infection or cancer in a patient under the age of 16 or older than 55, weight loss, fever, night sweats and trauma.

### What investigations are useful for assessment of a patient with back pain?

Bedside tests may not be directly relevant. Blood tests investigating infection or inflammatory markers may be useful to rule out differentials for back pain. Imaging is the main form, and an MRI scan is the recommended modality.

## Station 3.3    Shoulder

### Doctor Briefing

You are a junior doctor working in orthopaedics and have been asked to see Stephen O'Humeral, a 50-year-old non-binary person complaining of pain in and around their right shoulder. The pain is worse when trying to reach into his kitchen cupboards, and he has now been referred in by his primary care physician. Please examine Stephen's shoulder and present your findings.

### Patient Briefing

You started getting pain in your right shoulder 2 week ago, when you woke up you found it difficult to move your right arm. The pain is dull but constant and intense, and it is keeping you up at night. You have rested your shoulder since the pain began, but this hasn't helped. Your general health is good, and your only past medical history is diabetes, for which you take metformin.

You are concerned because the pain has not disappeared and you are worried it is something serious.

### Mark Scheme for Examiner

#### Introduction

| | | | | |
|---|---|---|---|---|
| Washes hands, introduces self, confirms patient identity and gains consent for examination | | | | |
| Ensures a chaperone is present | | | | |
| Appropriately exposes the patient's shoulders whilst keeping dignity at all times, and repositions into a suitable position for the examination | | | | |
| Asks if the patient has any pain currently | | | | |

#### General

| What are you looking for or examining? | Justification | Findings and evolving thought process | | | |
|---|---|---|---|---|---|
| General well-being | On initial glance, does the patient look well/unwell/in pain? | Patient looks comfortable at rest | | | |
| Obvious clues | Gives an indication of the patient's baseline health | Patient looks generally well, normal body habitus | | | |
| Surroundings | Look to see if the patient uses any mobility aids | No mobility aids | | | |

#### Orthopaedic Examination – Look

| | | | | | |
|---|---|---|---|---|---|
| Inspect from the front, side and back<br><br>Closer inspection of shoulder | Look for deformity, such as loss of normal contour of the deltoid muscle, or acromion prominence anteriorly or posteriorly seen in dislocation.<br>Assess for swelling, which is suggestive of inflammatory or infective pathology. Scars may indicate previous surgery or trauma to joint.<br>Assess for muscle wasting in the deltoid, pectoralis, supraspinatus and infraspinatus muscles, as seen in nerve injury or chronic inactivity.<br>Assess the scapula for winging, which would suggest long thoracic nerve palsy | No stigmata of shoulder pathology noted | | | |

| Orthopaedic Examination – Feel | | | | | | | |
|---|---|---|---|---|---|---|---|
| **What are you looking for or examining?** | **Justification** | **Findings and evolving thought process** | | | | | |
| Ask the patient if he has any pain and start palpation away from the pain. Observe the reaction on the patient's face at all times | Allows accurate assessment of pain and minimises discomfort/shock | Commence palpation away from the site of pain | | | | | |
| Assess temperature | Feel at the clavicle, acromioclavicular joint, scapular spine and biceps tendon, comparing both sides | Uniform and normal temperature around the shoulder | | | | | |
| Palpate the shoulder joint | Assess for tenderness, bony abnormalities, swelling and deformity at the:<br>• Sternoclavicular joint<br>• Clavicle<br>• Acromion<br>• Coracoid<br>• Scapular spine<br>• Biceps tendon<br>• Supraspinous tendon | No tenderness on palpation | | | | | |
| Palpate surrounding muscles, subacromial space and greater tuberosity | Assess for any tenderness | | | | | | |

| Orthopaedic Examination – Move | | | | | | | |
|---|---|---|---|---|---|---|---|
| Assess the cervical spine | Ask the patient to:<br>• Nod his head back and forth<br>• Look left, then right<br>• Try to touch his ear to each shoulder<br>Shoulder pain can be referred from neck pathology | No cervical spine pain noted | | | | | |
| Assess shoulder function | Ask the patient to perform:<br>• External rotation and abduction: put his hands up to his mouth, and then behind his head<br>• Internal rotation and adduction: ask patient to place each hand on his lower back, and then reach up his spine<br>• Circular 'stirring' movements with each upper limb | Patient is able to conduct compound movements of external rotation with abduction, and internal rotation with adduction but pain throughout movement | | | | | |

**Orthopaedic Examination – Move**

| What are you looking for or examining? | Justification | Findings and evolving thought process | | | | | | |
|---|---|---|---|---|---|---|---|---|
| Assess shoulder movements – actively and passively | Ask the patient to perform:<br>• Flexion: point his arms towards the celling. Normal is 0–180°<br>• Extension: stretch his arms out behind himself. Normal is 0–60°<br>• Abduction: raise his arms out to the side and up (normal is 0–150°), while the examiner palpates the inferior pole of the scapula with one hand<br>• Adduction: bring his arms down and across his body. Normal 0–30°<br>• External rotation: ask the patient to rotate his arm outwards, keeping the elbow flexed and by the side of the body<br>• Internal rotation: put his arm behind his back and move the thumb up the vertebrae, recording the highest level that can be touched. Normal is mid thoracic level.<br>• Passively move shoulder joint through the same movements, assessing for crepitus and pain, with one hand over the shoulder joint | Reduction of both passive and active movement globally, particularly external rotation.<br>No crepitus detected.<br>Clinical suspicion of frozen shoulder | | | | | | |

**Orthopaedic Examination – Special Tests**

| | | | | | | | | |
|---|---|---|---|---|---|---|---|---|
| Assess rotator cuff muscles | Each muscle of the rotator cuff needs to be assessed, so conduct special tests to isolate each one. Positive findings are loss of power and pain, which suggests a muscle injury/tear, or tendonitis respectively.<br>• Supraspinatus: Jobe's test is shoulder abduction against resistance with the thumb pointing downwards. Assess the first 15° of shoulder abduction against resistance<br>• Infraspinatus and teres minor: assess external rotation against resistance, with elbows flexed to 90°and arms adducted<br>• Subscapularis: perform Gerber's lift-off test by asking the patient to lift his hands off his back (internal rotation) against resistance | Resistance to external rotation. Other movements completed.<br>Pain on movement globally; no specific pathology identified | | | | | | |
| Perform impingement test | Assess for painful arc by asking the patient to passively abduct the shoulder and then release, then ask the patient to adduct it slowly. Positive when the patient has pain on abduction, usually between 60° and 120°.<br>Pain during the entire movement is indicative of a glenohumeral pathology; for example, osteoarthritis or frozen shoulder | Pain throughout entire movement | | | | | | |
| Perform scarf test | Ask the patient to place his hand on the opposite shoulder and apply force posteriorly over his flexed elbow.<br>Pain indicates acromioclavicular joint pathology | Pain globally. No evidence of specific acromioclavicular joint pathology | | | | | | |

**Orthopaedic Examination – Special Tests**

| What are you looking for or examining? | Justification | Findings and evolving thought process | | | | | |
|---|---|---|---|---|---|---|---|
| Assess for bicipital tendonitis | Supinate the forearm and flex the shoulder against resistance. Loss of power suggests a tear. Pain suggests tendonitis | Pain on movement. However, global pain on movement, not consistent with isolated biceps tendonitis | | | | | |
| Perform shoulder apprehension test | With the shoulder flexed and abducted at 90°, and fingers pointing to the ceiling, push forward on the shoulder with one hand and pull back on the elbow with your other hand. Apprehension to this manoeuvre is a positive test, suggesting previous dislocation | Increased pain on external rotation, which is more consistent with diagnosis of frozen shoulder. No evidence of previous shoulder dislocation | | | | | |
| Assess for winged scapula | Look at the scapula while the patient pushes his hands against the wall at shoulder height. A winged scapula is suggestive of long thoracic nerve palsy | No winging of scapula | | | | | |
| Neurovascular assessment | Assess sensation at the regimental badge area (skin over inferior region of the deltoid muscle), which is supplied by the axillary nerve and may be compressed in anterior shoulder dislocation. Assess dermatomes and myotomes C5–T1 and palpate the pulses in the upper limb | No neurovascular compromise identified | | | | | |

**Finishing**

| | | | | | | | |
|---|---|---|---|---|---|---|---|
| Check patient is comfortable, offer to help reposition himand give the privacy to change | Keeps the patient's dignity | Treating the patient with respect is important | | | | | |
| Remove your gloves and wash hands | Complying with hand hygiene is vital | No additional concerns | | | | | |

**Present Your Findings**

Stephen is a 50-year-old man presenting with sudden-onset pain in their right shoulder.

On examination he looked comfortable at rest. There was no tenderness on shoulder palpation. There was restricted range of movement and pain on movement globally in his right shoulder, particularly on external rotation. Special tests indicated global pain on movement but no weakness or muscle pathology.

I feel the most likely diagnosis is frozen shoulder/adhesive capsulitis, with differential diagnosis of calcific tendonitis.

To complete my examination, I would like to examine Mr O'Humeral fully, including examining the cervical spine and elbow. I would like to test the neurovascular status of the arm, provide adequate analgesia and refer to physiotherapy

**General Points**

| | | | | | |
|---|---|---|---|---|---|
| Polite to patient | | | | | |
| Maintains good eye contact | | | | | |
| Clear instruction and explanation to patient | | | | | |

## ❓ QUESTIONS FROM THE EXAMINER

### What role does imaging play in the diagnosis of frozen shoulder/adhesive capsulitis?

Imaging cannot assist in diagnosis, but it is useful to exclude other shoulder pathologies such as rotator cuff tear, particularly when diagnosis is not clear from history or examination.

### Mr Humeral is a diabetic, which is a risk factor for frozen shoulder. What other condition is associated with the disease?

Thyroid disease (both hypo- and hyperthyroidism) is associated with frozen shoulder.

### What is the most common mechanism of injury for posterior shoulder dislocation?

Posterior shoulder dislocation usually results from uncoordinated muscle contraction; for example, seizure or electric shock. It is much less common than anterior dislocation.

### Why would a patient with impingement syndrome have pain on raising the arms?

Lifting the arm causes the subacromial space to narrow, causing impingement of the supraspinatus muscle tendon, leading to an inflammatory response.

### If a patient presented with wasting of the deltoid muscle, several months following successful reduction of anterior shoulder dislocation, what complication would you suspect had occurred?

Axillary nerve injury.

### During a shoulder examination, a patient cannot put their arm behind their back. In this scenario, what alternative test can be used to assess the subscapularis muscle?

Instead of the lift-off test, the belly press can be used to test the subscapularis muscle for tear or dysfunction. This involves the patient pressing their palm into their upper abdomen with the elbow flexed. A positive test involves posterior movement of the elbow to compensate for subscapularis weakness.

### A 60-year-old woman presents with bilateral shoulder stiffness and associated hip pain. She has a past medical history of giant-cell arteritis. What is your clinical suspicion?

Polymyalgia rheumatica.

### What would a painless loss of external rotation of the shoulder indicate?

A subscapularis tear.

### What are the two main bursae of the shoulder joint?

The subacromial bursa (found deep to the deltoid and acromion, and superficial to the supraspinatus muscle) and the subscapular bursa (found between the subscapularis tendon and the scapula) are the two largest and most clinically relevant.

### How would a rotator cuff tear be managed?

Treatment of degenerative rupture, especially in elderly or inactive patients, can be conservative, consisting of physical therapy and analgesia. Surgical repair is indicated in cases of traumatic rupture, especially in physically active patients, with follow-up physical therapy.

## Station 3.4    Elbow

### Doctor Briefing

You are a junior doctor in orthopaedics and have been asked to see William Murray, a 35-year-old painter and decorator who has presented with right-elbow pain and reduced grip strength in the right hand. The pain has developed gradually over the last year, and now his elbow is causing him difficulty at work. He has been referred in by his primary care physician. Please examine Mr Murray and present your findings.

### Patient Briefing

Several months ago you developed pain in your right elbow that radiates down your forearm, and is getting progressively worse. Over the past few weeks you have noticed tingling and numbness in your right little and ring fingers, especially when you wake up in the morning. You have been struggling at work due to this and are finding it difficult to grip your tools. Your general health is good, and you keep fit and well.

You are concerned because the pain has not disappeared and you are worried it is something serious, and that you might lose your job.

### Mark Scheme for Examiner

#### Introduction

| | | | |
|---|---|---|---|
| Washes hands, introduces self, confirms patient identity and gains consent for examination | | | |
| Ensures a chaperone is present | | | |
| Appropriately exposes the patient's elbow whilst keeping dignity at all times, and repositions into a suitable position for the examination | | | |
| Asks if the patient has any pain currently | | | |

#### General Inspection

| What are you looking for or examining? | Justification | Findings and evolving thought process | | | |
|---|---|---|---|---|---|
| General well-being | On initial glance, does the patient look well/unwell/in pain? | Patient looks comfortable at rest | | | |
| Obvious clues | Gives an indication of the patient's baseline health | Patient looks generally well, normal body habitus | | | |

#### Orthopaedic Examination – Look

| | | | | |
|---|---|---|---|---|
| Inspect from the front, back, medial and lateral sides of the elbow<br><br>Closer inspection of the elbow | With the patient standing in the anatomical position:<br>• Note any fixed flexion deformity, asymmetry or scars<br>• Examine the carrying angle (5–15° of cubitus valgus is normal). More pronounced cubitus varus with the forearm towards the body suggests previous paediatric supracondylar fracture. Cubitus valgus suggests non-union of previous fracture<br>• Assess for biceps or triceps muscle wasting, as seen in lower motor neurone lesion or chronic inactivity<br>• Assess for skin changes, such as psoriatic plaques or rheumatoid nodules<br>Redness or swelling may indicate olecranon bursitis, gout or septic arthritis | No stigmata of elbow pathology noted | | |

**Orthopaedic Examination – Feel**

| What are you looking for or examining? | Justification | Findings and evolving thought process | | | | | |
|---|---|---|---|---|---|---|---|
| Ask the patient if he has any pain and start palpation away from the pain. Observe the reaction on the patient's face at all times | Allows accurate assessment of pain and minimises discomfort/shock | Commence palpation away from the site of pain | | | | | |
| Assess temperature | Feel at, above and below the elbow, comparing both sides | Uniform and normal temperature | | | | | |
| Palpate elbows | Assess for tenderness, bony abnormalities, swelling and deformity at the olecranon process, medial and lateral epicondyle and the radial head. Palpate the distal biceps tendon, with the elbow flexed to 90°, and feeling over the anterior crease | No tenderness on palpation | | | | | |

**Orthopaedic Examination – Move**

| | | | | | | | |
|---|---|---|---|---|---|---|---|
| Determine the range of active, then passive movements | Feel the elbow joint for crepitus whilst assessing movement, which is associated with osteoarthritis | No crepitus observed | | | | | |
| Elbow flexion | Ask the patient to bend his elbows. Normal is 0–150° | Full range of active and passive flexion | | | | | |
| Elbow extension | Ask the patient to straighten out his arms as far as possible. Normal is 0° | Full range of active and passive extension | | | | | |
| Pronation | With his elbows flexed at his side, ask the patient to turn his forearm so that the palm is facing the ground. Normal is 70° | Full range of active and passive pronation | | | | | |
| Supination | With his elbows flexed at his side, ask the patient to turn his forearm so that the palm is facing the ceiling. Normal is 90° | Full range of active and passive pronation | | | | | |

**Orthopaedic Examination – Special Tests**

| | | | | | | | |
|---|---|---|---|---|---|---|---|
| Assess elbow function | Assess function by asking the patient to:<br>• Raise the hands to the mouth: 'eating'<br>• Reach the hands to the buttocks: 'toileting' | Patient able to carry out movements without difficulty | | | | | |
| Cozen's test for lateral epicondylitis (tennis elbow) | Tests active wrist extension against resistance.<br>• Stabilise the elbow and palpate the lateral epicondyle<br>• Ask the patient to clench his hand into a fist and extend the wrist<br>• Push down gently on the extended wrist, whilst asking patient to continue extending.<br>Positive finding would be if the test reproduces pain | No pain elicited; no evidence of lateral epicondylitis | | | | | |

**Orthopaedic Examination – Special Tests**

| What are you looking for or examining? | Justification | Findings and evolving thought process | | | | |
|---|---|---|---|---|---|---|
| Test for medial epicondylitis (golfer's elbow) | Tests for medial epicondylitis or golfer's elbow. Tests active wrist flexion against resistance. With the patient's elbow at 90° flexion, feel the medial epicondyle with one hand. Ask the patient to make a fist and flex the wrist. Gently try to extend the wrist with your other hand, asking the patient to continue flexing. Positive finding would be if the test reproduces pain | No pain elicited; no evidence of medial epicondylitis | | | | |
| Neurovascular assessment | Perform a full peripheral nerve examination on the upper limbs. Perform a vascular assessment of the upper limbs | The patient displays wasting of the hypothenar eminence, right hand, altered sensation of the right little and ring finger, and weakened grip strength in the same hand | | | | |

**Finishing**

| | | | | | | |
|---|---|---|---|---|---|---|
| Check patient is comfortable, offer to help reposition him and give the privacy to change | Keeps the patient's dignity | Treating the patient with respect is important | | | | |
| Remove your gloves and wash hands | Complying with hand hygiene is vital | No additional concerns | | | | |

**Present Your Findings**

Mr Murray is a 35-year-old man with persistent right-elbow pain and reduced grip strength in his right hand. On examination he looked comfortable at rest. There was no tenderness on elbow palpation. He had a full range of active and passive movement. Special tests showed no evidence of medial or lateral epicondylitis. On neurovascular examination, there was altered sensation of the little and ring fingers, wasting of the hypothenar eminence and weakened grip strength all in the right hand.

I feel the most likely diagnosis is ulnar nerve entrapment at the elbow, with differential diagnosis of elbow osteoarthritis.

To complete my examination, I would like to examine Mr Murray fully, including examining the hand and shoulder. I also would like to document the neurovascular status of the arm. As initial treatment, I would tell Mr Murray to avoid resting on this elbow where possible, provide analgesia and offer a brace to wear at night

**General Points**

| | | | | |
|---|---|---|---|---|
| Polite to patient | | | | |
| Maintains good eye contact | | | | |
| Clear instruction and explanation to patient | | | | |

## ? QUESTIONS FROM THE EXAMINER

### If conservative management does not resolve nerve entrapment, what would be the next option?

Surgical decompression.

### What clinical test for nerve entrapment can be used at both the elbow and the wrist?

Tinel's test, where you attempt to provoke tingling and numbness of the fingers by tapping at the cubital tunnel at the elbow, or the carpal tunnel at the wrist.

### What muscles are responsible for flexion and extension of the elbow?

Triceps brachii and anconeus muscles facilitate elbow extension. Brachialis, biceps brachii, brachioradialis muscles facilitate elbow flexion.

### What classic hand deformity is associated with ulnar nerve damage?

Claw hand/ulnar claw. Palsy of the third and fourth lumbricals with preserved function of extrinsic flexors, appearing as clawing of the fourth and fifth fingers.

### What term describes ulnar nerve entrapment at the wrist?

Guyon canal syndrome.

### Describe the classic appearance of psoriasis at the elbow.

A rash consisting of red patches of plaque with silvery-white coating over the extensor surface of the elbow.

### What is the rationale for using a night splint for nerve entrapment syndromes such as carpal tunnel?

A night splint worn during the night, such as one worn on the wrist for carpal tunnel, prevents wrist flexion during the night when patients may not be aware of the action. This prevents pressure over the affected nerve and leads to improvement of symptoms in many patients.

### What is the most common mechanism of injury for a posterior elbow dislocation?

A fall onto an outstretched hand (also known as a FOOSH) is the classic mechanism of injury in posterior elbow dislocation.

### What are the clinical signs of a successful reduction of a dislocated elbow?

Return of the normal orientation of the three bony prominences of the elbow, the medial and lateral epicondyles and the tip of the olecranon, with an associated decrease in pain. This should be confirmed by X-ray imaging.

### How are radial head fractures classified?

Radial head fractures are classified according to the degree of displacement and intra-articular involvement, using the Mason classification.

## Station 3.5   Hand and Wrist

### Doctor Briefing

You are a junior doctor in orthopaedics and have been asked to see Caitlyn King, a 45-year-old woman who has presented with pain and stiffness of the finger joints. This has been an ongoing problem for the past year, and she has been referred in by her primary care physician. Please examine Mrs King and present your findings.

### Patient Briefing

Over the past year you have been experiencing increasing pain and stiffness in the joints of your hands. They affect both your hands, but your right one is usually worse. You have also noticed redness and swelling around the joints. The stiffness is worse in the morning, and after a few hours the stiffness begins to settle. You usually take ibuprofen for the pain, and it helps slightly. Your health is normally good, but you do smoke and drink regularly.

You are concerned because this stiffness is stopping you from working, as you need to type for extended periods of time.

### Mark Scheme for Examiner

| Introduction | | | | | | | |
|---|---|---|---|---|---|---|---|
| Washes hands, introduces self, confirms patient identity and gains consent for examination | | | | | | | |
| Ensures a chaperone is present | | | | | | | |
| Appropriately exposes the patient's hands, wrists and elbows whilst keeping dignity at all times, and repositions into a suitable position for the examination | | | | | | | |
| Asks if the patient has any pain currently | | | | | | | |

| General Inspection | | | | | | | |
|---|---|---|---|---|---|---|---|
| **What are you looking for or examining?** | **Justification** | **Findings and evolving thought process** | | | | | |
| General well-being | On initial glance does the patient look well/unwell/in pain? | Patient looks comfortable at rest | | | | | |
| Obvious clues | Gives an indication of the patient's baseline health | Patient looks generally well, normal body habitus | | | | | |

| Orthopaedic Examination – Look | | | | | | | |
|---|---|---|---|---|---|---|---|
| Inspects from the front, side and back | Inspect for splints, muscle wasting and asymmetry. Assess for muscle wasting, secondary to joint pathology or nerve injury. Look for cushingoid features, such as thin, easily bruising skin indicative of long-term steroid use. Look for gouty tophi and skin changes behind the back of the ear, seen in psoriasis and eczema. Observe for tremor with the patient's hands outstretched | Pale scaly rash behind the ears | | | | | |
| Inspect the elbow and ulnar border | Inspect the elbows for rheumatoid nodules, psoriasis, scars | Pale scaly rash on the extensor surface of the elbow, consistent with psoriasis | | | | | |

## Orthopaedic Examination – Look

| What are you looking for or examining? | Justification | Findings and evolving thought process | | | | |
|---|---|---|---|---|---|---|
| Inspect the dorsal aspect of the hands and wrist | Shortening or telescoping of the joints is seen in advanced psoriatic arthritis. Swelling and erythema may indicate infection or inflammation. Radiocarpal subluxation, ulnar deviation and subluxation are features of rheumatoid arthritis. Bouchard's nodes at the proximal interphalangeal (PIP) joints and Heberden's nodes at the distal interphalangeal (DIP) joints are seen in osteoarthritis. Swan neck deformity consisting of DIP flexion and PIP hyperextension, and boutonnière deformity, consisting of PIP flexion with DIP hyperextension, are both associated with advanced rheumatoid arthritis. Look for Z-thumb deformity (flexion at the metacarpophalangeal (MCP) joint and hyperextension at the PIP joint), which is also associated with rheumatoid arthritis. Wasting of the first dorsal web space is seen in ulnar nerve palsy. Look for mallet finger (involuntary flexion of the distal phalanx of a finger). Nail pitting and onycholysis are both seen in psoriasis. Nail fold infarcts are associated with rheumatoid vasculitis | Nail pitting observed. Redness and swelling of DIP joints | | | | |
| Inspect the palmar aspect of the hands and wrist | Scars from carpal tunnel release operation may be visible on the wrist. Muscle wasting of the thenar eminence suggests median nerve damage, such as carpal tunnel syndrome. Hypothenar wasting suggests ulnar nerve injury | No stigma of pathology noted | | | | |

## Orthopaedic Examination – Feel

| | | | | | | |
|---|---|---|---|---|---|---|
| Ask the patient if she has any pain and start palpation away from the pain. Observe the reaction on the patient's face at all times | Allows accurate assessment of pain and minimises discomfort/shock | Commence palpation away from the site of pain | | | | |
| Palpate upper-limb pulses | Palpate radial pulses together and capillary artery refill time | Normal pulse and perfusion | | | | |

## Orthopaedic Examination – Feel

| What are you looking for or examining? | Justification | Findings and evolving thought process | | | | | |
|---|---|---|---|---|---|---|---|
| Palpate the palmar aspect of the hand | Dupuytren's contracture is fixed flexion contraction of hands, caused by thickening of the palmar aponeurosis. Feel the bulk of the thenar and hypothenar eminences for wasting | No fascial thickening | | | | | |
| Feel temperature of the palmar and dorsal aspects of the hand | Compare the temperatures of the patient's forearm, wrists and MCP joints | Normal temperature bilaterally | | | | | |
| Palpate joints for tenderness | Ask whether the patient is in pain and look at her whilst you squeeze the MCP joints, assessing for tenderness. Bimanually palpate the MCP, PIP and DIP joints for signs of active synovitis, such as swelling, tenderness, warmth or hard bony swelling | Tenderness on DIP palpation | | | | | |
| Run your hand up the patient's arms to her elbows | Looking for rheumatoid nodules or psoriatic plaques | Psoriatic plaques, as previously noted | | | | | |

## Orthopaedic Examination – Move

| | | | | | | | |
|---|---|---|---|---|---|---|---|
| Assess active and passive movements | Assess active movement. Repeat passively if there is limited range of movement, or pain, ensuring to look at the patient's face | As per each movement below | | | | | |
| Finger flexion | Ask the patient to make a fist | Normal flexion | | | | | |
| Finger extension | Ask the patient to straighten the fingers fully | Normal extension | | | | | |
| Active and passive abduction and adduction | Abduct and adduct fingers, and touch the tip of each finger with the thumb on the same hand | Full range of abduction and adduction | | | | | |
| Active and passive wrist flexion and extension | Make a prayer and reverse prayer sign Assess wrist extension and flexion passively | Full range of wrist flexion and extension | | | | | |
| Assess for ulnar deviation of the wrist | Stabilise the forearm with one hand. Then, while grasping the metacarpals from the radial side with the other hand, apply traction in the ulnar direction. Do the opposite for radial deviation. Ulnar deviation should be greater than radial | Ulnar is greater than radial deviation; no abnormality detected | | | | | |
| Supination and pronation | Problems turning the hand could be associated with radioulnar joint abnormality | Normal supination and pronation | | | | | |

**Orthopaedic Examination – Special Tests**

| What are you looking for or examining? | Justification | Findings and evolving thought process | | | | |
|---|---|---|---|---|---|---|
| Perform Phalen's test<br><br>Perform Tinel's test | Hold the wrist in forced flexion, reverse prayer position, for 60 s. Paraesthesia in the distribution of the median nerve suggests carpal tunnel syndrome.<br>Percuss over the carpal tunnel for 30 s. Positive results as with Phalen's test | No tingling or numbness | | | | |
| Assess function | Ask the patient to:<br>• Grip two of your fingers (power grip)<br>• Pinch your finger (pincer grip)<br>• Pick up a small object (precision grip)<br>• Bring her hands to her mouth (eating)<br>• Put her hands behind her head (dressing)<br>• Put her hands to her lumbar spine (toileting) | Normal power throughout<br>Functional actions carried out as normal | | | | |
| Neurovascular assessment | Assess sensation with the patient's eyes closed.<br>Compare on both sides:<br>• Radial: first dorsal web space<br>• Median: tip of index finger<br>• Ulnar: dorsolateral surface of hand<br>Assess power, comparing both sides:<br>• Radial: wrist extension against resistance<br>• Median: try to break the patient's pincer grip<br>• Ulnar: finger abduction against resistance | Neurovascularly intact | | | | |

**Finishing**

| | | | | | | |
|---|---|---|---|---|---|---|
| Check patient is comfortable, offer to help reposition her and give the privacy to change | Keeps the patient's dignity | Treating the patient with respect is important | | | | |
| Remove your gloves and wash hands | Complying with hand hygiene is vital | No additional concerns | | | | |

**Present Your Findings**

Mrs King is a 45-year-old woman who presented with bilateral painful and stiff finger joints. On examination there were psoriatic plaques at the extensor surface of the elbow, behind the ear, and pitting of the nails. There were tenderness and swelling of the DIP joints. She had a full range of active and passive movement. Special tests showed no evidence of carpal tunnel syndrome. There was no altered sensation or weakness.

I feel the most likely diagnosis is psoriatic arthritis, with differential diagnoses being rheumatoid arthritis and osteoarthritis.

To complete my examination, I would like to examine Mrs King fully, including examining the elbow, and perform relevant blood tests. I would also organise a senior rheumatologist review for further investigation

| General Points | | | | | |
| --- | --- | --- | --- | --- | --- |
| Polite to patient | | | | | |
| Maintains good eye contact | | | | | |
| Clear instruction and explanation to patient | | | | | |

## ? QUESTIONS FROM THE EXAMINER

### What lifestyle changes may improve Mrs King's symptoms?

Stopping smoking. It is reported that patients who continue to smoke will have poorer disease outcomes with regards to psoriatic arthritis. Drinking alcohol is also thought to be linked.

### What classification system is used to help make a diagnosis of psoriatic arthritis?

The CASPAR (Classification criteria for Psoriatic Arthritis) criteria. This involves components such as evidence of psoriasis (clinically or personal/family history), nail changes, negative rheumatoid factor and radiological signs, in the presence of arthropathy.

### What score is commonly used to monitor rheumatoid arthritis and what are its components?

The DAS 28, or disease activity score. It involves counting the number of swollen joints (out of 28), the number of painful joints (out of 28), either erythrocyte sedimentation rate (ESR) or C-reactive protein (CRP) as a blood measure of inflammation and the patient's global assessment of health.

### What complication of long-term hydroxychloroquine requires monitoring?

Hydroxychloroquine is a disease-modifying antirheumatic drug (DMARD). A rare but serious complication is retinal damage, so patients on long-term use are recommended to attend retinal screening.

### What term describes the clinical sign of severe inflammation of a digit that can occur in psoriatic arthritis?

Dactylitis, which is described as a 'sausage finger' appearance.

### What structure is released in carpal decompression surgery?

The transverse carpal ligament, also known as the flexor retinaculum of the hand, is cut to decompress the median nerve.

### What is de Quervain tenosynovitis?

Inflammation of the sheath surrounding the abductor pollicis longus and extensor pollicis brevis, presenting clinically as painful movement of the thumb. It is usually caused by repetitive movement.

### What is the clinical test for de Quervain tenosynovitis?

The clinical test is Finkelstein test, which involves exerting longitudinal traction of the thumb, across the palm of the hand towards the ulnar side. If this produces pain, the test is positive.

### What are gouty tophi?

Gouty tophi are painless hard nodules caused by deposits of monosodium urate.

### Where are gouty tophi most commonly found?

They can be deposited in bones, such as elbows and extensor surfaces of forearms. They can also be deposited in soft tissue, the pinna of the external ear, subcutaneous tissue and synovial bursae.

## Station 3.6   Hip

### Doctor Briefing

You are a junior doctor working a busy shift in the emergency department (ED). Andrew Trendelenburg is an 82-year-old man who has fallen at home. His left lower limb looks shorter than his right and it also looks rotated. Please examine his hips and present your findings.

### Patient Briefing

This morning, on the way to the bathroom, you tripped and fell onto your bent left knee. This caused sudden-onset severe pain over your left hip, and you feel your movement is restricted. You do not have pain anywhere else, and you felt fine before the fall. Since the fall you have not been able to bear weight on the left leg.

You had bilateral hip replacement a few months ago, due to osteoarthritis. Your mobility has improved since then and you have had no problems. You usually get around with a walking stick.

You are concerned because you don't know if you have damaged your hip and if you will need another operation.

### Mark Scheme for Examiner

#### Introduction

| | |
|---|---|
| Washes hands, introduces self, confirms patient identity and gains consent for examination | |
| Ensures a chaperone is present | |
| Appropriately exposes the patient's hips and knees whilst keeping dignity at all times, and repositions into a suitable position for the examination | |
| Asks if the patient has any pain currently | |

#### General Inspection

| What are you looking for or examining? | Justification | Findings and evolving thought process | |
|---|---|---|---|
| General well-being | On initial glance, does the patient look well/unwell/in pain? | The patient looks uncomfortable and in pain | |
| Obvious clues | Gives you an indication of the patient's baseline health, any obvious trauma | Left leg appears shorter than right and looks internally rotated. Clinical suspicion of traumatic injury (fracture or dislocation) | |
| Surroundings | Look to see if the patient uses any walking aids or mobility equipment | Patient's walking stick is by the bedside | |

#### Orthopaedic Examination – Look

| | | | |
|---|---|---|---|
| Inspect from the front, side and back | Look for alignment and obvious deformity while ensuring that the pelvis is level. You can also feel for the iliac crests as misalignment is a cause of apparent leg length discrepancy | Obvious asymmetry, with posterior deformity over left hip joint, consistent with posterior dislocation of femoral head. Pelvis is in line with shoulders | |

**Orthopaedic Examination – Look**

| What are you looking for or examining? | Justification | Findings and evolving thought process | | | | |
|---|---|---|---|---|---|---|
| | Assess gait by asking the patient to walk across the room. An antalgic gait is often an indication of osteoarthritis. Trendelenburg gait could suggest previous hip surgery or L5 radiculopathy | Patient is in too much pain to bear weight | | | | |
| Closer inspection of hip | Look for scars, bruising, swelling, muscle wasting and redness | 12-cm scar over the left hip, consistent with previous total hip replacement. Quadriceps and gluteus muscle wasting is suggestive of lack of use from known osteoarthritis | | | | |

**Orthopaedic Examination – Feel**

| | | | | | | |
|---|---|---|---|---|---|---|
| Ask the patient if he has any pain and start palpation away from the pain. Observe the reaction on the patient's face at all times | Allows accurate assessment of pain and minimises discomfort/shock | Patient describes pain over left hip joint, worsening with movement. Commence palpation away from the site of pain | | | | |
| Assess temperature | It may be difficult to detect any changes, as the hip is a deep joint | Temperature comparable to opposite hip and joints above and below | | | | |
| Palpate hip joint, with the patient lying supine | Palpate the greater trochanter and anterior superior iliac spine (ASIS) bilaterally. Tenderness over greater trochanter seen in trochanteric bursitis can be elicited by rolling the leg from side to side. Tenderness or bony abnormalities at the ASIS could indicate osteoarthritis | Generalised tenderness on palpation with posterior deformity of hip joint, consistent with dislocation | | | | |

**Orthopaedic Examination – Move**

| | | | | | | |
|---|---|---|---|---|---|---|
| Assess lumbar spine | Ask the patient to raise his leg straight off the couch. Hip pain may be referred spinal pain | Normal lumbar spine movement | | | | |

## Orthopaedic Examination – Move

| What are you looking for or examining? | Justification | Findings and evolving thought process | | | | | |
|---|---|---|---|---|---|---|---|
| Hip flexion (actively and passively) | Ask the patient to flex his knee to 90°, then to flex his hip fully. Normal range of movement is 120°.<br>Then passively flex the hip by taking another 20° with one hand stabilising the pelvis | Patient is unable to move his left hip joint due to pain. Normal flexion, rotation, abduction, adduction and extension in his right hip joint. No crepitus felt on movement | | | | | |
| Hip rotation (passively) | Hold the hip in flexion and test internal rotation by moving his foot laterally. Normal is 40°.<br>Then perform external rotation by moving it medially. Normal is 45° | | | | | | |
| Abduction and adduction (actively and passively) | Stabilise the pelvis by having the legs extended, and one hand on the iliac crest of the opposite side of the pelvis. Then abduct (normal is 45°), and adduct (normal is 30°) | | | | | | |
| Hip extension | If possible, ask patient to roll on to one side to assess extension. Normal is 20° | | | | | | |

## Orthopaedic Examination – Special Tests

| | | | | | | | |
|---|---|---|---|---|---|---|---|
| Measure true (from ASIS to medial malleolus) and apparent (from umbilicus to medial malleolus) leg length bilaterally | If there is true leg length discrepancy, ask the patient to flex his knees (if able) whilst keeping heels together, to assess whether the shortening is below or above the knee.<br>If abnormality is above the knee, feel for the tops of the greater trochanters to assess whether the pathology is proximal to the trochanters.<br>Hip dislocation is a cause of true leg shortening, proximal to the greater trochanter | Patient's true left-leg length is shorter than the right leg length proximally | | | | | |
| Neurovascular assessment | Assess sensation along branches of the sciatic nerve (dorsum and sole of the foot) and the femoral nerve (medial thigh and medial calf).<br>Palpate for the dorsalis pedis and posterior tibial arterial pulses.<br>Hip dislocation can compromise the sciatic nerve, leading to numbness in this region | Both legs are neurovascularly intact | | | | | |
| Perform Thomas's test | Place one hand under the lower back, to ensure that the resting lordosis is removed. Fully flex the non-test hip with your other hand until the lumbar spine touches the fingers of the hand under the back. Look at the opposite leg. If it is lifted off the couch as a result of this manoeuvre, there is a fixed flexion deformity in that hip | Thomas's test was not performed due to the patient's recent bilateral hip replacements, which increases risk of dislocation | | | | | |

**Orthopaedic Examination – Special Tests**

| What are you looking for or examining? | Justification | Findings and evolving thought process | | | | | |
|---|---|---|---|---|---|---|---|
| Perform Trendelenburg's test | With the patient standing, crouch in front of him and gently place one of your hands on each ASIS. Ask the patient to stand on each leg in turn. In a negative test, the pelvis remains level or the raised-leg side may rise. In a positive test, the pelvis will dip on the raised-leg side and the patient's body will move towards the supporting leg. This assesses for weakness in the hip abductor muscles | Unable to conduct as patient unable to weight bear | | | | | |

**Finishing**

| | | | | | | | |
|---|---|---|---|---|---|---|---|
| Check patient is comfortable, offer to help reposition him and give the privacy to change | Keeps the patient's dignity | Treating the patient with respect is important | | | | | |
| Remove your gloves and wash hands | Complying with hand hygiene is vital | No additional concerns | | | | | |

**Present Your Findings**

Mr Trendelenburg is an 82-year-old man who presented to the ED following a fall. On examination he looks uncomfortable, with his left leg appearing shorter and internally rotated. There was obvious posterior deformity over the joint, and a scar consistent with total hip replacement. The joint was tender, and movement was restricted due to pain. Gait and the Trendelenburg test could not be assessed, as the patient was unable to bear weight. Thomas's test was not conducted due to patient's bilateral hip replacements. His legs are neurovascularly intact. On measurement, his true left leg length is shorter than the right proximally.

I feel the most likely diagnosis is hip dislocation, with differential diagnoses being a neck of femur fracture or post-hip arthroplasty.

I would like to examine Mr Trendelenburg fully, including examining the spine and knee, and lower-limb neurological system. I would also organise a pelvis X-ray. It is likely he will need an urgent reduction of the joint

**General Points**

| | | | | | |
|---|---|---|---|---|---|
| Polite to patient | | | | | |
| Maintains good eye contact | | | | | |
| Clear instruction and explanation to patient | | | | | |

## ❓ QUESTIONS FROM THE EXAMINER

### Why would Mr Trendelenburg be at increased risk of hip dislocation?

Recent total hip replacement, disrupting the tissues of the joint, increases the risk of dislocation in falls. This would predispose him to dislocating his hip from a low-impact injury.

### What is important to consider in traumatic hip dislocation and how does this impact management?

Traumatic hip dislocations are often associated with fractures (such as of the femoral neck, head or acetabulum). This may necessitate an open reduction if fractures are displaced.

### How are hip dislocations classified?

Position of the femoral head in relation to the acetabulum, either posterior (most commonly) or anterior.

### Urgent reduction of a dislocated hip is required to reduce the risk of what complication?

Osteonecrosis of the femoral head.

### What is the most common mechanism of hip dislocation in native joints?

Road traffic accidents or other high-impact injury. Classically this is caused by the knee hitting the car dashboard, causing a posterior dislocation.

### A young adult, with no history of trauma, presents with a native joint hip dislocation and hypermobile joints on examination. What underlying condition do you suspect?

Ehlers–Danlos syndrome, and other connective tissue diseases, will increase the risk of native hip dislocation.

### What underlying condition is the cause of most hip dislocations in children?

Developmental dysplasia of the hip. This refers to hip instability and subluxation/dislocation of the femoral head, which can lead to acetabular dysplasia and abnormal hip growth.

### What joint disease is associated with morning stiffness that improves with activity?

Rheumatoid arthritis classically presents with morning stiffness that improves with movement, in comparison to osteoarthritis, where pain and stiffness worsen throughout the day.

### You suspect a patient has osteoarthritis of the hip joint. What investigations and subsequent findings would support this?

Plain X-ray of the affected joint. Changes in osteoarthritis include osteophyte formation, joint space narrowing, subchondral sclerosis and subchondral bone cysts.

### If you suspected a patient had septic arthritis of a joint, what would be your immediate management plan?

Sepsis 6: Give immediate broad-spectrum intravenous (IV) antibiotics, IV fluids and oxygen if required, take blood cultures, measure urine output and lactate, and joint aspiration for synovial fluid culture and microscopy for sensitivities.

## Station 3.7    Knee

### Doctor Briefing

You are a junior doctor on your orthopaedics rotation and have been asked to see Sara Emerald, a 68-year-old woman, who has presented with chronic right-knee pain and reduced walking ability. She has been referred by her primary care physician to an orthopaedic clinic. Please examine Mrs Emerald's knee and present your findings.

### Patient Briefing

Your knee has been painful over the past few months, making it difficult to walk. You experience stiffness, particularly in the morning, and it takes some time to improve. Sometimes the pain is better for a while, but it always seems to come back. Your general health is good and your only past medical history is dandruff and dry skin. You think your mother has some form of arthritis, but you are not sure what type.

You are concerned because of the impact this pain is having on your life, as you are struggling to get about.

### Mark Scheme for Examiner

#### Introduction

| | | | | |
|---|---|---|---|---|
| Washes hands, introduces self, confirms patient identity and gains consent for examination | | | | |
| Ensures a chaperone is present | | | | |
| Appropriately exposes the patient's knees and ankles whilst keeping dignity at all times, and repositions into a suitable position for the examination | | | | |
| Asks if the patient has any pain currently | | | | |

#### General Inspection

| What are you looking for or examining? | Justification | Findings and evolving thought process | | | | |
|---|---|---|---|---|---|---|
| General well-being | On initial glance, does the patient look well/unwell/in pain? | Patient looks comfortable at rest | | | | |
| Obvious clues | Gives an indication of the patient's baseline health | Patient looks generally well, normal body habitus | | | | |
| Surroundings | Look to see if the patient uses any walking aids or mobility equipment | No stigmata of knee pathology noted | | | | |

#### Orthopaedic Examination – Look

| | | | | | | |
|---|---|---|---|---|---|---|
| Inspect from the front, side and back | Note the alignment with the patient standing, as alignment can only be assessed when weight bearing. Look for any obvious deformity such as fixed flexion deformity | No valgus or varus deformity | | | | |
| Closer inspection of knees | Look for scars, bruising, swelling, muscle wasting, redness. Loss of dimples medial to the kneecap could be indicative of an effusion | Skin changes bilaterally on the extensor surfaces – well-demarcated erythematous scaly plaques with a silvery appearance, which is consistent with psoriasis. Right knee appears swollen compared to the left. Clinical suspicion of psoriatic arthritis | | | | |

**Orthopaedic Examination – Look**

| What are you looking for or examining? | Justification | Findings and evolving thought process | | | | |
|---|---|---|---|---|---|---|
| Gait assessment | A stiff knee gait could be suggestive of cerebral palsy.<br>An antalgic gait indicates pain on weight bearing | Patient exhibiting antalgic gait | | | | |
| Measure circumference of thigh | Measure quadriceps bulk, using a measuring tape 15 cm above the tibial tuberosity, which detects subtle muscle wasting | Equal and normal quadricep bulk bilaterally | | | | |

**Orthopaedic Examination – Feel**

| | | | | | | |
|---|---|---|---|---|---|---|
| Ask the patient if she has any pain and start palpation away from the pain. Observe the reaction on the patient's face at all times | Allows accurate assessment of pain and minimises discomfort/shock | Commence palpation away from the site of pain | | | | |
| Assess temperature | Feel at, above and below the knee joints bilaterally to compare | Uniform and normal temperature around the knee | | | | |
| Palpate knee joints, with the patient lying supine | Palpate the patellar border with the knee straight and note any bone deformity.<br>Flex the knee to 90° and palpate the patellar border, femoral condyles and tibial tuberosity.<br>Tenderness at tibial tuberosity (tendon attachment point) can be seen in psoriatic arthritis.<br>With the knee flexed, feel for swelling in the popliteal fossa, which could suggest a Baker's cyst | Tenderness of right knee at the tibial tuberosity is noted | | | | |

**Orthopaedic Examination – Feel**

| What are you looking for or examining? | Justification | Findings and evolving thought process | | | | |
|---|---|---|---|---|---|---|
| Assess for effusion, with knees extended | Patellar tap can be performed to assess for large effusions. Grip the quadriceps muscles and slide down. Hold your position above the patella, emptying the suprapatellar pouch. With your opposite hand, press down on the patella. Positive test if you feel the patella moving down, like a 'tap'. Another test for large effusions is the patellar blot. Empty the supra-patellar pouch as before, holding your left hand above the knee. Press on the patella firmly with the thumb towards the femur. It is a positive test if you feel bulging under your left hand. The patellar sweep test can be performed for smaller effusions. Sweep distally to proximally along the medial side of the knee, moving the synovial fluid. Quickly repeat along the lateral side, but proximally to distally. The test is positive if the fluid bulges medially | No signs of effusion noted | | | | |

**Orthopaedic Examination – Move**

| | | | | | | |
|---|---|---|---|---|---|---|
| Assess the lumbar spine | Ask the patient to raise her leg straight off the couch, to screen for referred spinal pain | No spine pain noted | | | | |
| Assess the hip | Ask the patient to flex her hip and with your hands, internally and externally rotate hip, to screen for any hip pain | No hip pain noted | | | | |
| Knee flexion (actively and passively) | Ask the patient to move her heel up to their bottom. Normal is 140°. Repeat this movement passively by taking the patient's knee and ankle with your hands | Universal range of movement restricted due to pain. No hyperextension. No crepitus on movement | | | | |
| Knee extension (actively and passively) | Ask the patient to straighten her leg fully so that her leg lies flat on the couch. Inability to extend fully indicates an extensor lag, suggesting a disruption of the extensor mechanism or quadriceps weakness. Passively flex then extend the knee with one hand over the knee, feeling for crepitus. Passively hyperextend the knees by raising both ankles off the couch. Greater than 10° is considered to be hyperextended | | | | | |

## Orthopaedic Examination – Special Tests

| What are you looking for or examining? | Justification | Findings and evolving thought process | | | | | | | |
|---|---|---|---|---|---|---|---|---|---|
| Perform patellar apprehension test | Fully extend the knee and apply lateral force to the patella whilst slowly flexing the knee. Positive test if the knee is painful or resistant to flexion, suggesting patellar dislocation | Negative patellar apprehension test | | | | | | | |
| Perform anterior and posterior drawer test | Flex knee to 90° and sit on the patient's foot. Make sure to ask if she has pain in her foot beforehand. Place both thumbs on the tibial tuberosity and your fingers in the popliteal fossa. Ensuring the patient is relaxed, apply anterior and posterior force in turn. Positive test if significant movement anteriorly away from the femur, suggesting anterior cruciate ligament (ACL), injury or if significant movement posteriorly, suggesting posterior cruciate ligament (PCL) injury | No laxity or tear of the ACL or PCL identified | | | | | | | |
| Perform Lachman's test | Flex the knee to 20°. Support the lower leg and grasp on to the top of the femur with the other hand. Attempt to pull the calf anteriorly while pushing the thigh posteriorly. If gliding occurs, this suggests ACL injury in the knee | No laxity or tear of the ACL identified. No additional concerns identified | | | | | | | |
| Perform medial collateral ligament (MCL) and lateral collateral ligament (LCL) stress tests | Extend the knee fully and place the distal tibia of the leg between your elbow and side. Place one hand on the medial calf and one hand on the lateral knee. Apply varus and valgus stress in turn. Extreme pain or laxity elicited during valgus stress application suggests MCL injury. If elicited during varus stress application, this suggests LCL injury. If the knee is stable during the tests above, repeat with the knee flexed to 30° to assess for presence of minor laxity | No laxity or tear of MCL or LCL identified | | | | | | | |

## Orthopaedic Examination – Special Tests

| What are you looking for or examining? | Justification | Findings and evolving thought process | | | | | |
|---|---|---|---|---|---|---|---|
| Performs McMurray's test | Flex the knee to 90° by holding the calf with one hand and place your fingers of the other hand on the joint line.<br>Externally rotate the foot whilst abducting the hip, then flex and extend the knee, to assess for medial menisci tears.<br>Internally rotate the foot whilst adducting the hip, then flex and extend the knee to assess for lateral menisci tears.<br>Positive if there is pain or clicking, which would suggest a meniscal injury | No evidence of meniscal injury | | | | | |
| Neurovascular assessment | Perform a full peripheral nerve and vascular examination of the lower limbs | No additional concerns | | | | | |

## Finishing

| | | | | | | | |
|---|---|---|---|---|---|---|---|
| Check patient is comfortable, offer to help reposition her and give the privacy to change | Keeps the patient's dignity | Treating the patient with respect is important | | | | | |
| Remove your gloves and wash hands | Complying with hand hygiene is vital | No additional concerns | | | | | |

## Present Your Findings

Mrs Emerald is a 68-year-old woman presenting with chronic right-knee pain and reduced walking ability. On examination she looks comfortable. She walks with an antalgic gait and has bilateral skin changes over the knees consistent with psoriasis. The joint was tender over the tibial tuberosity, and movement was restricted due to pain. There was no evidence of effusion, and special tests did not indicate any ligament laxity.

I feel the most likely diagnosis is psoriatic arthritis, with differential diagnoses being osteoarthritis or rheumatoid arthritis.

I would like to examine Mrs Emerald fully, including examining the hip, foot and ankle. I would also like to examine all peripheral joints for evidence of psoriasis or arthropathy. I would also organise blood tests and a rheumatological review for further investigation

## General Points

| | | | | | |
|---|---|---|---|---|---|
| Polite to patient | | | | | |
| Maintains good eye contact | | | | | |
| Clear instruction and explanation to patient | | | | | |

# ? QUESTIONS FROM THE EXAMINER

## Why is Mrs Emerald's past medical history of dandruff relevant?

It may be that she has psoriasis of the scalp that has been mistaken for dandruff. This can be common when flaking of the scalp is the only complaint.

## If Mrs Emerald was to re-present with a red, painful eye, what complication of psoriatic arthritis would you suspect?

Uveitis is associated with psoriatic arthritis, and can present with a red, painful eye.

## What is the characteristic sign of advanced psoriatic arthritis of the hands on X-ray imaging?

Psoriatic arthritis of the fingers is especially associated with the pencil-in-cup deformity of DIP joints on plain X-ray films.

## What would be the benefit of testing Mrs Emerald for rheumatoid factor?

Rheumatoid factor is a non-specific test and can be positive in people without rheumatoid arthritis. However, as many arthropathies can present similarly, a negative rheumatoid factor would be useful in distinguishing between rheumatoid and psoriatic arthritis.

## Which joints are mostly likely to be affected in psoriatic arthritis?

Though early psoriatic arthritis may begin with a single large joint affected (such as the knee), it is common for patients to develop an oligoarthritis, with the spine, DIP and PIP joints the most commonly affected joints.

## What would be the first-line management of psoriatic arthritis and how could this be further escalated?

First-line management would be non-steroidal anti-inflammatory drugs, which can be escalated to DMARDs to control symptoms if multiple joints are affected or resolution is not achieved.

## What is the single best investigation to differentiate psoriatic arthritis from gout?

Synovial aspiration of the joint and analysis. The presence of monosodium urate crystals would confirm a diagnosis of gout.

## What is the function of the menisci of the knee joint?

The medial and lateral menisci are fibrocartilage structures that act as 'shock absorbers' by increasing surface area to dissipate forces further.

## What tendon attaches to the tibial tuberosity, and how would a complete tear present on examination?

Patellar tendon, and a complete tear would prevent extension of the leg. This may be accompanied by patellar displacement, and difficulty walking due to the knee 'giving way'.

## What injury is classically associated with an ACL tear?

Twisting injuries to the knee, particularly after slips or falls, are consistent with ACL injury.

## Station 3.8   Foot and Ankle

### Doctor Briefing

You are a junior doctor working in the ED and have been asked to see John Weber, a 43-year-old man, who has presented with severe left-ankle pain. He was playing football this morning and suddenly felt pain in his ankle whilst on the pitch. Please examine Mr Weber and present your findings.

### Patient Briefing

You were playing football with friends this morning. When you were tackling another player, you lost your balance and went over on the lateral side of your left foot. You felt your ankle 'pop', with a sudden onset of intense pain. Since then, you have not been able to walk or put any weight on it, and you had to take your shoe off as your ankle got so swollen.

Your health is normally good. You work in an office and play football with your friends occasionally. You have 'strained' your ankle before, but never anything as bad as today.

You are worried you have seriously injured your ankle and will not be able to walk. Your main concern at the moment is the pain, which is becoming unbearable.

### Mark Scheme for Examiner

| Introduction | | | | | | |
|---|---|---|---|---|---|---|
| Washes hands, introduces self, confirms patient identity and gains consent for examination | | | | | | |
| Ensures a chaperone is present | | | | | | |
| Appropriately exposes the patient's feet, ankles and knees whilst keeping dignity at all times, and repositions into a suitable position for the examination | | | | | | |
| Asks if the patient has any pain currently | | | | | | |

| General Inspection | | | | | | |
|---|---|---|---|---|---|---|
| **What are you looking for or examining?** | **Justification** | **Findings and evolving thought process** | | | | |
| General well-being | On initial glance, does the patient look well/unwell/in pain? | Patient looks in pain and uncomfortable | | | | |
| Obvious clues | Gives an indication of the patient's baseline health | Patient looks generally well, normal body habitus | | | | |
| Surroundings | Look to see if the patient uses any mobility aids, such as crutches or a walking stick | Patient sitting on bed, with the left ankle raised. Patient was brought to the examination by wheelchair as unable to bear weight | | | | |

| Orthopaedic Examination – Look | | | | | | |
|---|---|---|---|---|---|---|
| Inspect from front, side and back | Note any obvious deformities, asymmetry or scars. Assess medial arches of the foot. High arches (pes cavus) are often a result of Charcot–Marie–Tooth disease. Flat feet (pes planus) are often congenital. Inspect the Achilles tendon for swelling or asymmetry | Bruising and swelling visible over the lateral aspect of the left ankle | | | | |

## Orthopaedic Examination – Look

| What are you looking for or examining? | Justification | Findings and evolving thought process | | | | | |
|---|---|---|---|---|---|---|---|
| Inspection of the forefoot<br><br>Inspect the plantar surfaces<br><br>Examine the patient's footwear | Look for:<br>• Nail changes or rashes, such as psoriasis<br>• Toe alignment, including claw toe, hammer toe, mallet toe<br>• Intrinsic muscle wasting, a feature of diabetes neuropathy<br>Calluses are often a result of ill-fitting footwear.<br>Ulcers could be due to diabetes<br>Note any abnormal sole patterns or comfort aids | No stigmata of disease | | | | | |

## Orthopaedic Examination – Feel

| | | | | | | | |
|---|---|---|---|---|---|---|---|
| Assess temperature | Feel the temperature at the ankle joint and down the forefoot | Uniform and normal temperature | | | | | |
| Palpate pulses | Feel for the dorsalis pedis and lateral tibial pulses, which may be absent or reduced in vascular pathology | Pedal pulses present bilaterally | | | | | |
| Ask the patient if he has any pain and start palpation away from the pain. Observe the reaction on the patient's face at all times | Allows accurate assessment of pain and minimises discomfort/shock | Commence palpation away from the site of pain | | | | | |
| Palpate feet | Squeeze along each individual toe. Metatarsal squeeze: using one hand, grasp the patient's foot at the metatarsal heads and squeeze together. Using a bimanual approach, hold the patient's foot and use both of your thumbs to palpate the tarsal and metatarsal bones | No tenderness on palpation of foot | | | | | |
| Palpate the ankle | Palpate the medial malleolus, anterior ankle joint and lateral malleolus.<br>Using your thumb and second and third finger, palpate the subtalar joints.<br>Using the palm of your hand and fingers, palpate the Achilles tendon, feeling for any thickness or tenderness | Tenderness on palpation of the left lateral malleolus | | | | | |

## Orthopaedic Examination – Move

| | | | | | | | |
|---|---|---|---|---|---|---|---|
| Determine the range of active, then passive movements | Feel for crepitus whilst assessing movement; this is associated with osteoarthritis | No crepitus observed | | | | | |

## Orthopaedic Examination – Move

| What are you looking for or examining? | Justification | Findings and evolving thought process | | | | | | |
|---|---|---|---|---|---|---|---|---|
| Inversion and eversion | Place your hand at the lateral and then medial borders of the foot and ask the patient to try to touch your hand. Normal range of movement is 30° for inversion and 20°for eversion | Reduced active and passive movement due to pain | | | | | | |
| Dorsiflexion and plantar flexion of the big toe | Ask the patient to 'point toes to ceiling' and to 'curl toes inwards'. Normal range of movement is 70° for dorsiflexion and 45° for plantar flexion | Full range of movement | | | | | | |
| Ankle dorsiflexion and plantar flexion | Ask the patient to 'try to point your foot towards me' and 'press down like pressing on a car pedal' respectively. Normal range of movement is 40° for dorsiflexion and 20° for plantar flexion | Reduced active and passive movement due to pain | | | | | | |
| Midtarsal joint movement | Holding the ankle joint with one hand and the forefoot with the other hand, apply a twisting motion | Full range of movement | | | | | | |
| Subtalar joint movement | Holding the ankle joint with one hand and the heel with the other hand, invert and evert the foot | Reduced active and passive movement due to pain | | | | | | |

## Orthopaedic Examination – Special Tests

| | | | | | | | | |
|---|---|---|---|---|---|---|---|---|
| Gait assessment | Ask the patient to walk across the room, turn and walk back. Look for symmetry and normal cycle of heel strike, toe off. High-stepping gait may be present if there is foot drop | Gait could not be assessed as the patient is unable to bear weight | | | | | | |
| Simmond's/ Thompson's test | Ask the patient to lie face down on the couch, with his feet hanging off the bed. With both hands, squeeze the calf muscle. In a normal examination, the foot should plantar flex. Test is positive if no movement occurs and indicates Achilles tendon tear or rupture | No evidence of Achilles tendon tear or rupture | | | | | | |
| Neurovascular assessment | Perform a full peripheral nerve examination on the lower limbs. Perform a vascular assessment of the lower limbs | There was reduced sensation over the lateral aspect of the left foot, ankle and heel. Circulation to the lower limbs was preserved | | | | | | |

| **Finishing** | | | | | |
|---|---|---|---|---|---|
| **What are you looking for or examining?** | **Justification** | **Findings and evolving thought process** | | | |
| Check patient is comfortable, offer to help reposition him and give the privacy to change | Keeps the patient's dignity | Treating the patient with respect is important | | | |
| Remove your gloves and wash hands | Complying with hand hygiene is vital | No additional concerns | | | |

## Present Your Findings

Mr Weber is a 43-year-old man with severe left-ankle pain following injury. On examination the left lateral ankle appears swollen and was tender on palpation of the lateral malleolus. Range of movement was limited on ankle movements due to pain. Gait could not be assessed due to inability to bear weight. Simmond's test was normal. On neurovascular examination, there was reduced sensation over the lateral aspect of the left foot, ankle and heel.

I feel the most likely diagnosis is an ankle fracture of the lateral malleolus, with differentials being an ankle ligamentous injury or other form of ankle fracture.

To complete my examination, I would like to examine Mr Weber fully, including the knees. I would like to take X-rays of the left ankle to confirm my diagnosis and organise an orthopaedic review. In the meantime, Mr Weber should be provided with adequate analgesia

## General Points

Polite to patient

Maintains good eye contact

Clear instruction and explanation to patient

## ❓ QUESTIONS FROM THE EXAMINER

### How would an ankle fracture be managed?

Stable ankle fractures can be managed conservatively with a short leg cast for 4–6 weeks. Unstable, displaced or open fractures require open reduction and internal fixation.

### Why would Mr Weber have reduced sensation over the lateral aspect of his foot, heel and ankle?

The sensory innervation for the lateral foot is supplied by the sural nerve, which passes behind the lateral malleolus and may be damaged in a lateral malleolus fracture.

### What structures hold the distal ends of the tibia and fibula together?

The syndesmosis, which consists of the distal anterior tibiofibular ligament, the distal posterior tibiofibular ligament, the transverse ligament and the interosseous ligament.

### What system is used to classify ankle fractures by location?

The Weber ankle fracture classification (or Danis–Weber classification). Fractures can be classified as type A, below the level of the syndesmosis; type B, at the level of the syndesmosis; and type C, above the level of the syndesmosis.

## What is the cause of foot drop?

Foot drop, where the patient is unable to dorsiflex the ankle, is caused by damage to the peroneal nerve.

## What are the Ottawa ankle rules?

The Ottawa ankle rules are a screening tool to determine whether X-ray imaging is needed following ankle injuries. An X-ray is recommended if there is bony tenderness along any of the following: the posterior edge of the fibula, tip of the lateral or medial malleolus, base of the fifth metatarsal, navicular, or if the patient is unable to bear weight following injury.

## What structures make up the Achilles tendon?

The Achilles tendon consists of tendons from the gastrocnemius, soleus and plantaris muscles.

## What are the risk factors for plantar fasciitis?

Foot deformities, including pes cavus and pes planus, excessive standing/running or sudden changes in exercise and obesity.

## What bones make up the mortise joint of the ankle?

The tibia, fibula and talus of the foot all articulate to form the mortise joint of the ankle.

## What is Charcot–Marie–Tooth disease?

Also known as hereditary motor and sensory neuropathy or peroneal muscular atrophy, it describes a group of inherited conditions that cause damage to the peripheral nerves. It is associated with high arches (pes cavus), hammer toe, foot drop and high-stepping gait.

## Station 3.9   Gait, Arms, Legs and Spine (GALS)

### Doctor Briefing

You are a junior doctor working in rheumatology and are asked to see Caroline Lamb, a 45-year-old woman, who has been referred by her primary care physician due to increasingly stiff joints. Please perform a GALS screen on her and present your findings.

### Patient Briefing

You have had stiffness in your joints for the last 5 years. You used to take ibuprofen, which relieved the pain, but you recently had to stop this due to side effects, and then the pain and stiffness have been bothersome. Your main complaint is stiffness in your lower back and pain in your buttock. The stiffness is worse in the morning and can waken you from sleep. It gets better as the day goes on, but relief takes a while. You find it difficult to bend down.

You have a past medical history of ulcerative colitis. You have a younger brother who was diagnosed with some form of spine arthritis about 10 years ago, but you don't know anything else about it.

Your main concern is that the pain is becoming unbearable and stopping you from functioning normally.

### Mark Scheme for Examiner

#### Introduction

| | | | | |
|---|---|---|---|---|
| Washes hands, introduces self, confirms patient identity and gains consent for examination | | | | |
| Ensures a chaperone is present | | | | |
| Appropriately exposes the patient as required whilst keeping dignity at all times, and repositions into a suitable position for the examination | | | | |
| Asks if the patient has any pain currently | | | | |

#### General Inspection

| What are you looking for or examining? | Justification | Findings and evolving thought process | | | | |
|---|---|---|---|---|---|---|
| General well-being | On initial glance, does the patient look well/unwell/in pain? | Patient looks uncomfortable | | | | |
| Obvious clues | Gives an indication of the patient's baseline health | Patient looks generally well, normal body habitus | | | | |
| Surroundings | Look to see if the patient uses any mobility aids (such as crutches or a walking stick) | No mobility aids | | | | |

#### GALS Examination – Gait

| | | | | | | |
|---|---|---|---|---|---|---|
| Screening questions | Ask the patient:<br>• Whether there is any pain or stiffness in the muscles, joints or back: common symptoms of many joint pathologies<br>• Whether the patient can dress herself completely without any difficulties: assesses fine motor skills<br>• Whether the patient can walk up and down stairs without difficulty: assesses gross motor control and mobility | Patient has stiffness on bending forward but no other concerns | | | | |

**GALS Examination – Gait**

| What are you looking for or examining? | Justification | Findings and evolving thought process | | | | | |
|---|---|---|---|---|---|---|---|
| Gait assessment | Assess the gait cycle by asking the patient to walk a few steps, turn and walk back. Look for: symmetry, smoothness and the ability to turn quickly, which all may be restricted with joint pain or stiffness | Normal gait noted | | | | | |

**GALS Examination – Inspection**

| | | | | | | | |
|---|---|---|---|---|---|---|---|
| Inspect from the front | Shoulder and quadriceps bulk and symmetry, as wasting can indicate disuse secondary to joint problems or nerve injury. Elbow extension (inspect carrying angle of the elbow). Look for forefoot abnormalities, midfoot deformities and foot arches, which may cause gait abnormality | No stigmata pathology noted | | | | | |
| Inspect from behind | Look for:<br>• Muscle bulk and symmetry of the shoulder, gluteus and calf muscles<br>• Spinal alignment, for evidence of scoliosis<br>• Levelling iliac crests may reveal evidence of leg length discrepancy or hip abductor weakness<br>• Popliteal swelling, such as an aneurysm or Baker's cyst<br>• Hind foot abnormalities | No stigmata of pathology | | | | | |
| Inspect from the side | Look for:<br>• Normal spinal curvature (cervical lordosis, thoracic kyphosis, lumbar lordosis). These may be lost or exaggerated in pathology<br>• Knee flexion or hyperextension may indicate ligament laxity or hypermobility | No stigmata of pathology | | | | | |

**GALS Examination – Arms**

| | | | | | | | |
|---|---|---|---|---|---|---|---|
| Assess shoulder function | Ask the patient to put her hands behind her head to assess:<br>• Shoulder abduction<br>• External rotation<br>• Elbow flexion | Full range of movement | | | | | |
| Inspection | Ask the patient to hold her arms out, palms down and fingers outstretched. Observe the back of the hands and wrists for swelling and deformity, which may be seen in inflammatory or osteoarthritis. Look for nail changes, such as pitting or onycholysis, seen in psoriatic arthritis Ask the patient to turn her hands over. Look for muscle bulk and symmetry over the thenar and hypothenar eminences | No stigmata of disease | | | | | |

| GALS Examination – Arms | | | | | | | |
|---|---|---|---|---|---|---|---|
| **What are you looking for or examining?** | **Justification** | **Findings and evolving thought process** | | | | | |
| Assess hand function | Assess grip strength by asking the patient to squeeze your fingers. Assess fine precision pinch by asking the patient to bring each finger in turn to meet the thumb. Both can be reduced by nerve injury, or secondary to pain | Normal grip strength | | | | | |
| Palpation | Gently squeeze across the MCP joints for tenderness suggesting inflammation. Be sure to tell the patient first and look at her face for pain | No MCP joint tenderness | | | | | |

| GALS Examination – Legs | | | | | | | |
|---|---|---|---|---|---|---|---|
| With the patient supine on the couch, examine her legs | Whilst feeling for crepitus, assess passive flexion and extension of both knees. With the patient's hips and knees flexed to 90°, hold the knee and ankle and internally rotate both hips | Full range of movement | | | | | |
| Perform a patellar tap | Patellar tap can be performed by gripping the quadriceps muscles and sliding your hand down. Hold your position above the patella, emptying the suprapatellar pouch. With your opposite hand, press down on the patella. Positive test if you feel the patella moving down, like a 'tap', which suggests fluid accumulation | No evidence of effusion | | | | | |
| Inspect the feet | Inspect the feet for calluses, swelling and deformity | No stigmata of disease | | | | | |
| Palpation | Perform a metatarsophalangeal (MTP) squeeze, assessing for tenderness, which suggests inflammation. Ensure to warn the patient first and look at her face for pain | No MTP joint tenderness | | | | | |

| Orthopaedic Examination – Spine | | | | | | | |
|---|---|---|---|---|---|---|---|
| With the patient standing, examine the spine | Inspect the spine from behind for scoliosis | Normal spinal alignment | | | | | |
| Assess neck movement | Ask the patient to bring her ear to her shoulder on either side to assess lateral flexion | Full range of movement | | | | | |
| Assess jaw movement | Examine the temporomandibular joint (TMJ) by asking the patient to open her mouth and move her jaw from side to side | No pain on movement of TMJ | | | | | |

**Orthopaedic Examination – Spine**

| What are you looking for or examining? | Justification | Findings and evolving thought process | | | |
|---|---|---|---|---|---|
| Perform Schober's test | Place your fingers on the patient's lumbar vertebrae and then ask the patient to bend and touch her toes to assess lumbar and hip flexion. Your fingers should move apart on flexion, and back together on extension. This distance may be reduced in pathology such as ankylosing spondylitis | Pain and reduced range of movement on lumbar flexion | | | |

**Finishing**

| | | | | | |
|---|---|---|---|---|---|
| Check patient is comfortable, offer to help reposition her and give the privacy to change | Keeps the patient's dignity | Treating the patient with respect is important | | | |
| Remove your gloves and wash hands | Complying with hand hygiene is vital | No new concerns | | | |

**Present Your Findings**

Mrs Lamb is a 45-year-old woman who has presented with early-morning pain and stiffness, affecting the lower lumbar spine. On examination her gait was normal. She showed pain on lumbar flexion of the spine, associated with reduced movement. Schober's test revealed pain and reduced range of movement on lumbar flexion. Her gait, upper- and lower-limb examinations are otherwise unremarkable.

My main differential diagnosis is spondylarthritis, with differential diagnosis being inflammatory back pain or ankylosing spondylitis.

To complete my examination, I would like to examine the spine fully, perform routine and autoimmune blood tests to aid diagnosis and refer for rheumatological review. I will also record my findings on a GALS scoring table

**General Points**

| | | | | |
|---|---|---|---|---|
| Polite to patient | | | | |
| Maintains good eye contact | | | | |
| Clear instruction and explanation to patient | | | | |

## ❓ QUESTIONS FROM THE EXAMINER

**What is the most common extra-articular manifestation of ankylosing spondylitis?**

Acute, unilateral anterior uveitis.

**What is an enthesitis?**

An inflammation of an enthesis, where a tendon attaches to a bone.

**What is the best initial test for ankylosing spondylitis?**

An X-ray of the pelvis, to confirm sacroiliitis.

## What initial blood tests would you request, and what would you expect them to show in a patient with ankylosing spondylitis?

You would expect raised inflammatory markers (CRP and ESR), and negative autoantibodies (rheumatoid factor and anti-cyclic citrullinated peptide).

## What is the importance of measuring chest expansion in ankylosing spondylitis?

It is a useful measure of disease severity, as chest expansion may be reduced due to decreased mobility of the spine and thorax in advanced disease.

## What are other forms of spondylarthritis?

Reactive arthritis, psoriatic arthritis and inflammatory bowel disease–associated arthritis can all affect the axial skeleton.

## What does the FABER test examine?

Flexion, abduction and external rotation of the hip. Positive test if the patient has hip or back pain or the range of movement is limited. This is seen in sacroiliitis and hip pathology.

## What does the term 'bamboo spine' refer to?

Bamboo spine is a pathognomonic X-ray feature seen in ankylosing spondylitis, created by widespread fusion of the vertebral bodies.

## How many vertebrae are in each section of the spinal column?

There are 7 cervical vertebrae, 12 thoracic, 5 lumbar, 5 sacral (fused) and 4 coccyges (fused).

## What are the features of a parkinsonian gait?

Parkinsonian gait is described as a shuffling gait with slow movement (bradykinesia), particularly on turning or changing direction.

# Communication Skills

4

## Outline

## Station 4.1  Explaining Hypertension

### Doctor Briefing

You are a junior doctor in a primary care practice and have been asked to see Sonya Patel, a 47-year-old woman who has presented with persistently high readings of 156/98 mmHg on home blood pressure monitoring. Investigations for diabetes and underlying kidney disease have been negative. Please take a brief history of potential risk factors and explain Mrs Patel's diagnosis to her.

### Patient Briefing

You have been called in by your doctor to discuss your latest blood pressure results. You have a good diet and are fairly active. You do not have any significant medical problems. You feel that your blood pressure is high as a result of stress, as you frequently get headaches when you are at work. To help with your stress, you smoke (10 cigarettes a day) and drink a glass of red wine every night.

You are concerned because your father had high blood pressure and he had to be take tablets for it; you are not currently on such medication.

### Mark Scheme for Examiner

#### Introduction

| | | | |
|---|---|---|---|
| Cleans hands, introduces self and confirms patient identity | | | |
| Checks the identity of others in the room and confirms that the patient is happy for them to be present | | | |
| Establishes current patient knowledge and concerns | | | |

#### Explaining Hypertension

| Statement/Question | Justification | Answer | |
|---|---|---|---|
| Your blood pressure is the amount of pressure the walls of your arteries are dealing with | Start with a general open phrase to guide the patient | 'Yes, I am aware' | |

**Explaining Hypertension**

| Statement/Question | Justification | Answer | | | | | | |
|---|---|---|---|---|---|---|---|---|
| If this is high, your heart has to pump harder to get the blood around the body. This can lead to your heart becoming weaker over time | Simple, easy-to-follow explanation of blood pressure and how it affects the heart | 'OK' | | | | | | |
| High blood pressure increases your risk of having a stroke, as well as creating problems for your heart and kidneys | Explaining the importance of controlling blood pressure allows the patient to appreciate the complications of high blood pressure | 'Oh, I didn't realise this. What can we do about it?' | | | | | | |
| Really good question but before we discuss your blood pressure results and what we can do, can I ask a few questions? | It is important to signpost throughout your consultation, especially to prepare your patient for incoming personal questions | 'Sure' | | | | | | |

**Discussing Risk Factors**

| | | | | | | | | |
|---|---|---|---|---|---|---|---|---|
| Your diet and other lifestyle factors can raise your blood pressure. What is your diet like? | Lifestyle factors such as a diet high in salt, inactive lifestyle, smoking and high alcohol intake can raise blood pressure | 'My diet is OK. I eat lots of fruit and vegetables and try to stay away from junk food' | | | | | | |
| How about exercise? | | 'I like to go on walks with my family in my spare time' | | | | | | |
| Do you smoke or drink alcohol? | | 'I smoke and drink a glass of wine every night' | | | | | | |
| How many cigarettes do you smoke a day? | Really useful to be able to quantify this | 'Probably around 10 a day usually' | | | | | | |
| What is your stress level like? | Stress can directly cause the blood pressure to be raised but doesn't usually cause long-standing hypertension | 'I'm stressed all the time because of work and find that I'm getting more and more anxious. I think this is why I have high blood pressure' | | | | | | |
| Do you have a history of high blood pressure, even during any previous pregnancies? | Diabetes and kidney and thyroid disease are all linked to hypertension. If a patient was hypertensive during pregnancy, this increases her likelihood of having it later in life | 'No, I'm quite a fit and healthy person' | | | | | | |
| Does anyone in the family have high blood pressure? | Hypertension is a condition that can run over generations | 'My dad had high blood pressure, and he was taking tablets for it' | | | | | | |

## Discussing Risk Factors

| Statement/Question | Justification | Answer | | | | | |
|---|---|---|---|---|---|---|---|
| Are you on any medication? | Many medications can increase blood pressure as a side effect, such as steroids, combined oral contraceptive pill, antidepressants | 'No, I don't take any regular medications' | | | | | |

## Explaining the Diagnosis

| | | | | | | | |
|---|---|---|---|---|---|---|---|
| Last week we were monitoring your blood pressure at home. Some patients who have high blood pressure recordings at the surgery can have normal readings at home, where they may be naturally more relaxed | Explanation of white-coat hypertension | 'Yes, that is correct. I did think I would be more relaxed at home too' | | | | | |
| The blood pressure monitoring that you had while you were at home has shown that your blood pressure is persistently high. Ideally, we want it to be around 120/80 mmHg, but yours is on average 156/98 mmHg | Simple and brief explanation | 'Oh dear, how did that happen? That sounds really high' | | | | | |
| In most cases, the cause of high blood pressure is unknown. Sometimes it can be due to an underlying problem; for example, diabetes, hormone or kidney problems. Lifestyle factors can also affect it, such as a sedentary lifestyle, smoking, high salt intake | Explain to the patient the main causes of hypertension | 'I understand. What should I do about it?' | | | | | |
| We need to aim to lower the blood pressure reading. To start with, you can try implementing lifestyle changes, such as stopping smoking, increasing your level of exercise and reducing salt intake and we can support you with this if you wish<br><br>If that doesn't satisfactorily control your blood pressure, we can then look at prescribing you some tablets that will help you to lower it | Explain to the patient the conservative and medical management of hypertension.<br>Give your information in chunks so that you do not overload the patient | 'Yes, that sounds like a good plan. I would really like some help to stop smoking as I have tried to do this in the past by myself and been unsuccessful' | | | | | |
| In the meantime, we need to clarify whether your blood pressure is high all the time, even at night. I will organise an ambulatory blood pressure monitoring (ABPM) for you, which is a machine that measures your blood 24 h a day | Explain to the patient the next step of investigation. It is important to explain this in lay terms but also to use the appropriate medical terminology | 'That's fine' | | | | | |

**Finishing the Consultation**

| Question | Justification | Answer | | | | |
|---|---|---|---|---|---|---|
| We have discussed a lot of things today. To summarise, your blood pressure readings at home have been high. You have agreed to make some changes to your lifestyle, and then we can review your blood pressure again, along with the results from your ambulatory blood pressure reading. Then, we can decide if you need any further treatment | Short summary of the key points discussed so far | 'Yes' | | | | |
| I will provide you with a leaflet with more information and am happy to assist in any way possible | Leaflets and other resources will help to refresh the patient's memory | 'That'd be helpful' | | | | |
| Do you have any other questions or things to add? I know that we have discussed a lot of new things; please take some time to digest the information | May identify useful information that has been missed. Will also allow you to address any questions or concerns | 'No, thank you' | | | | |

**Present Your Findings**

Mrs Patel is a 47-year-old woman who has presented today to discuss her home blood pressure monitoring, which was increased at 156/98 mmHg. She is normally fit and leads an inactive lifestyle but admits to smoking and drinking as a result of stress.

Today I have discussed the risks of high blood pressure. I have explained that she will require ABPM and I have counselled her on lifestyle changes to help improve her blood pressure control. I will see her again in approximately 2 weeks' time, along with the results from her ABPM

**General Points**

| | | | |
|---|---|---|---|
| Polite to patient | | | |
| Maintains good eye contact | | | |
| Appropriate use of open and closed questions | | | |

## ❓ QUESTIONS FROM THE EXAMINER

### What are the stages of hypertension?

Stage 1: Clinic blood pressure ranging from 140/90 mmHg to 159/99 mmHg and subsequent ABPM daytime average or HBPM average blood pressure ranging from 135/85 mmHg to 149/94 mmHg.
Stage 2: Clinic blood pressure of 160/100 mmHg or higher but less than 180/120 mmHg and subsequent ABPM daytime average or HBPM average blood pressure of 150/95 mmHg or higher.
Stage 3: Clinic systolic blood pressure of 180 mmHg or higher or clinic diastolic blood pressure of 120 mmHg or higher.

### What is a 'hypertensive emergency'?

Severe hypertension (usually above 180 mmHg systolic), with evidence of acute damage to target organs.

### Give four potential sequelae that can occur in a hypertensive emergency.

Papilloedema, stroke, acute coronary syndrome and acute pulmonary oedema.

## Give three examples of medications that can be used to lower the blood pressure acutely.

Amlodipine, labetalol, glyceryl nitrate (GTN) infusions.

## What is pre-eclampsia?

Pre-eclampsia is a complication of pregnancy, characterised by high blood pressure and proteinuria. It can progress to eclampsia, a life-threatening seizure.

## Name four underlying medical conditions that can cause hypertension (secondary hypertension).

Cushing's syndrome, acromegaly, renal artery stenosis, phaeochromocytoma.

## Give four examples of features that a patient with Cushing's syndrome may present with.

Truncal obesity, buffalo hump, facial fullness, proximal muscle wasting and weakness.

## Name three investigations you would perform in a newly diagnosed hypertensive patient.

Urine dipstick, urea and electrolytes (U&Es), 12-lead electrocardiogram (ECG).

## What is orthostatic hypotension?

It is a form of low blood pressure that can happen when patients stand up from a lying or sitting position. It is defined as a systolic blood pressure decrease of at least 20 mmHg or a diastolic blood pressure decrease of at least 10 mmHg within 3 min of standing.

## Give three causes of postural hypotension.

Antihypertensive medications, dehydration, Parkinson's disease.

## Station 4.2 Lifestyle Advice Post Myocardial Infarction

### Doctor Briefing

You are a junior doctor working on the cardiology ward and have been asked to speak to James Smith, a 55-year-old accountant, who was admitted with chest pain and underwent primary angioplasty for an ST elevation myocardial infarction (STEMI). He is now recovering well following his procedure and is about to be discharged from hospital. Please explore why he was at risk for developing heart disease and what lifestyle measures could be adopted to reduce his risk of another event.

### Patient Briefing

You were admitted to hospital following a heart attack, and stents were inserted during a procedure where a tube was passed through your wrist. You are now being discharged on aspirin, clopidogrel, ramipril, bisoprolol and GTN spray. You have no contraindications to these medications. You do not understand why you have been started on so many medications and would like someone to go through them with you.

You work as an accountant and don't have time to do physical exercise. You usually eat takeout food and rarely eat fruit and vegetables. You are aware that you are slightly overweight. You have been smoking since you were 20, approximately 15 cigarettes per day, and you drink alcohol socially.

Your medical history consists of heartburn, high blood pressure (conservatively managed) and this episode of heart attack. Your father also suffered from one in his 70s.

You are very worried that you will have another heart attack and want to know how you can reduce the risk of this happening.

### Mark Scheme for Examiner

**Introduction**

Cleans hands, introduces self and confirms patient identity

Checks the identity of others in the room and confirms that the patient is happy for them to be present

Establishes current patient knowledge and concerns

**Clarifying the Situation**

| Statement/Question | Justification | Answer | | | | |
|---|---|---|---|---|---|---|
| Have you or any one in your family ever had a heart attack prior to this? | Elicit any non-modifiable risk factors such as personal or family history of myocardial infarction (MI) | 'This was my first heart attack. However, my dad had one in his 70s' | | | | |
| Could you describe your typical diet? | It is important to explore any modifiable risk factors; for example, poor diet, sedentary lifestyle, smoking and alcohol increase the risk of MI | 'It's not great. I'm usually too busy to cook so just grab whatever I can from fast-food places' | | | | |
| How active are you? | | 'I am so busy at work that I never get the chance to exercise' | | | | |
| Do you smoke or drink alcohol? | | 'I have been smoking for over 30 years, around 15 cigarettes a day. I drink alcohol whenever I go out with friends' | | | | |

## Clarifying the Situation

| Statement/Question | Justification | Answer | | | | |
|---|---|---|---|---|---|---|
| Do you suffer from any medical conditions? | Certain conditions increase the risk of MI, such as dyslipidaemia, hypertension and obesity | 'I've been told that I have high cholesterol and high blood pressure, but I wasn't on any tablets' | | | | |

## Post-Discharge Plans and Advice

| | | | | | | |
|---|---|---|---|---|---|---|
| Now that you are ready for discharge, there's some advice that we offer to everyone who's suffered a heart attack. Would you like me to go through it with you? | It's best practice to ask patients if they want certain information before giving it to them, so that you know they are ready to take on your advice | 'Yes please, everything's happened so quickly' | | | | |
| Yes, it can definitely be overwhelming, so I hope to explain everything to you today. After you leave the hospital, you will be supported by the cardiac rehabilitation team to help you improve various aspects of your life to reduce your risk of further events, and to provide psychological support | Brief the patient on post-discharge plans and advice so that he knows what he should be engaging in. Also provide him with conservative management action points such as improving his lifestyle | 'Yes, I know. It can be so difficult with my work but the support team sounds good' | | | | |
| I'd also like to emphasise the importance of participating in regular exercise and maintaining a healthy balanced diet, in order to maintain a healthy weight | | | | | | |
| Stopping smoking and aiming to drink within the recommended limits are desirable | | | | | | |
| You have been started on four different types of medications which all work to prevent you having further heart attacks. You can think of each one addressing a particular factor. I will now go on to discuss them individually | You are introducing a structure to your conversation that your patient can follow. Signposting is a good way of keeping your explanations succinct and allows the patient to follow your explanations easily, especially when explaining multiple concepts | 'Yes please, it's all so confusing!' | | | | |
| The first set of drugs are called antiplatelets. These are aspirin and clopidogrel | Dual antiplatelet therapy is essential, especially in those who have had stents inserted. Emphasise to the patient the importance of continuing antiplatelet therapy | 'How do they work?' | | | | |
| They reduce your risk of further heart attacks by preventing clots forming, especially in the new stents that were inserted | | 'How long should I take them for?' | | | | |
| You should take them every day for a year. After that, only aspirin should be continued | | 'I understand' | | | | |

**Post-Discharge Plans and Advice**

| Statement/Question | Justification | Answer | | | | | |
|---|---|---|---|---|---|---|---|
| The second set of drugs helps to reduce your blood pressure. These are ramipril (angiotensin-converting enzyme (ACE) inhibitor) and bisoprolol (beta-blocker). High blood pressure is an important risk factor of having further heart attacks and these drugs help to reduce it | Hypertension is an important risk factor that is addressed by both ACE-inhibitors and beta-blockers. Explaining beta-blockers and ACE inhibitors together helps to keep things simple | 'If they both do the same thing, why do I need to take both?' | | | | | |
| As well as lowering blood pressure, each drug also helps your heart after a heart attack in different ways. Ramipril can help to prevent the symptoms of heart failure and can also protect your kidneys. Bisoprolol, on the other hand, lowers your heart rate, which can help to prevent the symptoms of angina | | 'I see' | | | | | |
| Your primary care doctor will regularly monitor your kidney function as ramipril can affect it initially. It can also make you feel dizzy following standing up. The doctor will also continue to monitor your blood pressure | It is important to address the side effects and monitoring required and how these drugs can be titrated | 'OK' | | | | | |
| The third type of tablet is called a statin. This helps to lower cholesterol, which can also contribute to having a heart attack | High-dose statins are required for secondary prevention of MI. In some cases, patients may resist taking statins. Be prepared to explain their risks and benefits and allow patients to decide for themselves | 'Yes, I've heard of that before' | | | | | |
| You should take it every night and you will have regular monitoring of your liver function | | 'OK' | | | | | |
| The final drug that you have been prescribed is a spray called GTN | Symptomatic relief in the event of further anginal chest pain is important. | 'What is it for?' | | | | | |
| This is a spray that goes under your tongue and you should give yourself two sprays whenever you get chest pain | It is important to clarify when medical help should be sought | 'Sounds good' | | | | | |
| You can use it any time, but if you find that your chest pain does not go after using it twice, you should call for medical help. This may be a sign that you are having another heart attack | | 'Oh gosh' | | | | | |
| To conclude, there are four types of medications that act on platelets, blood pressure, cholesterol and further chest pain. Is there anything that you would like me to explain again? | Chunking and checking the patient's knowledge is a key communication skill | 'No, that's been very helpful' | | | | | |

**Finishing the Consultation**

| Question | Justification | Answer | | | | | |
|---|---|---|---|---|---|---|---|
| We have discussed a lot of things today. To summarise, you have had a heart attack but can now go home with some regular medications that you need to take. You have agreed to make changes to your lifestyle to reduce the risk of you having another event | Short summary of the key points discussed so far | 'Yes' | | | | | |
| I will provide you with a leaflet with more information and am happy to assist in any way possible | Leaflets and other resources will help to refresh the patient's memory | 'That'd be helpful' | | | | | |
| Do you have any other questions or things to add? I know that we have discussed a lot of new things; please take some time to digest the information | May identify useful information that has been missed. Will also allow you to address any questions or concerns | 'No, thank you' | | | | | |

**Present Your Findings**

Mr Smith is a 55-year-old man who is recovering from a heart attack, for which he underwent primary angioplasty. He is now ready for discharge, and I have explained to him the newly commenced medications. We have also discussed lifestyle advice and ways to reduce his risk of another event, including stopping smoking and increasing his physical activity

**General Points**

| | | | | | |
|---|---|---|---|---|---|
| Polite to patient | | | | | |
| Maintains good eye contact | | | | | |
| Appropriate use of open and closed questions | | | | | |

## ❓ QUESTIONS FROM THE EXAMINER

**According to National Institute for Health and Care Excellence (NICE) guidelines, when should primary percutaneous coronary intervention be performed?**

It should be performed as soon as possible (within 120 min of the time when thrombolysis could be given) in adults with STEMI who present within 12 h of onset of symptoms.

**Give one example of a drug used to thrombolyse patients.**

Alteplase, streptokinase, reteplase, anistreplase, urokinase.

**Give three complications of an acute MI.**

Heart failure, cardiogenic shock, arrhythmias.

**In a cardiac arrest, name the two shockable rhythms.**

Ventricular fibrillation and (pulseless) ventricular tachycardia.

### What is Dressler's syndrome?

Pericarditis that presents approximately 4 weeks following an acute MI. It is often associated with pleural and pericardial effusions.

### Give three ECG findings that are suggestive of a posterior MI.

Horizontal ST depression, tall broad R waves and upright T waves in V1–V3.

### What is the purpose of the cardiac rehabilitation team?

The goal of the cardiac rehabilitation is to support the patient to regain strength, prevent worsening of the condition and reduce the risk of future heart problems. Programmes cover physical activity, education about lifestyle risk factors, relaxation and psychological support.

### Which healthcare professionals make up the cardiac rehabilitation team?

Cardiac specialist nurses, physiotherapists, dieticians, exercise specialists, occupational therapists, pharmacists, psychologists and cardiologists.

### What is the difference between a stent and angioplasty?

An angioplasty is a procedure performed to open narrowed or blocked coronary arteries. During or immediately after this procedure, a coronary artery stent can be inserted into the vessels to keep them patent.

### What is the term for the combination of coronary angioplasty with stenting?

Percutaneous coronary intervention.

## Station 4.3   Explaining Statins

### Doctor Briefing

You are a junior doctor working in a primary care practice and are asked to see Ken Adams, a 45-year-old man, who has undergone cardiovascular screening and, as a result, has been prescribed statins, as he has a 12% (moderate) risk of developing cardiovascular disease (CVD) in the next 10 years. Please take a brief history covering his cardiovascular risk factors and then counsel him about statin use.

### Patient Briefing

You are a 45-year-old man. At your last visit, the doctor asked you some questions, measured your blood pressure and took some bloods. You are a smoker, have a poor diet and do not exercise. You have come in to find out the results of your blood tests.

Your medical background consists of type 2 diabetes and gout.

When asked, you do not know much about cholesterol. Your wife is taking statins, but she hates taking them because they give her muscle cramps. You do not want to take statins because of this and would prefer to try a different approach first.

### Mark Scheme for Examiner

#### Introduction

| | |
|---|---|
| Cleans hands, introduces self and confirms patient identity | |
| Checks the identity of others in the room and confirms that the patient is happy for them to be present | |
| Establishes current patient knowledge and concerns | |

#### Explaining Cholesterol and QRISK

| Statement/Question | Justification | Answer | | | | | |
|---|---|---|---|---|---|---|---|
| The results of your blood tests and blood pressure are back. Do you want me to discuss them with you now? | Always invite the patient to the conversation, because he may not be keen to receive the information at that moment in time. Open with a clear statement of what will be covered in the consultation. The patient is aware that you will be discussing reducing his cardiovascular risk | 'Yes, please do' | | | | | |
| In combination with your history, it revealed that you are at an increased risk of having a heart attack or stroke. Is it OK if we discuss ways that you can reduce this risk? | | 'Absolutely. I thought you might say this' | | | | | |
| Your risk of a stroke or heart attack in the next 10 years is 12%. This means that in a group of 100 people with the same background as you, 12 will have a heart attack or stroke in the next 10 years | Instead of just quoting the percentage, expand and explain to the patient fully what the risk is to emphasise the importance | 'That's quite scary. Is there anything I can do?' | | | | | |
| Your blood tests have shown that your cholesterol levels are particularly high, so today I want to discuss ways in which we can reduce this. What do you know about cholesterol? | Make the patient aware that reducing cholesterol is one way to reduce overall cardiovascular risk | 'I think if it's high, it's bad. That is what my wife was told by her doctor' | | | | | |

**Explaining Cholesterol and QRISK**

| Statement/Question | Justification | Answer | | | | | |
|---|---|---|---|---|---|---|---|
| Yes, you are correct. In fact, there are two types of cholesterol – these are called high-density lipoprotein (HDL) and low-density lipoprotein (LDL). High levels of LDL can be harmful because they can lead to fatty material building up in the artery walls. This makes them narrower and can increase the chance of clots forming. If these clots form in the arteries to the brain or heart, the result may beo a stroke or heart attack | Acknowledge what the patient has said and expand on it. Briefly explain that there are two types of cholesterol and how high cholesterol can relate to an increased risk of cardiovascular disease | 'How do I bring my levels down?' | | | | | |

**Identifying Cardiovascular Risk Factors**

| Statement/Question | Justification | Answer | | | | | |
|---|---|---|---|---|---|---|---|
| Let's start by exploring your lifestyle habits. Could you describe your typical diet? | Explore any modifiable risk factors. A sedentary lifestyle, smoking and alcohol can all increase the cholesterol level | 'It's quite poor. I just order from restaurants usually and have chocolate-flavoured cereal for breakfast' | | | | | |
| How active are you? | | 'I find it difficult to get active, which is why I'm overweight. I do not enjoy exercise' | | | | | |
| Do you drink alcohol? | | 'Only socially when I go out with friends' | | | | | |
| Do you smoke? If so, how much? | If the patient smokes, calculate the amount as the number of pack years | 'Yes, I've smoked since I was 18 years old, around 10 a day' | | | | | |
| Do you suffer from any medical conditions? | Certain conditions, for example hypertension, diabetes, chronic kidney disease and previous heart attacks or strokes, all put a patient at risk of future cardiovascular events | 'I have gout and diabetes and take medication for this' | | | | | |
| Has any family member got high cholesterol? | Elicit any non-modifiable risk factors such as family history of hypercholesterolaemia | 'No' | | | | | |
| Lifestyle changes can help to reduce your risk. Stopping smoking, doing more exercise and improving your diet can all help to lower the cholesterol level. Having good control of your diabetes would help as well | Lifestyle interventions can help and conservative management of lowering cholesterol should be discussed with the patient | 'OK' | | | | | |

## Explaining Statins

| Statement/Question | Justification | Answer | | | | | |
|---|---|---|---|---|---|---|---|
| Medications to lower your cholesterol are also available. Are you aware of any? | Begin to counsel the patient about statin use by providing him with enough information on statins so that he can make an informed decision about taking them or not. Answer the patient's questions throughout and acknowledge what he is saying so that he feels listened to | 'Do you mean statins? Yes, my wife takes them' | | | | | |
| Yes, that's right. Statins are commonly used to lower cholesterol and are offered to patients at a risk of greater than 10% | | 'I see' | | | | | |
| Statins should be taken once a day, during the evening, and are usually lifelong | | 'OK' | | | | | |
| If you miss a dose, make sure you take it as soon as you remember, but do not double up the dose the next day to make up for a missed dose | | Are there any side effects I should know about? | | | | | |
| Most people can tolerate statins, but they can cause people to feel sick and tired and develop muscle cramps | Common and serious side effects, such as liver failure and rhabdomyolysis, should be explained to the patient. Give patients key medical terminology but explain the concept in lay terms as well | 'Yes, my wife has complained of cramps a lot recently. I do not want this' | | | | | |
| In very rare circumstances, they can cause muscle breakdown in a condition called rhabdomyolysis which can be life threatening. They can also lead to liver damage | | 'That sounds quite dangerous' | | | | | |
| To avoid this, you will have regular blood tests which will monitor your liver function | Baseline and regular monitoring of liver function tests (LFTs) whilst on statins is required and should be discussed with the patient | 'I understand' | | | | | |
| If you start to develop muscle pain whilst taking the statins, you should stop taking them and speak to your primary care doctor who will order urgent blood tests | Muscle pain may be the initial presentation of rhabdomyolysis and you must advise the patient to seek medical advice if he experiences this. Stopping the statin and checking CK and LFTs is required | 'OK, then they can find a different drug' | | | | | |
| Potentially, but they will also make sure it is safe for you to continue taking them. Statins can also interact with some food as well as some antibiotics. It is important that you tell a new doctor if you are taking statins | Statins are metabolised via the CYP450 pathway. The patient should be made aware of the interactions that statins may have with other medications | 'I'll be mindful' | | | | | |

## Finishing the Consultation

| Statement/Question | Justification | Answer | | | | | |
|---|---|---|---|---|---|---|---|
| So far, we have discussed the importance of reducing your cholesterol and how this can be done with statins. I have explained the key information you need to know whilst you are taking them, including the side effects and monitoring that you will need and what to do if you miss a tablet | Short summary of the key points discussed so far | 'I'm a bit worried about the side effects. My wife doesn't like taking statins because she gets cramps. Is there another way that I can reduce my cholesterol?' | | | | | |

**Finishing the Consultation**

| Statement/Question | Justification | Answer | | | | | |
|---|---|---|---|---|---|---|---|
| There are a number of lifestyle changes you can make, in particular with your diet. Here is a leaflet with more information about how you can adapt your diet. You can try those first to see whether they lower your cholesterol levels. If they do not, then we can talk about statins again | Lifestyle changes can have an impact and can be a good first step. It is good to give patients some time to trial this, especially if they are not keen on medication anyway, as they will likely have poor compliance with the medication. A compromise is made by trying lifestyle interventions first and then discussing statins again at a later date | 'That sounds good' | | | | | |
| I will also provide you with some leaflets to help you remember what we have been through today | Leaflets and other resources will help to refresh the patient's memory | 'Great' | | | | | |
| Do you have any other questions or things to add? I know that we have discussed a lot of new things; please take some time to digest the information | May identify useful information that has been missed. Will also allow you to address any questions or concerns | 'No, thank you' | | | | | |

**Present Your Findings**

Mr Adams is a 45-year-old man who is at a moderately high risk of developing cardiovascular disease and has elevated cholesterol levels. Today I have explained the outcome of his cardiovascular screening, as well as the importance of lowering his cholesterol.

I have counselled him regarding statin use but at the moment he is reluctant to start them. He has agreed to trial lifestyle interventions for now and we will revisit statin use in the future if they fail to reduce his cholesterol levels

**General Points**

| | | | | |
|---|---|---|---|---|
| Polite to patient | | | | |
| Maintains good eye contact | | | | |
| Appropriate use of open and closed questions | | | | |

## ❓ QUESTIONS FROM THE EXAMINER

**Which enzyme do statins primarily act on?**

HMG-CoA reductase – an enzyme involved in the synthesis of cholesterol.

**Why should short-acting statins (e.g. simvastatin) be taken at night?**

In order to reduce the peak cholesterol synthesis which occurs during morning as well as help to reduce the effect of muscle aches as the patient will be asleep.

**Name three drugs that can interact with statins.**

Some antibiotics (for example, clarithromycin), antiepileptics (for example, carbamazepine) and certain antifungals (for example, fluconazole) can all interact with statins.

## Statins can be used in the secondary prevention of which conditions?

Statins are often started following an MI or stroke or in those who have angina or transient ischaemic attack.

## Can statins be used in pregnancy?

No, they would be avoided in pregnancy – ideally discontinued 3 months before attempting to conceive.

## Name four medications that can lead to dyslipidaemia.

Thiazide diuretics, beta-blockers, antipsychotics, corticosteroids.

## Aside from lifestyle and genetic factors, name three medical conditions that can lead to dyslipidaemia:

Hypothyroidism, type 2 diabetes, anorexia nervosa.

## Very high levels of triglycerides can cause pancreatitis. True or false?

True. Very high triglyceride levels can compromise capillary circulation and cause ischaemic damage to pancreatic acinar cells.

## Give three factors that can increase a patient's risk of having side effects when taking statins.

History of liver disease, family history of myopathy, alcoholism.

## Which fruit juice should patients on statins avoid?

Grapefruit juice can increase the risk of side effects.

## Station 4.4    Explaining Inhaler Technique

### Doctor Briefing

You are a junior doctor working in a primary care practice and have been asked to see Rosie Johnson, a 24-year-old woman, who has come in for an asthma review. Rosie has recently been diagnosed with asthma and has been prescribed a salbutamol inhaler to manage her symptoms. Please review her symptom control and explain the correct way of using an inhaler both with a spacer and without.

### Patient Briefing

You have been recently diagnosed with asthma a few months ago. You picked up your medication and spacer from the pharmacy. There is a brown inhaler that you have to use every morning and evening, and a blue inhaler that you can use whenever you feel wheezy or short of breath. When asked, you admit that you are unsure about the proper way of using your inhaler.

You find that you are needing to take the blue inhaler every day. But when you do use the inhaler, you are still wheezy afterwards. You've never been shown how to use one before.

Your main concern is that you are using it wrong and not getting any of the medication in.

### Mark Scheme for Examiner

#### Introduction

| | | | | |
|---|---|---|---|---|
| Cleans hands, introduces self and confirms patient identity | | | | |
| Checks the identity of others in the room and confirms that the patient is happy for them to be present | | | | |
| Establishes current patient knowledge and concerns | | | | |

#### Brief Review

| Statement/Question | Justification | Answer | | | | |
|---|---|---|---|---|---|---|
| How has your asthma been since you've started your inhalers? | It is important to review the patient's symptom control and how it has impacted the patient's daily activities | 'I've not noticed any difference – my breathing is still problematic' | | | | |
| Have you had any wheeze, chest tightness or shortness of breath? | | 'I get wheezy every night before I sleep and my chest can feel tight randomly throughout the day' | | | | |
| How often do you use the blue inhaler? Have you had any side effects or problems? | | 'I've been using it roughly twice a day, but it's not really helped. I'm not sure if I'm using it correctly though' | | | | |
| It is vital that you have good inhaler technique to ensure that you are getting the medication into your lungs. Do you want me to show you how to use them? | Explain to the patient the importance of good inhaler technique and how it affects the efficacy of the medication. This is also useful for signposting onto inhaler technique | 'Yes, please. I think I've been using it wrong as things are not getting any better' | | | | |

## Explaining Correct Inhaler Technique – With Spacer

| Statement/Question | Justification | Answer | | | | | |
|---|---|---|---|---|---|---|---|
| What I will do first is talk you through the equipment. Then I will talk you through each step at a time. At the end, I will ask you to repeat the steps back to me | The patient now knows the structure of the conversation and what to expect. She is aware that she is expected to remember the steps | 'OK' | | | | | |
| This is the inhaler – it contains the medication. Before using it, make sure the cap is removed and shake the inhaler well before using it  This is the spacer – the inhaler attaches to the spacer. The spacer allows the drug to be absorbed more smoothly and helps it get where it needs to | Familiarise the patient with the equipment that she will be using. Often explaining the reason why she has certain equipment will help understanding and thus improve compliance | 'I understand' | | | | | |
| Before you use any medication, remember to check the expiry date | This is something that is often forgotten by patients | | | | | | |
| Then, sit or stand up straight and slightly tilt your chin forwards. Breathe out completely | This ensures that all of the medication can easily travel to the lungs | | | | | | |
| Then put your lips around the mouth-piece of the spacer to create a tight seal | This is an important step – without a seal, the medication will not be delivered adequately | | | | | | |
| Press the top of the inhaler once. Make sure that you take a slow deep breath in at the same time | Show the patient exactly where she is meant to press to deliver the dose | | | | | | |
| Once the lungs are full, take the inhaler out of the mouth and hold the breath for around 10 s or as long as you can | This allows for maximum absorption of the medication into the lungs | | | | | | |
| Afterwards, remove the inhaler and disconnect it from the spacer. If repeat puffs are required, shake the inhaler well before using it again. Once finished, replace the cap | Finish the final steps by informing the patient what to do with the inhaler and spacer | | | | | | |
| Would you be able to summarise and show me the steps for taking an inhaler with a spacer? | To ensure that the information has been received, as well as providing an opportunity to correct any misunderstanding | 'Yes' | | | | | |

**Explaining Correct Inhaler Technique – Without Spacer**

| Statement/Question | Justification | Answer | | | | | |
|---|---|---|---|---|---|---|---|
| Now, I'll talk you through using the inhaler without a spacer. It is very similar to what we have just done | This lets the patient know that you are moving on to a different concept | 'I'm ready' | | | | | |
| Again, first make sure that you are sat or stood up straight with your chin slightly tilted forward. Then breathe out completely | You are recapping what you have previously covered and adapting your instructions for use without a spacer | 'I understand' | | | | | |
| Next, you need to take the inhaler and remove the cap. Once you have done that, shake the inhaler | | | | | | | |
| This time, put your lips around the inhaler mouthpiece, instead of the spacer, to form a good seal | | | | | | | |
| Press the top of the inhaler to release one puff of medicine as you take a deep breath in slowly | | | | | | | |
| Once you have delivered the dose, remove the inhaler but continue to hold your breath for around 10 s or as long as you can | | | | | | | |
| Lastly, breathe out slowly. If repeat puffs are required, shake the inhaler well before using it again. Once finished, replace the cap | | | | | | | |
| Would you be able to summarise and show me the steps for taking an inhaler without a spacer? | It is important to ask the patient to relay this information back to ensure that she has fully understood | 'Of course' | | | | | |

**Finishing the Consultation**

| | | | | | | | |
|---|---|---|---|---|---|---|---|
| So today we've talked through using the inhaler both with the spacer and without it. Are you happy with both of them or would you like me to show you again? | Short summary of the key points discussed so far and ensuring that the patient is happy with the information | 'I'm happy with both, thank you' | | | | | |
| I will provide you with a leaflet with more information and am happy to assist in any way possible. | Leaflets and other resources will help to refresh the patient's memory | 'That'd be helpful' | | | | | |
| Do you have any other questions or things to add? I know that we have discussed a lot of new things; please take some time to digest the information. | May identify useful information that has been missed. Will also allow you to address any questions or concerns | 'No, thank you' | | | | | |

**Present Your Findings**

Rosie Johnson is a 24-year-old woman who has recently been diagnosed with asthma. She has been prescribed a 'reliever' inhaler but has found that her symptoms of shortness of breath and wheeze have persisted. Ms Johnson has been struggling with how to use her inhaler, and therefore I have explained and demonstrated the correct technique of using her inhaler, both with and without the spacer. I have addressed all of her questions and provided her with further written information on correct inhaler technique

**General Points**

Polite to patient

Maintains good eye contact

Appropriate use of open and closed questions

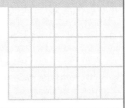

## ❓ QUESTIONS FROM THE EXAMINER

**Give three risk factors that are associated with asthma.**

Atopy, obesity, prematurity.

**Name two medications that are contraindicated in asthmatic patients.**

Non-steroidal anti-inflammatory drugs (NSAIDs) and beta-blockers are contraindicated in asthmatics.

**Give three differential diagnoses of a nocturnal cough.**

Heart failure, gastro-oesophageal reflux, asthma.

**A patient with suspected asthma undergoes spirometry. It shows an obstructive pattern. The patient is then given 400 mcg of salbutamol and spirometry is repeated after 15 min. There is no reversibility. What does this indicate?**

An obstructive pattern with no reversibility is suggestive of chronic obstructive pulmonary disease (COPD).

**Name three conditions that are associated with a restrictive pattern on spirometry.**

Pulmonary fibrosis, skeletal abnormalities such as kyphoscoliosis, neuromuscular disease (e.g. myasthenia gravis).

**In an asthmatic, what would the spirometry results show?**

Spirometry would show an obstructive pattern – reduced forced expiratory volume l s ($FEV_1$) (<80%), reduced forced vital capacity (FVC) and a reduced $FEV_1$/FVC ratio.

**What dose of prednisolone should be given to a patient with an acute asthma exacerbation?**

40 mg.

**What lifestyle changes can be recommended to patients with chronic asthma?**

Smoking cessation, weight loss in overweight patients, avoidance of asthma triggers.

**Name three common triggers of asthma.**

Tobacco smoke, dust mites, outdoor air pollution, pets and mould.

**What is occupational asthma?**

Asthma that is associated with substances that the patient is exposed to at work.

## Station 4.5    Smoking Cessation Counselling

### Doctor Briefing

You are a junior doctor working in a primary care practice and your next patient is Jennifer Roland, a 30-year-old woman, who wants help with quitting smoking. Please take a brief smoking history and counsel her regarding smoking cessation.

### Patient Briefing

You are a 30-year-old female who currently smokes around 20 cigarettes per day. You usually smoke alone and have been doing this since you were 17. Over the past 2 years, you have tried to quit a few times by yourself, but have been unsuccessful and end up smoking again within 3 weeks.

Recently, your dad has been diagnosed with lung cancer, which has really upset and frightened you. For that reason, you have decided to come and get professional help in stopping smoking and would like to stop for good.

### Mark Scheme for Examiner

#### Introduction

| | | | |
|---|---|---|---|
| Cleans hands, introduces self and confirms patient identity | | | |
| Checks the identity of others in the room and confirms that the patient is happy for them to be present | | | |
| Establishes current patient knowledge and concerns | | | |

#### Taking a Brief Smoking History

| Statement/Question | Justification | Answer | | | |
|---|---|---|---|---|---|
| How much do you currently smoke? | Gives an idea as to how dependent the patient is on smoking and allows for the number of pack-years to be calculated. One pack-year is equivalent to 20 cigarettes per day for 1 calendar year | 'About 20 cigarettes a day' | | | |
| What age did you start smoking? | | 'Since the age of 17' | | | |
| Who is around when you smoke? | This allows identification of certain factors that are preventing her from stopping, or factors that could be a motivation for her to stop; for example, children | 'I usually smoke alone' | | | |
| Have you previously tried to stop? If so, what did you do? | Establishes any previous attempts that the patient has made, how far she managed and if professional help was sought | 'On and off over the past 2 years. I've tried to quit by just stopping cold turkey. But it's never lasted more than 3 weeks and then I'd be smoking again' | | | |
| Why do you want to stop now? | Establishing the current reason can allow a more personalised and focused approach to helping the patient quit | 'My dad has recently been diagnosed with lung cancer, so it's scared and upset me quite a bit' | | | |
| I'm sorry to hear this. We can definitely help you with this | Empathy is important. Make sure you acknowledge anything that the patient discloses to you | 'Thank you' | | | |

**Smoking Cessation Advice**

| Question | Justification | Answer | | | | | |
|---|---|---|---|---|---|---|---|
| Smoking is associated with numerous serious illnesses that can reduce a person's life expectancy, such as lung and throat cancers, coronary heart disease, chronic obstructive pulmonary disease | It is important to explain to the patient the risks associated with smoking, both to her personal health and to others | 'Yes, it is really bad and I know that I must stop' | | | | | |
| Smoking also poses a threat to those who do not smoke themselves but are exposed to cigarette smoke by others. This is known as passive smoking and can be particularly harmful to children and pregnant woman | | 'I also want to be getting pregnant soon, so I'd definitely like to stop by then' | | | | | |
| It is really important to stop smoking if you are trying for a baby. It can be difficult to stop smoking, especially if you have been smoking for a while, as nicotine, one of the chemicals in cigarettes, is addictive | Acknowledging the difficulty of quitting smoking is vital. It can be helpful to use medical jargon, but you must explain in lay terms as well | 'I understand' | | | | | |
| Withdrawal symptoms (such as cravings to smoke, anxiety, irritability) tend to reach a peak after a day of stopping smoking. However, they gradually ease over 2–4 weeks | Counsel the patient on the withdrawal effects of quitting smoking and give examples of common ones to prepare her for what she may experience during the process | 'Yes, when I tried previously it made me feel very anxious, which is why I went back to smoking' | | | | | |
| Most people who have successfully stopped smoking have had multiple attempts | Noting this can reassure the patient that often more than one attempt is required and not to be discouraged if she does relapse. Some patients require continuous words of encouragement to push them through the obstacles and difficulties | 'That's good to hear, as I've tried so many times' | | | | | |
| To make the process easier for you, I'd advise that you get as much support as possible. This can be from family and friends, signing up to a local smoking cessation clinic or calling the Smokefree National Helpline to speak to trained advisors | Focus on ways that smoking cessation can be made easier by signposting the patient to helpful and professional resources | 'They all sound very helpful. I didn't think about them before' | | | | | |
| As an addition to helping you quit, you could also consider using nicotine replacement therapy (NRT), which a lot of people use when they quit smoking. Do you know what it is? | NRT can be a useful adjunct to willpower for people who are trying to quit smoking. Explain what is it and how it works | 'No, I've never heard of it' | | | | | |

## Smoking Cessation Advice

| Statement/Question | Justification | Answer | | | | | |
|---|---|---|---|---|---|---|---|
| NRT is a way of getting nicotine into the body without smoking, helping to stop smoking by reducing withdrawal symptoms. It comes in lots of forms, including patches, gum, inhalers and sprays. Doses vary depending on how much you smoke per day. Typically, it is used for 2–3 months, and then the patient is weaned off it. NRT should not be combined with other medications that are used to help with stopping smoking; for example, varenicline and bupropion | Can this row be on the same page as the row above, as the justification is meant to span across both rows? | 'That might be helpful. I'll bear that in mind. I'll take some information leaflets about it, if that is all right' | | | | | |

## Finishing the Consultation

| Statement/Question | Justification | Answer | | | | | |
|---|---|---|---|---|---|---|---|
| To summarise, you are motivated to stop smoking. I have informed you about some resources to help you and you are aware of some of the withdrawal effects. You also think that NRT may be beneficial to you. Is that correct? | Short summary of the key points discussed so far | 'Yes, this all sounds really helpful, thank you' | | | | | |
| I will provide you with a leaflet with more information and am happy to assist in any way possible | Leaflets and other resources will help to refresh the patient's memory | 'That'd be helpful' | | | | | |
| Do you have any other questions or things to add? I know that we have discussed a lot of new things; please take some time to digest the information | Allows any final concerns to be addressed | 'No, thank you' | | | | | |

## Present Your Findings

Miss Roland is a 30-year-old current smoker with a 13-pack-year history. She has tried to quit by herself on multiple attempts but has not been successful for longer than 3 weeks. She is seeking help to stop, as her father was recently diagnosed with lung cancer and she also wants to get pregnant soon.

Today I counselled her on the benefits of smoking cessation and have recommended that she use NRT whilst trying to quit. I have also signposted her to the smoking cessation clinic and provided her with the number of a smoking cessation helpline

## General Points

Polite to patient

Maintains good eye contact

Appropriate use of open and closed questions

## ❓ QUESTIONS FROM THE EXAMINER

### Name three differential diagnoses of a solitary round lesion seen on a chest X ray.

Abscess, granuloma, metastases.

### What is a Pancoast tumour?

A type of lung cancer that presents at the apex of the lung. As a result of pressure on the brachial plexus, symptoms include shoulder pain and weakness on the affected side.

### Give four causes of haemoptysis.

Pneumonia, lung cancer, pulmonary embolism, tuberculosis (TB), bronchitis, bronchiectasis, lung abscess.

### Name four cancers that commonly metastasise to the lungs.

Bladder, breast, prostate, kidney.

### What is mesothelioma?

A tumour of mesothelial cells, usually related to a previous exposure to asbestos.

### Aside from lung cancer, give four causes of clubbing.

Cystic fibrosis, lung abscess, bronchiectasis, infective endocarditis, liver disease, inflammatory bowel disease.

### Smoking is a major risk factor for bladder cancer. Why?

Carcinogens present in tobacco smoke are renally excreted and can therefore accumulate in the bladder.

### What is the most common presentation of bladder cancer?

Painless haematuria.

### Name three types of lung cancer.

Small-cell lung cancer, squamous cell carcinoma, adenocarcinoma, large-cell carcinoma, lung carcinoid tumours.

### Give three risk factors for lung cancer.

Smoking, COPD, exposure to radon, exposure to asbestos, previous radiation therapy to the lungs, air pollution, personal or family history of lung cancer.

## Station 4.6    Consent for Ascitic Drain

### Doctor Briefing

You are a junior doctor working on the medical admission unit and have been asked to see Perry Bard, a 59-year-old man, who has presented with increasing abdominal swelling and shortness of breath over the last 3 months. He is known to have liver cirrhosis. On examination of the abdomen, there is shifting dullness. Please take a brief history and gain Mr Bard's consent for an ascitic drain.

### Patient Briefing

You are a chronic alcoholic and have been diagnosed with liver cirrhosis for 5 years. You have noticed that your tummy is getting more and more distended over the last 3 months. It is gradually getting worse and feels quite tense. You are now also finding it difficult to walk long distances because you are getting short of breath. You have not got any abdominal pain, or swelling in your ankles.

You have never heard of an ascitic drain before but would be willing to find out more about it.

### Mark Scheme for Examiner

#### Introduction

| | | | | | |
|---|---|---|---|---|---|
| Cleans hands, introduces self and confirms patient identity | | | | | |
| Checks the identity of others in the room and confirms that the patient is happy for them to be present | | | | | |
| Establishes current patient knowledge and concerns | | | | | |

#### Taking a History

| Statement/Question | Justification | Answer | | | | |
|---|---|---|---|---|---|---|
| Before I discuss the procedure, I would like to ask some questions about your background. When did the swelling in your tummy begin? | This allows you to gauge the progression of the patient's condition. Worsening ascites and intra-abdominal pressure are likely to have contributed to the breathlessness | 'Over the last 3 months. It is getting worse and worse' | | | | |
| When did the breathlessness begin? | | 'Gradually over the last week' | | | | |
| Have you got any swelling in your ankles or lower back? | Heart failure is an important cause of both peripheral oedema and ascites and should be considered | 'No' | | | | |
| Have you got any abdominal pain? | Presence of pain with tense ascites can be a sign of spontaneous bacterial peritonitis (SBP) | 'No, just a bit uncomfortable' | | | | |
| Do you have any skin infections on your tummy or known blood clotting disorders or take any blood thinners? | Prior to the procedure, also ask the patient about potential contraindications. If the patient is female, enquire about the possibility of pregnancy as well | 'No' | | | | |

#### Explain and Obtain Consent for the Procedure

| | | | | | | |
|---|---|---|---|---|---|---|
| Have you ever had an ascitic drain before? | It may help to establish the patient's current knowledge about ascitic drains | 'Never. What is that?' | | | | |

## Explain and Obtain Consent for the Procedure

| Statement/Question | Justification | Answer | | | | | | |
|---|---|---|---|---|---|---|---|---|
| An ascitic drain involves passing a small needle through the abdominal wall to create a hole, through which a tube is then inserted, and it remains there. The abdominal fluid will drain through this tube to a collection bag, and it may take several hours or more for all the fluid to be drained | Introduce the patient to the procedure by explaining the main steps. Address any concerns or questions that the patient may have throughout | 'Will it hurt? It sounds painful' | | | | | | |
| Understandably, that's a common question. The procedure is carried out under local anaesthetic, therefore you may experience a small sharp scratch when the local anaesthetic is injected, but afterwards you should not feel pain. I can prescribe some painkillers for you to take after the procedure, if required | Some simple analgesia, such as paracetamol, can help the patient to overcome the immediate pain that he may experience post-ascitic drain. It is vital to give the patient reassurance and alleviate any concerns | 'That's good to know' | | | | | | |
| We will also send off samples of the fluid drained, which will hopefully provide us with more information about your condition. It may take several days for the results to return | Ask the patient for consent to send off the sample, and provide him with an estimated timeline | 'That's fine; these things always take a while it seems' | | | | | | |
| The benefit of having an ascitic tap is that it reduces the risk of infection of the inner lining of your tummy, to relieve your symptoms of breathlessness, and to find out what has caused the swelling | Carefully explain the risks and benefits of any procedure, as well as alternative options, to the patient so that he can make an informed decision | 'Are there risks?' | | | | | | |
| Although ascitic drains are commonly performed procedures, there are some risks associated with it, including: failure to insert the drain so it might not work, damage to surrounding structures during insertion such as your intestine, bleeding, drain leakage and infection | | 'Do I have any other options?' | | | | | | |
| If you do not want it, there are other options. We could continue to monitor and only drain if you are getting problematic symptoms. Alternatively, we could manage with salt restriction and water tablets. We could also consider other procedures, such as, putting a shunt into the vessels of your liver | | 'I see' | | | | | | |

**Explain and Obtain Consent for the Procedure**

| Statement/Question | Justification | Answer |
|---|---|---|
| What are your thoughts on having the procedure at the moment? | You should allow the patient plenty of time to make an informed decision and explore if there are ways that you could help.<br>It is important to obtain both written and verbal consent for such a procedure if the patient consents | 'I'd like a bit more time to think about it first' |

**Finishing the Consultation**

| | | |
|---|---|---|
| Of course. To summarise, we have discussed what an ascitic drain involves, as well as the risks and benefits. You would like some more time to consider this. In the meantime, I will provide you with a leaflet with more information and am happy to assist in any way possible | Short summary of the key points discussed so far | 'Fantastic. It would be useful to read some information, to help me decide what to do' |
| I will provide you with a leaflet with more information and am happy to assist in any way possible | Leaflets and other resources will help to refresh the patient's memory | 'That'd be helpful' |
| Do you have any other questions or things to add?<br>I know that we have discussed a lot of new things; please take some time to digest the information | May identify useful information that has been missed. Will also allow you to address any questions or concerns | 'No, thank you' |

**Present Your Findings**

Mr Bard is a 59-year-old man with known liver cirrhosis who has presented today with worsening ascites. I have explained why he needs an ascitic drain and have discussed the benefits and risks of having one inserted for symptomatic relief. I have also informed him of the alternative management options and he would like some more time to consider this. In the meantime, I have offered him an information leaflet to read through and have offered to support him if he requires assistance

**General Points**

Polite to patient

Maintains good eye contact

Appropriate use of open and closed questions

## ❓ QUESTIONS FROM THE EXAMINER

**What are the indications for an ascitic tap?**

To investigate new-onset ascites, suspected SBP or secondary bacterial peritonitis.

**Give three cautions when performing an ascitic tap.**

Overlying skin infection at the puncture site, pregnancy, coagulopathy.

**Although an ascitic tap is not contraindicated in patients with abnormal clotting profiles, when would it be advisable to give pooled platelets?**

In severe thrombocytopenia, when platelet count is less than 40,000/µL of blood.

**What is post-paracentesis circulatory dysfunction?**

A complication that can occur in large-volume (>5 L) paracentesis, leading to hyponatraemia, kidney injury and reaccumulation of ascites.

**Ascitic fluid that contains more than 250/mL of white cells is suggestive of what condition?**

SBP.

**How long should an abdominal drain stay in?**

In most cases, an abdominal drain should be removed after 6 h, but always check local guidelines as advice may vary.

**Aside from ascites, what are the features of decompensated liver disease?**

Hepatic encephalopathy, coagulopathy and jaundice.

**When is a transjugular intrahepatic portosystemic shunt (TIPS) indicated?**

Patients with refractory ascites who require more than three paracentesis procedures per month may benefit from TIPS.

**Why is ultrasound guidance used during an ascitic tap?**

It ensures that the procedure is performed as safely and successfully as possible, and it can provide information on the distance from skin to fluid and from skin to the midpoint of the collection.

**If ultrasound guidance is not available, where should the ascitic tap be inserted?**

In that case, the insertion site for an ascitic tap is approximately 15 cm laterally to the umbilicus (usually in either the right or left lower abdominal quadrant). Alternatively, you can insert it 2 cm below the umbilicus in the midline, through the linea alba.

## Station 4.7    Consent for Hernia Repair

### Doctor Briefing

You are a junior doctor working on the surgical ward and have been asked to see Benjamin Penneck, a 62-year-old man, who has recently been diagnosed with an inguinal hernia. Please take a brief, relevant history, explain to him the available management options as well as the risks and benefits of surgical repair of the hernia.

### Patient Briefing

You first noticed the lump in your groin after you helped your son move into his new house. The lump is not painful and gets smaller when you press it. You notice that it appears after coughing or if you are straining. It is not red or painful. You have had never had hernias before. You are overweight and do not do much exercise.

Your main concern is that the lump is unsightly and it bothers you that it appears every time you cough or strain.

### Mark Scheme for Examiner

#### Introduction

| | | | | |
|---|---|---|---|---|
| Cleans hands, introduces self and confirms patient identity | | | | |
| Checks the identity of others in the room and confirms that the patient is happy for them to be present | | | | |
| Establishes current patient knowledge and concerns | | | | |

#### Explaining the Procedure

| Statement/Question | Justification | Answer | | | |
|---|---|---|---|---|---|
| Before I discuss the procedure, I would like to ask some questions about your background. When did you first notice the lump? | This allows you to gauge the progression of the patient's condition and to rule out any serious complications, such as a strangulated hernia | 'Last week when I was helping my son move house' | | | |
| Does the hernia change size or appear spontaneously? | | 'It usually appears when I strain or cough' | | | |
| Can you push the lump back in? | | 'Sometimes I can push it back in' | | | |
| Is there any pain? | | 'No' | | | |

#### Management of a Hernia

| | | | | | |
|---|---|---|---|---|---|
| This sounds like a hernia. A hernia is like a weak spot in the wall of the tummy, where internal organs; for example, the gut, could come out, manifesting as a lump under the skin | Provide the patient with a basic explanation of what a hernia is so that you can explain the management options | 'OK, that sounds exactly like what I have' | | | |
| Hernias can potentially cause problems; for example, pain. The gut that is protruding can become kinked, compressed or blocked and if the blood supply is reduced, the gut may suffer and even burst | It is also important to warn the patient of potential complications from the hernia | 'That sounds dangerous. How do we treat it?' | | | |

**Management of a Hernia**

| Statement/Question | Justification | Answer | | | | | |
|---|---|---|---|---|---|---|---|
| Surgery can be performed to prevent the complications of hernias occurring. It can be done as an open procedure with a cut in the groin or laparoscopically with keyhole | The surgical management option depends on patient and hospital factors, but it is important to describe both to the patient. You should explain to the patient how a laparoscopic repair differs from open surgery in lay terms with the appropriate use of medical terminology | 'Oh gosh, I did not realise I would need an operation. What's the difference between them?' | | | | | |
| Keyhole surgery is where a camera and some instruments are inserted through small cuts in the tummy, and then tissues sticking out through the hernia are pulled back in through the hernia 'hole' and this 'hole' can be repaired. A patch is then put over the original site of the hernia, to help reduce the chances of a hernia happening again. This is usually done under general anaesthesia | | 'I understand' | | | | | |
| In open surgery, a cut is made in the groin, just above the lump. The protruding gut is pushed back in, the hole is stitched over and a patch is placed over the site of the hole to reduce the chances of recurrence. Open repair is commonly done under general anaesthetic, but can be done with anaesthetic just in the region | | | | | | | |
| Although a hernia repair is generally regarded as a common and safe procedure, it does have risks. Short-term risks include infection, bleeding, numbness at the surgical site, testicular pain and difficulty passing urine. Long-term risks include recurrence of hernia and possibility of developing chronic (abdominal or scrotal) pain | It is crucial that you explain both short- and long-term risks and benefits to the patient so that he can make an informed decision | 'Do I have any alternatives?' | | | | | |
| Hernias that do not cause any symptoms can be safely monitored under follow-up, without significant risk of complications. Once a hernia starts to cause discomfort, the risk of developing these complications increases and the risks of surgery are easier to justify | You should also offer alternative management options to the patient | 'I understand' | | | | | |

## Management of a Hernia

| Statement/Question | Justification | Answer | | | | | |
|---|---|---|---|---|---|---|---|
| Most patients are able to go home either the day of or the day after surgery.<br>As it is normal to experience discomfort around the incision sites for a few days after the operation, patients are discharged with pain relief.<br>Constipation may occur over the first few days; this can be prevented by drinking plenty of fluids and eating high-fibre foods. You may be able to return to work after 1–2 weeks, but you should avoid heavy lifting and strenuous activities for 4–6 weeks<br><br>If you experience any persistent abdominal swelling or pain, bleeding or redness around the surgical site, coughing, shortness of breath or difficulty passing urine, then you must seek further medical advice as it could be a complication from the surgery | It is important to detail the recovery process postoperatively so that the patient knows what to expect, and to safety net him appropriately of signs and symptoms to be wary of, that could be secondary to postoperative complications | 'That's fine' | | | | | |
| What are your thoughts on having the procedure at the moment? | It is important to obtain both written and verbal consent for such a procedure.<br>You should document the patient's wishes, and advise that he can change his mind at any point | 'I am very keen on surgery. I just want to get this sorted' | | | | | |

## Finishing the Consultation

| | | | | | | | |
|---|---|---|---|---|---|---|---|
| To summarise, we have discussed what a hernia is and how we can repair it surgically (keyhole or open). We have been through the risks and recovery process. You are happy to go ahead with the procedure. I will also provide you with a leaflet on hernia repairs | Short summary of the key points discussed so far | 'Fantastic' | | | | | |
| I will provide you with a leaflet with more information and am happy to assist in any way possible | Leaflets and other resources will help to refresh the patient's memory | 'That'd be helpful' | | | | | |
| Do you have any other questions or things to add?<br>I know that we have discussed a lot of new things; please take some time to digest the information | May identify useful information that has been missed. Will also allow you to address any questions or concerns | 'No, thank you' | | | | | |

## Present Your Findings

Mr Penneck is a 62-year-old man who has recently been diagnosed with an inguinal hernia. Today I have discussed with him the options of surgery and have explained the risks and benefits of having surgery to repair the hernia. I have obtained verbal consent for the hernia surgical repair and will get written consent now

| General Points | | | | | |
|---|---|---|---|---|---|
| Polite to patient | | | | | |
| Maintains good eye contact | | | | | |
| Appropriate use of open and closed questions | | | | | |

## ❓ QUESTIONS FROM THE EXAMINER

### What is the most common type of hernia?

Inguinal hernia.

### What are the contents of the inguinal canal in males?

Spermatic cord and the ilioinguinal nerve.

### What investigations are used in the diagnosis of a hernia?

Hernias are typically diagnosed clinically – however, if there is uncertainty, a patient may have an ultrasound.

### What is a parastomal hernia?

This is a type of incisional hernia that occurs following the formation of a stoma. Abdominal contents protrude through a defect in the abdominal wall around the site.

### Name three clinical features of a strangulated hernia.

Pain, unable to reduce, evidence of inflammation (erythema, but may also be dusky).

### Why are femoral hernias more likely to strangulate?

Femoral hernias tend to have narrow necks (where the sac emerges through the defect) compared to other hernias. Furthermore, as the femoral ring is rigid, the hernia is more likely to be irreducible and therefore at increased risk of strangulation.

### How should femoral hernias be managed?

As a result of an increased risk of strangulation, femoral hernias should be surgically managed.

### Name three risk factors for the development of an incisional hernia.

Overweight/obesity, steroid use, diabetes, wound infection, midline incisions, advanced age, pregnancy.

### What is Littre's hernia?

A rare type of hernia that contains a Meckel's diverticulum.

### What is a Richter's hernia?

A type of hernia where only a portion of the bowel wall herniates.

## Station 4.8    Dealing With an Agitated Patient

### Doctor Briefing

You are a junior doctor working in colorectal clinic and have been asked to see Bill Gates, a 65-year-old man. He is very angry because he was supposed to receive a computed tomography (CT) scan for bowel investigations over a month ago and hasn't heard anything about it. Please explore the concerns Mr Gates has.

### Patient Briefing

Over the past few months, you have had several camera and blood tests as you have had bleeding from your back passage and constipation for over a year. Your gut doctor diagnosed you with bowel cancer 2 months ago and he told you he would organise a full-body CT scan for you so that they could find out how advanced the disease is. He advised you to wait for a letter in the post. It has now been 7 weeks and you still haven't heard anything.

You are extremely worried that if you do have cancer, then this waiting is going to delay your treatment and worsen your outcome. It has had such a negative effect on your mental health that you have found it difficult to sleep and on occasions you have experienced panic attacks as well.

### Mark Scheme for Examiner

#### Introduction

| | |
|---|---|
| Cleans hands, introduces self and confirms patient identity | |
| Checks the identity of others in the room and confirms that the patient is happy for them to be present | |
| Establishes current patient knowledge and concerns. | |

#### Exploring the Patient's Emotions

| Statement/Question | Justification | Answer | |
|---|---|---|---|
| I understand that you are still waiting to have your CT scan and that this has been difficult to deal with | Show the patient that you understand his main concern and that you recognise his frustration. Allow the patient to vent his anger, if necessary, without interruption | 'Yes. I have been waiting for too long. It has been almost 2 months since my last appointment. Shouldn't I have had it by now?' | |
| Yes, you were due to have had your scan results by now so that we could discuss them today. I apologise that the scan has not happened | Acknowledge that there is an issue that is causing the patient distress. Patients may express themselves through other means, such as increasing their speech volume, swearing, restlessness, change in eye contact, change in facial expression. Look out for these non-verbal cues during the exam. | 'I don't need your apology, I need this scan to happen! You don't understand what this waiting around has done to me. It has only increased my stress levels' | |
| I understand how this would be causing you a lot of distress | Build rapport with the patient so that he feels comfortable sharing his concerns with you. Remain empathetic throughout the discussion. This builds rapport and may diffuse the situation | 'Finding out about my cancer and all this waiting have put a huge toll on my mental health! I was told this scan was important and it has not even happened yet' | |

**Exploring the Patient's Emotions**

| Statement/Question | Justification | Answer | | | | |
|---|---|---|---|---|---|---|
| Tell me more | Ask open questions to identify the main reason the patient is angry so that you can address the primary concern.<br>Active listening techniques; for example, maintaining eye contact, nodding and small verbal comments, are useful in encouraging the patient | 'I'm having panic attacks when I think about not knowing what is going to happen next and that I will be dead by the end of the year. I can't even sleep properly!' | | | | |
| You do look very worried. That must be distressing, and it is entirely reasonable that you feel that way | Pointing out the patient's emotion and that he appears upset can be helpful in allowing him to open up more | 'The thought of it all makes me feel sick. My daughter has convinced me that I need to get the scan, but all this delay is making me feel more nervous. What if it has spread to the rest of my body?' | | | | |
| Thank you for sharing this with me so that we can work together to help you. I apologise for the delay and that you are now having to go through this.<br>Some general ways that may help alleviate your anxiety include relaxation techniques and speaking to the oncology nurses for ongoing psychological support | It is important to validate the patient's feelings and it allows you to respond to the patient's emotion appropriately.<br>Apologise and explain the steps that you will take to rectify the situation | 'I just need you to deal with it as soon as possible' | | | | |
| I will chase up the scan and get it arranged as soon as possible and call you as soon as I have spoken to the scan department | Suggesting a plan to move forward with the situation shows acknowledgement of the patient's frustration | 'If you were in my position, would you make a complaint?' | | | | |
| I cannot say how I would respond but it is entirely within your rights to complain if that is something that you wish to do. I can provide you with some contact details for the correct department and will support you with this | Avoid becoming defensive as it can escalate the patient's anger. Provide the patient with the option to put in a formal complaint. In this situation, you should give the details of the Patient Advice and Liaison Service (PALS) | 'I'll take the information just in case. I think I will complain' | | | | |

**Finishing the Consultation**

| | | | | | | |
|---|---|---|---|---|---|---|
| In summary, you are upset that you are still waiting for your CT scan, which I am once again sorry about. I assure you that I will be chasing this so that there are no further delays. I have also provided you with the complaint team's details if you wish to make a complaint | It is helpful to summarise the patient's concerns and to reassure him of the actions that you will take to address them | 'I would really appreciate getting this sorted soon' | | | | |

**Finishing the Consultation**

| Statement/Question | Justification | Answer | | | | |
|---|---|---|---|---|---|---|
| Do you have any further questions or concerns that I can help with? | Allows any final concerns to be addressed | 'No, thank you' | | | | |

**Present Your Findings**

Mr Gates is a 65-year-old man who has been waiting for a staging CT scan of his bowel cancer. He has yet to receive an appointment, which is making him extremely anxious and frustrated. As a result, he now suffers from panic attacks and has difficulty sleeping.

To address this, I have apologised for the delay and will chase the appointment. We have also discussed relaxation techniques and psychological support which can help him come to terms with his diagnosis. By the end of the consultation, Mr Gates appeared more reassured and thanked me for my time

**General Points**

Polite to patient

Maintains good eye contact

Appropriate use of open and closed questions

## ❓ QUESTIONS FROM THE EXAMINER

### What are the main reasons for patient complaints?

Clinical care, poor/lack of doctor–patient communication and long waiting times are the main complaints received by the General Medical Council.

### Give four risk factors associated with colorectal cancer.

Inflammatory bowel disease, polyposis syndromes such as familial adenomatous polyposis, presence of hereditary non-polyposis colorectal cancer and a diet rich in meat and fat.

### Give three differential diagnoses of per rectum bleeding.

Diverticular disease, haemorrhoids, inflammatory bowel disease.

### What blood test results are suggestive of an iron deficiency anaemia?

Microcytic anaemia with low ferritin.

### Give three clinical features that may occur with right-sided colon cancers.

Occult bleeding/anaemia, abdominal pain, mass in right iliac fossa.

### What is the gold-standard investigation for the diagnosis of colon cancer?

Colonoscopy with biopsy.

### How can colorectal cancer be managed?

Surgery remains the only definitive curative option; however, chemotherapy and radiotherapy can be used as adjuvant treatments and in palliation.

### What is a Hartmann's procedure?

It involves complete resection of the rectosigmoid colon andformation of an end colostomy with closure of the rectal stump. It is usually performed in emergency bowel surgery.

### Where are the most common sites of metastases for colorectal cancer?

Liver is the most common site, but metastases can also be found in the lungs, bones, brain or spinal cord.

### Who is eligible for the National Health Service (NHS) Bowel Cancer Screening Programme?

Screening is offered every 2 years to those aged 60–75.

## Station 4.9    Blood Transfusion

### Doctor Briefing

You are a junior doctor on the phone to a ward nurse who has called you urgently about Janet Blatt, a 60-year-old patient, who started a blood transfusion 2 h ago. The patient's temperature is now 37.7°C, blood pressure is 99/60 mmHg, and the patient is anxious. Explore this further on the phone; identify what you would like the nurse to do and what you are going to do to further manage this patient.

### Patient Briefing

You are a nurse on the medical assessment unit and are looking after Mrs Blatt, a patient who has presented with symptomatic anaemia. The doctor prescribed a unit of blood for her.

As per protocol, you have started the transfusion, but after she has been on the infusion for 2 h, you repeat her observations and note that she is pyrexial. Her blood pressure has dropped to 99/60 mmHg. She feels quite unwell and appears anxious.

### Mark Scheme for Examiner

#### Introduction

| | |
|---|---|
| Cleans hands, introduces self and confirms patient identity | |
| Checks the identity of the patient | |
| Establishes current knowledge and concerns from the nurse | |

#### Managing Postoperative Complications

| Statement/Question | Justification | Answer | |
|---|---|---|---|
| Which blood products was the patient given and for what reason(s)? | Clarify details around the blood transfusion, including type of product, indication and symptoms the patient is currently experiencing. The patient was commenced on pack red cells, seemingly due to anaemia, but is now experiencing adverse effects after 2 h | 'She was given a unit of packed red cells because her haemoglobin level was low. It's been a long-standing problem; she's been in a few times for it' | |
| When was she started on the transfusion? | | 'Around 2 h ago' | |
| How is the patient now? | | 'She said that she felt really panicky and unwell' | |
| Have you got any previous and recent observations? | It is important to clarify any change in the observations, especially at the start of transfusion and any of the checkpoints during routine monitoring. Consider potential complications of blood transfusion, such as acute haemolytic reaction | 'Her observations were all normal prior to the transfusion, but now her temperature is 37.7°C and blood pressure 99/60 mmHg' | |
| Does she have any of the following: urticarial rash, breathing difficulty, swelling of her face or lips, pain or bleeding from the cannula site? | Enquire about other symptoms or signs suggestive of a specific complication of blood transfusion, such as anaphylaxis | 'None of those' | |
| Just to clarify, have any steps been taken to manage the patient yet? | The top diagnosis you should have currently is non-haemolytic febrile transfusion reaction. Clarify any management already implemented by nursing staff | 'No, I rang you as soon as we got the observation results' | |

## Managing Postoperative Complications

| Statement/Question | Justification | Answer | | | | | | |
|---|---|---|---|---|---|---|---|---|
| You need to stop the blood transfusion right now. You also need to check that the correct blood was given to the correct patient and this blood bag will need to be sent back to the laboratory | Prompt actions need to be taken to manage the patient safely. Give clear instructions to the nurse to avoid any delay in treatment | 'OK. Do we do anything about her blood pressure and temperature?' | | | | | | |
| You can give her some paracetamol for her fever, and we will need to insert a new giving set to give her some intravenous (IV) fluids. Can anyone do that? | | 'Yes, I can insert them' | | | | | | |
| Great. If you can take some bloods at the same time then that would be helpful. This includes full blood count (FBC), U&Es, coagulation screen, group and save | Consider any additional investigations that are needed | 'I will do that too' | | | | | | |
| I will reassess the patient as soon as I arrive on to the ward, but for now please continue to monitor her haemodynamic stability through regular observations and let me know if there are any concerns | Now that you have been through the management steps, inform the nurse if/when you will be attending to the patient. Remind the nurse that regular monitoring is required so that early interventions can be made if the patient deteriorates. Consider obtaining senior input if you cannot attend to the patient soon or if she deteriorates | 'Sure; thank you, doctor' | | | | | | |

## Finishing the Consultation

| Statement/Question | Justification | Answer | | | | | | |
|---|---|---|---|---|---|---|---|---|
| To conclude, Mrs Blatt was commenced on a blood transfusion 2 h ago, but now is slightly pyrexial and hypotensive. We are going to treat her as a non-haemolytic febrile transfusion reaction. For now, you need to stop the transfusion, take some bloods and commence IV fluids through a new giving set. You will also need to inform blood bank of this incident and return the sample to them. I am on my way now but please contact me again if you have any further concerns | It is helpful to summarise the management plan to the nurse and reassure the nurse that you will be attending to the patient soon | 'OK' | | | | | | |
| Do you have any other questions? | Allows any final concerns to be addressed | 'No, thank you' | | | | | | |

**Present Your Findings**

Mrs Blatt is a 60-year-old woman who was receiving a unit of red blood cells for likely chronic anaemia. Her temperature increased to 37.7°C and her blood pressure dropped to 99/60 mmHg, and she was feeling anxious.

I believe that she has had a non-haemolytic febrile transfusion reaction and have asked the nurses to stop the transfusion and give her IV fluids through a new giving set. The nurse will also take some bloods and administer paracetamol. We will be informing the blood bank of this incident and will send the blood bag back to the laboratory. I will make it my top priority to attend to the patient and have asked the nurse to escalate any concerns in the meantime

**General Points**

Maintains good eye contact

Appropriate use of open and closed questions

## ❓ QUESTIONS FROM THE EXAMINER

### If a pregnant woman is rhesus-negative, what medication can she be given to prevent rhesus disease?
Rhesus-negative pregnant patients can be given anti-ᴅ immunoglobulins.

### By how much will 1 unit of packed red cells increase the haemoglobin?
Generally, 1 unit of packed red cells should increase the haemoglobin by approximately 1 g/dL.

### Name three infections that may be transmitted via administering blood.
Hepatitis B, hepatitis C, human immunodeficiency virus (HIV), Creutzfeldt–Jakob disease, cytomegalovirus, parvovirus B19, West Nile virus.

### Give an indication for the transfusion of fresh frozen plasma.
Deficiency of coagulation factors, for example, in disseminated intravascular coagulation, is an indication for fresh frozen plasma.

### Who is at risk of developing fluid overload following a blood transfusion?
Patients with a history of cardiac failure and those with chronic anaemia who may be euvolaemic or hypervolaemic.

### Give three examples of delayed complications of blood transfusion.
Iron overload, graft-versus-host disease, delayed haemolysis.

### Give three types of patients that require irradiated blood.
Those who have received allograft bone marrow and stem cell transplants, those with Hodgkin's lymphoma, patients treated with purine analogue drugs (fludarabine, cladribine and deoxycoformycin).

### Iron overload can occur in those receiving regular red cell transfusion. True or false?
True.

### Which patients are more likely to have a febrile non-haemolytic transfusion reaction?
Women who have had multiple previous pregnancies or those who have received multiple transfusions in the past.

### What is posttransfusion purpura?
This is a severe adverse reaction where the body produces alloantibodies against the transfused platelet antigens, leading to thrombocytopenia.

## Station 4.10   Commencing Warfarin Therapy

### Doctor Briefing

You are a junior doctor working in a cardiology clinic and have been asked to see Peter Jacobs, a 70-year-old man who was recently diagnosed with atrial fibrillation (AF). He has been sent to your clinic with a view to potentially starting warfarin therapy. Please counsel him about warfarin therapy and its implications.

### Patient Briefing

You have recently been experiencing palpitations in your chest, and your doctor performed a heart tracing, which showed that you have an irregular heart rate. He diagnosed you with AF, for which he has prescribed you a new medication called warfarin.

You're generally fit and well. You sometimes experience angina, for which you have a GTN spray, but you haven't had to use this for a long time. You have never had a stroke or heart attack. You have not had any previous blood clots, heart operations, cancer, surgery or immobility. There is no personal or family history of bleeding disorders.

You're concerned because you know nothing about this medication or what it does.

### Mark Scheme for Examiner

#### Introduction

| | | | |
|---|---|---|---|
| Cleans hands, introduces self and confirms patient identity | | | |
| Checks the identity of others in the room and confirms that the patient is happy for them to be present | | | |
| Establishes current patient knowledge and concerns | | | |

#### Taking a Brief History

| Statement/Question | Justification | Answer | | | |
|---|---|---|---|---|---|
| Do you know why you have been started on warfarin? | Establish why the patient has been commenced on this medication | 'I was told that I have an irregular heart rate, but I don't know what this medication does' | | | |
| Before I go into the details of the medication, please can I ask some questions about your medical background?<br><br>Do you have a history of abnormal bleeding, heart attacks or strokes? | It is important to ask about past medical history, specifically relating to bleeding risk.<br>Warfarin can also affect fetal development; therefore you need to ask about the possibility of pregnancy in female patients of childbearing age | 'I've only got angina' | | | |
| Have you ever had blood clots in your legs or lungs/recent surgery/current cancer/immobility?<br><br>Have you got any valves in your heart, such as a mechanical prosthetic valve? | Elicit any previous history of venous thromboembolic events and risks of developing a clot | 'No, none of those' | | | |
| What medications are you currently on? | Warfarin has many interactions with other medications, including herbal medicine and supplements. It is also important to ask about other drugs that would increase bleeding risk, such as antiplatelets | 'I have a GTN spray, but I haven't used it for months' | | | |

**Counselling on Warfarin**

| Question | Justification | Answer | | | | | |
|---|---|---|---|---|---|---|---|
| You have been started on warfarin because of your recent diagnosis of AF, which is causing your heart palpitations | Introduce the patient to the consultation in an open way; for example, by explaining why he has been started on warfarin and what AF is. | 'I understand' | | | | | |
| AF is a condition that increases the risk of blood clots forming in the vessels supplying the heart and brain | You need to ensure that the patient understands the indication to improve patient compliance | 'How does it do that?' | | | | | |
| Warfarin is a medication that thins the blood, reducing the risk of blood clots forming in those vessels | Appropriately counsel the patient on warfarin, providing details of the medication such as what it is, when to take it, dosing and monitoring | 'I see' | | | | | |
| It is a medication that is taken daily, usually in the evening. As you are on it for AF, it is usually taken for life | | 'That's fine. I assumed as much' | | | | | |
| There are different doses of warfarin, and your daily dose may be adjusted by your doctor based on blood results | | 'That sounds very complicated' | | | | | |
| Your medication doses will be determined by the anticoagulation clinic. It is usually checked at least every 4 weeks, but may need to be checked more frequently if the international normalised ratio (INR), something that measures how 'thin' your blood is, goes out of its target range. Your INR results and warfarin doses will all be documented in a 'yellow anticoagulation' booklet that you can keep | Explain monitoring of INR and the role of the anticoagulation clinic and book | 'What do I do if I miss a dose? Will I get a blood clot then?' | | | | | |
| Take the missed dose as soon as possible and call your doctor or the anticoagulation clinic for advice. Do not double the dose the next day, as this may significantly increase your risk of bleeding | Explain what the patient should do if he misses a dose | That sounds scary. Is there anything else that I need to look out for? | | | | | |
| It can be scary but there is a lot of support available. Being on warfarin can affect your life in many ways and it's important that you are aware of this. You should avoid activities such as contact sports, due to an increased bleeding risk. Alcohol can increase the effects of warfarin, and it is recommended that you check that warfarin doesn't interact with any new medications that you may be started on in the future | Remember to inform the patient how warfarin will impact his daily life | 'I understand' | | | | | |

**Counselling on Warfarin**

| Statement/Question | Justification | Answer | | | | | |
|---|---|---|---|---|---|---|---|
| You must also notify someone immediately if you have any bleeding, severe bruising, prolonged nose bleeds, coughing or vomiting up blood, passing blood in your urine or if you pass foul-smelling, black stools. These may be signs that you are bleeding internally | Warn the patient of safety net advice and signs that may suggest that he is at an increased bleeding risk | I see | | | | | |

**Finishing the Consultation**

| | | | | | | | |
|---|---|---|---|---|---|---|---|
| We have discussed a lot of things today. To summarise, you have been started on warfarin, a blood thinner, because of your recent diagnosis of AF. You will be followed up in the anticoagulation clinic where they will regularly monitor your INR and let you know what dose you need to be on | You are coming towards the end of the consultation and need to ensure that the patient is happy with the information given | 'That's helpful, thank you' | | | | | |
| I will provide you with a leaflet with more information and am happy to assist in any way possible | Leaflets and other resources will help to refresh the patient's memory | 'That'd be helpful' | | | | | |
| Do you have any other questions or things to add? I know that we have discussed a lot of new things; please take some time to digest the information | May identify useful information that has been missed. Will also allow you to address any questions or concerns | 'No, thank you for taking the time to explain it to me' | | | | | |

**Present Your Findings**

Mr Jacobs is a 70-year-old man who was recently diagnosed with AF, after he presented with palpitations. He has had no previous strokes or heart attacks but has a history of angina, for which he is prescribed a GTN spray. Today I counselled Mr Jacobs on starting warfarin and have given him a 'yellow anticoagulation' book. He will be seen in the warfarin clinic next week, where we will monitor his INR

**General Points**

| | | | | |
|---|---|---|---|---|
| Polite to patient | | | | |
| Maintains good eye contact | | | | |
| Appropriate use of open and closed questions | | | | |

## ❓ QUESTIONS FROM THE EXAMINER

**What medication can be used to reverse warfarin?**

Vitamin K can be given to patients to reverse the anticoagulant effect of warfarin.

### Name three medications that may increase the effect of warfarin.

CYP-450 enzyme inhibitors such as omeprazole, valproate and erythromycin can increase the levels of warfarin and therefore its overall effect. Other medications include co-trimoxazole, fluconazole, isoniazid, metronidazole.

### Can warfarin and another direct oral anticoagulant (DOAC) be given at the same time?

Concurrent use of warfarin and another DOAC should be avoided due to the increased risk of bleeding that this poses.

### Apixaban, rivaroxaban and dabigatran are examples of DOACs. Which coagulation factor do both of these drugs impact?

Apixaban and rivaroxaban are both factor Xa inhibitors. Dabigatran is a factor IIa inhibitor.

### What kind of murmur does aortic stenosis produce?

An ejection systolic murmur.

### Do bioprosthetic (tissue) valve replacements require anticoagulation?

No, bioprosthetic valves do not require anticoagulation.

### Which DOACs have reversal drugs?

Reversal agents are available for some of the DOACs, such as dabigatran, apixaban and rivaroxaban.

### Give three risk factors that increase the risk of developing a pulmonary embolism/deep-vein thrombosis (DVT).

Pregnancy, dehydration, use of combined oral contraceptive pill, immobility, prolonged bed rest, recent major surgery, overweight/obesity, smoking, increased age.

### DOACs can be used with metallic heart valves. True or false?

False. At present, DOACs are not licensed for use in metallic heart valves.

### A patient developed a DVT after being on the combined oral contraceptive pill. How long should she be anticoagulated with warfarin?

Patients with a provoked DVT should be treated with warfarin for 3 months.

## Station 4.11   Sickle Cell Disease Diagnosis

### Doctor Briefing

You are a junior doctor working in primary care and have been asked to see Mrs Carr, mother of Jacob Carr. Jacob is a 7-week-old baby who was diagnosed with sickle cell anaemia following routine screening. His mother is keen to know more about the diagnosis. Please explain the diagnosis and answer any questions the parent may have.

### Patient Briefing

You have recently given birth to Jacob and have had no concerns with him. However, after he had a routine test when blood was taken from his heel, your doctor told you that he has sickle cell anaemia. You've never heard of this condition before and are unsure what this means for Jacob.

You are normally fit and well. You know that your husband's family has had some problems with anaemia, but are unsure of exact details.

You are concerned the sickle cell anaemia is going to be passed down to your future children, as you are hoping to expand your family.

### Mark Scheme for Examiner

#### Introduction

| | | | | |
|---|---|---|---|---|
| Cleans hands, introduces self and confirms patient identity | | | | |
| Checks the identity of others in the room and confirms that the patient is happy for them to be present | | | | |
| Establishes current patient knowledge and concerns | | | | |

#### Taking a Brief History

| Statement/Question | Justification | Answer | | | | |
|---|---|---|---|---|---|---|
| Has Jacob been unwell at all since his birth? | It is important to establish if the patient is symptomatic, as this will guide management | 'He's been well so far, thankfully' | | | | |
| Is there a family history of sickle cell disease? | The pattern of inheritance for sickle cell disease is autosomal-recessive, so bear in mind that some family members may have been carriers of the sickle cell trait without developing the disease | 'Not on my side, but I know that some of my husband's cousins have had anaemia problems before, although I don't know the exact details' | | | | |
| Did Jacob have any testing for sickle cell disease during your pregnancy? | In most cases, those affected by sickle cell disease will be identified via newborn screening. Early diagnosis may have been missed if the patient did not have the screening test | 'Only after he was born, when he had that blood test from his heel' | | | | |

**Counselling on Sickle Cell Disease**

| Question | Justification | Answer | | | | | | | |
|---|---|---|---|---|---|---|---|---|---|
| I just want to take this opportunity to explain sickle cell disease to you. Normal red blood cells are shaped like doughnuts and are very flexible. Sickle cell anaemia is a condition in which red blood cells become 'sickle'-shaped. These red blood cells are less flexible and are more likely to get stuck and block blood vessels, leading to pain as blood cannot reach the tissues. Sickle cells are more easily damaged than normal red blood cells and therefore do not last as long. This results in anaemia as the body is unable to keep up with the demand of producing new red blood cells | Explain the condition in lay terms, with the appropriate use of medical terminology | 'Oh dear, how has this happened to Jacob? Is it something that we should have known about?' | | | | | | | |
| Sickle cell disease is a genetic condition that is inherited in a recessive manner. This means that the child has inherited two copies of a faulty gene, one from each parent | Explain the cause of sickle cell disease and the pattern of inheritance | 'This means that I have it too! Does that mean that my future children will get it as well? I'm hoping to have more children' | | | | | | | |
| As two copies of the faulty gene are required to develop sickle cell anaemia, each of your children has a 25% chance of inheriting the condition | | 'I see' | | | | | | | |
| It is a serious condition which requires awareness of complications and early treatment to prevent life-threatening problems. Although the disease is very variable, most patients are able to lead normal lives | Explain the prognosis and potential complications | 'What kind of complications do you get? This all sounds so overwhelming' | | | | | | | |
| When sickle cells block a blood vessel, oxygen cannot reach the tissue. The lack of oxygen causes a sharp sudden pain; these are called 'sickle cell crises'. Common sites include legs, back, abdomen, fingers. Crises can be triggered by various things, such as being cold, dehydration and infections. Between episodes of sickle cell crises, patients are usually symptom-free | Explain sickle cell crises and other important complications that patients and their family need to be aware of. Be mindful to give information in chunks to make it easier for the patient to understand | 'This all sounds so serious and really scary. Is there a cure?' | | | | | | | |
| Blockages from sickle cells can also cause organ damage in the lungs, brain, kidneys, eyes and spleen, the latter of which can increase the risk of infection. Sickle cell disease can also contribute to severe anaemia | | | | | | | | | |
| That's a very valid question. Stem cell transplantation is the only known cure for sickle cell anaemia, but this is usually only for children who have had severe complications | Now that you have explained sickle cell crises, you need to explore treatment and management options. Carefully provide details on the management plan for the patient, both currently and potentially | 'So, what can be done for Jacob now?' | | | | | | | |
| To manage Jacob's sickle cell disease, he will be referred to the haematologists. These are doctors that specialise in looking at blood specifically | | 'What can they do?' | | | | | | | |

**Counselling on Sickle Cell Disease**

| Statement/Question | Justification | Answer | | | | |
|---|---|---|---|---|---|---|
| In general, they will aim to prevent crises occurring by avoiding known triggers and ensuring that Jacob receives his immunisations on time. He will also need to take antibiotics daily from the age of 3 months, and we could also consider prescribing another medication, called hydroxyurea, to reduce the occurrence of crises | You are not a specialist, but can provide the patient with an overview of what the likely management steps are | 'OK' | | | | |
| To manage a sickle cell crisis, we can use a combination of painkillers, antibiotics, oxygen and rehydration. In certain conditions involving the chest and severe anaemia, we can give a blood transfusion | Vital to explain to the parent how a sickle cell crisis can be managed | 'I understand' | | | | |

**Finishing the Consultation**

| | | | | | | |
|---|---|---|---|---|---|---|
| To summarise, as I have given you a lot of information, we have discussed what sickle cell disease is, as well as the complications and management options | Short summary of the key points discussed so far | 'Yes' | | | | |
| I will provide you with a leaflet with more information, as well as the contact details for the team who will look after Jacob. I am happy to assist in any way possible and more than happy to see you again if that would be useful, if you have further things you would like to go through | Leaflets and other resources will help to refresh the patient's memory | 'That'd be helpful, thank you so much' | | | | |
| Do you have any other questions or things to add?<br>I know that we have discussed a lot of new things; please take some time to digest the information | May identify useful information that has been missed. Will also allow you to address any questions or concerns | 'No, thank you' | | | | |

**Present Your Findings**

Jacob is a 7-week-old baby who has been diagnosed with sickle cell disease following the results of the heelprick test. There is no known family history of sickle cell disease; however, some of his paternal family members have suffered from anaemia to an unknown extent.

I explained the cause of sickle cell disease and its complications. I have emphasised the need to avoid any known triggers, complete all the childhood vaccinations and have daily antibiotics from 3 months old. Jacob's parent has been provided with an information leaflet and Jacob will be followed up by a haematologist in a couple of weeks

**General Points**

Polite to patient

Maintains good eye contact

Appropriate use of open and closed questions

## ❓ QUESTIONS FROM THE EXAMINER

**Those with sickle cell trait are relatively resistant to which infection?**

Falciparum malaria.

**Penicillin V is used prophylactically to protect patients with hyposplenism from which infection?**

Pneumococcal infection, which may be fatal in these patients.

**In a patient with sickle cell anaemia, what result of the FBC would you expect to find?**

Anaemia with reticulocytosis, and the blood film may also show sickle cells.

**Symptoms of sickle cell anaemia start at childbirth – true or false?**

False. Symptoms usually start at around 3 years old.

**Prenatal screening for sickle cell can be carried out – true or false?**

True. Testing can be done from 10 weeks of pregnancy.

**Which vitamin supplement can patients be given to help manage sickle cell anaemia?**

Folic acid is recommended to help the body make new red blood cells.

**Those with sickle cell trait are always asymptomatic – true or false?**

False. Though uncommon, those with sickle cell trait can develop symptoms in extreme conditions, such as low-oxygen conditions or if they are severely dehydrated.

**Aside from sickle cell disease, give three other diseases that the Guthrie test (newborn heelprick test) assesses.**

Cystic fibrosis, congenital hypothyroidism and inherited metabolic diseases such as homocystinuria.

**Haemoglobin S has the same oxygen-binding capacity as normal haemoglobin – true or false?**

False. It has reduced oxygen-binding capacity.

**How does haemoglobin S differ from normal haemoglobin?**

The mutation involves the replacement of valine instead of glutamate at position 6 of the beta globin chain.

## Station 4.12   Consent for HIV Testing

### Doctor Briefing

You are a junior doctor working in primary care and have been asked to see Anna Fredrick, a 19-year-old woman, who has attended asking for a human immunodeficiency virus (HIV) test. Please establish the level at which she is at risk of HIV and counsel her on HIV testing.

### Patient Briefing

You have recently entered university and met a male student, whom you have been regularly having sexual intercourse with for the past 2 months. You do not know anything about his past relationships. You have now decided that you would like to be in a relationship and both want to get a sexual health check. You do not have any other sexual partners. With your new boyfriend, you engage in oral and penetrative vaginal sex.

You have got multiple tattoos, with the last one being 1.5 years ago. It was performed in a clean environment. You do not have any piercings. You have never had a blood transfusion. You do not use any IV drugs. There is no family history of HIV and you are a healthy individual.

Your main concern is that you will be denied the test for HIV.

### Mark Scheme for Examiner

#### Introduction

| | | | |
|---|---|---|---|
| Cleans hands, introduces self and confirms patient identity | | | |
| Checks the identity of others in the room and confirms that the patient is happy for them to be present | | | |
| Establishes current patient knowledge and concerns | | | |

#### Brief History

| Statement/Question | Justification | Answer | | | |
|---|---|---|---|---|---|
| I understand that you have come here today for an HIV test | Confirm the patient's reason for attendance and explore the patient's reasons for requesting an HIV test | 'That's correct. I've recently got a new boyfriend and we both want to do a full sexual health check' | | | |
| That's very sensible. Before I offer the blood test, I would like to ask a few questions to gauge your risk. I apologise if some of the questions that I ask come across as offensive or too personal, but it is important for me to get the correct information | It is useful to give the patient a warning shot before you ask private questions about her life | 'I understand' | | | |

## Brief History

| Statement/Question | Justification | Answer | | | | | |
|---|---|---|---|---|---|---|---|
| Do you engage in sexual intercourse? If so, is it with males, females or both? | Take a detailed sexual history as HIV can be transmitted through sexual intercourse | 'I have sex with my boyfriend, but no one else' | | | | | |
| Do you know whether he has HIV or if his previous sexual partners have HIV? Where is he from? | | 'I'm not too sure about his past, to be honest. He's from the UK as well, though' | | | | | |
| What type of sex do you have, and do you use any contraception? | | 'We have penetrative vaginal and oral sex. We rarely use a condom' | | | | | |
| Have you had sex with anyone else recently, including sex workers or whilst abroad? | | 'No' | | | | | |
| Has there been any history of sexual assault? | | 'No' | | | | | |
| Have you had any previous diagnoses of sexually transmitted infections? | | 'I've had Chlamydia before but that was a long time ago and was treated with antibiotics' | | | | | |
| Have you had any invasive procedures such as piercings, tattoos or blood transfusions? | HIV is a blood-borne virus and can be transmitted through infected blood or bodily fluids | 'I have lots of tattoos but the last time I got one was over a year ago. I haven't had a piercing or blood transfusion' | | | | | |
| Do you use any IV drugs? | Needle sharing and accidental needlestick injuries are methods by which HIV can be transmitted | 'No' | | | | | |
| Is there a family history of HIV? | A mother can pass on HIV to her child during delivery via vertical transmission | 'Not that I'm aware of' | | | | | |
| How is your health overall? | HIV can lead to immunosuppression, which would make the patient more prone to opportunistic infections | 'I'm pretty healthy. I have never had any serious medical problems' | | | | | |

## Counselling on HIV Testing

| | | | | | | | |
|---|---|---|---|---|---|---|---|
| What is your understanding of HIV? | Establish what the patient currently knows about HIV | 'It's a really bad infection that you can get from having lots of sex, right?' | | | | | |

**Counselling on Sickle Cell Disease**

| Statement/Question | Justification | Answer | | | | |
|---|---|---|---|---|---|---|
| You're partially correct. HIV stands for human immuno-deficiency virus. Over time, it causes some of the white blood cells that fight off infection to drop to a dangerously low level, which means that you can become seriously ill and infected by other germs | Explain briefly what HIV is and its (potential) effect on the patient's life | 'It's deadly, isn't it?' | | | | |
| Although incurable, HIV is treatable with antiretroviral drugs, which allow people to lead a near-normal life | | 'I see' | | | | |
| As you are aware, we can do a blood test that will detect specific antibodies against HIV. If you have got HIV, then this will come back positive. We will take your blood today and inform you of the results when they return | Explain the process of HIV testing and provide the patient with an estimated time frame of when she may be informed of the results | 'Will I find out today?' | | | | |
| There is a fingerprick test that we can do, but it is not 100% accurate and we would still need to send a blood sample to the laboratories. The results from the laboratories usually take several weeks | | 'OK' | | | | |
| I also need to let you know what may happen if you test positive for HIV. Firstly, we may need to repeat the blood test to confirm the diagnosis. Secondly, we would strongly advise you to inform your current and previous sexual partners of the diagnosis for their benefit and they should get tested as well. Thirdly, we would have to consider how to prevent further spreading with different meas-ures. Finally, you should start treatment as soon as possible and we may refer you to a HIV special-ist to take over your care.<br>Are you still happy to consent to the blood test? | Discuss the implications of a positive test result, including further investigations, contact tracing and treatment | 'Yes, please' | | | | |

**Finishing the Consultation**

| Statement/Question | Justification | Answer | | | | | | |
|---|---|---|---|---|---|---|---|---|
| To summarise, we have discussed your risks of HIV, how to test for it and what it might mean to test positive. You have given us consent to perform the blood test | Short summary of the key points discussed so far | 'That's correct' | | | | | | |
| I will provide you with a leaflet and online resources for more information and am happy to assist in any way possible | Leaflets and other resources will help to refresh the patient's memory | 'That'd be helpful' | | | | | | |
| Do you have any other questions or things to add? I know that we have discussed a lot of new things; please take some time to digest the information | May identify useful information that has been missed. Will also allow you to address any questions or concerns | 'No, thank you' | | | | | | |

**Present Your Findings**

Miss Fredrick is a 19-year-old student who wants to have an HIV test as part of a full sexual health check. She has been engaging in regular unprotected sexual intercourse with her new boyfriend, penetrative and oral. She has no other sexual partners. Her last tattoo was 1.5 years ago. She does not have any other risk factors.

I have explained the HIV test and possible implications of a positive test. She is happy to undergo testing, and I have provided her with an information leaflet regarding HIV testing

**General Points**

Polite to patient.

Maintains good eye contact.

Appropriate use of open and closed questions.

## ❓ QUESTIONS FROM THE EXAMINER

**Give three symptoms that may occur during the seroconversion period.**

Fever, malaise, lymphadenopathy.

**In acute infection, which biochemical markers are present?**

Viral p24 antigen and HIV RNA levels will be elevated, whilst antibody tests may be negative.

**How is HIV staged?**

Staging is commonly based on assigning patients to a stage according to their CD4 count and clinical symptoms.

**When should a patient with HIV infection commence antiretroviral therapy?**

It is now recommended that all patients who have been newly diagnosed with HIV or those with established infection who have a reduced CD4 count should start antiretroviral therapy.

**Give three examples of antiretroviral drugs.**

Emtricitabine, lamivudine, efavirenz, abacavir, didanosine, lamivudine, tenofovir, atazanavir, stavudine.

## What is the goal of treatment when started on antiretroviral therapy?

The aim is to achieve a viral load of < 50 copies/mL within 4–6 months of treatment.

## Can pregnant women who are HIV-positive take antiretroviral therapy?

Treatment should be taken throughout pregnancy and postpartum.

## Should HIV-positive women breastfeed?

If possible, breastfeeding should be avoided unless there is no other alternative.

## Give three skin conditions associated with HIV infection.

Kaposi's sarcoma, recurrent and persistent *Candida* infection, cytomegalovirus ulcers.

## What is the duration of treatment in postexposure prophylaxis?

Treatment should be completed for 4 weeks.

## Station 4.13    Postmortem Discussion

### Doctor Briefing

You are a junior doctor speaking to Laura Parker, the daughter of one of your patients, Irene Parker. Mrs Parker died last week, and the cause of death was pneumonia. A number of abnormal lesions were noted on a previous CT scan, which are not thought to be related to the cause of death but are of unknown origin. The family and medical team are interested to explore this further, and your consultant has asked you to get authorisation for a hospital autopsy.

### Patient Briefing

Your mother had passed away last week after being admitted to hospital with pneumonia. You recall that she had a few scans in hospital before she died but you weren't sure what they were for and no one has discussed the results with you yet.

You've heard of autopsy (though not postmortem examination) but you're not really sure what it entails.

Your main concern is that you do not know if your mother would consent to an autopsy or not, and you don't want to make this decision by yourself, so you want to discuss it with your family first.

### Mark Scheme for Examiner

#### Introduction

| | | | | | |
|---|---|---|---|---|---|
| Cleans hands, introduces self and confirms patient identity | | | | | |
| Checks the identity of others in the room and confirms that the patient is happy for them to be present | | | | | |
| Ensure that you have a colleague present with you to act as a witness during the discussion, to sign the authorisation form | | | | | |

#### Gaining Consent for a Hospital Autopsy

| Question | Justification | Answer | | | | | |
|---|---|---|---|---|---|---|---|
| I'm very sorry about your mother's recent death. Can you please tell me what you know about it? | Establish the relative's level of knowledge regarding her mother's death. Do this sensitively and take into consideration the emotions that the relative may be experiencing | 'She passed away last week after contracting pneumonia. She'd been unwell for some time, to be honest' | | | | | |
| Yes, that's correct. Before she passed away, she had a CT scan. Has anyone talked to you about the results? | Recap the past events and explain the results in lay terms | 'Oh yes, I remember that she went for it, but no one discussed anything with us afterwards. I'm guessing it was the pneumonia. What did it show?' | | | | | |
| Her CT scan revealed a number of suspicious lesions in her lungs. We do not think that the lesions are related to her death, but we are unsure what they are | Explain the CT scan results to the relative clearly | 'So, you don't know what these lesions are?' | | | | | |
| Yes, unfortunately we cannot tell from the scan. That is why we would like to perform a postmortem examination | Explain why an autopsy is required | 'What's a postmortem examination?' | | | | | |

## Gaining Consent for a Hospital Autopsy

| Statement/Question | Justification | Answer | | | | | |
|---|---|---|---|---|---|---|---|
| A postmortem examination is also known as an autopsy. It is the examination of a body after death.<br>The aim of a postmortem examination is usually to determine the cause of death. In your mother's case, we already know that she died from pneumonia, but we think that it would be worth exploring what those lesions were | Explain what a postmortem examination is and the reason for performing it. Personalising it allows the relative to understand the rationale better | 'Oh yes, I've heard of an autopsy before. So, are you just going to go ahead with it? Do I have a say?' | | | | | |
| Firstly, we need consent for it. Do you know if Mrs Parker ever expressed any opinion about this when she was alive? | It is important to get consent for an autopsy requested by the hospital. If the autopsy was requested by a coroner, then consent isn't required, but it is still vital to have the discussion with the family | 'Not that I'm aware of' | | | | | |
| If we are to go ahead with an autopsy, we would need to obtain consent from you and your family. I would like to emphasise that it is not something that has to be agreed to and that permission can be refused.<br>Even if you do consent, you can withdraw it at any time up until the examination has started | Do not coerce the patient's relative into giving consent if she is not comfortable doing so, and advise her that she can change her mind | 'Can you give me more information about what happens?' | | | | | |
| The examination will be carried out in a manner that is respectful to Mrs. Parker and your family's wishes. Depending on what consent has been obtained, the examination can be limited to one area of the body or even to one organ, but this can prevent any comment being made on any other disease processes elsewhere. Organs will not be retained without specific permission from yourselves | Vital to explain how a postmortem examination is carried out. You must emphasise that consent can be given for examination of specific parts of the body, and not others, if that is their wish | 'I see, it's quite a big decision. I think I'll need to discuss it with the rest of my family' | | | | | |
| Of course, that is totally understandable. I will give you the details of whom to contact after you have discussed this decision with your family | Important to give the patient time, if appropriate | 'Thank you' | | | | | |

## Finishing the Consultation

| | | | | | | | |
|---|---|---|---|---|---|---|---|
| To summarise, we have discussed why it may be beneficial to perform a postmortem examination on Mrs Parker because her last CT scan showed abnormal lesions in her lungs and we don't know what they are. You would appreciate some more time to think and discuss this with your family, which is completely understandable.<br>I can meet with you again to discuss this at a later date, if you wish? | Short summary of the key points discussed so far and offer a follow-up appointment | 'Yes, I think it'd be useful to meet again' | | | | | |

**Finishing the Consultation**

| Statement/Question | Justification | Answer | | | | |
|---|---|---|---|---|---|---|
| I will provide you with a leaflet with more information and am happy to assist in any way possible | Leaflets and other resources will help to refresh the patient's memory | 'That'd be helpful' | | | | |
| Do you have any other questions or things to add? I know that we have discussed a lot of new things; please take some time to digest the information | May identify useful information that has been missed. Will also allow you to address any questions or concerns | 'No, thank you' | | | | |

**Present Your Findings**

Mrs Parker died last week from pneumonia, but her last CT scan showed lesions in her lungs which were of unknown origin. I discussed the prospect of a hospital postmortem with her daughter, Laura, and explained what happens at an autopsy. I have reassured Laura that her mother's body will be treated with respect at all times and have talked her through the consent process. She would like some time to think about it and discuss with the rest of her family. I have provided Laura with a patient information leaflet on postmortem examinations and have offered to have another meeting with her if she wants more information

**General Points**

| | | | | |
|---|---|---|---|---|
| Polite to patient | | | | |
| Maintains good eye contact | | | | |
| Appropriate use of open and closed questions | | | | |

## ❓ QUESTIONS FROM THE EXAMINER

**Once a family has consented to a postmortem, are they allowed to change their mind?**

Yes, a relative/partner should be given information on whom to contact in case they change their mind.

**Consent is required for a coroner's postmortem examination – true or false?**

False. Consent is not required.

**Once consented to a postmortem, the whole body of the deceased can be examined – true or false?**

False. Only those organs for which consent has been obtained can be examined.

**On a death certificate, what should be documented as the 1a cause of death?**

This should be the disease or condition that led directly to the patient's death.

**Give two conditions that need to be fulfilled in order for a diagnosis of brain death.**

Clear evidence of irreversible brain damage and failure to respond to outside stimulation.

**Who can make a diagnosis of brain death?**

This can only be confirmed by two senior doctors who will carry out a series of tests on the patient.

### Name three tests carried out in order to determine brainstem death.

Corneal reflex, gag reflex, disconnection from ventilator in order to assess apnoea.

### Name four organs that can be donated.

Kidney, liver, lung, heart, eyes, pancreas, small bowel.

### Name two conditions in which a person cannot donate their organs.

Creutzfeldt–Jakob disease (CJD), active cancer.

### Can a person who has HIV become an organ donor?

Rarely, those with HIV can donate their organs to those who have the same condition.

## Station 4.14 Opiate Counselling

### Doctor Briefing

You are asked to see Alan Smith, a 62-year-old man, who is suffering from severe pain. He has a diagnosis of inoperable pancreatic cancer. You have found it difficult to control his pain and now feel that his analgesia should be increased. Please counsel him on the risks and benefits of morphine therapy and discuss other adjuncts to improve his symptoms.

### Patient Briefing

You were diagnosed with pancreatic cancer 1 year ago after you started experiencing really bad pain in the centre of your tummy. The surgeons said that they cannot operate on you and will treat your symptoms only. The pain was initially relatively well controlled with paracetamol and codeine, but over the past few months even these medications haven't been able to control it. You are experiencing excruciating pain in your tummy and it sometimes causes shooting pain into your back as well. It is now having an impact on your quality of life because you cannot go out as often as you want.

You are here today to discuss the pain with your doctor. Previously, they have told you that there are other medications that could help in the later stages of your cancer, such as morphine, but you have some friends that have been on morphine and are essentially addicted to it, so you have been reluctant to start it.

### Mark Scheme for Examiner

#### Introduction

| | | | | | |
|---|---|---|---|---|---|
| Cleans hands, introduces self and confirms patient identity | | | | | |
| Checks the identity of others in the room and confirms that the patient is happy for them to be present | | | | | |
| Establishes current patient knowledge and concerns | | | | | |

#### Taking a Brief History

| Statement/Question | Justification | Answer | | | |
|---|---|---|---|---|---|
| I'm sorry to hear you are in pain. Can you explain the type of pain that you are experiencing now? | It is important to take a pain history so that you can appreciate what it is that you are trying to help the patient with | 'I've always had pain in the centre of my tummy because of my pancreatic cancer. But recently it's got really bad, present most of the day every day. I'm also getting pain going into my back now, which is unbearable' | | | |
| What painkillers have you used so far? | This helps to gauge previous analgesia use and its efficacy, which could be useful when looking at drugs from the same class | 'It was previously well controlled with paracetamol and codeine, but even this isn't touching the pain any more' | | | |
| Do you have any drug allergies? | As the prescriber, it is your duty to find out if the patient has any allergies before you prescribe anything | 'No, not that I am aware of' | | | |

#### Counselling on Morphine Use

| | | | | | |
|---|---|---|---|---|---|
| There are many uses of morphine-based medications, and in your case, we are suggesting it for pain relief | Explain why the patient is recommended to take morphine | 'How does it work exactly?' | | | |

## Counselling on Morphine Use

| Statement/Question | Justification | Answer | | | | |
|---|---|---|---|---|---|---|
| Morphine binds to specific receptors/proteins, to increase pain tolerance. It comes in different forms, including tablets and syrups | Explain what morphine is and how it works | 'I see' | | | | |
| Morphine can come in long- or short-acting preparations. Regular doses (long-acting) are used to control the pain, and sporadic doses (short-acting) can be used for breakthrough pain, when the pain suddenly becomes very severe | Explain when the drug should be taken | 'Will I become addicted to it? I have heard of people who have had it, but now cannot come off it. I don't want to be like that' | | | | |
| This is extremely rare when morphine is taken for the purpose of pain relief. Over time, patients may require a higher dose to achieve the same pain relief. Therefore, unlike with addiction, there is a rational reason for increasing analgesia. The concern is more regarding a patient who has been taking opiates for a long time and then suddenly stops, as they may suffer from withdrawal symptoms of opioids, such as anxiety and agitation. However, this can be prevented through gradual weaning off the medication | Explain the link between morphine and dependency, and warn the patient regarding withdrawal symptoms | 'OK, that's more reassuring' | | | | |
| People who take morphine often suffer from constipation, so we usually prescribe a laxative to help with that. They may also have nausea, which can be alleviated with an antiemetic. Other side effects to look out for include drowsiness, myoclonus and hallucinations. If these side effects occur, let us know and we can review | Explain the common side effects of morphine that the patient needs to be aware of | 'That's fine. If I take the morphine now, will it mean that it won't work when I really need it?' | | | | |
| When pain worsens, it is usually due to disease progression, not the morphine ceasing to work. Morphine can be given in the quantities needed to control the pain | Explain how morphine dose can be altered to accommodate pain level | 'Are there any alternatives?' | | | | |
| There are other medications that are not primarily used in pain relief but can have an analgesic role, such as radiotherapy or anticonvulsants. You have described to me something that sounds like nerve pain, which antidepressants such as amitriptyline could be used for. I must emphasise that we are using this as a painkiller only, and are not implying that you suffer from depression | Clearly state the reason for prescribing alternative medications that are used as pain relief. If the patient wants further details, you can explain the indication for various alternative medications used in pain relief and how they work | 'I understand' | | | | |

## Counselling on Morphine Use

| Statement/Question | Justification | Answer | | | | | |
|---|---|---|---|---|---|---|---|
| Other analgesic approaches that we can consider include emotional and spiritual support, relaxation techniques, creative therapies, acupuncture and transcutaneous electrical nerve stimulation. You can also be referred to the palliative care pain management team who could offer more specialist support service | Discuss alternative conservative management options and involve other relevant teams if the patient wishes to do so | 'I'm happy to give the morphine a go first. I will try anything. If it still doesn't work then I'd like to speak to the pain team' | | | | | |

## Finishing the Consultation

| | | | | | | | |
|---|---|---|---|---|---|---|---|
| To summarise, we have discussed what morphine is and how it works, discussed its side effects, including possible withdrawal symptoms when you wean off it and alternative methods that you can use. You are happy to trial morphine for now, but are open to getting the pain team involved as well | Short summary of the key points discussed so far | 'That's correct' | | | | | |
| I will provide you with a leaflet with more information and am happy to assist in any way possible | Leaflets and other resources will help to refresh the patient's memory | 'That'd be helpful. I like to read up on the medication I am being given' | | | | | |
| Do you have any other questions or things to add? I know that we have discussed a lot of new things; please take some time to digest the information | May identify useful information that has been missed. Will also allow you to address any questions or concerns | 'No, thank you' | | | | | |

## Present Your Findings

Mr Smith is a 62-year-old man who has been diagnosed with inoperable pancreatic cancer. His current pain regimen of codeine and paracetamol is ineffective, as he still has constant abdominal pain as well as intermittent episodes of shooting pain in his back.

As a result, I have counselled the patient on the commencement of morphine to manage his pain and have also suggested using amitriptyline as an adjuvant for the neuropathic pain. I have provided the patient with a leaflet on morphine and he is happy to trial with morphine to help him control his pain

## General Points

| | | | | |
|---|---|---|---|---|
| Polite to patient | | | | |
| Maintains good eye contact | | | | |
| Appropriate use of open and closed questions | | | | |

## ❓ QUESTIONS FROM THE EXAMINER

### How does patient-controlled analgesia provide a patient with pain relief?

Pressing a button gives a patient a preset dose of IV morphine via a pump.

### When is it appropriate to use syringe drivers?

In a palliative setting, syringe drivers may be started if the patient is no longer able to take oral morphine; for example, due to vomiting or swallowing difficulties.

### In renal impairment, why is it important to reduce the dose of opiates?

Opiates are renally excreted, therefore accumulation can occur in renal impairment, leading to increased sensitivity and a prolonged effect.

### Give three situations in which opiate doses may need to be reduced.

Impaired respiratory function, in elderly patients, patients with diseases of the biliary tract.

### Which drugs can be used in the management of opiate withdrawal?

Buprenorphine, naloxone and methadone can all be used.

### Why should opiates be used with caution in those presenting with head injury?

Opioids can affect the pupillary responses, which are part of your neurological assessment.

### Those taking opioids are not allowed to drive – true or false?

False. Patients who are taking opioids are allowed to drive; however, they should be warned that opioids may make them feel drowsy and they should not drive if they feel unfit to do so.

### Codeine should be avoided in children – true or false?

True. Codeine should be avoided in those under 12 because it is associated with respiratory side effects.

### What is phantom-limb syndrome?

Sensations that an amputated limb is still present or is experiencing pain can occur in amputees and usually occur within days to weeks after amputation.

### Give three examples of physical methods of pain management.

Joint injections, nerve blocks and acupuncture can be useful.

## Station 4.15    Breaking Bad News

### Doctor Briefing

You are a junior doctor working on the respiratory ward and have been asked to see Mrs Gardner. You admitted her husband last week; he was suffering from a chest infection, on a long-term background of colorectal cancer. Despite antibiotic therapy, he is now rapidly deteriorating and your consultant anticipates that Mr Gardner has days, if not hours, to live. Please have a discussion with Mrs Gardner regarding Mr Gardner's deterioration.

### Patient Briefing

You are Mrs Gardner, wife of Mr Gardner. As far as you're aware, he's been in hospital for a week being treated for a chest infection. Initially he just had a cough but now it seems to have worsened. The doctors have started him on a lot of antibiotics, but he doesn't seem to be responding well. When you visit him on the ward, he is sleeping most of the time and appears very weak. You think that he is coming to the end of his life but have not been wanting to accept it.

Your main concern is that he's currently suffering. If he is dying, you know that he would rather be kept comfortable.

### Mark Scheme for Examiner

#### Introduction

| | | | |
|---|---|---|---|
| Cleans hands, introduces self and confirms patient identity | | | |
| Checks the identity of the people present in the room and confirms that the patient is happy for them to be spoken to | | | |
| Ensure that you are in an appropriate setting to deliver bad news, preferably a quiet, private and bleep-free environment | | | |

#### Relative's Current Understanding

| Statement/Question | Justification | Answer | |
|---|---|---|---|
| Could you update me on what you know has been happening with Mr Gardner? | Establishes current knowledge and concerns from the relative | 'He's been in hospital for a week being treated for a chest infection but I think it's been getting worse' | |
| Yes, that has been the case. Mr Gardner has got a very bad chest infection. Over the week we've treated it with different types of strong antibiotics but unfortunately, he's still not getting better | You are summarising what the relative knows, while adding more information to provide more context | 'Yes, he looks very weak and is asleep most of the time' | |

#### Explaining the Situation

| | | | |
|---|---|---|---|
| Regrettably I have got some bad news. Would you like me to continue or would you like anyone with you? | When delivering bad news, it's important to give patients a warning shot so that they can prepare themselves for the news to come. It is also good to gauge whether they want to have the conversation right now or not | 'No, I'm all right by myself. Please go ahead. I think I know what you're about to say anyway' | |

**Explaining the Situation**

| Statement/Question | Justification | Answer | | | | | |
|---|---|---|---|---|---|---|---|
| From past experience and our observations of Mr Gardner, the impression that we have is that, sadly, he is dying despite all the treatment we are giving him | Information should be given in small, manageable pieces. Giving too much information in one go can be overwhelming and ineffective. Be straightforward in your delivery, such as by using the word 'dying' | 'Oh dear … I suspected this' | | | | | |
| Allow for a short period of silence and/or offer tissues if appropriate | In such circumstances, it is important to respond to the relative's reaction with empathy. If the relative falls silent, it is tempting to fill the space with more reassurance, but you should respect the silence for a while. This gives the relative some time to deal with her emotions and reaction | 'I knew it, but I just didn't want to accept it. Now hearing you say it makes it feel so much more real. How long do you think he has left?' | | | | | |
| It is difficult to say, and is different for every patient. In Mr Gardner's case, the team thinks that he has days, if not hours, to live regardless of what treatment is given | Address any concerns or questions that the relative may have. If you do not have an answer, don't make it up | 'Oh gosh, that's so soon! I'm really worried that he may be in pain or suffering' | | | | | |
| We believe that the best thing for Mr Gardner right now is to keep him as comfortable as possible and to make sure he is in no pain. Any further tests are unlikely to be beneficial and instead might cause him unnecessary distress. So, we feel that it is in his best interest not to do any more tests or to give him treatment | Be straightforward but sensitive when explaining to the patient's relative that you will be withdrawing treatment and the rationale behind it | 'Yes, I just want him to be painfree and comfortable. What about eating and drinking though?' | | | | | |
| Understandably, some people have concerns that not giving any active treatment to the patient means that their loved one will be left without any food or drink. That definitely isn't the case. Mr Gardner can eat and drink as he pleases, but from experience, we know that patients who are dying usually have a reduced appetite and don't want to eat or drink | A lot of relatives are concerned that when a patient is put on an end-of-life pathway, he is deprived of food and drink. Therefore, it is important to reassure them that this is not the case | 'OK' | | | | | |
| We will arrange for him to be moved into a side room so that he can spend his last moments with his family in privacy | Give patients at the end of their life their own space, preferably in their own room without other interferences | 'Yes, that would be good. I would like our children to be able to come and see him, if they want to' | | | | | |

**Finishing the Consultation**

| Question | Justification | Answer | | | | |
|---|---|---|---|---|---|---|
| Sorry to reiterate this, but I just want to ensure that the key details have been relayed to you. In summary, Mr Gardner has a severe chest infection that is not improving with treatment. He is now slowly dying. We think that he only has hours to days left. Our aim is to keep him comfortable and we will stop all active treatment | Short summary of the key points discussed so far. Given the circumstances, this needs to be done sensitively and with empathy. Your non-verbal communications here will be critical | 'Yes ... I just want to go and spend some time with Joe' | | | | |
| I am very sorry to be giving you such sad news and understand that you may need some time to take in everything. We can arrange another meeting at any time, but do you have any questions for me now? | | 'Not right now. I'll let you know if I do. Thank you for your support' | | | | |
| Of course. I will leave you with this leaflet that you can read in your own time. It details what to expect of someone who is approaching end of life. We are also more than happy to support you and your family in any way that we can | Provide the relative with written information and offer continuous support from the team | 'Thank you. Everyone has been very kind to us' | | | | |

**Present Your Findings**

Today I spoke with Mrs Gardner and explained that her husband has deteriorated over the last few days, despite being on antibiotics for a chest infection. I have informed her that the team believes that he is dying. She agrees that we should aim for him to be kept comfortable and will stop any active treatment. I will arrange for him to be moved to a side room so that they can have privacy and she is aware that she can speak to me again if she wants more support

**General Points**

| | | | | |
|---|---|---|---|---|
| Polite to patient | | | | |
| Maintains good eye contact | | | | |
| Appropriate use of open and closed questions | | | | |

## ❓ QUESTIONS FROM THE EXAMINER

**Where in the hospital is an appropriate place to speak to family members about private matters, such as in the above scenario?**

In most hospitals, each ward or clinical area will have its own family or relative's room. This is usually a private space where you can speak at length with the family without being disturbed.

**What is a 'living will'?**

A 'living will' is also known as an advanced decision. This is a decision that you can make ahead of time about a certain choice under certain circumstances and that would become relevant if you were to become unable to make or communicate your own decisions.

## Is a 'living will' legally binding?

Yes. This means that healthcare professions must respect your wishes and follow your instructions as outlined in your 'living will'.

## What can you not request in a 'living will'?

A 'living will' cannot be used to request certain treatment, nor can you request for your life to be ended.

## What is the main difference between an advanced statement and an advanced decision?

An advanced decision is legally binding, whereas an advanced statement is not.

## What information can you include on an advanced statement?

Any details about your wishes or preferences can be detailed in an advanced statement so that the best care can be provided to you. This includes your dietary requirements, where you would like to be cared for (home, hospice, care home), religious beliefs and values and which of your closest family and friends to discuss your care with.

## What is the difference between empathy and sympathy?

Empathy refers to the ability to understand and share someone else's feelings, whereas sympathy refers to the ability to feel sorrow for someone else.

## List three ways that you can display active listening skills.

Maintaining eye contact appropriately, having an open body language (uncrossed legs and arms, leaning slightly forward towards the patient), nodding your head to acknowledge what the patient is saying, not interrupting the patient throughout the consultation.

## What are 'warning shots' with respect to communication?

They are phrases that you can use to warn a patient that you are about to deliver some bad news; for instance, 'unfortunately I have some bad news for you'.

## What would you do if a patient asks a question about prognosis and you are unsure of the answer?

If you do not know the answer or the next step is unclear, then clearly state so! You should answer questions kindly and honestly, and you must not lie.

## Station 4.16   Ethics

### Doctor Briefing

You are a junior doctor working in the emergency department and you have been asked to assess Evelyn Beech, a 79-year-old woman who has presented with back pain. During your examination, you see that she has multiple bruises on her back. When questioned, she confides that sometimes her carer gets frustrated with her. Please discuss your options with the examiner and what you would do in this situation.

### Mark Scheme for Examiner

#### Introduction

| | | | |
|---|---|---|---|
| Cleans hands, introduces self and confirms that you are talking to the examiner | | | |
| Checks the identity of others in the room | | | |

#### Ethical Dilemma Considerations

| Statement/Question | Justification | | | | |
|---|---|---|---|---|---|
| Firstly, I would gather information from the patient, including: the length and frequency of the abuse, type(s) of abuse, severity of the abuse, effect on the patient and identifying other people at potential risk | It is important to find out as much information as possible from the patient in order to assess her risk, while doing so in a sensitive way. I would make sure I ask about physical, emotional, psychological, sexual and financial abuse | | | | |
| It may be that I have another healthcare professional present during this discussion who could act as a scribe, writing down everything the patient says | In cases of alleged abuse, it is vital to document clearly what the patient says, without suggestion or supposition | | | | |
| It may be appropriate to ask her to describe what happens in a usual day with her carer to ascertain the frequency and level of abuse | It is important to ask questions in a way that the patient understands. Gauging her answers to the first question will be able to guide you | | | | |
| Another possible question would be to ask her what is the worst thing the carer has done to her | This would give you an example of what the patient feels is the worst experience she has had | | | | |
| I would also need to assess and document whether, or not, I feel the patient has capacity | Documenting capacity is a vital part for any patient interaction | | | | |
| One option is to do nothing. This goes against the principles of non-maleficence (to do no harm) and beneficence (to do what's best for the patient). However, if the patient doesn't want you to disclose it, then it allows you to maintain confidentiality and respect the patient's autonomy, unless you think the patient is at risk | When discussing actions, it is important to relate the justification back to ethics principles such as the four key pillars, confidentiality, consent or capacity. Depending on the patient's wishes, respecting the patient's autonomy should be discussed with the relevant option | | | | |
| Another option is that I could encourage the patient to report the abusers, or to allow me to advocate for her. This will involve her in the decision making and also means that confidentiality is not broken | | | | | |
| Alternatively, I could report the carer against the patient's wishes. Confidential information can be disclosed against the patient's wishes if it is done to prevent a risk to national security or public health, crime or to protect others from death or serious harm. This option cannot be taken lightly as it may lead to a breakdown of the doctor–patient relationship | It would be important to warn the patient that if the healthcare professional feels that the patient or others are at risk of significant harm, then confidentiality may be broken | | | | |

**Ethical Dilemma Considerations**

| Statement/Question | Justification | | | |
|---|---|---|---|---|
| The decision regarding what to do is not one that I would make by myself. I would involve my seniors but also the hospital safeguarding team.<br>In some cases it may be appropriate to notify the police | Depending on which defence union you are with, they usually have a contact to whom you can speak regarding ethical scenarios such as this. You would not be expected to manage this alone | | | |
| In addition, I would inform and provide written information to the patient informing her where she would be able to access further support | In such a vulnerable patient, it is crucial that you signpost her to further resources that may be able to help her either in the present or the future | | | |
| Furthermore, it may not be safe to discharge the patient home to her usual package of care; it may be best to keep her in hospital as a place of safety | Keeping a patient in hospital as a place of safety is frequently performed in these situations, even if just whilst initial investigations are being undertaken | | | |
| I would also consider speaking to my defence union for more professional advice and information if I did not have immediate access to an adult safeguarding team | Depending on which defence union you are with, they usually have a contact to whom you can speak regarding ethical scenarios such as this | | | |

**Present Your Findings**

Mrs Beech is a 79-year-old woman who has reported that she has suffered physical abuse from her carer. I have discussed this case in detail, taking into consideration the actions that I could take as a junior doctor, relating it back to medical ethics

**General Points**

Maintains good eye contact

Appropriate use of open and closed questions

## ❓ QUESTIONS FROM THE EXAMINER

### What is 'elderspeak'?

'Elderspeak' refers to when healthcare professionals 'talk down' to older patients, often coming across as patronising and demeaning. Some describe it as being similar to 'baby talk' and it is often characterised by slow and loud speech.

### When can confidentiality be broken?

Under some circumstances, confidentiality can be broken, including: with the patient's consent, when it is justifiable in the public interest (to prevent a risk to national security or public health, protect others from death or other serious harm, to prevent serious crime) or when it is ordered under the court of law.

### How many stages does capacity assessment consist of?

Capacity assessment involves a two-stage test.

### What is paternalism and which ethical pillar does it conflict with?

Paternalism refers to when a healthcare professional makes decisions for a patient without asking the patient for their opinion first. The physician usually believes that they are making the decision in the patient's best interest. This conflicts with respecting the patient's autonomy.

## What does the term *primum non nocere* mean?

It is the Latin terminology for 'first, do no harm'.

## What is a best-interest meeting?

It is a multidisciplinary meeting that is arranged when a patient is deemed to lack the mental capacity for a specific decision around a patient's care or treatment.

## When is a patient deemed unable to make a decision?

If a patient is unable to understand the information given to make the decision, retain the information for long enough to make the decision, weigh up the benefits and risk and communicate their decision, then they are deemed unable to make a decision.

## What is the HARK framework?

The HARK framework consists of four questions and was developed to identify those who are victims of abuse.

## What is the Mental Health Act 1983?

It is the main piece of legislation that covers the assessment, treatment and rights of people with a mental health disorder.

## What is Deprivation of Liberty Safeguards?

It is a procedure that is aimed to protect a person's rights, if they become deprived of their liberty in a hospital or care home setting, and they lack mental capacity to consent to those arrangements.

# Data Interpretation

5

## Outline

## Station 5.1 Full Blood Count

### Doctor Briefing

You are a junior doctor on a primary care placement and have been asked to see Mrs Brown, a normally active 75-year-old woman, who has presented with an 8-week history of increasing lethargy. She appears quite pale. You take some blood tests, and the results are reported as below. Please review the blood tests, explain the findings to Mrs Brown and formulate an appropriate management plan.

### Patient Briefing

You have seen your general practitioner (GP) for tiredness, and they took some blood. You have not noticed any other symptoms that you are aware of; however, when asked, you confirm that you have very dark stools and are slightly short of breath when walking up stairs. When the GP talks to you about low iron levels, you become very upset and distressed, as you associate this with cancer.

### Results

| Components | Results | Reference ranges with units |
|---|---|---|
| Haemoglobin (Hb) | 88 ↓ | Males:130–180 g/L<br>Females: 115–165 g/L |
| Haematocrit (Hct) | 0.3 ↓ | Males: 0.4–0.54 L/L<br>Females: 0.37–0.47 L/L |
| Red cell count (RCC) | 3 ↓ | Males: 4.5–6.5 × 10$^{12}$/L<br>Females: 3.8–5.8 × 10$^{12}$/L |
| Mean cell volume (MCV) | 50 ↓ | 80–95 fL |
| Mean corpuscular haemoglobin (MCH) | 24 ↓ | 27–34 pg/cell |
| Mean corpuscular haemoglobin concentration (MCHC) | 275 ↓ | 300–350 g/L |
| White cell count (WCC) | 4 | 3.6–11.0 × 10$^9$/L |
| Platelets (Plt) | 200 | 140–400 × 10$^9$/L |

| Components | Results | Reference ranges with units |
|---|---|---|
| Neutrophils | 2 | $1.8–7.5 \times 10^9$/L |
| Lymphocytes | 3 | $1.0–4.0 \times 10^{92}$/L |
| Eosinophils | 0.3 | $0.1–0.4 \times 10^9$/L |
| Basophils | 0.07 | $0.02–0.10 \times 10^9$/L |
| Monocytes | 0.5 | $0.2–0.8 \times 10^9$/L |

## Mark Scheme for Examiner

### Introduction

| | | | | | |
|---|---|---|---|---|---|
| Cleans hands, introduces self and confirms patient identity | | | | | |

### Establishes Current Patient Knowledge

| Statement/Question | Justification | Answer | Thoughts | | | | |
|---|---|---|---|---|---|---|---|
| I understand you have been feeling tired but not noticed anything else that concerns you | Start with a general open phrase to guide the patient and to clarify the consultation | 'Yes, I have been a bit tired for a while now – but I think I'm fine' | The patient describes a potentially long-standing issue but denies any other symptoms | | | | |
| Have you noticed any other symptoms, like breathlessness or change in the colour of your stools, for example? | Important to ensure that the patient hasn't got any more concerning features. Remember, this is an interpretation station, not a history station, so a full history is not expected but checking for red flags is pertinent | 'Now you mention it, I do become a bit breathless after going up the stairs and my stool is darker than usual – this is new. I didn't have this before my blood test' | Really useful for you to be able to determine a change in the patient's presentation | | | | |

### Data Interpretation and Discussion

| | | | | | | | |
|---|---|---|---|---|---|---|---|
| I have done a blood test to look at the iron levels in your blood, known as haemoglobin | Explain what the blood test is for and why we are doing it | 'OK' | Establish a baseline of what the blood test is looking at | | | | |
| As I suspected, your tests show that you have a low haemoglobin, known as anaemia | Clarifying the test results to the patient | 'OK' | The patient has not asked anything at this point, so you can carry on with your explanation. Some patients may start asking all sorts of questions at this point | | | | |

## Data Interpretation and Discussion

| Statement/Question | Justification | Answer | Thoughts | | | | |
|---|---|---|---|---|---|---|---|
| Some medical problems can cause us to have low iron levels. This can cause many symptoms, including the ones you describe | Important to validate the patient's symptoms and clarify to her that you think the low haemoglobin level is contributing to how she is feeling | 'Do you know what is causing it?' | Nearly always the patient will ask what the cause is. It is all right not to have an answer and to explain that further investigation is required | | | | |
| I cannot tell you exactly what the cause is at the moment but we know the type of anaemia you have and this will help guide our investigations | It is vital to discuss things in lay terms but also to let the patient know the medical terminology | 'What type is it?' | Be prepared to have to explain yourself further when you offer information to patients | | | | |
| It is called microcytic anaemia, a common type of anaemia that has many causes | This is explaining the diagnosis and also reassuring the patient that it is commonly found | 'OK. What happens next?' | The patient does not seem to want to know any more about the anaemia and instead is focused on the investigations | | | | |
| I would like to do another blood test to measure the iron stores in your body | Need to explain that further tests are needed | 'All right' | The patient has accepted the blood test | | | | |
| I would also like to investigate the change in your stool colour a bit further by referring you to my colleagues who specialise in the gut | You are explaining that you suspect a gastrointestinal cause for her anaemia | 'OK, what will they do?' | The patient understandably wants to know more | | | | |
| We would send them your story and all the blood test results to review – they would then decide the best investigations but it usually involves a camera test of the throat and stomach | You are explaining that the specialist makes specific decisions regarding invasive investigations but you will be giving them your thoughts | 'What do you think is wrong with my insides – is this cancer?' | The patient is giving you their concerns. Remember, this is a data interpretation station and not a communication one, so breaking bad news or spending a long time on this won't be expected. However, acknowledging the concerns is vital and will be marked positively | | | | |

## Data Interpretation and Discussion

| Statement/Question | Justification | Answer | Thoughts | | | | |
|---|---|---|---|---|---|---|---|
| I really cannot tell you what it is now, as I don't know. With any patient we are always making sure we don't miss a potential cancer, but there are also a lot of other things this could be. When we have further results back I'll be able to give you more information | You have acknowledged the patient's concerns, you have explained you cannot answer her question now but you have also reassured her that as you know more, you will share your thoughts with her | 'Thank you doctor, that makes sense' | The patient is happy with your explanation | | | | |

## Finishing the Consultation

| | | | | | | | |
|---|---|---|---|---|---|---|---|
| Would you mind please repeating what I have just told you? | Checking that the patient was listening and understands the information | 'I have low iron levels in the blood. You don't know what is causing this at the moment but will find out why' | You have a patient who has listened and correctly interpreted what you have told her | | | | |
| I understand there is a lot to take in. Do you have any immediate questions for me? | May identify useful information that has been missed | 'No, I understand' | This patient is happy with the plan | | | | |
| I will organise the blood test for you now and I expect the hospital gut doctors to get in touch soon regarding further tests | Recapping the plan to yourself, the examiner and the patient is always important | 'Thank you' | The patient is satisfied with your management | | | | |

## Present Your Findings

This is Mrs Brown, a normally active 75-year-old woman, who has presented with lethargy and on further questioning divulged shortness of breath on exertion and dark stools.

An FBC was taken; it demonstrates microcytic anaemia, with a Hb of 88 g/L and MCV of 0.3 fL.

I have explained the findings to Mrs Brown and she is aware I would like to check her ferritin level and have referred her to gastroenterology for further investigation

## General Points

Polite to patient

Maintains good eye contact

Appropriate use of open and closed questions

# ? QUESTIONS FROM THE EXAMINER

### Define polycythaemia.

Poylcythaemia is also known as erythrocytosis and means an abnormally high level of red blood cells in the blood.

### What is the MCV measuring?

It is a measure of the average size of the red cells present in the blood sample.

### Name three causes of microcytic anaemia.

Iron deficiency anaemia, thalassaemia syndrome, hookworm infection, sideroblastic anaemia and lead poisoning. Anaemia of chronic disease can be microcytic but is more often normocytic.

### What does the haematocrit measure and what factors can affect its value?

It is the percentage of the blood sample that is made up of red cells and can be affected by either the number of red blood cells or the volume of blood plasma.

### What is hyperviscosity syndrome?

It refers to any state in which the blood has an increased viscosity, secondary to a raised haematocrit or increased levels of circulating plasma components.

### What are plasma cells?

Plasma cells are a type of white blood cell that is produced in the bone marrow. They produce antibodies and immunoglobulins that help to fight infection.

### Describe haematopoesis.

It is the process by which all of the cellular components of blood and blood plasma are developed and formed.

### What are the four main types of leukaemia?

Acute myeloid leukaemia, chronic myeloid leukaemia, acute lymphocytic leukaemia and chronic lymphocytic leukaemia.

### How does steroid use affect the results of FBCs?

Typically, glucocorticosteroid use, such as dexamethasone and prednisolone, increases white blood cells.

### What are the diagnostic criteria for neutropenic sepsis?

A neutrophil count equal to or less than $0.5 \times 10^9$/L, plus either a temperature greater than 38.0°C or other signs and symptoms consistent with sepsis.

## Station 5.2    Urea and Electrolytes

### Doctor Briefing

You are a junior doctor on a general medicine placement and have been asked to see Mrs Smith, a 70-year-old woman, who was admitted with gastroenteritis. The nursing staff are concerned that she has not passed urine in 12 h. She has a background of type 2 diabetes, hypertension and osteoarthritis in her spine. You take some blood tests, and the results are reported as below. Please review the results, explain the findings to Mrs Smith and formulate an appropriate management plan.

### Patient Briefing

You have been brough to hospital with a stomach bug and are finding it really hard to drink a lot, despite the nurses asking you to. The doctors have told you that you have not been passing enough urine; you cannot remember when you last did. You are told that the doctors are worried about your kidneys.

You are concerned that your tablets may be damaging your kidneys.

### Results

| Components | Result | Reference ranges with units |
|---|---|---|
| Sodium | 136 | 135–145 mmol/L |
| Potassium | **5.7** ↑ | 3.5–5.5 mmol/L |
| Chloride | 100 | 95–110 mmol/L |
| Bicarbonate | 25 | 22–29 mmol/L |
| Urea | **10** ↑ | 2.5–6.5 mmol/L |
| Creatinine | **130** ↑ | 60–120 µmol/L |
| Estimated glomerular filtration rate | **45** ↓ | >60 mL/min/1.73 m² |

### Mark Scheme for Examiner

#### Introduction

| | | | | |
|---|---|---|---|---|
| Cleans hands, introduces self and confirms patient identity | | | | |

#### Establishes Current Patient Knowledge

| Statement/Question | Justification | Answer | Thoughts | | | |
|---|---|---|---|---|---|---|
| I understand you have had a stomach bug and have not passed urine in a while | Start with a general open phrase to guide the patient | 'I'm not really sure. The nurses have told me I have not passed urine all day' | You know the patient understands the situation and is aware there are concerns | | | |
| How are you feeling now? | Important to ensure that the patient hasn't become more unwell since presentation | 'I feel a bit better. I have stopped being sick now and managed to eat some soup for lunch' | Before you start explaining something to a patient, it is important to determine her knowledge as it will help you pitch your discussion | | | |

## Data Interpretation and Discussion

| Statement/Question | Justification | Answer | Thoughts | | | | |
|---|---|---|---|---|---|---|---|
| I have done a blood test to look at how well your kidneys are working at the moment | Explain what the blood test is for and why we are doing it | 'OK' | Establish a baseline of what we are looking at with renal function testing | | | | |
| Some medical problems can cause our kidneys not to work as we expect. This is usually a temporary issue | Important to explain that something abnormal has been found and to highlight that this is not a permanent issue | 'What is causing it?' | When explaining things to patients, try not to over-load them. It is useful to give them small chunks of information and then allow them to ask questions | | | | |
| This is due to reduced blood flow to the kidneys when you are unwell with an upset stomach. This causes a derangement in the salts in our blood stream | It is vital to discuss things in lay terms | 'How can I increase the blood flow?' | Address the patient's concerns by answering any questions that she has | | | | |
| While you are poorly and dehydrated, we gave you fluid through a drip to help. Now you are feeling better, eating and drinking will help rehydrate you and increase the blood flow | It is vital to explain the steps of treatment and management | 'OK. Do I need to stay in hospital?' | The patient understandably wants to know more detail | | | | |
| You need to stay in until we know your blood results are improving and you start passing urine | Need to explain to the patient that this is something that can be managed but that more monitoring is needed before discharge | 'Are my tablets causing a problem with my kidneys?' | The patient is asking appropriate questions and has concerns regarding her medication. It is vital to acknowledge her concerns | | | | |
| Really good question. We actually temporarily stopped one of your medications when you were admitted as it can make kidney function worse. However your GP will be able to restart this once your kidneys begin to work as usual | You are explaining to the patient that the medication is not the cause of her problems but you are aware of the renal impact. You have also made her aware that you expect her to be able to take the medication again | 'Fine' | No additional concerns | | | | |

## Finishing the Consultation

| | | | | | | | |
|---|---|---|---|---|---|---|---|
| Would you mind please repeating what I have just told you? | Checking that the patient was listening and understands the information | 'My kidneys are not working well due to dehydration but you expect it to get better' | You have a patient who has listened and correctly interpreted what you have told her | | | | |

**Finishing the Consultation**

| Statement/Question | Justification | Answer | Thoughts | | | | |
|---|---|---|---|---|---|---|---|
| I understand there is a lot to take in. Do you have any immediate questions for me? | May identify useful information that has been missed | 'When will the GP see me to start my medication?' | The patient is thinking about the next steps. It is important she is aware of these | | | | |
| We will write to your GP and put a plan in your discharge summary so you know when to see them | Recapping the plan to yourself, the examiner and the patient is always important | 'Perfect. Thank you' | The patient is happy with your management | | | | |

**Present Your Findings**

Mrs Smith is a 70-year-old woman who presented with gastroenteritis and oliguria. Serum U&Es have demonstrated an acute kidney injury (AKI), which has been managed with intravenous fluids.

I feel that Mrs Smith understands the diagnosis of AKI and is aware that we have temporarily withheld some of her nephrotoxic medication.

We will closely monitor her renal function and repeat in 12 h. If her potassium rises further she will need an electrocardiogram (ECG) and further management

**General Points**

| | | | | |
|---|---|---|---|---|
| Polite to patient | | | | |
| Maintains good eye contact | | | | |
| Appropriate use of open and closed questions | | | | |

## ❓ QUESTIONS FROM THE EXAMINER

### What is the difference between creatinine and creatine?

Creatine is a very important substance used to produce energy needed for muscle action. Creatinine is a waste product from the breakdown of creatine.

### What happens to serum creatinine in pregnancy?

Serum creatinine falls in pregnancy. The reference range of AKI in pregnant women is therefore different to the non-pregnant population.

### What happens during the urea cycle?

Ammonia is converted into urea in the liver.

### Name three indications for kidney dialysis.

Intractable acidosis, electrolyte abnormalities (such as hyperkalaemia, hyponatraemia or hypercalcaemia), intoxicants, overload and uraemia.

### What are the three types of AKI?

The three types are prerenal, renal and postrenal. Examples are hypotension, glomerulonephritis and renal stone, respectively.

## What is the most common intrinsic cause of AKI?

Acute renal tubular necrosis, where there is reduced blood flow and oxygen supply to the kidneys, leading to kidney damage.

## Is AKI reversible?

Yes. AKI can be reversed with correct identification and management. However, it can be life-threatening and can cause irreversible kidney injury.

## Why do we perform venous blood gas in patients with suspected AKI?

The venous blood gas is useful to check for metabolic acidosis and a low bicarbonate level. It also promptly reveals electrolyte levels, of which potassium and sodium are most important to note.

## What are the two mechanisms that lead to renal artery disease?

Atherosclerosis involving the renal arteries from the aorta and fibromuscular dysplasia involving the distal renal arteries.

## What is stage 2 of the Kidney Disease Improving Global Outcomes (KDIGO) AKI staging?

It is when serum creatinine is 2–2.9 times of its normal baseline.

## Station 5.3   Liver Function Tests

### Doctor Briefing

You are a junior doctor on a general surgery rotation and have been asked to see Mrs King, a 44-year-old woman, who was admitted with constant right-upper-quadrant pain, fever and vomiting. Over the past few months she has noticed colicky pain after eating fatty food. Her husband noticed that her skin and sclera now look quite yellow. You take some blood tests, and the results are reported as below. Please review the blood test results, explain the findings to Mrs King and formulate an appropriate management plan.

### Patient Briefing

You are in hospital with tummy pain that seems to be getting worse. You are also feeling very sick and have vomited several times. You have noticed it is worse after eating food. You are scared you need to have an operation.

### Results

| Component | Results | Reference ranges with units |
|---|---|---|
| Total bilirubin | **38** ↑ | < 20 mg/dL |
| Alanine aminotransferase (ALT) | 35 | 5–40 U/L |
| Aspartate aminotransferase (AST) | 22 | 5–40 U/L |
| Gamma-glutamyl transferase (GGT) | **270** ↑ | <65 U/L |
| Alkaline phosphatase (ALP) | **350** ↑ | 25–130 U/L |
| Albumin | 42 | 35–50 g/dL |

### Mark Scheme for Examiner

#### Introduction

| | |
|---|---|
| Cleans hands, introduces self and confirms patient identity | |

#### Establishes Current Patient Knowledge

| Statement/Question | Justification | Answer | Thoughts | |
|---|---|---|---|---|
| I understand you now have constant abdominal pain. Have you noticed anything else that concerns you? | Start with a general open phrase to guide the patient and to clarify the consultation | 'Yes, the pain is now there all the time and unbearable. My husband says my eyes look a bit yellow too' | The patient confirms her symptoms and clarifies them with you. It is important that you gauge the patient's understanding before you continue | |
| Have you or anyone in your family had a pain like this? | Important to check the patient's history, and this will determine her understanding | 'No, this has never happened to me before, or anyone I know. Can you make it go away?' | The patient is keen to focus on managing her pain | |

## Data Interpretation and Discussion

| Statement/Question | Justification | Answer | Thoughts | | | | |
|---|---|---|---|---|---|---|---|
| I have done a blood test to look at your how your liver is functioning | Explain what the blood test is for and why we are doing it | 'OK' | Establish a baseline of what the blood test is looking at | | | | |
| This shows some abnormalities in the salts and enzymes in the liver | Clarifying the test results to the patient | 'OK' | The patient has not asked anything at this point, so you can carry on with your explanation. Some patients may start asking all sorts of questions at this point | | | | |
| Taking into consideration your symptoms and your blood test results, we suspect you have a gallstone blocking the drainage system of the liver | Explain your working diagnosis in lay terms | 'Do I have to have an operation?' | The patient is understandably concerned about an operation, so it is important to recognise this and explain the next steps | | | | |
| Now I cannot tell you for certain just yet. What we need to do is a scan of your tummy to see if the stones are there and how many you have. Often there is more than one stone; they can sit anywhere along the draining system of the liver | It is important to acknowledge the patient's concerns but key also to explain that further investigation is needed to confirm the diagnosis | 'If you do see stones, how will I be treated?' | The patient seems really keen to understand the management plan | | | | |
| At first, we will try conservative management. This means treating you with fluid, antisickness medication and pain relief into the veins. If we think there is an infection, you may need antibiotics too | This is explaining in lay terms what conservative management is. Patients will not know what this entails, so it is important to describe all aspects of the management plan | 'OK. What happens next?' | The patient wants to know all possible management plans | | | | |
| If there is a stone that is stuck or you do not get better with the initial management plan we may need to perform a procedure to release the stone from the tube it is stuck in | Need to explain to the patient the next steps in the treatment ladder | 'That makes sense. Thank you. Can I please ask how you will know if I need antibiotics?' | The patient has accepted your explanation and has a further valid question | | | | |
| If you have a temperature and further blood tests demonstrate signs of infection then we will start antibiotics | You have explained to the patient clearly the criteria for requiring antibiotics | 'OK, thank you. I'm not very good at swallowing tablets' | The patient wishes you to know she has trouble taking tablets | | | | |

## Data Interpretation and Discussion

| Statement/Question | Justification | Answer | Thoughts | | | | |
|---|---|---|---|---|---|---|---|
| Thank you for letting me know. If you need antibiotics they would be given into a vein at first and then tablets or a liquid solution can be given after a few days | You acknowledge her concern and show her that there are ways around not having to take tablets by mentioning liquid preparations. Her aversion to taking tablets can be explored further down the line, as she may not need antibiotics | 'OK' | The patient is happy with this explanation | | | | |

## Finishing the Consultation

| | | | | | | | |
|---|---|---|---|---|---|---|---|
| Would you mind please repeating what I have just told you? | Checking that the patient was listening and understands the information | 'I have abnormal liver tests which are probably because I have a stone stuck' | You have a patient who has listened and correctly interpreted what you have told her | | | | |
| I understand there is a lot to take in. Do you have any immediate questions for me? | May identify useful information that has been missed | 'No, I understand. Can I have some stronger pain relief?' | This patient is happy with the plan and indicates that her pain may not be adequately controlled | | | | |
| Yes. Let me look at your drug chart. I will also organise the scan for you and we can take things from there | Recapping the plan to yourself, the examiner and the patient is always important | 'Thank you' | The patient is satisfied with your management | | | | |

## Present Your Findings

Mrs King, a 44-year-old woman, was admitted with constant right-upper-quadrant pain, fever and vomiting.

LFTs were taken and demonstrate cholestasis with raised bile acids, GGT and ALP. Combined with her presentation I suspect she has a biliary stone.

I have explained the findings to Mrs King, and she is aware we have ordered her an ultrasound scan

## General Points

Polite to patient

Maintains good eye contact

Appropriate use of open and closed questions

## ? QUESTIONS FROM THE EXAMINER

### What is measured using ALT, AST, GGT and ALP in comparison to using bilirubin and albumin?

The enzymes ALT, AST, GGT and ALP are used to distinguish between hepatocellular damage and cholestasis. On the other hand, bilirubin and albumin are used to assess the liver's synthetic function.

## Where does the conjugation of bilirubin occur?

Bilirubin is conjugated in the hepatocytes and is then secreted into the bile.

## What might a high ALT suggest?

ALT is an enzyme found primarily in hepatocytes, and also in the kidney, skeletal muscles and myocardium. If raised, it suggests hepatocellular damage.

## What might a high AST suggest?

AST is an enzyme found primary in hepatocytes, and also in the myocardium, skeletal muscle, kidneys and brain. It is less specific to liver disease than ALT and if raised, it could be due to cardiac and hepatic pathology, as well as muscle injury.

## Describe Wilson's disease.

It is a autosomal-recessive genetic disorder than leads to excessive accumulation of copper in the body.

## What changes to ALP might you observe during pregnancy?

In a pregnant woman, ALP may be raised during the third trimester.

## Where do cholangiocarcinomas arise and what is the prognosis?

From the epithelial cells of intrahepatic and extrahepatic bile ducts. Typically, cholangiocarcinomas have a very poor prognosis.

## What might a raised ALP but normal GGT suggest and what subsequent blood test would you request?

There may be underlying bone disease such as osteomalacia, Paget's disease or malignancy. In this case it would be useful to obtain a bone profile to determine the underlying cause.

## How can the AST/ALT ratio be used to interpret LFTs?

If ALT is greater than AST, this is often associated with chronic liver disease. If AST is greater than ALT, this is often associated with cirrhosis and acute alcoholic hepatitis.

## What is the difference between gluconeogenesis and glycogenesis?

Gluconeogenesis is the production of glucose, whereas glycogenesis is the process of formation of glycogen from glucose.

## Station 5.4    Coagulation Screen

### Doctor Briefing

You are a junior doctor in the emergency department (ED) and have been asked to see Mr Barr, a 73-year-old man, with a background of atrial fibrillation (for which he is on warfarin) and ischaemic heart disease. He was commenced on antibiotics for a urinary tract infection (UTI) 3 days ago. He has presented with lethargy, dizziness and haematemesis. You did some blood tests, the results of which are now back. Please review the blood tests, explain the findings to Mr Barr and formulate an appropriate management plan.

### Patient Briefing

You are in the ED and feeling very unwell. You have been vomiting up blood and are scared it is related to your warfarin. You are really careful about taking your tablets on time and getting your bloods checked with the nurse at your GP surgery.

### Results

| Component | Results | Reference ranges with units |
|---|---|---|
| Prothrombin time (PT) | **22 ↑** | 11–13 s |
| Activated partial thromboplastin time (APTT) | **40 ↑** | 23–32 s |
| Fibrinogen | 4 | 1.5–4.0 g/L |

### Mark Scheme for Examiner

#### Introduction

| | | | |
|---|---|---|---|
| Cleans hands, introduces self and confirms patient identity | | | |

#### Establishes Current Patient Knowledge

| Statement/Question | Justification | Answer | Thoughts | |
|---|---|---|---|---|
| I understand you are being sick a lot and feel very unwell. Is this correct? | Start with a general open phrase to guide the patient and clarify the consultation | 'Yes – and I think there is blood in my vomit as well' | The patient confirms his symptoms and the worrying presentation of haematemesis | |
| I understand you are on warfarin for an irregular heart beat? | Important to check key facts related to the station | 'Yes – It has been really well controlled for a long time. I take 2 mg a day and have done for ages' | Really useful for you to know that historically, the patient has had a stable international normalised ratio (INR) | |

#### Data Interpretation and Discussion

| | | | | |
|---|---|---|---|---|
| I have done a blood test to look at how quickly your blood clots | Explain what the blood test is for and why we are doing it | 'OK' | Establish a baseline of what the blood test is looking at | |
| As I suspected, your tests show that your blood is taking longer than usual to clot | Clarifying the test results to the patient | 'OK' | The patient has not asked anything at this point, so you can carry on with your explanation. Some patients may start asking all sorts of questions at this point | |

## Data Interpretation and Discussion

| Statement/Question | Justification | Answer | Thoughts | | | | | | |
|---|---|---|---|---|---|---|---|---|---|
| This is why you have noticed blood in your vomit | Important to validate the patient's symptoms and clarify why he has the symptoms he is presenting with | 'Do you know what is causing it?' | The patient will nearly always ask what the cause is | | | | | | |
| We think it may be due to an interaction between your antibiotics for your UTI and your warfarin tablets | It is vital to discuss causes with the patient | 'Why did the other doctor give me the antibiotics then?' | Be prepared to be appropriately challenged by patients. Remember, it is all right not to have all the answers straight away | | | | | | |
| I'm not sure, but this is something that we will investigate. For now, we will change the antibiotic for your UTI to one that we know does not interact with warfarin | This is being honest with the patient and informing him that the prescribing issue will be addressed but also explaining what will happen now | 'OK. Will that make my blood clot quicker?' | The patient is keen to understand how the clotting will return to normal | | | | | | |
| We would like to treat you with medication into the vein called vitamin K to reverse the action of warfarin to ensure your clotting returns to normal | Describe the initial management plan | 'All right' | The patient has accepted this course of action | | | | | | |
| I would like to keep you in hospital and take regular blood tests to ensure your blood clotting levels return to normal | You are explaining the need for an inpatient stay – this needs to be clarified with the patient | 'OK. Do you know how long I will be in hospital?' | The patient understandably wants to know more detail | | | | | | |
| We would expect you to stay in for a couple of days but, as you know, everyone's bodies reacts to warfarin differently so we may need to keep you in for longer | You are being honest and giving the patient an answer but also explaining that the reality may be slightly different to this | 'Thank you, doctor. I appreciate your help' | The patient seems to be happy with the plan you have given | | | | | | |

## Finishing the Consultation

| | | | | | | | | | |
|---|---|---|---|---|---|---|---|---|---|
| Would you mind please repeating what I have just told you? | Checking that the patient was listening and understands the information | 'The antibiotic I was given for my waterworks infection has reacted badly with my warfarin, meaning that my blood is not clotting as usual' | You have a patient who has listened and correctly interpreted what you have told him | | | | | | |
| I understand there is a lot to take in. Do you have any immediate questions for me? | May identify useful information that has been missed | 'No, I understand' | This patient is happy with the plan | | | | | | |

**Finishing the Consultation**

| Statement/Question | Justification | Answer | Thoughts | | | | | |
|---|---|---|---|---|---|---|---|---|
| I will organise the treatment to reverse the warfarin straight away and arrange further blood tests for you | Recapping the plan to yourself, the examiner and the patient is always important | 'Thank you' | The patient is satisfied with your management | | | | | |

**Present Your Findings**

This is Mr Barr, a 73-year-old man, who has presented with lethargy, dizziness and haematemesis. He is on a new antibiotic for a UTI and currently takes warfarin.

A clotting screen was taken and demonstrates a prolonged clotting time with PT of 22 s and APTT of 40 s.

I have explained the findings to Mr Barr, and he is aware we need to change his antibiotic and start a vitamin K infusion

**General Points**

Polite to patient

Maintains good eye contact

Appropriate use of open and closed questions

## ❓ QUESTIONS FROM THE EXAMINER

**Define thrombocytopenia.**

Thrombocytopenia refers to a low platelet count.

**How many factors are there in the clotting cascade?**

Thirteen factors, from I to XIII.

**What are the three pathways that, combined, make up the classical blood coagulation pathway?**

The intrinsic, extrinsic and combined pathways.

**Which pathway is measured by PT and APTT?**

PT measures the extrinsic pathway whereas APTT measures the intrinsic pathway of the coagulation cascade.

**Which factor is fibrinogen also known as and what is its role in the coagulation cascade?**

Fibrinogen is also factor I, which is converted, by thrombin, into fibrin.

**Which test measures how fast fibrinogen is converted to fibrin?**

Thrombin time.

**How are clots dissolved?**

The fibrin mesh of fibrin clots is broken down by plasmin, whose precursor is plasminogen.

## What are the inheritance patterns of haemophilia A, B and C?

Haemophilia A and B are inherited in an X-linked recessive pattern, and haemophilia C is inherited in an autosomal-recessive pattern.

## What is Virchow's triad?

It consists of stasis, endothelial injury and hypercoagulability, and is used to describe the risk factors and aetiology of thrombosis.

## What are the clinical manifestations of antiphospholipid syndrome during pregnancy?

Maternal thrombosis, recurrent miscarriage, late miscarriage, stillbirth, premature birth, pre-eclampsia. Placental complications and fetal growth restriction.

## Station 5.5    Thyroid Function Tests

### Doctor Briefing

You are a junior doctor on a primary care placement and have been asked to see Mx Freesia, a 46-year-old non-binary person, who has presented feeling tired all the time with a history of unintentional weight gain. She saw your colleague last week who took some blood, and the results are now back. She is known to have hypertension. Please review the blood tests, explain the findings to Mrs Freesia and formulate an appropriate management plan.

### Patient Briefing

You have seen your GP for tiredness and weight gain. When they first saw you, they took some blood. You are very distressed about the weight gain, especially as you have been eating healthy and exercising more.

### Results

| Component | Results | Reference ranges with units |
|---|---|---|
| Thyroid-stimulating hormone (TSH) | 14 ↑ | 0.5–5.7 mU/L |
| Free thyroxine (T$_4$) | 28 ↓ | 70–140 mmol/L |

### Mark Scheme for Examiner

#### Introduction

| Cleans hands, introduces self and confirms patient identity | | | | |
|---|---|---|---|---|

#### Establishes Current Patient Knowledge

| Statement/Question | Justification | Answer | Thoughts | |
|---|---|---|---|---|
| I understand you have been feeling tired and noticed unintentional weight gain, is this correct? | Start with a general open phrase to guide the patient and to clarify the consultation | 'Yes, and it is really frustrating me' | The patient describes a potentially long-standing issue but denies any other symptoms | |
| Have you noticed any other symptoms like change in your menstrual periods, dry skin or constipation? | Important to ensure that the patient hasn't got any more features of your presumed diagnosis | 'Actually, I have been really constipated for several months and nothing I have been doing seems to help' | Really useful for you to be able to clarify all the patient's symptoms at the beginning of the station | |

#### Data Interpretation and Discussion

| We did a blood test to see if we can find the cause of your symptoms | Explain what the blood test is for and remind the patient of the context | 'Yes, something to do with my neck' | Establish a baseline of what the blood test is looking at and the patient's understanding | |
|---|---|---|---|---|
| Yes, there is a gland in our necks called the thyroid gland. It is responsible for producing hormones to maintain the systems in our bodies | Clarifying the understanding of the patient and ensuring that you provide a clear lay explanation | 'OK' | The patient has accepted your explanation and has not asked for further details | |

## Data Interpretation and Discussion

| Statement/Question | Justification | Answer | Thoughts | | | | | |
|---|---|---|---|---|---|---|---|---|
| When we checked the functioning of your thyroid gland we found that it is underactive, so not working as well as we expect | Important to explain the blood results in lay terms. Many people will not know what an underactive thyroid means | 'Can you fix it?' | Patients often just want to know a treatment plan. Be adaptable in your consultation to react to the patient's questions | | | | | |
| Yes. An underactive thyroid, known as hypothyroidism, is common and easily treated with tablets | It is good to let the patient know it is a common condition and the management | 'How long do I need to take the tablets for?' | Be prepared to have to explain yourself further when you offer a management plan | | | | | |
| Usually, it is lifelong medication. The tablets replace the vital hormone that your thyroid is not producing enough of. | This is explaining the diagnosis a little more and making the patient aware of what is in the medication | 'OK. Do you know why I have this condition?' | The patient seems to be content with the management plan but keen to know more about the underlying diagnosis | | | | | |
| The most common cause is an autoimmune disorder, where cells in your body attack the thyroid gland, causing it not to function as well. We will investigate the cause for you | Important to state the cause of the diagnosis but also really key to explain that other causes are also possible | 'OK. Thank you. Will my children get this?' | The patient has accepted what you have told her but still has further valid questions | | | | | |
| We know that it can run in families, but it does not always | You are explaining that there is a genetic component to a condition | 'OK – is it associated with anything else?' | The patient understandably wants to know more | | | | | |
| If the cause of your underactive thyroid is autoimmune, as we suspect, it can be linked with other autoimmune conditions. We can talk about this once we have confirmed the cause | You are explaining that there could be potential links with other conditions, but before you go into more detail, you need to confirm the diagnosis | 'That makes sense. What happens next?' | The patient is currently happy with the plan and keen to know the next steps | | | | | |
| I will start you on a tablet called thyroxine. We will carefully monitor your thyroid levels, so we know we are giving you the correct dose | You have described the management plan and made the patient aware that it involves monitoring | 'OK. Thank you' | The patient is happy with your explanation | | | | | |

## Finishing the Consultation

| | | | | | | | | |
|---|---|---|---|---|---|---|---|---|
| Would you mind please repeating what I have just told you? | Checking that the patient was listening and understands the information | 'A gland in my neck is not working well enough and it will be treated with tablets for the rest of my life' | You have a patient who has listened and correctly interpreted what you have told her | | | | | |

**Finishing the Consultation**

| Statement/Question | Justification | Answer | Thoughts | | | | |
|---|---|---|---|---|---|---|---|
| I understand there is a lot to take in. Do you have any immediate questions for me? | May identify useful information that has been missed | 'No, thank you. Will you give me the medication today?' | This patient is happy with the plan | | | | |
| I will give you a prescription today and arrange your follow-up blood test | Recapping the plan to yourself, the examiner and the patient is always important | 'Thank you' | The patient is satisfied with your management | | | | |

**Present Your Findings**

This is Mx Freesia, a 46-year-old non-binary person, who has presented with lethargy, unintentional weight gain and constipation.

TFTs were taken and demonstrate hypothyroidism with a TSH of 14 mU/L and $T_4$ of 28 mmol/L.

I have explained the findings to Mx Freesia, and she is aware of the need for lifelong thyroxine

**General Points**

Polite to patient

Maintains good eye contact

Appropriate use of open and closed questions

## ❓ QUESTIONS FROM THE EXAMINER

**Where is TSH released from?**

The anterior pituitary gland.

**How long is the approximate half-life of $T_4$?**

One week.

**What does the presence of high levels of thyroid peroxidase antibodies mean?**

It suggests that the cause of the thyroid disease is caused by an autoimmune disorder, such as Graves' disease.

**Name three common causes of primary hypothyroidism.**

Autoimmune thyroiditis, iodine deficiency or excess, thyroidectomy, radioactive iodine therapy, external radiotherapy and medications.

**What do you expect to see in the TFT results of someone with subclinical hypothyroidism?**

A normal $T_4$ and a raised TSH level.

**What do you expect to see in the TFTs of a pregnant patient?**

During the first trimester, TSH is often lower than in the non-pregnant state. This is due to beta-human chorionic gonadotrophin (beta-HCG) having similar effects to TSH. During the second and third trimesters, the TSH level is closer to non-pregnant levels as the level of beta-HCG decreases.

### What blood test should you order if a patient on carbimazole has a suspected infection?

FBC should be obtained due to the risk of bone marrow suppression induced by carbimazole. If there is clinical or laboratory evidence of neutropenia, then carbimazole should be stopped immediately.

### For which condition are cells with 'orphan Annie eye' nuclei pathognomonic?

Papillary carcinoma, which is the most common type of thyroid cancer.

### Embryologically, how do the thyroid glands develop?

They originate at the base of the tongue and then migrate to the anterior neck.

### Anatomically, where are the parathyroid glands positioned relative to the thyroid glands?

There are four parathyroid glands that are located on the posterior surface of the thyroid gland.

## Station 5.6   Bone Profile

### Doctor Briefing

You are a junior doctor on a primary care placement and have been asked to see Mrs Stone, a 68-year-old woman, who has presented with fatigue, constipation and dyspepsia. She saw your colleague last week who took some bloods, and the results are now back. Please review the blood tests, explain the findings to Mrs Stone and formulate an appropriate management plan.

### Patient Briefing

You have seen your GP for tiredness and new constipation. They took some blood. You are very concerned there is something wrong with your bowels and are anxious to know the diagnosis.

### Results

| Component | Results | Reference ranges with units |
|---|---|---|
| Adjusted calcium | 2.95 ↑ | 2.2–2.6 mmol/L |
| ALP | 130 ↑ | 35–120 U/L |
| Phosphate | 0.6 ↓ | 0.8–1.4 mmol/L |
| Albumin | 40 | 35–50 |

### Mark Scheme for Examiner

#### Introduction

| | | | | | | | |
|---|---|---|---|---|---|---|---|
| Cleans hands, introduces self, confirms patient identity | | | | | | | |

#### Establishes Current Patient Knowledge

| Statement/Question | Justification | Answer | Thoughts | | | | |
|---|---|---|---|---|---|---|---|
| I understand you have been feeling tired and came to see a colleague recently | Start with a general open phrase to guide the patient and to clarify the consultation | 'Yes, but also I have been really struggling with constipation which is new for me' | The patient confirms her symptoms but also confirms her constipation | | | | |
| Yes, I note this from the notes that my colleague made. How long has constipation been a problem for you? | Important to acknowledge the patient's concerns and get a grasp of the timeline if possible | 'I'm not really sure, but I have never had it before. It can be 7–10 days before I can go to the toilet and I have tried many over-the-counter treatments' | Really useful for you to be able to determine the prescribed or over-the-counter medications to treat her symptoms. These may have unwanted side effects | | | | |
| What treatments have you tried? | Important to make sure you ask about any non-prescribed medication to ensure there are no side effects | 'I cannot remember the names but some gentle laxatives and I have been eating a lot of prunes and flaxseed' | The patient has clarified with you what she has been taking, and you can make an assessment as to whether these may be related to her presentation. In this case, unlikely | | | | |

## Establishes Current Patient Knowledge

| Statement/Question | Justification | Answer | Thoughts | | | | |
|---|---|---|---|---|---|---|---|
| We performed blood tests following your last appointment. One of these measures the levels of some minerals in your blood | Explain what the blood test is for and why we are doing it | 'OK, what minerals?' | Establish a baseline of what the blood test is looking at. This also helps you to gauge the patient's understanding | | | | |
| Specifically, the calcium levels in your blood are high | Clarifying the test results to the patient | 'OK – what does this mean?' | The patient wants to know more. It is important that you can explain the findings in lay terms | | | | |
| Calcium is very important for bone health as well as the health of our nerves and muscles. However, too much can be harmful | Important to explain the role of the mineral and that high levels can be dangerous | 'Are the high calcium levels causing my constipation?' | The patient is very concerned about this symptom, so it is important to acknowledge it and explain the implication of the blood test on this symptom | | | | |
| Constipation is a common symptom when someone has high calcium levels | It is vital to discuss things in lay terms and explain that the findings and symptoms are related | 'How can we lower the calcium levels?' | Patients often want to know the treatment straight away. You may or may not be able to give this straight away. Be honest when providing the patient with the next steps | | | | |
| The treatment to lower the calcium levels depends on the cause, and we need to do a little bit more investigating before we can tell you that | This is letting the patient know that treatment is available but it needs to be tailored to her specific case | 'OK. What happens next?' | The patient is happy with your explanation so far | | | | |
| There are two things. Firstly, I would like to discuss with you some medication to help with your constipation whilst we are investigating the cause of your high calcium levels | You are putting the patient first and offering treatment for a symptom she is finding distressing | 'Thank you, I would really appreciate this' | The patient is grateful. Remember that this is a data interpretation station, so more details about the prescription do not need to be given here | | | | |
| Secondly, these changes in blood minerals are often caused by a change in hormone released from a gland in your neck called the parathyroid gland | You are explaining that you suspect a hormonal cause, where that hormone is and given the patient the name | 'OK, how do we check this?' | The patient understandably wants to know more | | | | |

## Data Interpretation and Discussion

| Statement/Question | Justification | Answer | Thoughts | | | | |
|---|---|---|---|---|---|---|---|
| We would send another blood test to check the level of hormone. If this is high then we would organise a scan on your neck, where the parathyroid gland sits, to look at it more closely | You are explaining that the next blood test may not have all the answers but making the patient aware of the most likely course of action | 'Thank you. If there is a problem with this thing in my neck, will I need an operation?' | The patient is giving you her concerns. Remember this is a data interpretation station and not a communication one, so spending a long time on this won't be expected – however, acknowledging the concerns is vital and will be marked positively | | | | |
| I really cannot tell you for definite as we need to do several checks but often, if there is a problem with the parathyroid gland, patients need an operation to remove it | You have acknowledged the patient's concerns, you have explained you cannot answer her question now, but you have also explained the likely course of action | 'Thank you doctor, that makes sense' | The patient is happy with your explanation | | | | |

## Finishing the Consultation

| | | | | | | | |
|---|---|---|---|---|---|---|---|
| Would you mind please repeating what I have just told you? | Checking that the patient was listening and understands the information | 'I have high levels of calcium in my blood. This is making me constipated. You will give me something to help with this. Also, you need to do more blood tests to see if it is something to do with a gland in my neck' | You have a patient who has listened and correctly interpreted what you have told her | | | | |
| I understand there is a lot to take in. Do you have any immediate questions for me? | May identify useful information that has been missed | 'No, I understand' | This patient is happy with the plan | | | | |
| I will organise the blood test for you now and will be in contact as soon as the results come back to us | Recapping the plan to yourself, the examiner and the patient is always important | 'Thank you' | The patient is satisfied with your management | | | | |

## Present Your Findings

This is Mrs Stone, a 68-year-old woman, who has presented with fatigue, constipation and dyspepsia. She saw a colleague last week who took some bloods, and the results are now back.

A bone profile was taken and demonstrates hypercalcaemia, with an adjusted calcium of 2.95 mmol/L, raised ALP at 130 U/L and a slightly low phosphate at 0.6 mmol/L.

I have explained the findings to Mrs Stone, and she is aware I would like to check her parathyroid levels. She is happy with this plan, and we will call her as soon as the results are back

| General Points | | | |
|---|---|---|---|
| Polite to patient | | | |
| Maintains good eye contact | | | |
| Appropriate use of open and closed questions | | | |

## ❓ QUESTIONS FROM THE EXAMINER

### How is the release of parathyroid hormones controlled?

By the negative feedback of calcium levels in the blood to the parathyroid glands.

### Why are the parathyroid hormone and serum calcium checked in all patients post-thyroid surgery?

The parathyroid glands are at high risk of being injured or removed unintentionally during thyroid surgery, due to its location. Therefore, it is standard to check parathyroid hormone and serum calcium levels to aid the early detection of such complications.

### To which protein is calcium most commonly bound?

Most calcium is found to be bound to albumin.

### What are the roles of osteoblasts and osteoclasts?

Osteoclasts are cells that are responsible for bone resorption by degrading bone to initiate normal bone remodelling. Osteoblasts are cells that are responsible for new bone formation.

### What is Trousseau's sign and what does it indicate?

It refers to the involuntary contraction of the muscles in the hand and wrist secondary to the inflation of a blood pressure cuff. It is suggestive of hypocalcaemia.

### How is phosphate typically excreted?

The kidneys excrete most (90%) of the daily phosphate load while the gastrointestinal tract excretes the rest.

### What condition may children be at risk of if they are deficient in vitamin D?

If children do not have an adequate supply of vitamin D, they can develop bone deformities, such as rickets.

### What sources have a high amount of vitamin D?

Oily fish, red meat, liver, egg yolks, fortified foods, sunlight.

### Name five possible signs and symptoms of hypercalcaemia.

Arthritis, osteomalacia, osteoporosis, renal calculi, uraemia, constipation, nausea and vomiting, peptic ulcer disease, pancreatitis, lethargy, confusion, coma.

### What is the mechanism of action of bisphosphonates?

Bisphosphonates reduce the rate of bone turnover by adsorbing on to hydroxyapatite crystals in bone, which slows the rate of bone growth and dissolution.

## Station 5.7 Arterial Blood Gas

### Doctor Briefing

You are a junior doctor in the ED and have been asked to see Mrs Freesia, a 72-year-old woman who presented with shortness of breath and swollen legs. On examination, you note that she is tachypnoeic and has a raised jugular venous pressure (JVP) and fine bibasal crepitations on chest auscultation. She had a myocardial infarction (MI) 5 years ago. You have obtained an ABG. Please review the result, explain the findings to Mrs Freesia and formulate an appropriate management plan.

### Patient Briefing

You have been brought to the ED by your family and they are concerned that you are getting more and more breathless with swollen legs. You have had lots of blood tests taken and are waiting to speak to the doctor to find out what is wrong.

You are concerned that you are having another heart attack.

### Results On Air

| Component | Results | Reference ranges with units |
|---|---|---|
| pH | 7.36 | 7.35–7.45 |
| Arterial oxygen partial pressure ($PaO_2$) | 8.0 | 10–14 kPa |
| Arterial carbon dioxide partial pressure ($PaCO_2$) | 4.7 | 4.6–6.0 kPa |
| Oxygen saturation ($SaO_2$) | 88% | > 94% |
| Bicarbonate ($HCO^{3-}$) | 25 | 24–28 mmol/L |
| Base excess (BE) | 1.0 | –2.0–+2.0 |

### Mark Scheme for Examiner

#### Introduction

| | | | | | | | | |
|---|---|---|---|---|---|---|---|---|
| Cleans hands, introduces self and confirms patient identity | | | | | | | | |

#### Establishes Current Patient Knowledge

| Statement/Question | Justification | Answer | Thoughts | | | | | |
|---|---|---|---|---|---|---|---|---|
| I understand you have been very breathless with swollen legs | Start with a general open phrase to guide the patient | 'Yes, I have been feeling steadily worse for the past week' | You know the patient is listening and there have been no changes to her symptoms | | | | | |
| How are you feeling now? | Important to ensure that the patient hasn't become more unwell since presentation | 'I feel just the same' | Before you start explaining something to a patient, it is important to determine her knowledge, as it will help you pitch your discussion | | | | | |

#### Data Interpretation and Discussion

| | | | | | | | | |
|---|---|---|---|---|---|---|---|---|
| I have done a blood test to look at your oxygen and carbon dioxide levels | Explain what the blood test is for and why we are doing it | 'OK' | Establish a baseline of what we are looking at with the ABG | | | | | |

## Data Interpretation and Discussion

| Statement/Question | Justification | Answer | Thoughts | | | | | |
|---|---|---|---|---|---|---|---|---|
| Some medical problems can make our oxygen levels too low and make us feel very breathless. Your oxygen levels are lower than we would normally expect | Important to explain that something abnormal has been found and is causing the symptoms | 'What is causing it?' | When explaining things to patients, try not to overload them. It is useful to give small chunks of information and then allow them to ask questions | | | | | |
| This is due to fluid in the lungs. It looks like your heart is not pumping well and the fluid has backed up to your lungs and legs and is leaking out – this is called oedema | It is vital to discuss things in lay terms but also to let the patient know the medical terminology | 'Can you treat it?' | Address the patient's concerns by answering any questions that she has | | | | | |
| We will treat you with medication that will get rid of this fluid, first through a drip and then in tablet form (water tablets or diuretics). You also need supplemental oxygen. You will need further blood tests, a heart tracing and a scan of your heart | It is vital to explain the steps of treatment and management | 'OK. Do I need to stay in hospital?' | The patient understandably wants to know more | | | | | |
| You need to stay in until you improve and no longer need the oxygen. It is likely that you will need to be on water tablets long-term when you leave hospital | Need to explain to the patient that this is something that can be managed but is a long-term problem | 'Why is my heart not pumping well?' | The patient is asking appropriate questions | | | | | |
| It would be useful to know more about your past medical history to try to work out why your heart is not pumping well | You are explaining to the patient that you may not have all of the answers immediately | 'Fine' | No additional concerns | | | | | |

## Finishing the Consultation

| | | | | | | | | |
|---|---|---|---|---|---|---|---|---|
| Would you mind please repeating what I have just told you? | Checking that the patient was listening and understands the information | 'My heart isn't pumping well so there is fluid on my legs and lungs. You are going to treat it and look for a cause' | You have a patient who has listened and correctly interpreted what you have told her | | | | | |
| I understand there is a lot to take in. Do you have any immediate questions for me? | May identify useful information that has been missed | 'No, I understand' | This patient is happy with the plan | | | | | |

### Finishing the Consultation

| Statement/Question | Justification | Answer | Thoughts | | | | |
|---|---|---|---|---|---|---|---|
| I will start you on the med-ications now, and request a scan of your heart to see how well it is pumping | Recapping the plan to yourself, the examiner and the patient is always important | 'Perfect. Thank you' | The patient is satisfied with your management | | | | |

### Present Your Findings

Mrs Freesia is a 72-year-old woman who presented with shortness of breath and leg swelling. ABG showed a type 1 respiratory failure with $PaO_2$ of 8.0 kPa.

I feel that Mrs Freesia understands the diagnosis of pulmonary oedema and will start her on intravenous (IV) diuretics, which she will continue in tablet form post-discharge.

After reviewing her other blood results and chest X-ray (CXR) I will request an echocardiogram and ECG

### General Points

Polite to patient

Maintains good eye contact

Appropriate use of open and closed questions

## ❓ QUESTIONS FROM THE EXAMINER

### What would you expect to see on an ABG in type 2 respiratory failure?

Low $PaO_2$ (< 8.0 kPa) and high $PaCO_2$ (> 6.9 kPa), possibly increased $HCO_3^-$ as metabolic compensation.

### Name three causes of a type 2 respiratory failure.

Hypoventilation, life-threatening asthma exacerbation, chronic obstructive pulmonary disease (COPD), pneumonia, pulmonary oedema, obesity, myasthenia gravis, Guillain–Barré syndrome, pulmonary embolism.

### Name two cardiac causes of pulmonary oedema.

Acute coronary syndrome, valvular heart disease (aortic stenosis, aortic regurgitation and mitral regurgitation, acute arrhythmia, hypertensive crisis, cardiomyopathy and cardiac tamponade.

### What are some CXR signs of pulmonary oedema?

Kerley B lines, increased cardiothoracic ratio (cardiomegaly), upper-lobe venous diversion, airspace opacification in batwing dis-tribution and pleural effusion.

### Name three causes of a metabolic alkalosis.

Vomiting, burns, diarrhoea, hypokalaemia, Conn's syndrome.

### How do you assess a JVP?

Position the patient at 45° and turn head slightly to the left. Look for the JVP above the clavicle between the sternal and clavicular heads of the sternocleidomastoid muscle. Measure the vertical distance between the top of the pulsation point and the sternal angle.

### Is COPD a restrictive or obstructive lung disease? What would the forced expiratory volume in 1 s ($FEV_1$)/forced vital capacity (FVC) ratio show?

Obstructive, reduced $FEV_1$/FVC ratio compared to predicted.

### What is paroxysmal nocturnal dyspnoea?

Sudden episode of shortness of breath at night.

### Do you know any classification systems for heart failure symptoms and level of function?

New York Heart Association (NYHA) is most commonly used.

### Name two causes of metabolic acidosis with a normal anion gap.

Diarrhoea, Addison's disease, renal tubular acidosis and pancreatic fistula.

## Station 5.8    Electrocardiogram

### Doctor Briefing

You are a junior doctor on an emergency medicine placement and have been asked to see Mr Fredrickson, a 65-year-old man who has presented with central crushing chest pain and diaphoresis. He has type 2 diabetes, and his mother had stents inserted due to 'heart trouble'. Glyceryl trinitrate (GTN) spray has not helped the patient. An electrocardiogram (ECG) performed by the ambulance crew which arrived with Mr Fredrickson showed ST depression in leads $V_2$–$V_6$. They performed a second ECG on route to the hospital, which is shown below. Please review the ECG, explain the findings to Mr Fredrickson and formulate an appropriate management plan.

### Patient Briefing

You are petrified. You suddenly developed chest pain in the middle of your chest that did not go away. Your wife called an ambulance. You remember the ambulance crew giving you some medicine in your mouth but that did not seem to help. You think you are going to die.

### Results (Fig. 5.1)

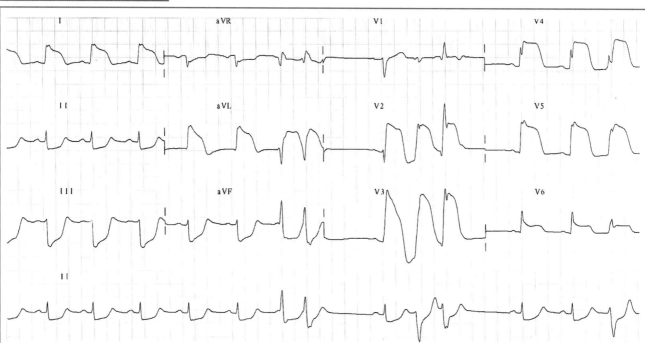

**Fig. 5.1** ECG for Mr Fredrickson. $FEV_1$, forced expiratory volume in 1 s; $FEF_{25-75}$, forced expiratory flow from 25 to 75% of vital capacity; FVC, forced vital capacity.

### Mark Scheme for Examiner

#### Introduction

| | | | | |
|---|---|---|---|---|
| Cleans hands, introduces self and confirms patient identity | | | | |

#### Establishes Current Patient Knowledge

| Statement/Question | Justification | Answer | Thoughts | |
|---|---|---|---|---|
| I understand you have been brought in to us by ambulance with chest pain | Start with a general open phrase to guide the patient and clarify the consultation | 'Yes – am I going to die?' | The patient confirms the presentation and voices his immediate concern | |

**Establishes Current Patient Knowledge**

| Statement/Question | Justification | Answer | Thoughts | | | | |
|---|---|---|---|---|---|---|---|
| I'm sorry to hear this. There is a lot we can do to help treat the pain and make you feel better | Important to let the patient know that there are treatments for this. You can never say a patient is not going to die; there are different ways to approach this, but acknowledging treatment plans is a subtle way of suggesting it is unlikely they will die | 'That medicine they gave me in the ambulance did nothing' | The patient may think that the GTN he has already had was the treatment. It is important to let him know that this is not the only treatment | | | | |
| That is only one of the medications we can give you. I have prescribed some strong painkillers and antisickness medication for you that will help with the pain | Reassure the patient that there are medications you can give now to help. This is a data interpretation question, so you do not need to get into detail here | 'Thank you, doctor, I would appreciate that' | The patient appears happy with this initial plan | | | | |

**Data Interpretation and Discussion**

| Statement/Question | Justification | Answer | Thoughts | | | | |
|---|---|---|---|---|---|---|---|
| As you may remember, the ambulance crew performed an ECG. Do you know what this is? | You are explaining the test to the patient and checking his understanding before moving forwards with the consultation | 'Is that the thing with all the leads? It has something to do with my heart...' | The patient understands that the ECG was an assessment of the heart but not really any specifics | | | | |
| That is correct. An ECG assesses the electrical impulses in the heart; these impulses cause the heart to beat | Confirm to the patient that his understanding is correct and give a little more information | 'OK' | The patient has not asked anything at this point, so you can carry on with your explanation. Some patients may start asking all sorts of questions at this point | | | | |
| ECGs can show us if there are any problems with the electrical impulses. Your ECG shows changes associated with a heart attack | Important to tell the patient the diagnosis if you know one, but also to give some time to process the information | 'I thought it was a heart attack. What happens now?' | Nearly always the patient will ask what the treatment or next steps will be. Be prepared for this | | | | |
| A heart attack happens when one or more arteries in your heart is blocked. When this happens blood with oxygen and nutrients cannot reach that part of the heart, causing damage and chest pain | It is really important to explain how the diagnosis fits with the patient's symptoms of the patient so he can understand the disease process | 'Can you treat it?' | The patient is keen to know the next steps | | | | |

## Establishes Current Patient Knowledge

| Statement/Question | Justification | Answer | Thoughts | | | | |
|---|---|---|---|---|---|---|---|
| Yes. You will be seen by the heart doctors, called cardiologists, who will perform a procedure to unblock any blocked arteries with something called a stent | This is explaining the management plan using lay terminology but also using a few of the terms they may hear, such as cardiologist and stent | 'My mum had to have this. Will it happen today?' | The patient does not seem to want to know any more now and has acknowledged that he may have some understanding of the procedure. He is are now focused on the timeframe | | | | |
| I would expect you to have this done today, likely in the next few hours | This has given the patient an approximate time frame, but you are not the specialist so cannot give them any certainties | 'OK. Thank you' | The patient has accepted this course of action | | | | |

## Finishing the Consultation

| | | | | | | | |
|---|---|---|---|---|---|---|---|
| Would you mind please repeating what I have just told you? | Checking that the patient was listening and understands the information | 'I have had a heart attack and need to have stents put in. You think this will be done today' | You have a patient who has listened and correctly interpreted what you have told him | | | | |
| I understand there is a lot to take in. Do you have any immediate questions for me? | May identify useful information that has been missed | 'Yes – how long is the recovery?' | This is a commonly asked question when discussing procedures. You aren't expected to know all the answers but should be able to guide the patient | | | | |
| I cannot tell you precisely as I am not the specialist, but I know that people usually make a quick and healthy recovery. Write these questions down and make sure you ask the heart team when you see them | Here you are not dismissing the patient but reassuring him and advising him to make a note of questions he may have | 'Thank you' | The patient is satisfied with the consultation | | | | |

## Present Your Findings

Mr Fredrickson, a 65-year-old man, has presented with central crushing chest pain and diaphoresis.

An ECG has been performed demonstrating an anterior ST elevation MI (STEMI).

I have explained the findings to Mr Fredrickson, and he is aware he has been referred to cardiology for stenting. We have made him comfortable with analgesia and antiemetics

| General Points | | | | |
|---|---|---|---|---|
| Polite to patient | | | | |
| Maintains good eye contact | | | | |
| Appropriate use of open and closed questions | | | | |

## ❓ QUESTIONS FROM THE EXAMINER

### What is meant by reciprocal changes?

Typically, this term is used to describe ST changes. For example, you see ST elevation in one territory and ST depression in another territory.

### How many millimetres does one large square represent?

One large square represents 5 mm on the ECG paper, which is equivalent to 0.2 s or 200 ms.

### How do you determine cardiac axis and what is normal?

There are different ways to do this. One way is to look at the QRS complexes in lead I and aVF. If both are positive, then the axis is normal. Normal QRS axis measures between −30° and +90°. If they are both negative, then there is extreme axis. A positive QRS complex in lead I but negative in aVF suggests possible left-axis deviation, and the opposite in both would suggest a right-axis deviation.

### Which leads look at the lateral aspects of the heart?

Leads I, aVL, V5 and V6.

### What are considered adverse features in the resuscitation arrhythmia algorithms?

Shock, syncope, myocardial ischaemia and heart failure.

### What management steps can be performed for a patient with regular narrow QRS tachycardia?

Vagal manoeuvres and administer adenosine intravenously (6 mg initially, then 12 mg if no effect, and another 12 mg if no further effect).

### What does the left coronary artery divide into?

The left anterior descending artery and the left circumflex arteries.

### Typically, how does the ECG of a patient whose heart is paced by a pacemaker look like?

Features of the paced ECG are pacing spikes, which appear as vertical spikes of short duration. Depending on the pacing mode and other factors, the pacing spikes can precede the P wave, the QRS complex or both.

### Name three causes of sinus bradycardia.

Myocarditis, hypothyroidism, extreme fitness, MI and medications.

### What arrhythmia is usually described as having a 'saw-toothed' appearance on the ECG?

Atrial flutter.

## Station 5.9    Cerebrospinal Fluid

### Doctor Briefing

You are a junior doctor on an emergency medicine placement and have been asked to see Mr Smith, a 19-year-old man who has presented with fever, headache, muscle aches, photophobia and general malaise. After a computed tomography (CT) brain was carried out, you performed a lumbar puncture. On inspection, the CSF was clear. The results of the CSF are now back, as is the plasma glucose you sent. Please review them, explain the findings to Mrs Ranson and formulate an appropriate management plan.

### Patient Briefing

You have been sent to the ED by your GP who is worried you have a serious infection. You have no idea where you have got the infection and feel scared. You are normally fit and well. When the doctor tells you that you have meningitis, ask them where you caught the bacteria from.

### Results

| Components | Results | Reference ranges with units |
|---|---|---|
| Predominant cell type | Lymphocytes | Lymphocytes |
| WCC | 95 | 50–1000/µL |
| Protein | 0.5 | 0.2–0.4 g/L |
| Glucose | 4 | Half to two-thirds of plasma glucose |

Plasma glucose: 6.0 mmol.

### Mark Scheme for Examiner

#### Introduction

| | | | | | | | | |
|---|---|---|---|---|---|---|---|---|
| Cleans hands, introduces self and confirms patient identity | | | | | | | | |

#### Establishes Current Patient Knowledge

| Statement/Question | Justification | Answer | Thoughts | | | | |
|---|---|---|---|---|---|---|---|
| I understand you have been feeling unwell with a fever and muscle aches | Start with a general open phrase to guide the patient and to clarify the consultation | 'Yes, I have suddenly become really unwell. My GP thinks I have an infection but I have no idea where I caught anything' | The patient confirms his symptoms with you | | | | |
| Have you noticed any other symptoms – headaches, vomiting, blurred vision or an aversion to light? | Important to ensure that the patient hasn't got any more concerning features such as raised intracranial pressure. Remember, this is an interpretation station, not a history station, so a full history is not expected but checking for red flags is pertinent | 'Yes. I told the GP I really do not like being in bright rooms at the moment and have an awful head-ache. I haven't been sick or noticed any change in my vision' | Really useful for you to be able to determine a change in the patient's presentation; he could have developed raised intracranial pressure | | | | |

## Data Interpretation and Discussion

| Statement/Question | Justification | Answer | Thoughts | | | | |
|---|---|---|---|---|---|---|---|
| You understand that we did a special test called a lumbar puncture on the fluid that sits around the brain | If you were not the person taking the test, it is important to ensure that the patient understands what it was and what you were looking for | 'Yes' | The patient understands the test that was performed | | | | |
| The fluid is called cerebrospinal fluid or CSF and we can test it for infection | Clarifying the reason for performing the test to the patient | 'OK' | The patient has not asked anything at this point, so you can carry on with your explanation. Some patients may start asking all sorts of questions at this point | | | | |
| We have the results back and they have confirmed what we suspected. You have an infection in the fluid around the brain. This is called meningitis | Important to explain the test results clearly and to use the lay and medical terms for any diagnosis | 'Meningitis! People die from that, don't they?' | This patient is understandably shocked and upset by this news. Communication is key here | | | | |
| Yes, people can become poorly with meningitis. However, the good thing in your case is that you came to hospital early, we have diagnosed it quickly and we have started antibiotics | It is vital to be truthful to patients but to also put their condition into context | 'Where did I get the bacteria from?' | This question is testing you. This patient has viral meningitis, not bacterial | | | | |
| That is a good question. We actually think your infection has come from a virus and not a bacteria | Important not to belittle the patient and just state 'it isn't a bacteria' but to validate the question and explain the findings | 'OK. Do I know where I got the virus?' | The patient is keen to find out he they contracted the virus causing them meningitis | | | | |
| Now we are unsure of the exact virus, but we will take a detailed history from you which will help us determine the cause | Need to explain that we do not know now but that also this is a data interpretation/communication station, not a history-taking one | 'OK, that makes sense' | The patient has accepted this information | | | | |
| Importantly, meningitis caused by a virus is usually much less severe than meningitis caused by bacteria | You are reassuring the patient regarding the diagnosis and prognosis | 'Thank you, and the antibiotics will help?' | The patient understandably wants to understand the management plan | | | | |

**Data Interpretation and Discussion**

| Statement/Question | Justification | Answer | Thoughts | | | | |
|---|---|---|---|---|---|---|---|
| Now we know it is a viral cause we can actually stop the antibiotics. Antibiotics are only useful against bacteria. We start them on everyone as someone with a bacterial meningitis can become very poorly very quickly | You are explaining the reasoning behind starting and stopping antibiotics so rapidly to the patient, which can be a hard concept to understand | 'OK. What is the treatment for me now?' | The patient is keen to know the management plan | | | | |
| We will give you fluid into your vein, pain relief and antisickness medication. We will keep you in hospital and maintain a close eye on you | You have acknowledged the patient's question and answered it appropriately | 'Thank you, doctor, that makes sense' | The patient is happy with your explanation | | | | |

**Finishing the Consultation**

| | | | | | | | |
|---|---|---|---|---|---|---|---|
| Would you mind please repeating what I have just told you? | Checking that the patient was listening and understands the information | 'I have meningitis, but not the bad type. I need to stay in hospital and have medication – but not antibiotics' | You have a patient who has listened and correctly interpreted what you have told him | | | | |
| I understand there is a lot to take in. Do you have any immediate questions for me? | May identify useful information that has been missed | 'No, I understand' | This patient is happy with the plan | | | | |

**Present Your Findings**

This is Mr Smith, a 19-year-old man who has presented with fever, headache, muscle aches, photophobia and general malaise.

A lumbar puncture was performed and demonstrates viral meningitis with prominent lymphocytes, slightly raised protein and elevated glucose levels.

I have explained the findings to Mr Smith, and he is aware we will stop antibiotic treatment and be managed supportively at the moment

**General Points**

Polite to patient

Maintains good eye contact

Appropriate use of open and closed questions

# ❓ QUESTIONS FROM THE EXAMINER

## What produces CSF?

The choroid plexus in the lateral, third and fourth ventricles.

## What is considered as normal opening pressure?

10–20 cm of CSF.

## Name three potential complications from a lumbar puncture.

Post-lumbar puncture headache, pain or tenderness at the puncture site, bleeding, infection, nerve damage, blood clots.

## In chronological order, what are the main structures that are pierced through/into by the lumbar puncture needle?

Skin, subcutaneous tissue, supraspinous ligament, intraspinous ligament, ligamentum flavum and lastly the epidural space (where CSF is located).

## What condition is suggested if oligoclonal bands are seen on electrophoresis?

Guillain–Barré syndrome.

## If you suspect bacterial meningitis, what other investigations might you consider in addition to CSF analysis?

CSF Gram stain and culture, CSF polymerase chain reaction (PCR), CSF bacterial antigens, blood cultures and FBC.

## Define xanthochromia.

Xanthochromia translates to yellow colour and refers to the yellow appearance of CSF that is usually seen in subarachnoid haemorrhage.

## Name three causes of viral meningitis.

Herpes simplex virus, enteroviruses, varicella-zoster virus, mumps, human immunodeficiency virus (HIV) and adenovirus.

## What is the first-line investigation in suspected subarachnoid haemorrhage?

CT head is usually the first-line investigation for suspected subarachnoid haemorrhage. However, its sensitivity reduces after the first 12 h. Therefore, lumbar puncture is used to rule it out.

## Name some clinical features of meningitis.

Headache, fever, confusion, nausea and vomiting, neck stiffness and photophobia.

## Station 5.10    Pleural Fluid

### Doctor Briefing

You are a junior doctor on the respiratory ward and have been asked to see Mr Green, a 76-year-old man who has worsening dyspnoea and tachypnoea. On examination you note reduced left-sided expansion in addition to a stony dull percussion note and reduced breath sounds on the left side. You sent some blood tests and a sample of pleural fluid for analysis. Please review the results, explain the findings to Mr Green and formulate an appropriate management plan.

### Patient Briefing

You have been in hospital for a few days and think that your breathing is getting worse. You have had pneumonia before, about 5 years ago, and were in hospital for a week or so. You are usually active and fit for your age. Before admission you were feeling generally unwell with a fever and cough.

### Results

| Component | Results | Reference Range with units |
|---|---|---|
| Pleural fluid protein | 35 | 10–20 g/L |
| Serum protein | 60 | 60–80 g/L |
| Pleural fluid lactate dehydrogenase (LDH) | 98 | <50% of plasma LDH (u/L) |
| Serum LDH | 150 | 100–250 u/L |
| Cell count and differential count | 900/mm$^3$ | <1000 white cells/mm$^3$ |
| Gram stain | Nil | Nil |
| Cytology | Nil | – |
| Glucose | 2.2 | 4–6 mmol/L |
| pH | 7.2 | 7.60–7.66 |

### Mark Scheme for Examiner

#### Introduction

| Cleans hands, introduces self and confirms patient identity | | | | | | | |
|---|---|---|---|---|---|---|---|

#### Establishes Current Patient Knowledge

| Statement/Question | Justification | Answer | Thoughts | | | | |
|---|---|---|---|---|---|---|---|
| How have you been feeling since being in hospital, Mr. Green? | Start with a general open phrase to guide the patient and clarify the consultation | 'Everyone is being so kind looking after me, but I must say I think my breathing is getting worse' | The patient describes a possible deterioration in his condition | | | | |
| I'm sorry to hear this | It is important to acknowledge the patient's condition and not to dismiss such a comment | 'Thank you' | There is nothing to add here; you can carry on with the consultation | | | | |

## Data Interpretation and Discussion

| Statement/Question | Justification | Answer | Thoughts |
|---|---|---|---|
| You understand we took a sample of the fluid around your lungs to help assess exactly what is causing you to feel unwell | Explain what the blood test is for and why we are doing it | 'Yes' | Establish a baseline of why the investigation was being performed |
| There are many tests we can perform on the fluid; all of these can help us understand what is going on | Clarifying that it is not one single thing that the investigation is looking at | 'OK – the other doctor said something about checking it is infection and not cancer' | The patient has recalled a previous consultation – it is important you address these points |
| Yes, you are correct. The tests can help us determine if the excess fluid is caused by an infection or cancer or something else | Important to confirm the patient's knowledge if correct | 'So, do you know what is causing it?' | The patient is essentially asking you whether he has cancer, but indirectly. It is important to share what you know with him |
| All the tests on the fluid around your lungs suggests this is a bad infection and not caused by cancer | It is vital to discuss things in lay terms but to give an indication of whether this is a mild or severe infection | 'I'm so glad it isn't cancer. That was worrying me' | Allow the patient to share his concerns with you |
| I can imagine. It can be a stressful time, waiting for test results to come back. Now we know it is an infection we can make sure that we tailor the treatment correctly | This is explaining that the findings of the test may mean modification of the treatment plan | 'OK. That makes sense. What will you do now?' | The patient is keen to learn the treatment plan |
| As I said to you before, this appears to be a severe infection, which is why your breathing is becoming more difficult | Always relate things back to the presentation of the patient if you can. Recapping on the diagnosis is also useful | 'Hmm…' | The patient has nothing to ask at this moment so you can carry on |
| We need to continue the antibiotics you are on, the ones that we are giving through the vein | You are explaining that you plan to continue the treatment that has already been started | 'OK' | Again, the patient has no questions at this point. You can carry on |
| With severe infections such as yours, antibiotics alone are unlikely to remove the infection that you have. We also need to insert a little tube into the area of infection and fluid to drain it away | You are explaining that simple medication won't treat all the symptoms. You have introduced the concept of a chest drain | 'OK – that makes sense. If there is stuff there, you need to get rid of it' | The patient seems happy with the management plan and has no immediate questions. Remember this is a data interpretation station and not a practical skills station, so you do not need to go into detail about chest drains here |

### Data Interpretation and Discussion

| Statement/Question | Justification | Answer | Thoughts | | | | |
|---|---|---|---|---|---|---|---|
| We will also keep you on oxygen and nebulisers for as long as you need. The physiotherapy team will continue to see you to help with your breathing | You have spent a little time confirming the management plan with the patient | 'Thank you, doctor, I appreciate everything you are all doing for me' | The patient is happy with your consultation so far | | | | |

### Finishing the Consultation

| Statement/Question | Justification | Answer | Thoughts | | | | |
|---|---|---|---|---|---|---|---|
| Would you mind please repeating what I have just told you? | Checking that the patient was listening and understands the information | 'I have a really bad infection around my lungs. You need to put a tube in to remove it and keep me on the drip' | You have a patient who has listened and correctly interpreted what you have told him | | | | |
| I understand there is a lot to take in. Do you have any immediate questions for me? | May identify useful information that has been missed | 'No, I understand' | This patient is happy with the plan | | | | |
| I will organise someone to come and speak to you about the chest drain in more detail later on. In the meantime, please keep rested | Recapping the plan to yourself, the examiner and the patient is always important | 'Thank you' | The patient is satisfied with your management | | | | |

### Present Your Findings

This is Mr Green, a 76-year-old man who has worsening dyspnoea and tachypnoea.

A sample of pleural fluid was taken for analysis which demonstrated a complex parapneumonic effusion.

I have explained the findings to Mr Green, and he is aware he will be continued on IV antibiotics and likely have a chest drain sited

### General Points

| | | | |
|---|---|---|---|
| Polite to patient | | | |
| Maintains good eye contact | | | |
| Appropriate use of open and closed questions | | | |

## ❓ QUESTIONS FROM THE EXAMINER

### What is the minimum amount of pleural fluid that has accumulated for CXR and clinical signs to be present?

Usually there is at least 300 mL of pleural fluid before CXRs can detect a pleural effusion, and to detect clinical signs such as dullness to percussion and diminished breath sounds.

## If there is a large effusion, to which direction may the trachea deviate?

In large pleural effusions, there may be tracheal deviation away from the effusion.

## What criteria can be used to distinguish between transudate and exudates?

Light's criteria, which outlines that the effusion is an exudate if pleural fluid protein is serum protein ratio greater than 0.5, or if pleural fluid LDH to serum LDH ratio is greater than 0.6 or if pleural fluid LDH is greater than two-thirds of the upper limit of normal serum LDH.

## Name two causes of blood-stained pleural fluid.

Pneumonia, trauma, malignancy, pulmonary embolism and haemothorax.

## What are the commonest causes of transudates?

Heart failure, liver failure, such as in cirrhosis, and nephrotic syndrome.

## Describe Meigs' syndrome.

Meigs' syndrome is the presence of ascites and pleural effusion in association with a benign ovarian tumour.

## How is pleural fluid produced and removed?

Pleural fluid is primarily produced by the parietal pleura and reabsorbed by the pleural lymphatics.

## Define 'chylothorax'.

Chylothorax is when chyle (lymph formed in the digestive system) accumulates in the pleural cavity.

## Which part of the pleura is the only part that can detect and sense painful stimuli?

The parietal pleura.

## What is the innervation to the visceral pleura?

The vagus nerve and sympathetic fibres.

## Station 5.11    Ascitic Fluid

### Doctor Briefing

You are a junior doctor on a hepatology placement and have been asked to see Mr Can, a 65-year-old man who has presented with abdominal swelling. One of your colleagues performed an ascitic tap and sent the fluid for analysis. The results are now back. He is known to have alcoholic liver disease. Please review the results, explain the findings to Mr Can and formulate an appropriate management plan.

### Patient Briefing

You are an alcoholic and have had multiple health problems for a long time. You have never been into hospital with tummy swelling before; your GP has always managed any aliments for you. You have heard of people who have got infections in their liver that can cause tummy swelling – you think your symptoms are probably due to an infection.

### Results

| Components | Results | Reference ranges with units |
|---|---|---|
| Ascitic fluid albumin | 3 | <4 g/dL |
| Serum albumin | 5 | 3.5–5.5 g/dL |
| Total protein | 3.5 | <4 g/dL |
| Glucose | 7 | 7–10 g/L |
| Amylase | 150 | 140–400 u/L |
| Bilirubin | 0.7 | 0.7–0.8 mg/dL |
| Triglycerides | 10 | <110 mL/dL |
| Differential WCC | 150 | <300 cells/mm³ |

### Mark Scheme for Examiner

#### Introduction

| Cleans hands, introduces self and confirms patient identity | | | | | | | |
|---|---|---|---|---|---|---|---|

#### Establishes Current Patient Knowledge

| Statement/Question | Justification | Answer | Thoughts | | | | |
|---|---|---|---|---|---|---|---|
| I understand that you came to us with new tummy swelling that is caused by an increase of fluid in your tummy | Start with a general open phrase to guide the patient and clarify the consultation. Use lay terminology where possible | 'Yes, I have never had this before. My tummy is massive' | The patient confirms that this is a new symptom and that he feels it is a significant change to his normal abdominal appearance | | | | |
| It must be uncomfortable for you. I also understand that my colleague took a sample of fluid to try and see what is causing this fluid to build up in your tummy | Important to acknowledge any pain, discomfort or distress the patient may be in. Also, take a moment to corroborate with the patient what he has had done | 'Yes. They said they would be able to work out what the problem is with this test. It wasn't the nicest thing to have done' | Really useful for you to be able to confirm the patient's understanding | | | | |

## Data Interpretation and Discussion

| Statement/Question | Justification | Answer | Thoughts | | | | | |
|---|---|---|---|---|---|---|---|---|
| As you are aware, we look at lots of different things in the fluid to see what the problem is | Explain that the ascitic fluid sample is not just providing one result but a host of results to determine the diagnosis | 'Yes. They said something about this. I think it is an infection' | The patient has likely surprised you by providing his suspected diagnosis. It is important not to dismiss this, even though you know it is not correct | | | | | |
| We don't think it is caused by an infection. What makes you think it is an infection? | It is important to explore the ideas of the patient, as it may provide further information | 'Well, I know a few people who have had these liver infections, fluid and such like … so just thought it was the same' | The patient has not given you any specific reasons to consider infection, such as pyrexia or rigors | | | | | |
| You are right, sometimes symptoms such as yours can be caused by infection, but not in your case | Important to recognise the patient's ideas but also acceptable to correct them if they are incorrect | 'Do you know what is causing it?' | A logical question for the patient to ask next | | | | | |
| Yes. The results show that the fluid in your tummy is caused by a lot of scar tissue in your liver. This is a result of damage to your liver caused by alcohol | It is vital to be explicit with the patient. The patient will know his alcohol intake will cause liver damage; it is important to state this and not be afraid to bring this up. The opening statement to the station specified the patient has chronic liver disease | 'Oh. I have really cut down over the last few days' | Be supportive towards the patient in this setting but know that this is data interpretation and not a communication station about reducing alcohol intake | | | | | |
| Well done, that is good. What this does show is that your liver is quite badly damaged and working really hard to function normally | You are confirming to the patient the severity of the condition | 'OK. How do you get rid of the fluid?' | The patient has not mentioned alcohol intake at the moment and is concerned about the management plan | | | | | |
| We will firstly give you a medication which will help remove the fluid by causing you to pass more urine. We will also reduce your salt intake as this helps | Ensure you give the management plan in small chunks | 'OK. I don't really eat much salt anyway' | The patient has nothing to ask at this point | | | | | |
| If these steps do not work well enough, we may have to put a drain, or small tube, into your tummy to remove the fluid that is there | You are explaining that the management plan you listed initially is the first step but that you may have to do more | 'That doesn't sound very nice' | The patient is making an appropriate response to what you have just said | | | | | |

## Data Interpretation and Discussion

| Statement/Question | Justification | Answer | Thoughts | | | | |
|---|---|---|---|---|---|---|---|
| It doesn't, no. Hopefully we won't have to do this, but it depends on how your body responds to the medication | You are acknowledging the patient's concerns and reiterating the management plan | 'OK. Thanks' | The patient has accepted your diagnosis and management | | | | |
| I think it is really important you seriously consider stopping drinking alcohol and I would like to talk to you about this when you feel better | You have restated your main concern to the patient and given a warning shot that a discussion about alcohol cessation needs to be had | 'OK' | The patient does not want to engage with this conversation at the moment | | | | |

## Finishing the Consultation

| Statement/Question | Justification | Answer | Thoughts | | | | |
|---|---|---|---|---|---|---|---|
| Would you mind please repeating what I have just told you? | Checking that the patient was listening and understands the information | 'The fluid in my tummy is not caused by infection but because my liver is not working properly. You are going to give me some medication to make it better but if that doesn't work you will shove a tube into my tummy' | You have a patient who has listened and correctly interpreted what you have told him | | | | |
| I understand there is a lot to take in. Do you have any immediate questions for me? | May identify useful information that has been missed | 'No' | This patient seems content with the plan and does not want to engage any further | | | | |
| I will come and see you later to check how you are getting on | At this point you can either recap information to the patient or close with an appropriate interaction, such as explaining that you will review him later | 'Thank you' | The patient is satisfied with your plan | | | | |

## Present Your Findings

This is Mr Can, a 65-year-old man who has presented with abdominal swelling. He is known to have alcoholic liver disease.

An ascitic tap was taken and the results demonstrate a high serum–ascites albumin gradient (SAAG) and no other abnormal biomarkers, in keeping with cirrhosis.

I have explained the findings to Mr Can, and he is aware that if initial treatment measures fail he will require an ascitic drain

## General Points

| | | | | |
|---|---|---|---|---|
| Polite to patient | | | | |
| Maintains good eye contact | | | | |
| Appropriate use of open and closed questions | | | | |

## ❓ QUESTIONS FROM THE EXAMINER

### Name three possible causes of ascitic fluid with a milky appearance.

Tuberculosis, parasitic infection, malignancy, cirrhosis and lymphatic obstruction.

### Normally, how much ascitic fluid is present before it is clinically detected?

At least 500 mL.

### What are the clinical features of ascites?

Shortness of breath, weight gain, abdominal distension and/or discomfort and loss of appetite.

### How is the SAAG calculated?

SAAG is serum albumin minus ascitic fluid albumin.

### Give three causes of ascites with a high SAAG.

Cirrhosis, congestive heart failure, nephrotic syndrome, hepatic metastases, chronic hepatitis, Budd–Chiari syndrome and portal vein thrombosis.

### What is Budd–Chiari syndrome?

It is a condition in which the hepatic veins are occluded or stenosed by a blood clot.

### If there is an increased level of ALP in the biochemistry of the ascitic fluid, what should you consider?

It would be important to rule out small-bowel perforation and strangulation.

### What is the most common bacteria causing spontaneous bacterial peritonitis?

*Escherichia coli*, *Klebsiella pneumoniae* and *Streptococcus pneumoniae* are the most common pathogens responsible for spontaneous bacterial peritonitis.

### If you suspect that your patient's ascites is related to the pancreas, what other laboratory investigations would you request?

Serum amylase level.

### How is the patient normally positioned during paracentesis?

Either the supine (with a slight tilt or rotation) or the lateral decubitus position. If the patient's head is slightly elevated at 45–60°, this will allow the fluid to accumulate in the lower abdomen.

## Station 5.12    Synovial Fluid

### Doctor Briefing

You are a junior doctor in the ED and have been asked to see Mr Brady, a 65-year-old man who has presented with a red, hot and swollen knee. One of your colleagues obtained a synovial fluid aspirate from the knee and sent it for analysis. The results are now back. He is overweight and takes medication for hypertension. Please review the results, explain the findings to Mr Brady and formulate an appropriate management plan.

### Patient Briefing

You are normally fit and well. You take tablets for high blood pressure, and doctor says you are overweight but you don't think that you really are. Overnight you noticed your knee becoming hot and sore. It is hard to bend your knee and walk. You are worried that you have a bad infection.

### Results

| Components | Results | Reference range with units |
| --- | --- | --- |
| Crystals | Monosodium urate | Nil |
| WCC | 2000 | <200/mm$^3$ |
| % Polymorphonuclear neutrophils | 56 | <25% |
| Colour | Yellow | Colourless |
| Clarity | Cloudy | Clear |
| Viscosity | Low | High |
| Gram stain | Negative | Negative |

### Mark Scheme for Examiner

#### Introduction

| Cleans hands, introduces self and confirms patient identity | | | | | | |
| --- | --- | --- | --- | --- | --- | --- |

#### Establishes Current Patient Knowledge

| Statement/Question | Justification | Answer | Thoughts | | | |
| --- | --- | --- | --- | --- | --- | --- |
| I understand you have come to us with a really sore and hot knee. Have you ever had anything like this before? | Start with a general open phrase to guide the patient and clarify the consultation | 'Yes, that's right. It suddenly came, it is getting worse and it is really uncomfortable to walk on. I have never had any-thing like this before' | The patient describes an acute presentation of a hot, swollen joint | | | |

## Establishes Current Patient Knowledge

| Statement/Question | Justification | Answer | Thoughts | | | | |
|---|---|---|---|---|---|---|---|
| Do you otherwise feel well? Have you noticed any fevers, shivers or any other sore joints? | Important to ensure that the patient hasn't got any more concerning features. Remember, this is an interpretation station, not a history station, so a full history is not expected but checking for red flags such as sepsis is pertinent | 'No, I feel fine otherwise. It is really strange' | Really useful for you to be able to determine if the patient is stable or not | | | | |

## Data Interpretation and Discussion

| Statement/Question | Justification | Answer | Thoughts | | | | |
|---|---|---|---|---|---|---|---|
| As you are aware, we took a small sample of fluid from around the knee to try and work out what is going on | Explain what the investigation is for and clarify what sample you took | 'Yes – I'm worried I have a bad infection' | The patient understands what investigation was performed and has shared his concerns with you | | | | |
| It is really worrying when something like this happens to our bodies. I can confirm that there is currently no sign of infection in the knee joint | Here you are acknowledging the concerns of the patient but also stating that the results show no infection | 'That is a relief – what is it then?' | The patient is reassured that he doesn't have an infection and now is ready for more information | | | | |
| What the results show is that you have something called gout – have you heard of this before? | Important to give a small amount of information here. Not everyone will know what gout is. It is vital to pause and check understanding | 'No – I have never heard of it. Is it serious?' | This patient doesn't know what gout is, so it is really good that you have paused here to check understanding. You can now explain the condition in lay terms | | | | |
| Gout is a type of arthritis, or inflammation of the joints, that can cause pain and swelling | It is vital to discuss things in lay terms but also to let the patient know the medical terminology too. Providing the common presentation helps the patient to relate the condition to himself | 'Oh – that's interesting. I never knew it existed. Is it because I'm getting older?' | Be prepared to have to explain yourself further when you offer information to patients | | | | |
| Partly, but gout is not only inflammation but also an increase of crystals in your joints. We think that lifestyle factors make having gout more likely | This is explaining the diagnosis in more detail and alluding to the management plan | 'That sounds strange. What lifestyle things?' | The patient is keen to know more about the condition | | | | |

## Data Interpretation and Discussion

| Statement/Question | Justification | Answer | Thoughts | | | | | |
|---|---|---|---|---|---|---|---|---|
| Well, firstly, we need to treat the condition now. We will give you anti-inflammatory medication, like ibuprofen, in the first instance, if that is safe for you to have | Need to explain the first-line management | 'OK. I'm fine with ibuprofen' | The patient has confirmed that anti-inflammatory medication should be all right for them to take | | | | | |
| I'll get the specialist team to come and talk to you about lifestyle factors but these include dietary changes, reducing alcohol intake and checking the medication you are taking | You are explaining that there are other measures that can reduce gout attacks as well as confirming that a more detailed conversation needs to be had | 'OK, thank you. Will I need an operation?' | The patient accepts what you have told him regarding lifestyle factors but wants to clarify the management plan | | | | | |
| No – this condition rarely needs an operation and can be managed with medication and lifestyle changes | You are answering his question and clarifying the management plan to the patient and examiner | 'That is good to hear. Thank you' | The patient seems happy | | | | | |

## Finishing the Consultation

| | | | | | | | | |
|---|---|---|---|---|---|---|---|---|
| Would you mind please repeating what I have just told you? | Checking that the patient was listening and understands the information | 'I have a funny arthritis in my knee – not an infection – I don't need an operation' | You have a patient who has listened and correctly interpreted what you have told him | | | | | |
| I understand there is a lot to take in. Do you have any immediate questions for me? | May identify useful information that has been missed | 'No, I understand' | This patient is happy with the plan | | | | | |
| We start you on some pain medication and ask the bone and joint doctors to come and speak to you | Recapping the plan to yourself, the examiner and the patient is always important | 'Thank you' | The patient is satisfied with your management | | | | | |

## Present Your Findings

Mr Brady, a 65-year-old man, has presented with a red, hot and swollen knee.

A synovial fluid aspirate was taken and indicates a flare of gout. There are monosodium crystals in the sample with a raised WCC and an increased polymorphonuclear neutrophil count of 56%. The sample was yellow and cloudy.

I have explained the findings to Mr Brady, and he is aware of the immediate and longer-term management plan

| General Points | | | | |
|---|---|---|---|---|
| Polite to patient | | | | |
| Maintains good eye contact | | | | |
| Appropriate use of open and closed questions | | | | |

## ❓ QUESTIONS FROM THE EXAMINER

### Name three inflammatory causes of joint effusion.

Rheumatoid arthritis, psoriatic arthritis, Reiter's syndrome, acute gout, acute pseudogout, systemic lupus erythematosus and viral arthritis.

### Define 'haemarthrosis' and state its most common cause.

Haemarthrosis is haemorrhage into a joint space and is most often caused by trauma. Other causes include bleeding disorders, anticoagulation, tumours and vascular damage.

### What is the most common pathogen responsible for septic arthritis and what is the first-line antibiotic?

Usually, septic arthritis is caused by *Staphylococcus*, which can be treated with flucloxacillin.

### What are the clinical features of osteoarthritis?

Osteoarthritis is more common in women than men. It is typically worse at the end of the day and on movement/weight bearing. There may also be stiffness and pain at rest.

### What is a bursa and what is its function?

A bursa is a closed, fluid-filled sac. Its purpose is to reduce the friction between the bony prominences and the other surrounding structures, such as muscles, tendons and joints.

### In psoriatic arthritis, what is the most common joint affected?

Psoriatic arthritis generally affects small joints of the hand and wrist, most commonly the distal interphalangeal joints.

### What is the intended puncture site in a knee joint aspiration using the lateral approach?

The needle should be inserted at the intersection between the lateral and proximal borders of the patella.

### What are the therapeutic and diagnostic reasons for performing a knee joint aspiration?

For therapeutic reasons, a knee joint aspiration can be obtained for haemarthrosis and effusions. For diagnostic reasons, it is indicated in cases of suspected septic arthritis, gout and pseudogout.

### Which knee bursae are most susceptible to inflammation (bursitis)?

Prepatellar bursa, infrapatellar bursa, pes anserinus bursa and suprapatellar bursa.

### Name three common triggers of a gout attack.

Red meat, shellfish, offal, alcohol, dehydration, sugary drinks and food high in fructose.

## Station 5.13 Peak Flow and Spirometry

### Doctor Briefing

You are a junior doctor on a respiratory placement and have been asked to see Mrs Smith, a 60-year-old woman who has presented with shortness of breath, chronic cough and reduced exercise tolerance. She has smoked 30 cigarettes a day for 45 years. She saw your colleague last week who ordered some investigations, and the results are now back. Please review the results, explain the findings to Mrs Smith and formulate an appropriate management plan.

### Patient Briefing

You are known to have COPD. For the past few weeks, you have been feeling increasingly breathless and you were referred for specialised tests. You do not know why are you feeling like this but are worried that your lungs are getting weaker.

### Results (Fig. 5.2)

| | Results (% predicted) | Reference range (% predicted) |
|---|---|---|
| Forced expiratory volume in 1 s ($FEV_1$) | 60% | >80% |
| Forced vital capacity (FVC) | 90% | >80% |
| $FEV_1$/FVC | 0.67 | >0.7 |
| Peak expiratory flow rate (PEFR) | 85% | >80% |

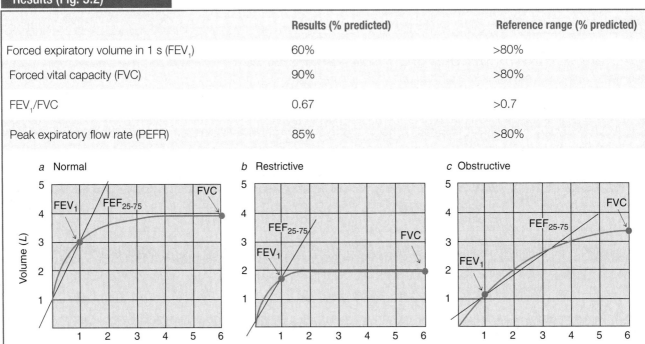

Fig. 5.2 Graphs demonstrating spirometry seen in (left) normal, (middle) restrictive and (right) obstructive conditions. Source: http://what-when-how.com/acp-medicine/lung-function-assessment-and-thoracic-diagnostic-techniques- part-2/

### Mark Scheme for Examiner

| Introduction | | | | |
|---|---|---|---|---|
| Cleans hands, introduces self and confirm patient identity | | | | |

| Establishes Current Patient Knowledge | | | | |
|---|---|---|---|---|
| **Statement/Question** | **Justification** | **Answer** | **Thoughts** | |
| I understand you recently saw my colleague as you had breathing difficulties | Start with a general open phrase to guide the patient and clarify the consultation | 'Yes, I have had it for a while actually' | The patient describes a potentially long-standing issue | |

## Establishes Current Patient Knowledge

| Statement/Question | Justification | Answer | Thoughts | | | | |
|---|---|---|---|---|---|---|---|
| Remind me what your other issues are? | Important sometimes to clarify with the patient the presenting complaint, if it feels appropriate | 'Well, just breathless really, even more when trying to walk upstairs or something like that. I have also had a dry cough for months. My family says it is to do with my smoking' | Really useful for you to be able to confirm symptoms but also here the patient has started to give you her ideas and concerns, which are important to acknowledge | | | | |
| What do you think your breathing problems are due to? | Sometimes it feels right to ask the patient directly what she thinks is happening | 'Well, it is probably is the smoking, isn't it? Everyone tells you how bad it is for you, but that is what the tests will show, isn't it?' | The patient has confirmed that she has a suspicion her smoking history is related to the presentation, but has put the onus back on you to explain further | | | | |

## Data Interpretation and Discussion

| Statement/Question | Justification | Answer | Thoughts | | | | |
|---|---|---|---|---|---|---|---|
| Yes, as you are aware, we ordered some breathing tests to show us how your lungs are working | Important to clarify the investigation with the patient | 'Yes, I had to do a lot of breathing down these funny tubes' | Good to clarify the investigation to the patient | | | | |
| These tests have shown us that you are not able to blow air out of your lungs as quickly as you should | Providing the test results to the patient in small chunks | 'OK, I did find that bit hard in the test.' | The patient has not asked anything at this point so you can carry on with your explanation | | | | |
| We see this problem in people who have a chest condition called COPD or chronic obstructive pulmonary disease. Have you heard of this before? | Important to explain the diagnosis to the patient, to let her hear the lay term and to ask if she has any prior knowledge of the condition | 'No, I have not. Do you know why I have this?' | Nearly always the patient will ask what the cause is. Here you can relate back to the patient's own ideas | | | | |
| We commonly see this chest condition in people who smoke. One of the most important things you can do to help your chest is to stop smoking | It is vital to discuss the diagnosis, if known, with the patient and to touch on the management plan | 'Oh dear, I'm not sure I'll be able to stop. I have smoked for so long' | The patient has concerns; always address these in the exam | | | | |
| I can imagine. I have given you a lot of information today. If you want, I can make an appointment with our stop-smoking team and you can make a plan together | This is supporting and signposting the patient appropriately | 'Thank you. That sounds like a good idea. Is there anything I can do now to help?' | The patient is keen to know if any further lifestyle choices can help | | | | |

## Data Interpretation and Discussion

| Statement/Question | Justification | Answer | Thoughts | | | | |
|---|---|---|---|---|---|---|---|
| That is a really good question. Apart from stopping smoking, keeping active and healthy is always beneficial. We can also help with some medication | Here you are taking the opportunity for health promotion but also informing the patient that there is medical management as well | 'OK. What sort of medication?' | The patient wishes to explore the management plan further | | | | |
| We often start with inhalers, medication that you breathe into your lungs that will help with your symptoms | You are explaining inhalers in lay terms | 'Oh, my friend uses them' | The patient shares an awareness of inhaler use | | | | |
| They are really commonly used for lots of chest conditions. We have a specialist nurse who will go through how to use them with you | You are explaining that inhaler use is widespread and that the patient will be supported when starting medication | 'Thank you. Will you make an appointment or do I have to do that?' | Patients often ask about the logistics of further appointments | | | | |
| We can make the appointment now if you want, so you can choose a time that suits you. At the same time the nurse will talk to you about getting vaccinations such as the flu vaccine, to help prevent you getting chest infections | You have explained the importance of vaccinations but not overwhelmed the patient in one consultation | 'Thank you, doctor, that makes sense' | The patient is happy with your management plan | | | | |

## Finishing the Consultation

| | | | | | | | |
|---|---|---|---|---|---|---|---|
| Would you mind please repeating what I have just told you? | Checking that the patient was listening and understands the information | 'I have a chest condition because of my smoking – you want me to stop. I also need to take inhalers which will help me' | You have a patient who has listened and correctly interpreted what you have told her | | | | |
| I understand there is a lot to take in. Do you have any immediate questions for me? | May identify useful information that has been missed | 'No, I understand' | This patient is happy with the plan | | | | |
| We will organise the two appointments for you now: one with the stop-smoking team and one with the chest nurses | Recapping the plan to yourself, the examiner and the patient is always important | 'Thank you' | The patient is satisfied with your management | | | | |

## Present Your Findings

Mrs Smith, a 60-year-old woman, has presented with shortness of breath, chronic cough and reduced exercise tolerance. She has a strong smoking history.

Spirometry and peak flow investigations were undertaken. She has a low $FEV_1$ of 60% with a reduced $FEV_1$/FVC ratio.

I have explained the findings to Mrs Smith, and she is aware that we have given her a diagnosis of COPD. I have advised her to stop smoking but also referred her to the smoking cessation nurse as well as the chest nurse to initiate inhaler treatment

| General Points | | | | |
|---|---|---|---|---|
| Polite to patient | | | | |
| Maintains good eye contact | | | | |
| Appropriate use of open and closed questions | | | | |

## ❓ QUESTIONS FROM THE EXAMINER

### In what group of patients is the PEFR typically higher?

Male patients and taller patients tend to produce a high peak flow reading.

### How many times should you repeat the peak flow for an accurate single reading?

The peak flow should be attempted at least three times and the highest value is the one to be recorded for that occasion.

### What is the hygiene hypothesis in relation to asthma?

The hygiene hypothesis suggests that young children who are brought up in an environment that is 'too clean' may be less able to develop a fully mature immune system. This is thought to be due to the lack of exposure to certain viruses, bacteria or parasites. Therefore, the body is less able to differentiate between harmless and harmful substances, which results in the immune system 'overreacting', and this can trigger asthma.

### Define 'residual volume'.

It is the volume of air remaining in the lungs after maximum forceful expiration.

### What is the normal tidal volume in men and women?

Normally, the tidal volume in an average health adult male is approximately 500 mL and in an average healthy female it is approximately 400 mL.

### Name the different groups of inhaler devices.

Nebulisers, inhalers with spacer devices, pressurised metered-dose inhalers, dry-powder inhalers, soft-mist inhalers.

### What tool can be used to assess the severity of dyspnoea?

The Medical Research Council dyspnoea scale, which is often used in monitoring COPD.

### Name two causes of obstructive lung disease.

COPD, asthma, emphysema, bronchiectasis and cystic fibrosis.

### Prior to spirometry, how long should bronchodilator therapy be omitted?

Short-acting beta-2-agonists should be stopped 6 h prior to testing, and long-acting beta-2-agonists should be stopped 12 h prior.

### Is there an age restriction for the use of the peak flow meter?

There is no strict cut-off for using the peak flow meter. As long as the patient is able to understand and perform the instructions to obtain an accurate reading, then it can be used.

## Station 5.14    Chest X-Ray

### Doctor Briefing

You are a junior doctor on a medical placement and have been asked to see Mrs Black, a 63-year-old woman, with a history of COPD. She has had a sudden onset of increased shortness of breath and right-sided pleuritic chest pain. A CXR was carried out and the results have returned. Please review the film, explain the findings to Mrs Black and formulate an appropriate management plan.

### Patient Briefing

You have had COPD for years and never had any real change in your symptoms apart from when you get chest infections. You are worried that this is another infection and that you need antibiotics. When asked, explain that the right-sided chest pain is getting worse and worse.

### Results (Fig. 5.3)

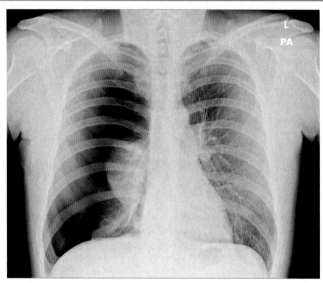

**Fig. 5.3** Mrs Black's chest X-ray.

### Mark Scheme for Examiner

#### Introduction

| Cleans hands, introduces self and confirms patient identity | | | | |
|---|---|---|---|---|

#### Establishes Current Patient Knowledge

| Statement/Question | Justification | Answer | Thoughts | | | | |
|---|---|---|---|---|---|---|---|
| I understand you came into hospital feeling suddenly short of breath with some pain in the right-hand side of your chest | Start with a general open phrase to guide the patient and clarify the consultation | 'Yes. It suddenly came on, out of the blue' | The patient confirms her acute presentation | | | | |

## Establishes Current Patient Knowledge

| Statement/Question | Justification | Answer | Thoughts | | | | |
|---|---|---|---|---|---|---|---|
| Have you noticed any other symptoms? | Important to ensure that the patient hasn't got any more concerning features. Remember this is an interpretation station, not a history station, so a full history is not expected but checking for red flags is pertinent | 'No, not really, just the breathing is getting worse and worse' | Really useful for you to be able to determine a change in the patient's presentation or if there are any other concerns | | | | |

## Data Interpretation and Discussion

| Statement/Question | Justification | Answer | Thoughts | | | | |
|---|---|---|---|---|---|---|---|
| As you are aware, we have done an X-ray of your chest to see if we can find a cause for your symptoms | Explain what the investigation was and why it has been performed | 'Yes. I'm really worried this is another infection' | The patient has immediately shared her concerns with you. It is important to address this immediately | | | | |
| Have you had a recent infection? | Exploring the concerns of the patient, asking an open question to allow her to share her thoughts | 'It was about a year ago now, but I was really poorly. I had to have antibiotics in the drip and was in hospital for several days' | The patient is sharing her concerns and recent history with you. This is really important information | | | | |
| I'm sorry to hear that; it must have been really scary. The CXR actually does not show any sign of an infection at the moment | Important to acknowledge the patient's concerns and also to reassure her if appropriate | 'Oh, so if it is not an infection, then what is it?' | The patient has appropriately asked this question, the answer to which you were likely to give anyway | | | | |
| It looks like there is an air leak in your chest. We see this commonly in people with COPD | This is complex information for a patient, so make sure you chunk it up | 'OK' | The patient has not asked any more at this point, so you can continue with your explanation | | | | |
| In COPD, as you probably know, the air sacs in the lungs are enlarged. Sometimes these can burst, causing an air leak. This can cause the breathlessness and pain you are experiencing | This is explaining the diagnosis to the patient in lay terms and relating it to her symptoms | 'OK' | The patient still has no questions, so you can continue | | | | |
| We cannot see anything else concerning on your CXR | Good to clarify that there are no other abnormalities | 'OK. What is the treatment for this air leak?' | The patient understandably wants to know the management plan | | | | |

**Data Interpretation and Discussion**

| Statement/Question | Justification | Answer | Thoughts | | | | | |
|---|---|---|---|---|---|---|---|---|
| We will continue giving you oxygen through the mask. Have you noticed that this helps? | You are chunking up the management plan to the patient and checking whether the oxygen therapy is providing any symptomatic relief | 'Yes. It really is. My breathing feels a lot better with it' | The patient has confirmed that the oxygen therapy is beneficial | | | | | |
| We will also have to put a small tube into your chest, through your lungs to drain the air that is in the wrong place away. This is done by the specialist lung team | You are explaining that the specialist performs the more complicated procedure of a chest drain | 'That sounds really painful. Will I be awake for this?' | The patient is sharing with you her concerns and asking appropriate questions | | | | | |
| I can imagine it does sound scary. We perform this procedure regularly under local anaesthetic, meaning you will be awake but you will not feel any pain. The lung team will explain it fully to you when they see you | You have acknowledged the patient's concerns, you have answered her immediate question and made her aware that nothing will be done unless she is fully informed | 'Thank you, doctor, that makes sense' | The patient is happy with your explanation and plan | | | | | |

**Finishing the Consultation**

| | | | | | | | | |
|---|---|---|---|---|---|---|---|---|
| Would you mind please repeating what I have just told you? | Checking that the patient was listening and understands the information | 'I have a popped lung and not an infection. You need to put a drain in to make me better' | You have a patient who has listened and correctly interpreted what you have told them | | | | | |
| I understand there is a lot to take in. Do you have any immediate questions for me? | May identify useful information that has been missed | 'No, I understand' | This patient is happy with the plan | | | | | |
| I will speak to the chest team now and get them to come and see you as soon as possible | Recapping the plan to yourself, the examiner and the patient is always important | 'Thank you' | The patient is satisfied with your management | | | | | |

**Present Your Findings**

Mrs Black, a 63-year-old woman, has a history of COPD and has had a sudden onset of increased shortness of breath and right-sided pleuritic chest pain.

A CXR was performed and demonstrates a right-sided pneumothorax.

I have explained the findings to Mrs Black, and she is aware of her diagnosis and that we will continue oxygen therapy and will need to insert a chest drain

| General Points | | |
|---|---|---|
| Polite to patient | | |
| Maintains good eye contact | | |
| Appropriate use of open and closed questions | | |

## ❓ QUESTIONS FROM THE EXAMINER

### How is cardiomegaly defined on a CXR?

Cardiomegaly is when the maximal transverse cardiac diameter is greater than 50% of the maximal transverse internal thoracic diameter.

### Name two possible causes of widening of the mediastinum.

Technical factors (such as an anteroposterior projection), vascular structures, masses and haemorrhage.

### If the costophrenic angles are not sharp, what may this indicate?

There is likely to be pleural fluid in the lung bases.

### How would surgical emphysema be seen on a CXR?

You may see gas in the soft tissues, which would appear as black areas, as gas is the least dense.

### What is the most common site of insertion for central lines and where should the tip be located?

Central lines are most commonly placed in the internal jugular veins. Their tips should be in the mid or lower superior vena cava.

### What are air bronchograms?

They refer to bronchioles that contain air, running through a consolidated lung.

### Which part of the lungs is in contact with the right and left heart borders?

The right heart border is in contact with the right middle lobe, while the left heart border is in contact with the lingula (part of the left upper lobe).

### What is the immediate management for a tension pneumothorax?

Needle thoracocentesis in the second intercostal space, midclavicular line.

### What is the Luftsichel sign and when would you see it?

The Luftsichel sign is demonstrated as radiolucency in the left upper zone (around the aortic arch) due to compensatory hyperinflation of the left lower lobe. It may be seen in left-upper-lobe collapse.

### Name three signs on a CXR that suggest loss of lung volume; for instance, in the case of a lobar collapse.

A raised hemidiaphragm ipsilaterally, tracheal and mediastinal shift towards the collapsed side, displacement of the hila and narrowing of the space between the ribs (relative to the contralateral side).

## Station 5.15    Abdominal X-Ray

### Doctor Briefing

You are a junior doctor on a surgical placement and have been asked to see Mr Adams, a 65-year-old man, who has presented with abdominal pain and distension, vomiting and no bowel movements for 3 days. He has a history of an appendectomy at 22 years old. An abdominal X-ray was carried out and the results are back. Please review the film, explain the findings to Mr Adams and formulate an appropriate management plan.

### Patient Briefing

You feel very unwell. You cannot stop vomiting, no matter what medication you have been given by the doctors. You are concerned you have something seriously wrong with you and will die. If asked, you share that your wife passed away from bowel cancer last year.

### Results (Fig. 5.4)

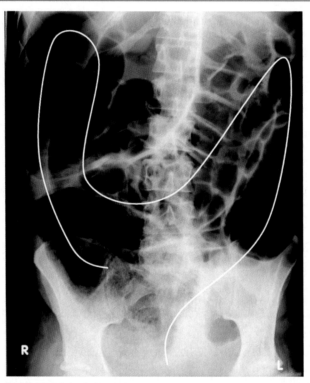

Fig. 5.4  Mr Adam's X-ray.

### Mark Scheme for Examiner

**Introduction**

Cleans hands, introduces self and confirms patient identity

**Establishes Current Patient Knowledge**

| Statement/Question | Justification | Answer | Thoughts | | | | |
|---|---|---|---|---|---|---|---|
| I understand you have been feeling really unwell and came into hospital with vomiting and tummy pain | Start with a general open phrase to guide the patient and clarify the consultation | 'Yes. It is getting worse and worse. I seem to be getting more bloated, with more pain and vomiting as time passes' | The patient confirms his symptoms with you | | | | |

## Establishes Current Patient Knowledge

| Statement/Question | Justification | Answer | Thoughts | | | | |
|---|---|---|---|---|---|---|---|
| Have you noticed any blood in your vomit? | Important to ensure that the patient hasn't got any more concerning features. Remember, this is an interpretation station, not a history station, so a full history is not expected but checking for red flags is pertinent | 'No, nothing like that. It is more like bile. I haven't been able to go to the toilet for about 3 days now' | Really useful for you to be able to check for red flags but also the patient is confirming that there are obstructive features to the presentation | | | | |
| When you say 'go to the toilet', do you mean to pass urine or to pass a bowel motion? | It is important to check what the patient means. You must never assume and will never lose marks for clarifying symptoms | 'I mean opening my bowels. It is just like there is nothing there. I'm passing urine just fine' | This clarification is really useful | | | | |

## Data Interpretation and Discussion

| | | | | | | | |
|---|---|---|---|---|---|---|---|
| You are aware that we have done an X-ray of your tummy to see if we can work out what is causing your symptoms | Explain what the investigation is for, confirming this to both the patient and the examiner | 'Yes' | Good to establish the facts and see whether the patient has any immediate questions to ask | | | | |
| As I suspected, the X-ray shows there is a blockage in your bowel – something we call bowel obstruction | Clarifying the investigation results to the patient | 'OK' | The patient has not asked anything at this point, so you can carry on with your explanation. Some patients may start asking all sorts of questions at this point | | | | |
| We can see that the blockage appears to be in your small bowel. This causes all the symptoms that you are experiencing | Important to validate the patient's symptoms | 'Do you know why I have this blockage?' | Nearly always the patient will ask what the cause is. It is all right not to have an answer and to explain that further investigation is required | | | | |
| I cannot tell you exactly what the cause is now. Have you had any operations on your tummy before? | It is vital to check for the leading differentials | 'Yes. I had my appendix taken out a long time ago. It had burst so I had to have a big cut on my tummy' | This information makes adhesions the most likely cause of small-bowel obstruction, but without a full examination and further investigations you cannot confirm this yet | | | | |

**Data Interpretation and Discussion**

| Statement/Question | Justification | Answer | Thoughts | | | | | |
|---|---|---|---|---|---|---|---|---|
| Thank you. The most likely cause of the blockage will be scar tissue from your previous operation. Sometimes this scar tissue can cause problems years after an operation | This is explaining the most likely diagnosis to the patient | 'I never knew that. So it isn't cancer?' | The patient has shared with you his concerns, it is important to address these | | | | | |
| What makes you think it is cancer? At the moment, I cannot say it definitely isn't, but, from what you have told me so far, it is unlikely | You are exploring the patient's concerns | 'All right. I guess that makes sense. It is just that my wife died from bowel cancer' | The patient shared with you the reason for his concerns | | | | | |
| I am very sorry to hear this and can understand why you are worried. The most likely cause in your case is previous scar tissue from your operation but we will be performing investigations to confirm the cause | You are explaining that further tests are required | 'OK, what will those be?' | The patient understandably wants to know more | | | | | |
| At first we will order some blood tests and an X-ray of your chest but also we will make sure you are more comfortable | You are explaining the ongoing investigations and also reminding the patient that you will treat him as well | 'Is there something you can do to make me feel better then?' | The patient is wanting to know the possible management plan | | | | | |
| We will make sure you have pain relief and antisickness medication through a drip, so you don't have to swallow anything. We will also give you fluid through the drip to keep you hydrated | You are sharing the management plan with the patient in lay terms | 'Thank you doctor, that makes sense' | The patient is happy with your explanation | | | | | |
| We will also put a fine tube through your nose into your tummy to drain the contents of your stomach. This will make the pain and bloating go away and allow your tummy to have some rest | You have chunked up the management information for the patient, allowing him to take on small amounts of information and making sure he isn't overwhelmed | 'That doesn't sound very nice, but I guess if it makes me feel better …' | The patient is relaying his thoughts to you. It is important to acknowledge these | | | | | |

## Data Interpretation and Discussion

| Statement/Question | Justification | Answer | Thoughts | | | | |
|---|---|---|---|---|---|---|---|
| It doesn't, but it is something that will help and something we do routinely | You are reassuring the patient | 'OK, thank you' | The patient is satisfied at the moment with your plan | | | | |

## Finishing the Consultation

| Statement/Question | Justification | Answer | Thoughts | | | | |
|---|---|---|---|---|---|---|---|
| Would you mind please repeating what I have just told you? | Checking that the patient was listening and understands the information | 'There is a blockage in my tummy, you think caused by my previous operation' | You have a patient who has listened and correctly interpreted what you have told him | | | | |
| I understand there is a lot to take in. Do you have any immediate questions for me? | May identify useful information that has been missed | 'No, I understand' | This patient is happy with the plan | | | | |
| I will order the further investigations and arrange for this tube to be placed into your tummy for you. You should feel a lot better after this | Recapping the plan to yourself, the examiner and the patient is always important | 'Thank you, doctor' | The patient is satisfied with your management | | | | |

## Present Your Findings

Mr Adams, a 65-year-old man, has presented with abdominal pain and distension, vomiting and no bowel movements for 3 days. He has a history of an appendectomy performed via laparotomy at 22 years old.

An abdominal X-ray was performed and demonstrated a small-bowel obstruction, likely from previous adhesions.

I have explained the findings to Mr Adams, and he is aware I would like to place a nasogastric tube to relieve his symptoms as well as perform further blood tests and a chest X-ray

## General Points

| | | | | |
|---|---|---|---|---|
| Polite to patient | | | | |
| Maintains good eye contact | | | | |
| Appropriate use of open and closed questions | | | | |

## ❓ QUESTIONS FROM THE EXAMINER

### What is the projection of a standard abdominal X-ray?

An anteroposterior X-ray with the patient in the supine position.

### The large bowel should be no wider than **6 cm, except which part?**

The caecum can be up to 9 cm.

## What are valvulae conniventes and in what part of the bowel are they seen?

Valvulae conniventes are lines that traverse the full width of the small bowel.

## What is Rigler's sign and what might it suggest?

Rigler's sign is when both sides of the bowel wall are clearly visible (normally, only the inner wall of the bowel is visible due to the contrast of the inner wall against air present inside the bowel). If noted, this may indicate a pneumoperitoneum.

## What type of X-ray is best for detecting a pneumoperitoneum?

CXRs are best at detecting a pneumoperitoneum. Even if there are no suggestive signs on the abdominal X-ray, if you are suspecting a pneumoperitoneum, make sure you request an erect CXR.

## What other imaging modalities might you request if you noted gas within the portal system or biliary tree?

Consider obtaining an abdominal ultrasound or CT, as they are more accurate compared to X-rays.

## What is the normal diameter for the abdominal aorta?

The abdominal aorta should measure less than 3 cm. If it is greater, then this could suggest an aneurysm and further investigation and/or monitoring may be necessary.

## What are the most common causes of a small-bowel obstruction?

Either adhesions or a hernia.

## What must you rule out in a patient with background of inflammatory bowel disease, presenting with abdominal pain?

It is vital to rule out inflammatory bowel disease-related toxic megacolon. On the abdominal X-ray, you may note an enlarged colon with thumbprinting (thickening of the bowel wall caused by oedema, haemorrhage or tumour).

## Define a sigmoid volvulus.

A sigmoid volvulus refers to when the sigmoid colon twists on its own mesentery, which can cause obstruction and restrict blood flow to that part of the colon.

## Station 5.16   Orthopaedic X-Ray

### Doctor Briefing

You are a junior doctor on an emergency placement and have been asked to see Mrs Cotton, an 84-year-old woman, who has presented with left-hip pain, shortening and internal rotation following a fall in her garden. She has a history of polymyalgia rheumatica. A hip X-ray was carried out and the results are back. Please review the film, explain the findings to Mrs Cotton and formulate an appropriate management plan.

### Patient Briefing

You are normally fit and well and don't require any care or help at home. You were out in the garden trimming some of your plants when you lost your footing and fell. You didn't hit your head. You remember tripping over and being unable to get back up. Your foot seemed to be pointing at an odd angle. Your husband came to help you and called an ambulance. You are concerned that you may need an operation. You are worried about this, as you are older and unsure as to the recovery. You help care for your husband so are keen to get home as soon as possible.

### Results (Fig. 5.5)

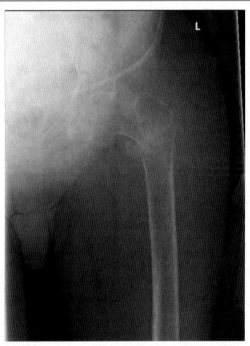

**Fig. 5.5** Mrs Cotton's hip X-ray.

### Mark Scheme for Examiner

#### Introduction

| Cleans hands, introduces self and confirms patient identity | | | | |
|---|---|---|---|---|

#### Establishes Current Patient Knowledge

| Statement/Question | Justification | Answer | Thoughts | | | | |
|---|---|---|---|---|---|---|---|
| I understand you fell over in the garden and have a sore hip | Start with a general open phrase to guide the patient and clarify the consultation | 'Yes, I can't believe I did it. I have never fallen before. I think I must have tripped' | The patient describes what happened to her and confirms that her mobility is not usually an issue | | | | |

## Establishes Current Patient Knowledge

| Statement/Question | Justification | Answer | Thoughts | | | | | |
|---|---|---|---|---|---|---|---|---|
| Did you hit your head or lose consciousness when you fell over? | Important to ensure that the patient hasn't got any further injuries that would require assessment | 'No, not at all. I remember falling and I landed in a strange position on my side' | Really useful for you to be able to determine no loss of consciousness or head injury | | | | | |

## Data Interpretation and Discussion

| Statement/Question | Justification | Answer | Thoughts | | | | | |
|---|---|---|---|---|---|---|---|---|
| We have performed an X-ray to look at your sore hip on the right side | Explain what the investigation is for | 'OK' | Remind the patient of the investigation she had | | | | | |
| As I suspected, it sadly shows that you have a break, or fracture, in one of the bones in your hip joint on the right-hand side | Confirming the test results with the patient | 'Really, I cannot believe that, from a simple fall' | The patient is shocked at the X-ray report. Spend some time acknowledging this | | | | | |
| I can understand this has come as a shock. We often see these sorts of injuries from a simple trip | Important to recognise and address the patient's concern | 'So what happens now? Do I have to have it in plaster?' | The patient has asked a very sensible question about her management plan | | | | | |
| That is a really good thought. I think we may need to do a little more than put a plaster on it | This is a warning shot to the patient that the management plan is likely to be more complex | 'Oh, OK' | Now you have given the patient a warning shot that the management plan isn't what she suspected, you can continue | | | | | |
| We know that these breaks in the hip joint don't really respond to being in plaster like some other breaks in bones in the arm or leg. In breaks such as yours, we would recommend an operation to fix it | This is explaining the management plan in a clear and simple way. You are spelling out why a simple plaster is not the correct management | 'Oh dear. An operation ... I'm not sure I can stay away from my husband' | The patient has shared her concerns about being away from her husband. You will need to explore this further in order to be able to make a shared management plan with her | | | | | |
| I can imagine it is a bit scary being told you need an operation. Is there any reason why you need to be with your husband? | Here you are sensitively exploring her concerns in more detail | 'Well, I help care for him, you see. We have carers once a day but I do a lot of the help' | The patient has shared her concerns with you | | | | | |
| I understand. The really important thing is that without this operation, you will not be able to stand on your sore leg, let alone walk or be able to care for your husband. So, for both of you, it is really important we fix it as soon as possible | You are explaining that without an operation her mobility will be severely compromised | 'I guess so. What will I do about his care though?' | The patient understandably wants to ensure that her husband is cared for | | | | | |

## Data Interpretation and Discussion

| Statement/Question | Justification | Answer | Thoughts | | | | |
|---|---|---|---|---|---|---|---|
| We will speak to your family and liaise with the carers to ensure that he has the appropriate care and support whilst you are in hospital | You are reassuring the patient that you will help her organise the care for her husband | 'Thank you doctor, it is just so worrying' | The patient sounds reassured but still apprehensive and scared | | | | |
| I can understand. We will take good care of you and ensure your husband is looked after as well. The bone doctors, called orthopaedic doctors, will come along shortly to explain more about the operation to you | You have acknowledged the patient's concerns, you have reassured her and explained that she will be seen by the specialists | 'Thank you doctor, I appreciate your help' | The patient is happy with the plan | | | | |

## Finishing the Consultation

| | | | | | | | |
|---|---|---|---|---|---|---|---|
| Would you mind please repeating what I have just told you? | Checking that the patient was listening and understands the information | 'When I tripped in the garden, I landed in a funny position and have broken my hip. I have to have an operation' | You have a patient who has listened and correctly interpreted what you have told her | | | | |
| I understand there is a lot to take in. Do you have any immediate questions for me? | May identify useful information that has been missed | 'No, I understand' | This patient is happy with the plan | | | | |
| I will speak to the other doctors now and get you seen as quickly as possible. It was a pleasure to meet you | Recapping the plan to yourself, the examiner and the patient is always important | 'Thank you' | The patient is satisfied with your management | | | | |

## Present Your Findings

Mrs Cotton, an 84-year-old woman, has presented with left-hip pain, shortening and internal rotation following a fall in her garden.

A left-hip X-ray demonstrates a displaced intracapsular neck-of-femur fracture.

I have explained the findings to Mrs Cotton, and she is aware that she needs an operation to fix the fracture. I have referred her to the orthopaedic team

## General Points

Polite to patient

Maintains good eye contact

Appropriate use of open and closed questions

## ❓ QUESTIONS FROM THE EXAMINER

### Name three signs that you might see on an orthopaedic X-ray that may suggest degenerative joint changes.

Loss of joint space, subchondral sclerosis, subchondral cysts and osteophytes.

### Name two signs that you might see on an orthopaedic X-ray that may suggest inflammatory joint changes.

Periarticular osteoporosis, soft-tissue swelling and bony erosions.

### What might the presence of posterior and elevated anterior fat pads suggest?

Potential joint effusion, which has many possible causes. An elbow effusion in the context of trauma suggests a possible underlying fracture.

### Define an 'impacted fracture'.

A fracture that involves the bone fragments being driven into each other.

### How might you expect the bones of a patient with osteopenia to appear?

Most of the bone may be radiolucent (looks black) and the cortices appear thinned.

### What is the difference between subluxation and dislocation?

Subluxation refers to the normal anatomy of the joint being disrupted, but there is still some contact between the articular surfaces of the joint. Dislocation refers to complete disruption of the joint with no contact between the joint surfaces.

### In the context of trauma and a patient presenting with neck pain, what are the minimum views of the cervical spine that are necessary?

Lateral view (which must show all seven cervical vertebrae and the top of the first thoracic vertebra), anteroposterior view, and open-mouth anteroposterior/peg view (to view C1 and C2).

### At what level do most cervical spine injuries occur?

C1–C2 or C5–T1 region.

### What is a Monteggia fracture?

A Monteggia fracture is when there is an ulnar shaft fracture with associated radial head dislocation.

### What is the Garden classification?

It is the classification system used for intracapsular neck-of-femur fractures, with a total of four classes.

## Station 5.17   CT Head

### Doctor Briefing

You are a junior doctor on an emergency medicine placement and have been asked to see Mr May, an 84-year-old man, who has presented with a headache of sudden onset, left-sided hemiparesis and left-sided brisk reflexes. A CT head has been performed. Please review the scan, explain the findings to Mr May and formulate an appropriate management plan.

### Patient Briefing

You were sitting down watching TV when you suddenly developed a headache. You have never had a headache like this before. You had migraines when you were a teenager but never anything like this. You take warfarin. Your wife said you couldn't really move the left side of your body. You don't really understand what happened. All you know is that you couldn't walk. You suspect you have had a stroke, and are not surprised when the doctor tells you this.

### Results (Fig. 5.6)

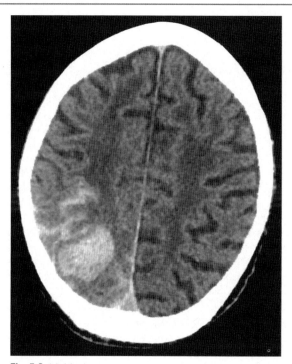

Fig. 5.6  Mr May's computed tomography (CT) scan.

### Mark Scheme for Examiner

#### Introduction

| | | | |
|---|---|---|---|
| Cleans hands, introduces self and confirms patient identity | | | |

#### Establishes Current Patient Knowledge

| Statement/Question | Justification | Answer | Thoughts | | | | | |
|---|---|---|---|---|---|---|---|---|
| I understand you developed a severe headache and some difficulty walking; is this correct? | Start with a general open phrase to guide the patient and clarify the consultation | 'Yes, one minute I was fine and then the next I was in this state' | The patient describes a potentially long-standing issue but denies any other symptoms | | | | | |

**Establishes Current Patient Knowledge**

| Statement/Question | Justification | Answer | Thoughts | | | | | |
|---|---|---|---|---|---|---|---|---|
| Have you ever had anything like this before? | Important to clarify whether the patient has experienced symptoms like this before | 'No, never. I have had migraines before but they have never stopped me walking' | Really useful for you to be able to determine that this is the first presentation of these symptoms | | | | | |

**Data Interpretation and Discussion**

| Statement/Question | Justification | Answer | Thoughts | | | | | |
|---|---|---|---|---|---|---|---|---|
| We performed a special scan of your head called a CT scan. This allows us to see if we can find any cause for your symptoms | Explain what the investigation was and why you were doing it. Always useful to let the patient know the name of the investigation | 'Yes, someone said that' | Important to establish a baseline with the patient | | | | | |
| Unfortunately, the scan of your head shows us that you have had a bleed in your brain. We call this a stroke | Using the word 'unfortunately' at the beginning of the sentence prepares the patient for bad news | 'OK' | The patient has not asked anything at this point, so you can carry on with your explanation. Some patients may start asking all sorts of questions at this point | | | | | |
| Do you know what I mean when I say that you have had a stroke? | Crucial to gauge the patient's understanding. Most people have heard of a stroke but they may come with very preconceived ideas or concerns | 'Yes. It is where you can have funny speech and when your arms and legs don't work properly' | The patient has demonstrated to you that he hase some understanding of what a stroke is | | | | | |
| That is exactly right. There are a few causes for a stroke but in your case we think it has happened because of bleeding in the brain | It is vital to make the patient aware of the cause, if it is known | 'Is this because of those blood-thinning tablets?' | Be prepared to have to explain yourself further when you offer information to patients | | | | | |
| The tablets you are taking, warfarin, do thin the blood and make bleeding more likely. It is important that we reverse the warfarin in your blood which will help stop any further bleeding | This is explaining the management plan to the patient | 'OK. What happens next?' | The patient does not seem to want to know any more about the warfarin and is keen to understand the next steps | | | | | |
| When you came into hospital you had high blood pressure. We need to reduce this slowly with some medication. This will help reduce further bleeding as well | Need to explain that there are several aspects to the management of his stroke | 'I thought I was already on blood pressure tablets?' | The patient has asked you to clarify your plan to him | | | | | |

## Data Interpretation and Discussion

| Statement/Question | Justification | Answer | Thoughts |
|---|---|---|---|
| Yes, you are correct, you are on blood pressure tablets. Sometimes, despite taking these tablets, your blood pressure can still be high, so we will be giving you more medication to lower this | You are explaining that the patient was correct regarding the medication but that he does need to do more to control the blood pressure | 'OK. Thank you for explaining that. I knew I was taking blood pressure medication' | The patient is grateful for your explanation and has no further questions, so you can carry on with your consultation |
| I will contact the doctors who look after people who have strokes. They will look after you whilst you are in hospital. I will also need to speak to the brain surgeons, called neurosurgeons, who will want to review you | You are explaining the next steps for the patient. This suggests that he will be staying in hospital, will be looked after by a specialist team, and you have suggested the prospect of surgery. The patient may or may not pick up on this | 'Crikey, do I need surgery?' | The patient has picked up on what you said. Be prepared to explain yourself if you provide the patient with suggestions such as this |
| There is a possibility you may need an operation, but I cannot say for sure. Not everyone who has a bleed in the brain needs an operation but it is important that the right specialists review you to decide the best management | You have acknowledged the patient's concerns, you have explained you cannot answer his question now, but that he will be looked after by the specialist team who will make these decisions | 'Thank you doctor, that makes sense' | The patient is happy with your explanation |

## Finishing the Consultation

| Statement/Question | Justification | Answer | Thoughts |
|---|---|---|---|
| Would you mind please repeating what I have just told you? | Checking that the patient was listening and understands the information | 'I have had a stroke. I will be looked after in hospital and may need an operation' | You have a patient who has listened and correctly interpreted what you have told him |
| I understand there is a lot to take in. Do you have any immediate questions for me? | May identify useful information that has been missed | 'Can my wife come in and visit me?' | This patient understandably wishes to know if he can have visitors |
| Of course. As soon as you are on the ward, I will ask one of the nurses to call her for you | Being empathetic and helping the patient is very important | 'Thank you doctor, I would really appreciate that' | The patient is grateful and happy with your plan and care |

## Present Your Findings

Mr May, an 84-year-old man, has presented with a headache of sudden onset, left-sided hemiparesis and left-sided brisk reflexes.

A CT head was performed and demonstrated an intraparenchymal haemorrhage.

I have explained the findings to Mr May, and he is aware of his stroke diagnosis. I have informed him of the initial management plan and that his case will be discussed with the neurosurgeons

| General Points | | | | | |
|---|---|---|---|---|---|
| Polite to patient | | | | | |
| Maintains good eye contact | | | | | |
| Appropriate use of open and closed questions | | | | | |

## ❓ QUESTIONS FROM THE EXAMINER

### How is the attenuation of tissues represented on CT scans?

Either as the CT number or Hounsfield unit.

### What are the three routes through which contrast can be administered?

Orally, intravenously and rectally.

### What is the equivalent ionising radiation dose as a CXR for a single CT head scan?

The amount of dosage received from 75 CXRs is equivalent to the amount of ionising radiation dose received during a single CT head.

### Where is the site of bleeding in an acute subdural haemorrhage?

Between the arachnoid mater and dura mater.

### What is the most common vessel to bleed in an acute extradural haemorrhage?

The middle meningeal artery in the temporal region.

### Name three causes of an intra-axial haemorrhage.

A haemorrhagic stroke, a bleed into an underlying lesion (such as a tumour or vascular malformation), trauma and venous sinus thrombosis.

### After how long are CT findings of an ischaemic stroke usually visible?

CT findings of an ischaemic stroke are usually only visible at least 6 h after the stroke started. An ischaemic stroke is normally diagnosed on clinical suspicion once a CT head has ruled out a haemorrhagic stroke or alternative causes.

### How many phases, and what are they, of contrast-enhanced CT head scans?

There are three phases: the arterial phase scan/angiogram, venous phase scan/venogram and delayed phase.

### Which primary tumours most commonly metastasise to the brain?

Lung cancer, breast cancer, genitourinary tract tumours and melanoma.

### What might you see on a CT head if mass effect is present?

There may be effacement of the normal CSF spaces (such as the ventricles or sulci), midline shift to the opposite side and herniation (such as cerebellar tonsillar herniation).

# Practical Skills

6

## Outline

## Station 6.1    Intermediate Life Support

### Doctor Briefing

You are the junior doctor working in the emergency department (ED). You have been asked to follow up on Mr Bencini, a 33-year-old man, who was admitted following a motor vehicle accident. You notice that the patient has suddenly become unresponsive, and the senior emergency nurse asks you to help resuscitate him. Please carry out intermediate life support (ILS) and follow any instructions given by your examiners throughout this station.

### Patient Briefing

You are one of the senior nurses working in the ED. You were looking after one of the patients in a bay, Mr Bencini.

He is a 33-year-old man who had a motor vehicle accident about 2 h ago. He was brought into the ED and has been in the department for 10 min. You have not had the chance to do any observations on him yet. You approached him to ask a few questions and he suddenly became unresponsive. You quickly grab the junior doctor nearby and ask him/her to help resuscitate the patient.

### Mark Scheme for Examiner

| Introduction | | | | | |
|---|---|---|---|---|---|
| Cleans hands, introduces self and confirms patient identity | | | | | |
| Establishes current knowledge and concerns (from team members) | | | | | |
| **Life Support** | | | | | |
| Looks for danger | | | | | |
| Checks for responses and asks questions down both ears | | | | | |
| Shouts for help | | | | | |
| Checks the airway for signs of obstruction | | | | | |
| If no concerns regarding spinal injury, performs head tilt, chin lift manoeuvre | | | | | |
| Checks breathing by looking for chest movement and listening for breath sounds for 10 s | | | | | |
| Checks circulation by feeling for the carotid pulse for 10 s | | | | | |

**Life Support**

| | | | |
|---|---|---|---|

If the patient is not breathing and has no pulse, calls 2222

Commences cardiopulmonary resuscitation (CPR) – starts chest compressions directly over the distal sternum, at a rate of 100–120/min to a depth of approximately 5–6 cm

After 30 chest compressions, gives two breaths using a bag valve mask device connected to high-flow oxygen

Asks helper(s) to continue chest compressions and ventilations at a ratio of 30:2. If there is more than one person on chest compressions, then they rotate at least every 2 min

Turns on the defibrillator and applies self-adhesive pads – one below the right clavicle, one in the left midaxillary line in the V6 position. Ensures the CPR continues while pads are placed

Once pads have been applied, asks the team to stop CPR in order to assess the rhythm

**Management of Shockable Rhythms**

Correctly identifies the rhythm – pulseless ventricular tachycardia or ventricular fibrillation – and clearly states it to the team

Immediately instructs team member to continue chest compressions

Commands team to 'Stand clear, oxygen away, charging defibrillator now', while informing the person performing chest compression to continue

Charges the defibrillator to 150–200 J biphasic

Once charge is complete, commands the remaining team member on chest compressions to 'Stand clear'

While looking at the patient and his surroundings, presses the 'shock' button while saying to the team 'Shocking now'

Once shock has been administered, immediately instructs the team to restart chest compressions and ventilations at a ratio of 30:2 for 2 min without pausing for reassessment

After 2 min, stops chest compressions again and performs a second rhythm check

If still in a shockable rhythm, then repeats management steps above

Administers adrenaline 1 mg intravenously (IV) or interosseously (IO) and amiodarone 300 mg IV after the third shock. Then continues to give adrenaline 1 mg IV every other shock, and gives amioderone 150mg IV/IO after 5th shock

**Management of Non-Shockable Rhythms**

Correctly identifies the rhythm – pulseless electrical activity or asystole – and clearly states it to the team

Immediately instructs team member to continue chest compressions

Immediately administers adrenaline 1 mg IV/IO

Continues chest compressions and ventilations at a ratio of 30:2 for 2 min without pausing for reassessment

After 2 min, stops chest compressions again and performs a second rhythm check

If still in a non-shockable rhythm, then repeats management steps above

Administers adrenaline 1 mg IV/IO every other shock

| During the 2-Min Cycles | | | | |
| --- | --- | --- | --- | --- |
| Obtains IV or intraosseous access | | | | |
| Performs an arterial blood gas (ABG) and obtains blood samples | | | | |
| Excludes the reversible causes – '4 Hs and 4 Ts' | | | | |
| **Post-Resuscitation Care** | | | | |
| Initiates post-resuscitation care once the patient is displaying a rhythm consistent with organised electrical activity and has a pulse | | | | |
| Administers oxygen | | | | |
| Administers fluids | | | | |
| Performs electrocardiogram (ECG) | | | | |
| Performs a full set of observations | | | | |
| Contacts high dependency unit or intensive therapy unit | | | | |
| **Finishing** | | | | |
| Dispose of equipment safely, ensuring that you are adhering to the local infection control guidelines | | | | |
| Remove your gloves and wash your hands | | | | |
| Offer to update family on the incident and document the events in the notes | | | | |
| **General Points** | | | | |
| Maintains good communication with team throughout | | | | |

## ❓ QUESTIONS FROM THE EXAMINER

### What is the normal PR interval?

Normal PR interval is expected to be 0.12–0.20 s. This is also equivalent to 3–5 small squares on an ECG paper.

### When attempting to perform tracheal intubation, what is the maximum amount of time that chest compression should be interrupted for?

Aim for less than 5-s interruption in chest compression.

### Which structure in the heart stimulates atrial contraction?

The sinoatrial node, which is also known as the 'physiological pacemaker', as it generates normal electrical activity in heart.

### Define bradycardia.

Bradycardia is a heart rate less than 60 bpm.

## What is the Beck triad?

The Beck triad is a combination of three clinical signs: hypotension (weak pulse or narrow pulse pressure), muffled heart sounds and raised jugular venous pressure. These signs collectively are associated with pericardial tamponade, which is secondary to an excessive accumulation of fluid within the pericardial sac.

## Where is a pericardiocentesis needle inserted?

Typically, the needle insertion site is the fifth left intercostal space, close to the sternal border. The needle is directed at approximately 40° angle to the skin.

## What is the role of insulin in the treatment of hyperkalaemia?

Insulin can help to lower the potassium concentration in the blood by stimulating the uptake of potassium into the cells.

## What must you do during resuscitation to minimise the risk of a fire incident?

You must remove any oxygen mask or nasal cannulae and place them at least 1 m away from the patient's chest during defibrillation.

## What system is implemented in hospitals for the early identification of patients who are critically ill or at risk of clinical deterioration?

The track-and-trigger early-warning score system. It takes into consideration seven parameters: respiratory rate, heart rate, blood pressure, oxygen saturation, any supplemental oxygen, level of consciousness and temperature.

## Amiodarone is indicated in ventricular fibrillation and pulseless ventricular tachycardia in cardiac arrest refractory to defibrillation. What is an alternative to amiodarone?

Lidocaine.

## Station 6.2   Venepuncture

### Doctor Briefing

You are the junior doctor in primary care. Your next patient is Mr Fredrick, a 50-year-old man, who is having his renal function monitored after having recently started a diuretic medication. Please prepare your equipment and perform a venepuncture, explaining your steps to the examiner.

### Patient Briefing

You have come to see the general practitioner today for a blood test. You have recently started a 'water tablet' for your high blood pressure. You know that the blood test is to check how well your kidneys are working.

You are concerned because you are scared of needles. However, you understand that you need to have the blood test.

### Mark Scheme for Examiner

#### Introduction

| | | | | |
|---|---|---|---|---|
| Cleans hands, introduces self and confirms patient identity | | | | |
| Establishes current patient knowledge and concerns | | | | |
| Asks for arm preference, if the patient has any allergies and whether he has any contraindications (such as lymphoedema, mastectomy, arteriovenous (AV) fistula) | | | | |

#### Explaining the Procedure

| Statement/Question | Justification | Answer | Thoughts | | | |
|---|---|---|---|---|---|---|
| I would like to take a blood sample from you. Have you had one of these before? | Start with a general open phrase to guide the patient | 'Yes' | You know the patient is listening | | | |
| This involves putting a needle into a vein near the surface of your skin and taking a small amount of blood out | Important to explain the procedure in detail so that the patient knows what to expect. You need to check that the patient understands the procedure in full | 'I understand. I'm a bit scared of needles though' | If a patient says no, you need to decide if he has capacity and if you have given him enough information to understand what you are suggesting. This allows you to accommodate if he has a fear of needles | | | |
| We will then analyse the blood. This will help us check that the new medication isn't having a negative effect on your kidneys | It is important the patient knows why the procedure is happening | 'That's fine with me' | | | | |
| Are you on any blood-thinning medication that you know of? | Checking the patient's bleeding risk | 'No, not that I know of' | Make sure you fully explain the procedure | | | |
| Sometimes you have some bruising at the site we take blood from. There is also the chance that I can't get any blood and will need to reattempt at another site | It is vital to discuss complications with a patient | 'That's fine' | | | | |

**Performing Venepuncture**

**Equipment Checklist**

| Statement/Question | Justification | Answer | Thoughts | | | | | |
|---|---|---|---|---|---|---|---|---|
| I am just gathering the equipment I need, checking sterility and expiry dates | Explaining to the examiner you are following routine practice | 'OK' | The patient is aware you are preparing for the procedure | | | | | |

**Preparation**

Decontaminates hands

Cleans tray according to local policy

Assembles all equipment in the clean tray

Opens packaging, attaches Vacutainer to venepuncture needle, places bottles in draw order and cuts tape to size

**Drawing Blood**

Cleans hands, dons non-sterile gloves and applies a single-use disposable apron

| I am going to position your arm. Is this comfortable? | Important to check that the patient is comfortable throughout the procedure | 'That's fine, thank you' | No additional concerns |
| I am going to tie a tight band around your arm for a bit to help me feel for a vein I wish to take the sample from. Is that OK? | You are warning the patient you are about to examine him | 'Fine' | No additional concerns |

Places the tourniquet 7–10 cm proximal to the proposed insertion site

Selects a vein. It should feel 'bouncy'. If not, it is either inadequately filled or if rigid, it may be thrombosed

Loosens the tourniquet

**Skin Preparation**

| I am now going to clean your arm. It needs a while to dry so please keep still if you can | Explaining to the patient the reason why you may not take the blood sample immediately | 'OK' | No additional concerns |

Cleans the site: cleans for 30 s using an up-and-down, back-and-forth friction technique. Allows to dry fully

**Taking the Sample**

Retightens tourniquet

**Performing Venepuncture**

*Taking the Sample*

| Statement/Question | Justification | Answer | Thoughts | | | | |
|---|---|---|---|---|---|---|---|
| Just to warn you, I am about to take the sample. You should expect a sharp scratch. I know that you are afraid of needles, so please let me know if you need me to stop | It is usually good to forewarn the patient, unless they ask you not to. This patient is also needle-phobic, so it's good to acknowledge this concern | 'OK, I will let you know' | No additional concerns | | | | |
| Punctures the vein using a non-touch technique (NTT), warning the patient as above | | | | | | | |
| Collects blood in the order of draw and inverts the bottles an appropriate number of times | | | | | | | |
| Removes the tourniquet and immediately disposes of any sharps into the sharps bin at the bedside | | | | | | | |
| That is all done. Please will you press down on this cotton wool whilst I dispose of the needle | You have told the patient the procedure is finished and you are prioritising safety by disposing of the sharp | 'That's fine' | No additional concerns. You need to be sure that your patient is able to press down on the puncture site himself. Some people may not be able to and you will need to offer your assistance in this case | | | | |
| Are you allergic to tape? If not, I will just secure that cotton wool | Checking for allergies and ensuring some safety to the puncture site | 'No, I have no allergies' | No additional concerns | | | | |
| I am going to label up the blood samples by your bedside | You are labelling the bottles at the bedside to ensure they are not confused with another patient's blood bottles | 'OK' | No additional concerns | | | | |

*Finishing*

| | | | | | | | |
|---|---|---|---|---|---|---|---|
| Dispose of equipment and clean the tray, ensuring that you are adhering to the local infection control guidelines | | | | | | | |
| Please let a member of staff know if the puncture site bleeds, becomes painful or you have any concerns. You can remove the dressing after a couple of hours | It is vital to make sure the patient is aware when to call for help | 'I will do, thank you' | No additional concerns | | | | |
| Remove your gloves and wash your hands | | | | | | | |
| Explain to the examiner that you would send the samples to the pathology laboratory and chase the results | | | | | | | |

| General Points | | | |
|---|---|---|---|
| Polite to patient | | | |
| Maintains good eye contact | | | |
| Appropriate use of open and closed questions | | | |

## ❔ QUESTIONS FROM THE EXAMINER

### If you were to give yourself a needlestick injury during this procedure, what should you do?

Encourage the wound to bleed underneath a tap and wash the wound with soap and water. Contact the hospital's occupational health team or present to accident and emergency if you require urgent blood testing. Remember to follow local hospital guidelines for reporting the needlestick injury.

### What is the order of draw for taking full blood count (FBC), group and save and liver function tests (LFTs)?

LFTs, FBC, then group and save.

### What would you look for on the bloods to diagnose macrocytic anaemia and what other tests would you order afterwards?

High mean corpuscular volume and low haemoglobin would suggest macrocytic anaemia. I would also measure folate and vitamin $B_{12}$.

### What is INR and how is it calculated?

INR stands for international normalised ratio. It is a measure of the patient's prothrombin time (PT) compared to a normal PT, taking into account the type of analytical system employed so as to standardise results.

### In a patient with acute viral hepatitis A, what would you expect to see in the results?

Very raised aspartate aminotransferase/alanine aminotransferase, mildly raised gamma-glutamyl transferase, mildly raised alkaline phosphatase, positive for immunoglobulin M (IgM) anti-hepatitis A virus.

### Name three causes of hyponatraemia.

Diuretic use, adrenocortical failure, gastrointestinal losses (vomiting and diarrhoea), burns, syndrome of inappropriate antidiuretic hormone secretion, hypothyroidism, cirrhosis, congestive heart failure and nephrotic syndrome can all contribute towards hyponatraemia.

### What blood tests would you order for someone with suspected coeliac disease?

Anti-tissue transglutaminase and IgA levels.

### Name some blood tests that are analysed in the red blood bottle.

Hepatitis screening, virology, coeliac screening, CA125 and rubella serology.

### What blood tests can be ordered to help rule out a pulmonary embolism or deep-vein thrombosis?

D-dimer. If this comes back negative and risk stratification score (for example, Wells or Geneva score) is low, then we can be somewhat confident in excluding deep-vein thrombosis/pulmonary embolism.

### What is meant by 'left shift' on a blood film?

A 'left shift' refers to an increase in the number of immature white blood cells. This usually indicates that there is an infection or inflammation, and that the bone marrow is producing more white blood cells that are released into the blood before they have the chance to mature fully.

## Station 6.3   Intravenous Cannulation and Setting Up a Giving Set

### Doctor Briefing

You are the junior doctor on call and the surgical ward has contacted you to see Mrs Jones, a 50-year-old woman, who was admitted with small-bowel obstruction. She is dehydrated and requires IV fluid; however, she does not have a cannula sited. Please prepare your equipment, site an intravenous (IV) cannula and start intravenous fluids, explaining your steps to the examiner.

### Patient Briefing

You are in hospital being treated for bowel obstruction. Your stomach is distended and you have been vomiting for days. You have been told that you are listed for surgery, so you are 'nil by mouth', which the nurses explained means that you cannot eat or drink anything until after the surgery. You feel really thirsty, and your skin and mouth are both really dry. The nurses also feel that you are dehydrated so they have asked a doctor to come and put a cannula into one of your veins to give you some fluid.

You're worried that this may be really uncomfortable and you will be unable to use your arm when you have a cannula in.

### Mark Scheme for Examiner

#### Introduction

| | | | | |
|---|---|---|---|---|
| Cleans hands, introduces self and confirms patient identity | | | | |
| Establishes current patient knowledge and concerns | | | | |
| Asks for arm preference, if the patient has any allergies and whether she has any contraindications (such as lymphoedema, mastectomy, AV fistula) | | | | |

#### Explaining the Procedure

| Statement/Question | Justification | Answer | Thoughts | | | | |
|---|---|---|---|---|---|---|---|
| I would like to put a cannula into one of your veins. Have you had one of these before? | Start with a general open phrase to guide the patient | 'No, and I'm not really sure what it is' | You know that the patient is listening and has some questions | | | | |
| This involves putting a needle into a vein near the surface of your skin and then I will remove the needle but a very small piece of flexible plastic tube will be left in the vein | Important to explain the procedure in detail so that the patient knows what to expect. You need to check that the patient understands the procedure in full | 'OK, I understand' | If a patient says no, you need to decide if she has capacity and if you have given her enough information to understand what you are suggesting. This allows you to accommodate if the patient has a fear of needles | | | | |
| Then through this tube, we will be able to give you some fluids for rehydration | Important that the patient knows why the procedure is happening | 'That's fine with me' | | | | | |
| Are you on any blood-thinning medication that you know of? | Checking the patient's bleeding risk | 'No' | Make sure you fully explain the procedure | | | | |
| Sometimes, as in venepuncture, you may have bruising from the site that we insert the cannula into. There is also the chance that the first attempt misses, and I will need to reattempt at another site | It is vital to discuss complications with a patient | 'That's fine. Would I be able to use my arm afterwards?' | | | | | |

## Explaining the Procedure

| Statement/Question | Justification | Answer | Thoughts | | | | | |
|---|---|---|---|---|---|---|---|---|
| You will still be able to use your arm afterwards. Depending on where the cannula is placed, you may need to be a bit careful of the movement that you make with your arm, as the cannula may come out or become kinked, in which case we'd have to put another one in | Address any questions or concerns the patient has | 'That makes sense' | You have answered the questions | | | | | |

## Performing Cannulation

### *Equipment Checklist*

| I am just gathering the equipment I need, checking sterility and expiry dates | Explaining to the examiner you are following routine practice | 'OK' | The patient is aware you are preparing for the procedure | | | | | |
|---|---|---|---|---|---|---|---|---|

### *Preparation*

Washes hands

Cleans tray according to local policy

Assembles all equipment in the clean tray

Opens packaging and cuts tape to size

### *Preparing the Flush and the Cannula*

Cleans hands, dons non-sterile gloves and applies a single-use disposable apron

Attaches the 21G needle to the 10-mL syringe

Draws up saline and immediately discharges the needle

Expels any air and attaches the sterile bung/cap to the syringe for storage

Removes gloves and washes hands

### *Performing the Procedure*

Cleans hands, dons non-sterile gloves and applies a single-use disposable apron

Removes the cannula from its packaging and opens the sterile dressing pack

| I am just going to position your arm. Is this comfortable for you? | Important to check that the patient is comfortable throughout the procedure | 'That's fine, thank you' | No additional concerns | | | | | |
|---|---|---|---|---|---|---|---|---|
| I am going to tie a tight band around your arm for a bit to help me feel for a vein I wish to take the sample from. Is that OK? | You are warning the patient you are about to examine her | 'Fine' | No additional concerns | | | | | |

**Performing Cannulation**

*Performing the Procedure*

| Statement/Question | Justification | Answer | Thoughts | | | | | |
|---|---|---|---|---|---|---|---|---|
| Places the tourniquet 7–10 cm proximal to the proposed insertion site | | | | | | | | |
| Selects a vein. It should feel 'bouncy'. If not, it is either inadequately filled or, if rigid, it may be thrombosed | | | | | | | | |

**Loosen the tourniquet**

| Washes hands and puts on a new pair of non-sterile gloves and apron | | | | | | | | |
|---|---|---|---|---|---|---|---|---|

*Skin Preparation*

| I am now going to clean your arm. It needs a while to dry so please keep still if you can | Explaining to the patient the reason why you may not take the blood sample immediately | 'OK' | No additional concerns | | | | | |
|---|---|---|---|---|---|---|---|---|
| Cleans the site: clean for 30 s in an up-and-down, back-and-forth friction technique. Allow to dry fully | | | | | | | | |

*Taking the Sample*

| Retightens tourniquet | | | | | | | | |
|---|---|---|---|---|---|---|---|---|
| Just to warn you, I am about to insert the cannula. You should expect a sharp scratch | It is usually good to forewarn the patient, unless she asks you not to | 'No problem' | No additional concerns | | | | | |
| Inserts the cannula at approximately 45° using an NTT, warning the patient as above | | | | | | | | |
| Advances the cannula until flashback is seen, then advances the cannula further (while holding the needle in place) until it is all the way into the vein | | | | | | | | |
| Removes the tourniquet | | | | | | | | |
| Occludes the vein and cannula with firm pressure whilst removing the needle, then immediately disposes of the needle straight into the sharps bin | | | | | | | | |
| Attaches a bung/cap to the cannula, cleans any leakage of blood and applies a (prelabelled) sterile adhesive dressing | | | | | | | | |
| The cannula is in now. Please keep your arm in a comfortable position for now. Next, I will flush the cannula | You have told the patient that part of the procedure is finished and that you are moving on to the next step of the procedure | 'That's fine' | No additional concerns. Ensure that your patient doesn't make big movements with her arm while you are finishing off the procedure | | | | | |

*Flushing the Cannula*

| Removes the cap/bung from the cannula | | | | | | | | |
|---|---|---|---|---|---|---|---|---|
| Removes the cap/bung from the saline flush syringe | | | | | | | | |

**Loosen the tourniquet**

*Flushing the Cannula*

| Statement/Question | Justification | Answer | Thoughts | | | | | |
|---|---|---|---|---|---|---|---|---|
| Now I'm going to push the flush through. You might feel something cold running up the arm | Update the patient on what you are doing and what she should expect | 'OK' | No additional concerns | | | | | |
| Attaches the pre-prepared flush to the cannula and flush 1 mL at a time (up to a total of 5–10 mL) and check that the fluid does not leak into the surrounding tissues | | | | | | | | |
| Removes the syringe, replaces the cap on the cannula and immediately disposes of the syringe into the sharps bin | | | | | | | | |
| The cannula is now ready for use. Lastly, I am going to prepare the fluids that we will be giving to you through the cannula. Has everything been fine so far? | You are checking on the patient to see how she is doing and you can also address any concerns she may have | 'Yes, I'm fine' | No additional concerns | | | | | |

*Setting Up a Giving Set*

| | | | | |
|---|---|---|---|---|
| Washes hands | | | | |
| Cleans the tray according to local policy | | | | |
| Washes hands again and puts on a pair of non-sterile gloves | | | | |
| Checks the appearance and integrity of the fluid bag, and cross-checks with the examiner details, including:<br>• Type and volume of fluid on the bag match the prescription<br>• Any additives required<br>• Expiry date | | | | |
| Removes the fluid from the outer packaging and hangs it on the drip stand | | | | |
| Removes the giving set from the outer packaging and rolls the flow control wheel down to the 'off' position | | | | |
| Removes the cap from the fluid bag and exposes the trocar of the giving set. Then inserts the trocar into the fluid bag | | | | |
| Prepares the chamber of the giving set by squeezing it, then slowly opens the flow control wheel until fluid flows to the end of the line | | | | |
| Resets the flow control wheel to the closed position and hangs the fluid bag back on the drip stand | | | | |

| Everything is ready now. Are you happy for me to connect the fluids to your cannula? | You are asking the patient if she is comfortable with this and giving her autonomy | 'Yes, go ahead' | No additional concerns | | | | | |
|---|---|---|---|---|---|---|---|---|
| Removes the bung/cap from the cannula and connects the line from the giving set. Once secured, rolls the flow control wheel to the 'on' position | | | | | | | | |
| Removes gloves and washes hands | | | | | | | | |

**Finishing**

| Statement/Question | Justification | Answer | Thoughts | | | | |
|---|---|---|---|---|---|---|---|
| Disposes of equipment and clean the tray, ensuring that you are adhering to the local infection control guidelines | | | | | | | |
| *Please let a member of staff know if the puncture site becomes painful or red, or you have any concerns* | It is vital to make sure the patient is aware when to call for help | *'I will do, thank you'* | No additional concerns | | | | |
| Removes gloves and wash your hands | | | | | | | |
| Explains to the examiner that you would complete a cannula insertion record (including the date and time of start of infusion) and place it in the notes | | | | | | | |

**General Points**

| | | | | | | |
|---|---|---|---|---|---|---|
| Polite to patient | | | | | | |
| Maintains good eye contact | | | | | | |
| Appropriate use of open and closed questions | | | | | | |

## ❓ QUESTIONS FROM THE EXAMINER

**What is the smallest-gauge cannula recommended for blood transfusion?**

20-gauge can be used, but 18-gauge is preferred.

**What is the current maximum duration recommended for a peripheral cannula to remain in situ, to reduce the incidence of *Staphylococcus aureus* bacteraemia?**

Peripheral cannulas should be resited every 72–96 h.

**In an emergency, apart from IV access, what other routes are acceptable for adrenalin?**

The intraosseous (IO) route is acceptable.

**What is the maximum number of cannulation attempts that a clinician can make, after which they should seek assistance from a more senior colleague?**

It is recommended that clinicians make no more than two attempts at cannulation before seeking assistance from a more experienced clinician, or gaining IO access.

**Why should the use of steel needles for cannulation be avoided?**

Due to the risk of extravasation and needlestick injuries.

**What factors need to be taken into consideration when choosing the size of the cannula?**

Age, condition of the target vein, degree of cardiovascular stability and medical or surgical interventions.

**On the dorsal forearm, which veins are the preferred sites for cannulation?**

The basilic or cephalic veins.

**Why should the use of veins on the ventral forearm be avoided in patients with chronic kidney disease?**

These patients may need for renal dialysis, therefore you should preserve upper-extremity veins for fistula or graft implantation. For these patients, the dorsum of the hand is the recommended site of peripheral IV cannulation.

**When selecting the site for cannulation, why should you avoid areas of flexion?**

This may predispose to phlebitis due to excessive movement causing vessel wall trauma.

**How often should cannulas be reviewed?**

The insertion site of cannulas should be visually inspected hourly if there is a continuous infusion, and at least 8-hourly if there is no infusion.

## Station 6.4   Arterial Blood Gas

### Doctor Briefing

You are the junior doctor on call, and the respiratory ward has contacted you to see Mr Frederick, a 60-year-old patinet, who was admitted with infective exacerbation of chronic obstructive pulmonary disease. He is unwell with a high temperature and respiratory rate. His oxygen saturations have fallen. You are asked to do an ABG, for which he has given you verbal consent. Please prepare your equipment and complete this procedure, explaining your steps to the examiner.

### Patient Briefing

You have been admitted to hospital several times with respiratory problems. You have always been treated with oxygen and nebulisers. You cannot remember having this blood test before.

You are concerned because you don't know why you need this special test and are worried that it may mean something is seriously wrong.

### Mark Scheme for Examiner

#### Introduction

| | | | |
|---|---|---|---|
| Cleans hands, introduces self and confirms patient identity | | | |
| Establishes current patient knowledge and concerns | | | |
| Identifies current respiratory support | | | |

#### Explaining the Procedure

| Statement/Question | Justification | Answer | Thoughts | | | |
|---|---|---|---|---|---|---|
| I would like to take a blood gas sample, which allows us to identify, amongst many things, how much oxygen is in your body | Start with a general open phrase to guide the patient | 'OK. What is it?' | You know the patient is listening | | | |
| It is similar to a routine blood test, but we take blood from an artery instead of a vein | Important to reassure patients with regard to what the procedure is | 'OK' | If a patient says no, you need to decide if he has capacity and if you have given him enough information to understand what you are suggesting | | | |
| We usually take the blood sample from your wrist using a small needle. You should expect it to be more painful than a normal blood test | Check that the patient understands the procedure in full | 'That sounds fine to me' | | | | |
| Are you on any blood-thinning medications? | Check the patient's bleeding risk | 'Not that I know of' | No increased risk of bleeding | | | |
| Sometimes, as in a normal blood test, you may have some bruising at the site that we take blood from | Vital to discuss complications with the patient | 'Fine' | You have fully explained the procedure | | | |

### Explaining the Procedure

| Statement/Question | Justification | Answer | Thoughts | | | | | |
|---|---|---|---|---|---|---|---|---|
| Before I take any blood from your wrist, I just want to make sure that the blood supply to the hand is adequate, by performing a quick test | You must perform (modified) Allen's test before taking a radial arterial blood sample to check the patency of the radial and ulnar arteries | 'Sure' | If the test result is abnormal, then the radial arterial blood sampling cannot be safely performed in that hand | | | | | |

### Equipment Checklist

| | | | | | | | | |
|---|---|---|---|---|---|---|---|---|
| I am just gathering the equipment I need, checking sterility and expiry dates | Explain to the examiner you are following routine practice | 'OK' | The patient is aware you are preparing for the procedure | | | | | |

### Preparation

| | | | | |
|---|---|---|---|---|
| Decontaminates hands | | | | |
| Cleans tray according to local policy | | | | |
| Places all equipment in the clean tray | | | | |
| Opens packaging and safely attaches the needle on to the ABG syringe | | | | |

### Palpating the Radial Artery

| | | | | | | | | |
|---|---|---|---|---|---|---|---|---|
| I am just going to position your arm correctly. Is this comfortable? | Very important to check that the patient is comfortable throughout the procedure | 'That's fine, thank you' | No additional concerns | | | | | |
| Now I am going to feel for the artery I wish to take the sample from | You are warning the patient that you are about to examine him | 'Fine' | No additional concerns | | | | | |

### Skin Preparation

| | | | | | | | | |
|---|---|---|---|---|---|---|---|---|
| Please could keep your arm in that position whilst I put on gloves and an apron | Explain to the patient what you are about to do | 'Yes' | No additional concerns | | | | | |
| I am now going to clean your arm. It needs a while to dry so please keep still if you can | Explain to the patient the reason why you are not taking the blood sample immediately | 'OK' | No additional concerns | | | | | |
| Clean the site: clean for 30 s in an up-and-down, back-and-forth friction technique. Allow to dry fully | | | | | | | | |

**Taking the Sample**

| Statement/Question | Justification | Answer | Thoughts | | | | |
|---|---|---|---|---|---|---|---|
| Just to warn you, I am about to take the sample | It is usually good to fore-warn the patient, unless he asks you not to | 'OK' | No additional concerns | | | | |
| Places the index and middle fingers proximally to the puncture site by 1–2 cm. Alternatively, separates the index and middle fingers by 2–4 cm over the intended puncture site | | | | | | | |
| Holds the needle and syringe like a pencil, with the bevel up | | | | | | | |
| Inserts the needle at 45° just distal to the index finger. If using the alternative method, the needle should be inserted at 45° between the index and middle fingers | | | | | | | |
| Advances the needle into the radial artery and obtains a sample (approximately 3 mL) | | | | | | | |
| Withdraws the needle and immediately applies pressure to the puncture site using cotton wool | | | | | | | |
| That is all done now. Please can you press down on this cotton wool whilst I dispose of the needle | You have told the patient the procedure is finished and you are prioritising safety by disposing of the sharp | 'Of course' | No additional concerns. You need to be sure that your patient is able to press down on the puncture site himself. Some people may not be able to | | | | |
| Disposes of equipment and clean the tray, ensuring that you are adhering to the local infection control guidelines | | | | | | | |
| Are you allergic to tape? If not, I will secure the cotton wool | You are checking for allergies and ensuring safety to the puncture site | 'No, not allergic to anything as far as I know' | No additional concerns | | | | |

**Finishing**

| | | | | | | | |
|---|---|---|---|---|---|---|---|
| I am going to process this sample now; the results come back very quickly | You have explained to the patient the timeline for getting the results | 'Thank you' | No additional concerns | | | | |
| Please let a member of staff know if the puncture site bleeds, becomes painful or you have any concerns. You can remove the dressing after a couple of hours | Vital to ensure that the patient is aware of when to call for help | 'I will do, thank you' | No additional concerns | | | | |
| Removes gloves and washes hands once the sample has been processed | | | | | | | |
| Documents the procedure and findings in the notes | | | | | | | |

| **General Points** | | | | |
|---|---|---|---|---|
| Polite to patient | | | | |
| Maintains good eye contact | | | | |
| Appropriate use of open and closed questions | | | | |

## ❓ QUESTIONS FROM THE EXAMINER

### What are the indications for performing an ABG puncture?

Assessment of acid–base balance, oxygenation status or ventilator status, or if you need to check electrolyte or haemoglobin levels quickly.

### Can you use local anaesthetic (LA) before taking the ABG puncture?

Yes. Some people choose to infiltrate the superficial skin with LA before taking the sample, to aid with pain relief.

### How does profuse vomiting lead to metabolic alkalosis?

When people vomit excessively, they can lose a significant amount of stomach acid, which results in a net loss of hydrogen ions. This means that there is less hydrogen ion available for bicarbonate ions to bind to. Volume depletion also triggers the release of hormones and corticosteroids, which increase the reabsorption of bicarbonate ions by the kidneys. Overall, there is a greater amount of free bicarbonate ion, which explains the metabolic alkalosis.

### What are the signs and symptoms of hypercapnoea (high carbon dioxide level)?

Hypercapnoea can be associated with confusion, reduced consciousness level, asterixis and a bounding pulse.

### Why does sepsis usually present as metabolic acidosis?

In severe cases of sepsis, the patient may suffer from reduced end-organ perfusion, resulting in tissue hypoxia, which forces the cells to respire anaerobically to generate energy. Lactic acid is a by-product of anaerobic respiration; therefore there is a greater amount of acid in the patient's blood, leading to metabolic acidosis.

### How does hyperventilation lead to perioral and peripheral paraesthesia?

Hyperventilation usually presents with respiratory alkalosis. When serum blood becomes more alkalotic, the bound hydrogen ions unbind from serum albumin, resulting in more albumin for ionised calcium to bind to, which in turn decreases the level of freely ionised calcium. Hypocalcemia is the cause of paraesthesia often seen with hyperventilation.

### Why does diabetic ketoacidosis (DKA) usually present as a metabolic acidosis?

DKA occurs secondary to a lack of insulin in the body. Glucose cannot be accessed, therefore the body finds another energy source by breaking down adipose tissue and converting fatty acids into ketone bodies. The ketone bodies make the blood more acidic, leading to metabolic acidosis.

### Can any peripheral artery be used for an ABG?

Technically yes, any peripheral artery that you can access will provide the same results.

### Can you perform a venous blood gas (VBG) instead of an ABG?

No, not always. The VBG can give you useful information regarding the pH, lactate and electrolytes but will not tell you specifically about ventilation and oxygenation.

### Is a venous gas as accurate?

No, be cautious when using the VBG to assess electrolytes as they can be deranged. For example, haemolysis can cause high K levels.

## Station 6.5   Male Urethral Catheterisation

### Doctor Briefing

You are the junior doctor on call, and the surgical ward has contacted you to see Mr Miller, a 70-year-old man, who was admitted with abdominal pain and an inability to pass urine. Following an examination, you diagnose acute urinary retention. He has given you verbal consent for catheterisation. Please prepare your equipment and complete this procedure, explaining your steps to the examiner.

### Patient Briefing

You have been admitted to hospital after you started experiencing lower tummy pain and have not been able to pass urine for the entire day. You've also noticed that your lower belly appears slightly bloated. One of the doctors has come to examine you and told you that you've got urinary retention, which is a condition where you cannot empty your bladder completely. The doctor wants to put a catheter in, but you've never had this done before.

You are concerned because you are in a lot of pain and are worried that the procedure that the doctor is going to do will make the pain worse.

### Mark Scheme for Examiner

#### Introduction

| | | | | | |
|---|---|---|---|---|---|
| Cleans hands, introduces self and confirms patient identity | | | | | |
| Establishes current patient knowledge and concerns | | | | | |
| Positions the patient and provides him with a blanket to maintain dignity | | | | | |
| Asks for a chaperone/assistant | | | | | |
| Selects appropriate catheter | | | | | |

#### Explaining the Procedure

| Statement/Question | Justification | Answer | Thoughts | | | |
|---|---|---|---|---|---|---|
| A catheter is a flexible plastic tube that is inserted through the urethra at the tip of the penis and goes directly into your bladder | Start with a general open phrase to guide the patient | 'OK' | No initial concerns on process being explained | | | |
| The reason we are doing this is because you are in acute urinary retention, which means that your bladder cannot empty completely and is filling up with urine | Important to explain the purpose of the procedure and to obtain consent | 'OK' | If a patient says no, you need to decide if he has capacity and if you have given him enough information to understand what you are suggesting | | | |
| Hopefully this will help to ease the abdominal pain you are having | You need to check that the patient understands the procedure in full | 'That sounds good to me' | | | | |
| There will be another member of staff present, who will act as a chaperone/assistant | You need to make the patient aware that someone else will be in the room as well during the procedure | 'I'm happy with that but I'm worried that it will be really sore having this done' | | | | |

## Explaining the Procedure

| Statement/Question | Justification | Answer | Thoughts | | | | |
|---|---|---|---|---|---|---|---|
| It may be uncomfortable, but it should be a quick procedure. The main risks are trauma and infection, but we will regularly monitor and review the catheter once it is in situ | It is vital to discuss potential complications with a patient and explain how we will minimise the risk | 'Fine' | Make sure you fully explain the procedure | | | | |

## Performing Catheterisation

### Equipment Checklist

| | | | | | | | |
|---|---|---|---|---|---|---|---|
| I am gathering the equipment I need, checking sterility and expiry dates | Explaining to the examiner you are following routine practice | 'OK' | The patient is aware you are preparing for the procedure | | | | |

### Preparation

| | | | | |
|---|---|---|---|---|
| Decontaminates hands | | | | |
| Cleans tray according to local policy | | | | |
| Assembles all equipment in the clean tray | | | | |

### Preparing the Procedure Trolley

| | | | | |
|---|---|---|---|---|
| Washes hands | | | | |
| Cleans the trolley according to trust policy | | | | |
| Places the sharps bin on the bottom of the trolley | | | | |
| Attaches the disposable rubbish bag to the side of the trolley | | | | |
| Opens the catheterisation pack using an NTT | | | | |
| Using an NTT, opens the outer packing and drops the LA gel, gloves and catheter on to the aseptic field | | | | |
| If sterile water is pre-drawn, then drops this on the aseptic field as well. If not provided with the catheter set, draws up 10 mL sterile water using a green needle and immediately disposes of the sharp into the sharps bin | | | | |
| Opens the packaging of the catheter bag | | | | |

### Prepare the Patient

| | | | | | | | |
|---|---|---|---|---|---|---|---|
| Takes trolley to the bedside | | | | | | | |
| Please can I ask you to put this pad under your bottom? | This is to ensure that urine does not leak on to the patient's bed | 'Sure' | No additional concerns | | | | |

**Performing Catheterisation**

*Prepare the Patient*

| Statement/Question | Justification | Answer | Thoughts | | | | | |
|---|---|---|---|---|---|---|---|---|
| Now that I've got everything ready, I would like to prepare you properly for the procedure. Please can you lie down flat and keep this blanket over you until I ask you to remove it | Ensure that the patient is correctly positioned and keep him covered until just before the procedure to maintain patient dignity | 'OK' | No additional concerns | | | | | |
| Washes hands, puts on a single-use apron and pair of sterile gloves | | | | | | | | |
| Is it OK for my assistant to remove your blanket now, exposing you from belly button to knee? | For such procedures we must ensure that we maintain the patient's dignity and respect his consent/autonomy throughout | 'Go ahead' | Ask your assistant to expose the patient from umbilicus to knees | | | | | |
| Places a sterile drape with a central hole over the penis, leaving the penis exposed | | | | | | | | |

*Asepsis and Anaesthesia*

| | | | | | | | | |
|---|---|---|---|---|---|---|---|---|
| Asks assistant to empty the sterile water sachets into a plastic pot on the trolley, then soaks the swabs with water | | | | | | | | |
| I am now going to gently position your penis with one of my hands and clean it with cotton wool with the other hand. Then, I am going to put some anaesthetic gel into the penis to make the procedure less uncomfortable | Always ensure that a patient is aware of what you are doing next, especially when handling such an intimate area | 'That's fine' | The patient is aware of the indication | | | | | |
| Holds the penis with the non-dominant hand and retracts the prepuce/foreskin *This hand is contaminated and should now not touch the aseptic trolley* | | | | | | | | |
| With the dominant hand, cleans the penis in circles, beginning at the urethra and moving progressively outwards. Repeats this at least three times | | | | | | | | |
| Disposes of the swabs in the disposable rubbish bag | | | | | | | | |
| Warns the patient again as above, and with the non-dominant hand, applies some upwards traction to the penis and administers the entire LA gel syringe into the urethral meatus, using the dominant hand | | | | | | | | |
| Leaves the gel for 5 min to take effect | | | | | | | | |
| Removes gloves, washes hands and puts on a second pair of sterile gloves | | | | | | | | |

## Performing Catheterisation

### Inserting the Catheter

| Statement/Question | Justification | Answer | Thoughts | | | | |
|---|---|---|---|---|---|---|---|
| Please put this dish between your legs. It's to catch the urine that comes out from the catheter | Explaining to the patient the reason why you need to put the dish there will help him to understand the process | 'OK' | No additional concerns | | | | |
| Now I am going to insert the catheter. It may be a bit uncomfortable, but please bear with me for a few moments. If you really want me to stop, then please let me know. Is that OK? | You are warning the patient of the next step and giving the patient his autonomy | 'Sure' | No additional concerns | | | | |
| Holds the base of the penis with the non-dominant hand and applies gentle upward traction | | | | | | | |
| Holds the catheter between the thumb and the forefinger of the dominant hand. Gently inserts the catheter into the urethral meatus using a NNT but touching only the packaging | | | | | | | |
| Advances the catheter using steady and gentle pressure, until urine is seen, then advances the catheter by a further 2–3 cm | | | | | | | |
| Attaches the sterile water syringe to the balloon port of the catheter and inserts 10 mL slowly. Stops if there is pain or high resistance | | | | | | | |
| Attaches the catheter to the catheter bag | | | | | | | |
| Replaces the prepuce | | | | | | | |
| If there is a leg bag, attaches this to the patient. If there are larger collection bags, then attaches this to the patient's bed | | | | | | | |
| Cleans the patient, removes the incontinence pad, drape and replaces the blanket | | | | | | | |
| Disposes of waste and gloves, then washes hands | | | | | | | |
| Cleans the trolley, then washes hands again | | | | | | | |

### Finishing

| | | | | | | | |
|---|---|---|---|---|---|---|---|
| That is all done and you can now get dressed again. Do you need any help with that? | You have told the patient the procedure is finished and given the patient privacy to get dressed again | 'I'll be fine, thank you' | No additional concerns | | | | |
| Please let a member of staff know if you have any concerns about the catheter or the catheter bag | It is vital to make sure the patient is aware when to call for help and remember to inform a member of the nursing staff that the patient now has a urinary catheter in situ | 'I will do, thank you' | No new concerns at present | | | | |
| Explains to the examiner that you would document the procedure in the notes | | | | | | | |

| General Points | | | | |
|---|---|---|---|---|
| Polite to patient, continually talking to patient throughout the procedure | | | | |
| Maintains good eye contact | | | | |
| Appropriate use of open and closed questions | | | | |
| Avoided patient contamination by using NTT throughout | | | | |
| Disposes of all sharps immediately | | | | |

## ❓ QUESTIONS FROM THE EXAMINER

### How much urine can a bladder typically hold?

300–500 mL.

### What is paraphimosis?

Paraphimosis is when the retracted foreskin is unable to be replaced over the head of the penis.

### What is the difference between paraphimosis and phimosis?

Paraphimosis is when the retracted foreskin is unable to be replaced over the head of the penis, which is a urological emergency. Phimosis is when the foreskin cannot be retracted from the tip of the penis, and this rarely requires emergency intervention.

### What is the minimum urine output that you should expect?

0.5 mL/kg/h.

### Define priapism.

Priapism is persistent painful erection (longer than 4 h) in the absence of sexual desire.

### Define hypospadias.

Hypospadias is when the urethra meatus opens on the ventral aspect of the penile shaft, at a point proximal to the normal site.

### Why might bladder spasms occur in a patient with a catheter in situ?

Bladder spasms occur when the smooth muscle of the bladder contracts and does not allow for complete expansion of the bladder as it fills with urine. It can be due to a urinary tract infection (UTI), traction on the bladder neck, a blocked catheter or irritation from the balloon holding the catheter in place.

### What is the difference between an indwelling catheter and an intermittent catheter?

Both catheters are inserted in the same way, but an indwelling catheter is left in place (usually changed every 3 months), whereas an intermittent catheter is removed immediately after the bladder has been emptied on that single occasion.

### Why is a non-distended bladder a contraindication to suprapubic cystostomy being performed via a percutaneous approach?

A non-distended bladder puts the patient at significant risk of inadvertent bowel or vascular injury.

### Three-way catheters have three channels. What is the purpose of each of them?

One is used for each of the following purposes: inflation of the balloon, urine drainage and irrigation.

## Station 6.6    Urinalysis

### Doctor Briefing

You are the junior doctor in primary care. Your next patient is Mrs Manpreet, a 35-year-old woman, who presents with abdominal pain and vomiting. She has been going to the toilet more often than normal and is concerned that her urine is foul-smelling. She has brought a urine sample with her. Please prepare your equipment, perform a urine dipstick and then discuss the results with her.

### Patient Briefing

Over the past week, you have been going to the toilet more often than normal, including in the middle of the night. You've noted that your urine looks darker and is foul-smelling. A couple of days ago, you started getting tummy pain and vomited on one occasion. Therefore, you have come to see your primary care physician today.

You are concerned because you've had similar symptoms before and needed antibiotics for a waterworks infection.

### Mark Scheme for Examiner

#### Introduction

| | | | | |
|---|---|---|---|---|
| Cleans hands, introduces self and confirms patient identity | | | | |
| Establishes current patient knowledge and concerns | | | | |

#### Explaining the Procedure

| Statement/Question | Justification | Answer | Thoughts | | | |
|---|---|---|---|---|---|---|
| If it's OK with you, I would like to take your urine sample and dip an agent strip into it in order to find out more about the substances present in your urine | Start with a general open phrase to guide the patient | 'That's fine' | You know the patient is listening | | | |
| Ideally this should be a fresh, midstream urine sample | Important to confirm for the accuracy of results | 'Yes, I did it just before I came here' | If you are concerned about the urine sample, ask the patient to provide you with another one and give her instructions on obtaining a midstream urine sample if required | | | |
| The reason we are doing this is because your symptoms could be due to an infection, so this test will provide us with more information | Important to explain the purpose of the procedure and to obtain consent | 'I understand. I have had something like this before' | The patient is aware of the indication | | | |

#### Equipment Checklist

| | | | | | | |
|---|---|---|---|---|---|---|
| I am just gathering the equipment I need, checking sterility and expiry dates | Explaining to the examiner you are following routine practice | 'OK' | The patient is aware you are preparing for the procedure | | | |
| Decontaminates hands | | | | | | |
| Places all equipment in tray | | | | | | |
| Checks expiry date of reagent sticks | | | | | | |

**Performing Urine Dipstick**

| Statement/Question | Justification | Answer | Thoughts | | | | |
|---|---|---|---|---|---|---|---|
| I am going to start by making some general observation points about the urine sample, then I will dip one of the reagent strips into the sample | Always ensure that the patient is aware of what you are doing next | 'Go ahead' | No additional concerns | | | | |
| Inspects sample | | | | | | | |
| Removes cap and notes odour | | | | | | | |
| Removes a single dipstick from container and dips the urine for 2–3 s | | | | | | | |
| Places dipstick on a flat surface and leaves for specified time | | | | | | | |

**Interpreting the Urine Dipstick**

| | | | | | | | |
|---|---|---|---|---|---|---|---|
| Uses the colour chart of dipstick container to analyse results | | | | | | | |
| Comments on each component of the urine dipstick result (blood, ketones, nitrites, leukocytes, protein, glucose, specific gravity and pH) | | | | | | | |

**Finishing**

| | | | | | | | |
|---|---|---|---|---|---|---|---|
| The test has been completed. Your urine does seem to suggest that you have a waterworks infection. We can treat this with antibiotics | You have explained to the patient the results and treatment options | 'Thank you' | No additional concerns | | | | |
| Is it OK if we send the sample to the laboratory for further analysis? | Important to gain consent before sending samples to the laboratory | 'Of course' | If the urine is clear, then it can be disposed of into the sluice | | | | |
| Please let a member of staff know if your symptoms persist once you have completed your course of antibiotics | It is vital to make sure the patient is aware when to call for help | 'I will do, thank you' | Safety net advice provided to the patient | | | | |
| Removes gloves and washes hands | | | | | | | |
| Disposes of equipment and cleans work surface | | | | | | | |
| Documents the procedure and findings in the notes | | | | | | | |

**General Points**

| | | | | | | | |
|---|---|---|---|---|---|---|---|
| Polite to patient | | | | | | | |
| Maintains good eye contact | | | | | | | |
| Appropriate use of open and closed questions | | | | | | | |

## ❓ QUESTIONS FROM THE EXAMINER

**On examining a patient with cystitis, what sign might you elicit when examining the abdomen?**

Suprapubic tenderness.

**Why are women more prone to UTIs than men?**

In females, the urethra is relatively short (3 cm) compared to that of males.

**In acute uncomplicated UTIs, what is the most common pathogen?**

*Escherichia coli* accounts for up to 80% of all UTIs.

**Name three pathogens that could be responsible for a complicated UTI.**

*Pseudomonas aeruginosa, Staphylococcus epidermidis, Klebsiella, Enterobacter* and *Proteus*.

**If the urine sample has a faeculent smell or appearance, what may this suggest?**

Colovesical fistula or a contaminated sample.

**If you were concerned about bladder malignancy, what investigation would you consider performing?**

Cystoscopy.

**What does 'pyuria' mean?**

White blood cells present in the urine.

**The urine dipstick is most sensitive for which ketone?**

Acetoacetic acid.

**Name two causes of ketonuria.**

DKA, alcoholic ketoacidosis and starvation ketosis.

**How does multiple myeloma lead to proteinuria?**

In multiple myeloma, an excess of paraprotein is filtered through the glomerulus and overloads the filtering capacity of the kidneys.

## Station 6.7   Instruments

### Doctor Briefing

On this table are a number of instruments. Please take each one in turn, tell me its name and what you know about it.

### Mark Scheme for Examiner

| | | | | |
|---|---|---|---|---|
| Cleans hands, introduces self | | | | |
| Correctly names the instrument | | | | |
| Clearly gives indication for use | | | | |
| Gives description of how to use instrument | | | | |
| Lists potential complications (at least three) from the use of the instrument | | | | |
| Gives contraindications to the use of the instrument | | | | |

#### Oropharyngeal/Gueduel Airway

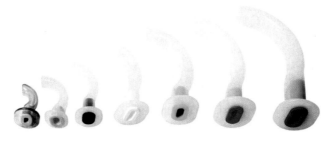

**Fig. 6.1** Oropharyngeal airway.

| | | | | | |
|---|---|---|---|---|---|
| Name | This is an oropharyngeal/Guedel airway. It is an example of a non-definitive airway adjunct | | | | |
| Indication | It is used to maintain a patent airway in an unconscious patient to facilitate ventilation | | | | |
| How to use the instrument | The correct size is chosen by measuring the distance from the incisors to the angle of the mandible. It is then held with two forefingers and a thumb at the thick plastic attached to the oval disc. During insertion, the Guedel airway is held in a position where the spout points towards the operator and the bend in the device is away from the operator. The device is rotated 180° as it descends past the hard palate. The approach reduces the risk of pushing the tongue backwards | | | | |
| Complications | Complications include trauma to the oropharynx, upper-airway obstruction and stimulation of the gag reflex, resulting in vomiting | | | | |
| Contraindications | Contraindications include active airway reflexes and active bleeding | | | | |

**Endotracheal Tube**

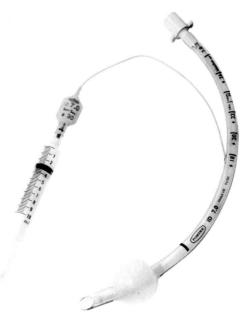

Fig. 6.2 Endotracheal tube.

| | |
|---|---|
| Name | This is a cuffed endotracheal tube and is an example of a definitive airway |
| Indication | It is used in anaesthetics and in intensive care patients during intubation and ventilation of unconscious patients |
| How to use the instrument | It is inserted into the trachea under direct vision using a laryngoscope to identify the glottis. After insertion the balloon cuff is inflated with the use of air and a syringe to keep the tube in place, and to prevent aspiration of gastric contents into the respiratory tract |
| Complications | Complications include tube misplacement, trauma to teeth, gums or lips, pulmonary aspiration of gastric contents, oesophageal or tracheal perforation, subglottic stenosis and vocal cord paralysis |
| Contraindications | Contraindications include cervical spine injury |

**Nasogastric Tube**

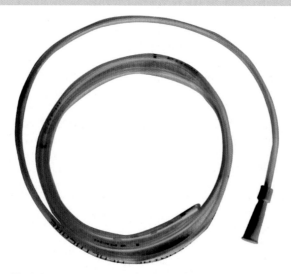

Fig. 6.3 Nasogastric tube.

| Name | This is a nasogastric (NG) tube: there are fine and wide-bore types |
|---|---|
| Indication | Fine-bore NG tubes are typically used for enteral feeding. Wide-bore NG tubes are typically used to provide gastric decompression in patients with bowel obstruction or following upper gastrointestinal surgery |
| How to use the instrument | The distance required to insert the tube is sized by measuring the distance of the tube from the nostril to the xiphisternum, passing via the tragus of the ear. The leading 10 cm is lubricated and advanced along the base of the nasal cavity in an upright patient. The patient is asked to sip water using a straw when the tube reaches the posterior pharynx. Drinking helps the introduction of the tube into the oesophagus. The tube is inserted the sized distance and then a little more to ensure correct positioning. Position is confirmed by testing some aspirate with pH paper and taking a chest X-ray |
| Complications | Complications include damage to the nasal turbinates and malposition |
| Contraindications | Contraindications include base-of-skull fracture, severe mid-face trauma, recent nasal surgery, oesophageal varices, oesophageal obstruction and coagulation abnormalities |

## Bag Valve Mask

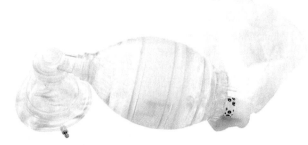

Fig. 6.4 Bag valve mask.

| Name | This is a bag valve mask |
|---|---|
| Indication | It is used to provide positive-pressure ventilation. It is used to oxygenate and ventilate patients who are not breathing or breathing inadequately |
| How to use the instrument | The bag valve mask can be connected to oxygen but also works independently and is self-filling. The mask is triangular in shape and its tip should be placed just over the bridge of the patient's nose. The larger portion of the mask should be placed between the lower lips and the chin to provide a good seal. Although one person can operate the device, it is better with two – one person holding the mask in place and the other squeezing the bag to provide ventilation |
| Complications | Complications include aspiration, hypoventilation and hyperventilation |
| Contraindications | Contraindications include complete upper-airway obstruction and facial fractures |

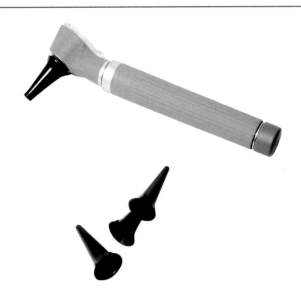

**Fig. 6.5** Otoscope.

| | |
|---|---|
| Name | This is an otoscope, of which there are four different types: direct, indirect, pneumatic and operating |
| Indication | It is used to examine the external auditory canal and tympanic membrane |
| How to use the instrument | It is typically held in the same hand as the side of the face that the ear is on. It is held in the same way as a pen, with the fingers placed on its neck next to the eyepiece and the speculum facing away from the operator. After activating the light source and inspecting the external auditory canal and surrounding areas, the pinna is manually retracted superiorly and posteriorly with the other hand. The otoscope is gently introduced into the ear canal |
| Complications | Complications include trauma to the ear canal |
| Contraindications | There are no contraindications |

## ❓ QUESTIONS FROM THE EXAMINER

**Which laparoscopic port site is most associated with complications?**

The umbilical port.

**What is a proctoscope used for?**

A proctoscope is a hollow tube used to examine the inside of the rectum and anus (proctoscopy).

**Which veins are most commonly used for central line placement?**

The internal jugular, femoral and subclavian veins.

**Why is the Sim's speculum preferred over the Cusco's speculum for gynaecological surgeries?**

The Sim's speculum is inserted into the vagina to retract the posterior vaginal wall, allowing for greater visualisation of the vaginal walls.

## What is the Pipelle tube used for?

The Pipelle tube is used to obtain biopsy samples for the endometrium, most commonly to investigate for endometrial cancer in women who present with postmenopausal bleeding.

## Which sigmoidoscope is longer – the rigid or the flexible?

A flexible sigmoidoscope (approximately 60 cm long) is longer than a rigid sigmoidoscope (approximately 25 cm long) and can therefore reach further.

## Why is the ventouse not suitable if the patient is less than 34 weeks' gestation?

Babies who are premature have a softer head and if the ventouse is attached and pulled, there is an increased risk of bruising, brain haemorrhage and jaundice.

## Why are dynamic hip screws designed to be sliding?

Historically, fixed plates matched the angle of the femoral head. However, they did not allow any compression across the fracture site, resulting in stress failures and frequent non-union. Therefore, dynamic hip screws with sliding barrels were designed to allow for controlled compression across the fracture site, which is vital for bone healing.

## Why is it difficult for patients with a tracheostomy to generate speech and what solution can be offered?

Speech is generated when air passes over the vocal cords at the back of the throat, but when a tracheostomy is in situ, most of the air breathed out passes through the tracheostomy tube instead of over the vocal cords. One method to overcome this is to use a speaking valve, which is a temporary attachment to the end of the tracheostomy, to prevent the leakage of air out of it.

## What is Swan-Ganz catheterisation?

Swan-Ganz catheterisation is also known as right-heart catheterisation or pulmonary artery catheterisation. It is when a catheter is passed into the right side of the heart and into the pulmonary arteries.

## Station 6.8   Suturing

### Doctor Briefing

You are a junior doctor in the ED. You have been asked to see Mr Harrison, a 27-year-old man, who has a small wound to his right forearm that requires suturing. Please prepare your equipment and complete this procedure, explaining your steps to the examiner.

### Patient Briefing

You have come to the ED because you injured yourself when you were doing some housework this evening. On your right forearm, you have a small open wound, and the doctor has examined it. He/she has told you that it is too big to close with glue or Steri-Strips, therefore it will need stitching, which you have never had before. The wound is not bleeding at the moment. As far as you are aware, there is no foreign body inside the wound. You have all feeling in your fingers and can move them freely. You have not got any other wounds.

You do not have any allergies.

You are concerned because you are scared that the suturing is going to hurt and that it will leave a huge ugly scar.

### Mark Scheme for Examiner

#### Introduction

| | | | | |
|---|---|---|---|---|
| Cleans hands, introduces self and confirms patient identity | | | | |
| Establishes current patient knowledge and concerns | | | | |
| Assesses the wound and neurovascular supply and determines if senior involvement or plastic surgery referral is warranted | | | | |

#### Explaining the Procedure

| Statement/Question | Justification | Answer | Thoughts | | | | |
|---|---|---|---|---|---|---|---|
| *Your wound requires suturing, which is when we use a needle and a piece of thread-like material to close your wound up. Have you had this done before?* | Start with a general explanation and establish if the patient has previously had sutures | 'No, I've never had it before, and it sounds quite scary' | You know the patient is listening | | | | |
| *Some people describe it as being comparable to sewing the wound up. Before I suture, I will apply LA at the wound site to numb the area so that the procedure is not painful* | You need to check that the patient understands the procedure in full | 'That sounds fine to me' | If a patient says no, you need to decide if he has capacity and if you have given him enough information to understand what you are suggesting | | | | |
| *After suturing, there is the possibility that your wound might reopen, get infected and there could be a residual scar* | It is vital to discuss complications with a patient, especially as this patient is worried about the development of a scar. This needs to be explicitly warned about prior to suturing | 'I'm a bit worried about the scar' | You should address any questions or concerns that the patient has | | | | |
| *I'll do my best to make the suture as small as possible. If I take smaller gaps and you keep it clean afterwards, the wound usually heals nicely* | Address any questions or concerns that the patient has | 'I appreciate that, thank you' | You have answered the questions | | | | |

## Suturing

### Equipment Checklist

| Statement/Question | Justification | Answer | Thoughts | | | | | | |
|---|---|---|---|---|---|---|---|---|---|
| I am just gathering the equipment I need, checking sterility and expiry dates | Explaining to the examiner you are following routine practice | 'OK' | The patient is aware you are preparing for the procedure | | | | | | |
| Decontaminates hands | | | | | | | | | |
| Cleans tray according to local policy | | | | | | | | | |
| Places all equipment in tray | | | | | | | | | |

### Wound Preparation and Local Anaesthetic Administration

| | | | | | | | | | |
|---|---|---|---|---|---|---|---|---|---|
| I am going to clean your wound and apply some LA. Do you have any allergies? | Important to establish the patient's allergy status before administering medication | 'Not that I know of' | No additional concerns | | | | | | |
| Washes hands and puts on a single-use apron and pair of sterile gloves | | | | | | | | | |
| Removes any large visible debris from the wound | | | | | | | | | |
| Soaks the gauzes in sterile water and uses them to clean the wound gently | | | | | | | | | |
| Checks the LA dose and expiry date with a second person | | | | | | | | | |
| Draws up 5 mL of LA into the syringe using the 21G needle | | | | | | | | | |
| Detaches the 21G needle without resheathing it and immediately discards it into the sharps bin | | | | | | | | | |
| Now I am going to inject the LA around the wound, it might sting a bit at the start but then the area should feel numb | Important to inform the patient what you are doing at each stage and prepare him for the LA | 'No problem' | No additional concerns | | | | | | |
| Attaches the 25G needle to the syringe and inject the LA subcutaneously, using the 'aspirate and filtrate' technique to ensure that LA is not administered IV | | | | | | | | | |
| Waits 5–10 min for LA to take effect, then tests it with the forceps | | | | | | | | | |
| Cleans the wound again with gauze soaked in iodine solution | | | | | | | | | |
| Dries the wound with clean gauze | | | | | | | | | |
| Removes the first pair of sterile gloves | | | | | | | | | |

### Suturing

| | | | | | | | | | |
|---|---|---|---|---|---|---|---|---|---|
| I am going to position your arm to get it ready for suturing. Is this comfortable? | Suturing can take a long time, therefore it is essential that the patient is comfortable throughout the procedure | 'Yes' | No additional concerns | | | | | | |

## Suturing

| Statement/Question | Justification | Answer | Thoughts | | | | | |
|---|---|---|---|---|---|---|---|---|
| Dons a new pair of sterile gloves | | | | | | | | |
| *Just to warn you, I am about to start suturing now* | It is usually good to fore-warn the patient, unless he asks you not to | 'OK' | No additional concerns | | | | | |
| Inserts the needle perpendicular to the skin at 5 mm from the wound edge, advances the needle through the wound in a circular arc and exits in the middle of the wound | | | | | | | | |
| Reinserts the needle in the middle of the wound, exiting 5 mm from the wound edge | | | | | | | | |
| Ties three surgical knots and ensure that they are not lying over the wound | | | | | | | | |
| Cuts the ends of the suture, leaving 5 mm on each end | | | | | | | | |
| Repeats the suturing and knot-tying steps down the wound, with 5–10-mm gaps, until the entire wound is closed | | | | | | | | |
| Immediately disposes of the needle into the sharps bin when suturing is finished | | | | | | | | |
| Removes gloves and washes hands | | | | | | | | |

## Finishing

| | | | | | | | | |
|---|---|---|---|---|---|---|---|---|
| *I have finished the suturing now and will apply a dressing over the wound. The sutures are non-dissolvable therefore they need to be removed in 7–14 days. Remember to keep the wound dry in the meantime* | You have explained to the patient the aftercare for the wound | 'Thank you' | No additional concerns | | | | | |
| *Look out for signs of infection, including redness, soreness, discharge or swelling at the wound site* | It is vital to make sure the patient is aware when to call for help | 'I will do' | | | | | | |
| *When was your last tetanus vaccination?* | Consider administering a tetanus booster if the patient has not had one in the past 10 years or if the wound is contaminated | 'I can't remember' | Consult trust and/or national guidelines or speak to a senior for advice | | | | | |
| Documents the procedure and findings in the notes | | | | | | | | |

## General Points

| | | | | | | | | |
|---|---|---|---|---|---|---|---|---|
| Polite to patient | | | | | | | | |
| Maintains good eye contact | | | | | | | | |
| Appropriate use of open and closed questions | | | | | | | | |
| Never handles the needle with own hands | | | | | | | | |

## ❓ QUESTIONS FROM THE EXAMINER

### What is a fasciotomy, and when would you use it?

Fasciotomy is surgery to relieve swelling and pressure in a compartment of the body, such as in compartment syndrome.

### What is meant by asepsis?

Asepsis is the absence of microorganisms, such as pathogenic bacteria, viruses, fungi and parasites.

### What are the stages of wound healing?

Haemostasis, inflammation, proliferation and remodelling.

### How many types of wound healing are there and what are they?

There are three main types of wound healing: primary, secondary and tertiary.

### What is the definition of a 'chronic wound' and how do they normally present?

A wound that has failed to heal in 4 weeks is defined as a chronic wound and most commonly it is an ulcer.

### What are the four main classifications of chronic wounds outlined by the Wound Healing Society?

Pressure ulcers, diabetic foot ulcers, venous ulcers and arterial insufficiency ulcers.

### Name three factors that can affect wound healing.

Infection, ischaemia, lack of oxygenation, age, metabolic conditions, immunosuppression, smoking and malnutrition.

### When should X-rays be performed when a patient presents with a wound?

If there is suspicion of a fracture or foreign body.

### How does the number prefix of the suture thread relate to its diameter?

The larger the number prefix, the smaller the diameter of the thread.

### What are the most common reasons for using steel sutures?

Although not one of the most commonly used suture materials, steel still plays a role in orthopaedic surgeries (such as for cerclage and tendon repairs) and in the closure of the sternum.

# Obstetrics and Gynaecology

# 7

## Outline

## Station 7.1   History: Headache in Pregnancy

### Doctor Briefing

You are a junior doctor on labour ward and have been asked to see Leanne Jones, a 36-year-old woman who has presented with a headache. She is 36 weeks pregnant. Please take a history from Miss Jones, present your findings and formulate an appropriate management plan.

### Patient Briefing

You are a 36-year-old woman, in your first pregnancy. You have come to the labour ward because you have been experiencing a severe headache. The pain is on both sides of your head and feels like it is pulsing. Your vision is normal, and you are not sensitive to light. You have tried paracetamol at home, but this has not helped. You have no nausea, vomiting or weakness, but you do have some upper abdominal discomfort.

You have had an uncomplicated pregnancy so far and have not needed any growth scans. You have no medical problems and no family history of note. Your baby is moving normally.

You live with your husband, who is supportive, and you don't smoke.

You are concerned because you don't know what is causing the headache, and you are scared you have developed pre-eclampsia and that your baby will be affected.

### Mark Scheme for Examiner

| Introduction | | | | | |
|---|---|---|---|---|---|
| Cleans hands, introduces self, confirms patient identity and gains consent for history taking | | | | | |
| Establishes current patient knowledge and concerns | | | | | |

## History of Presenting Complaint

| Question | Justification | Answer | Thoughts | | | | | | |
|---|---|---|---|---|---|---|---|---|---|
| When did you first notice the headache, and has it happened before? | This helps to determine if this is acute or chronic. A headache that has been present in early pregnancy or before conception will not be pre-eclampsia | 'It started a few hours ago, I've never felt anything like it' | A bit concerning, as new-onset headache in pregnancy can be caused by serious pathology | | | | | | |
| Where in your head is the pain worst? | A sudden-onset occipital headache could suggest subarachnoid haemorrhage | 'I can feel it on both sides of my head' | More consistent with pre-eclampsia | | | | | | |
| What does the pain feel like? | A pulsing headache may suggest migraine or pre-eclampsia; a tight headache may be tension | 'It feels like it is pulsing in my head' | | | | | | | |
| Do you feel like the light is hurting your eyes? | Photophobia can suggest migraine or meningeal irritation | 'No, I just want it to go away' | No additional concerns | | | | | | |
| Can you think of anything that might have brought it on? | To assess if there are any specific triggers | 'I've been very busy at work today, and might not have eaten much' | No additional concerns | | | | | | |
| Do you have any pain at the top of your tummy or vision changes? | Classical symptoms of pre-eclampsia | 'The top of my tummy feels uncomfortable' | Could point to pre-eclampsia | | | | | | |
| Does your neck hurt or feel stiff? | Important to elicit signs of meningeal irritation | 'No' | Likely rules out meningism | | | | | | |
| How bad is the pain on a scale of 1–10? | A subarachnoid haemorrhage is described as the worst pain imaginable | 'I'd say it's about 7 or 8' | Although severe pain, it is reassuring that it is not 10 | | | | | | |
| Have you tried anything for the pain? | Can help to assess degree of pain | 'I had some paracetamol which hasn't helped' | This can be usual for headaches, as it is important to know what medication a patient has tried before prescribing anything | | | | | | |
| Is your baby moving normally? | Pre-eclampsia can be associated with risks to the fetus, including stillbirth | 'Yes, it has been moving all day' | No additional concerns | | | | | | |

## Past Medical and Obstetrics History

| | | | | | | | | | |
|---|---|---|---|---|---|---|---|---|---|
| Do you have any chronic medical conditions? | Comorbidities have implications for both diagnosis and management | 'No' | No additional concerns | | | | | | |

## Past Medical and Obstetrics History

| Question | Justification | Answer | Thoughts | | | | |
|---|---|---|---|---|---|---|---|
| Have you had a baby before? | Pre-eclampsia is more likely if it has occurred in a previous pregnancy | 'No' | No additional concerns | | | | |
| How many pregnancies have you had? | Note the patient's parity and gravidity | 'This is my first' | Patient is a primip | | | | |

## Drug History

| Question | Justification | Answer | Thoughts | | | | |
|---|---|---|---|---|---|---|---|
| Are you on any medication at the moment, or have any allergies? | Important to check, as people may not disclose their whole medical history. You must always check for allergies | 'No medications and no allergies' | No additional concerns | | | | |
| Have you had all your immunisations? | Important to check pregnant women have had relevant vaccinations; for example, influenza and whooping cough | 'Yes' | No additional concerns | | | | |

## Family History

| Question | Justification | Answer | Thoughts | | | | |
|---|---|---|---|---|---|---|---|
| Are there any diseases that run in the family, including pre-eclampsia? | Pre-eclampsia is more likely if it has occurred in a first-degree relative | 'Not that I know of' | No additional concerns | | | | |

## Social History

| Question | Justification | Answer | Thoughts | | | | |
|---|---|---|---|---|---|---|---|
| Who is currently at home? Are you working? | Find out if there are any social concerns or if wider support is needed | 'I live with my husband and work full-time in a café' | No social concerns at present | | | | |
| Do you feel supported and safe with your husband? | Important to consider domestic violence in pregnant women | 'We are happy and have no problems' | No additional concerns | | | | |
| Do you smoke? | Find out a patient's wider risk factors | 'No, I have never smoked.' | No additional concerns | | | | |
| What is your average weekly alcohol consumption? | | 'I haven't had any since I found out I was pregnant and rarely drank before' | No additional concerns | | | | |
| Have you recently travelled abroad? | Ensure no tropical infections as a cause of the symptoms | 'No, not for several years' | No travel concerns at present | | | | |

**Systems Review**

| Question | Justification | Answer | Thoughts | | | | |
|---|---|---|---|---|---|---|---|
| Just to check, have you had any problems with bladder or bowel function? | Find out if there are any wider concerns that have not arisen yet | 'No, they have been normal' | No additional concerns | | | | |
| Have you had any recent night sweats, fever, weight loss or fatigue? | It is essential to ask about B symptoms to rule out certain causes, such as infection | 'No' | No additional concerns | | | | |

**Finishing the Consultation**

| Question | Justification | Answer | Thoughts | | | | |
|---|---|---|---|---|---|---|---|
| Is there anything that you would like to tell me? | May identify useful information that has been missed and helps to build rapport with the patient | 'I'm really worried I'm getting pre-eclampsia, I've heard of that and it sounds awful. I'm worried for my baby' | Take the time to explain what will happen from here | | | | |
| Do you have any questions? | Allows any final concerns to be addressed | | | | | | |

**Present Your Findings**

Mrs Jones is a 36-year-old woman who is 36 weeks pregnant. She presents with a new-onset headache, which started today and has not been helped by analgesia. This is her first pregnancy, and it has been low risk to date. Her fetal movements are normal. She has no significant medical history and is not taking any medication.

My main diagnosis would be pre-eclampsia, with a differential of migraine.

I am going to perform a urine dip to look for proteinuria, and take her observations, including blood pressure. If these are abnormal, I will send bloods, including a full blood count, renal function and liver function tests

**General Points**

| | | | | |
|---|---|---|---|---|
| Polite to patient | | | | |
| Maintains good eye contact | | | | |
| Appropriate use of open and closed questions | | | | |
| Acknowledges patient's concern about baby | | | | |

## ❓ QUESTIONS FROM THE EXAMINER

### What is pre-eclampsia?

A multiorgan disease specific to pregnancy, which typically manifests as hypertension and proteinuria.

### What effects can pre-eclampsia have on the mother?

Raised blood pressure can lead to eclampsia (seizures) if untreated. Another serious sequalae is HELLP syndrome (haemolysis, elevated liver enzymes and low platelets). The disease can be fatal if not managed.

## What effects can pre-eclampsia have on the fetus?

Fetal growth restriction or stillbirth can occur from placental insufficiency or abruption.

## How is pre-eclampsia managed?

Treating hypertension is the immediate priority to prevent eclampsia. Delivery is the only definitive treatment.

## What is the likelihood of pre-eclampsia occurring in a future pregnancy?

At least 16% of women will get it again. If the delivery was before 34 weeks' gestation, then 33% of women will get it again.

## What are the long-term effects of pre-eclampsia for women?

They are up to three times more likely to suffer a major adverse cardiovascular event in the future.

## How is a tension headache managed?

Simple analgesia, rest and relaxation aids.

## How would you diagnose a subarachnoid haemorrhage?

Computed tomography (CT) scan as the initial investigation, with lumbar puncture to look for blood if index of suspicion is still high.

## How would you assess fetal well-being to reassure Mrs Jones?

Cardiotocograph (CTG) and consider a growth scan if there are any concerns about growth.

## If this was a migraine, what would you advise for the rest of the pregnancy?

Avoid known triggers and get adequate sleep. Paracetamol and codeine can be used. If needed, beta-blockers may be used for prophylaxis. Sumatriptan should be avoided as safety is unknown.

## Station 7.2    History: Reduced Fetal Movements

### Doctor Briefing

You are a junior doctor on the Obstetric Assessment Unit and have been asked to see Carol Grant, a 35-year-old woman who has presented with reduced fetal movements. She is 34 weeks pregnant. Please take a history, present your findings and formulate an appropriate management plan.

### Patient Briefing

You are 35 years old and this is your first pregnancy. You are 34 weeks pregnant. This was a planned pregnancy, and you and your husband and very excited about it. You have not felt your baby move for the last 6 h and have attended the unit after calling for advice.

You have no medical problems and no family history of note.

You are worried because your baby has never done this before and frightened that something is wrong with it.

### Mark Scheme for Examiner

#### Introduction

| | | | |
|---|---|---|---|
| Cleans hands, introduces self, confirms patient identity and gains consent for history taking | | | |
| Establishes current patient knowledge and concerns | | | |

#### History of Presenting Complaint

| Question | Justification | Answer | Thoughts | | | | |
|---|---|---|---|---|---|---|---|
| How long has your baby not been moving for? | The longer it has been going on, the more concerning for a stillbirth | 'I last felt it move about 6 h ago' | While not completely reassuring, better than 24 h | | | | |
| Has this ever happened before? | Recurrent reduced movements can be associated with worse outcomes | 'No, this is the first time' | No additional concerns | | | | |
| What triggers usually make your baby move and have you tried them? | Most fetuses respond to stimuli by this gestation | 'Usually I have a cold drink or poke my tummy, but neither has worked' | Concerning that there is not a usual response | | | | |
| Have you got any abdominal pain or vaginal bleeding? | To rule out placental abruption | 'No, I feel well otherwise' | Does not rule out pathology but makes it less likely | | | | |
| Have you been unwell recently, with diarrhoea or vomiting? | Dehydration and intercurrent illness can affect movements | 'No, I have been well' | Makes a medical cause less likely | | | | |

#### Past Medical and Obstetrics History

| | | | | | | | |
|---|---|---|---|---|---|---|---|
| Do you have any chronic medical conditions? | Comorbidities have implications for both diagnosis and management | 'No' | No further concerns | | | | |
| How many pregnancies have you had? | Note the patient's parity and gravidity | 'This is my first' | Patient is a primip | | | | |

## Drug History

| Question | Justification | Answer | Thoughts | | | | |
|---|---|---|---|---|---|---|---|
| Are you on any medication at the moment, or have any allergies? | Drugs such as opioids can affect movements. You must always check for allergies | 'No medications and no allergies' | No additional concerns | | | | |
| Have you had all your immunisations? | Important to check pregnant women have had relevant vaccinations; for example, influenza and whooping cough | 'Yes, I had them earlier in pregnancy' | No additional concerns | | | | |

## Family History

| | | | | | | | |
|---|---|---|---|---|---|---|---|
| Are there any diseases that run in the family, including pre-eclampsia? | Important always to check for relevant heritable conditions | 'Not that I know of' | No additional concerns | | | | |

## Social History

| | | | | | | | |
|---|---|---|---|---|---|---|---|
| Who is currently at home? Are you working? | Find out if there are any social concerns or if wider support is needed | 'I live with my husband and work in a clothes shop' | No social concerns at present | | | | |
| Do you feel supported and safe with your husband? | Important to consider domestic violence in pregnant women | 'We are happy and have no problems' | | | | | |
| Do you smoke? | Increases the risk of stillbirth and fetal growth restriction | 'No, I have never smoked' | No additional concerns | | | | |
| What is your average weekly alcohol consumption? | Alcohol and withdrawal can affect fetal movements | 'I haven't had any alcohol while I have been pregnant' | No additional concerns | | | | |
| Have you recently travelled abroad? | Ensure no tropical infections as a cause of the patient's symptoms | 'No, not for several years' | No travel concerns at present | | | | |

## Systems Review

| | | | | | | | |
|---|---|---|---|---|---|---|---|
| Just to check, have you had any problems with bladder or bowel function? | Find out if there are any wider concerns that have not arisen yet | 'No, they have been normal' | No additional concerns | | | | |
| Have you had any recent night sweats, fever, weight loss or fatigue? | It is essential to ask about B symptoms to rule out certain causes, such as infection | 'No' | No additional concerns | | | | |

### Finishing the Consultation

| Question | Justification | Answer | Thoughts | |
|---|---|---|---|---|
| Is there anything that you would like to tell me about? | May identify useful information that has been missed and helps to build rapport with the patient | 'I'm just really scared something has happened to my baby' | Take the time to explain what will happen from here | |
| Do you have any questions? | Allows any final concerns to be addressed | | | |

### Present Your Findings

Mrs Grant is a 35-year-old primiparous woman who is 34 weeks pregnant. She presents today with 6 h of reduced fetal movements. She has not had any other symptoms. She has tried her usual methods of getting her baby to move but these have been unsuccessful. She is fit and well, and has had an uncomplicated pregnancy to date. She does not take any medication and does not smoke or drink alcohol.

I am going to check fetal heart action is present and then perform a CTG if it is. I would also like to examine Mrs Grant and perform observations to assess for any underlying pathology. If I have any concerns about growth, I will arrange an ultrasound scan

### General Points

| General Points | |
|---|---|
| Polite to patient | |
| Maintains good eye contact | |
| Appropriate use of open and closed questions | |
| Acknowledges patient's concerns | |

## ❓ QUESTIONS FROM THE EXAMINER

### From what gestation should women feel fetal movements?

Most women can feel movements by 24 weeks' gestation.

### How many times a day should a fetus move?

There is no set number of movements, but they should follow a pattern of movement instead.

### What drugs can affect fetal movements?

The most common drugs to affect movements are opioid drugs, such as codeine. They can also be affected by drugs such as heroin, or replacements such as methadone.

### What is a placental abruption, and how can it cause a stillbirth?

It is the separation of the placenta from the uterine wall before birth, leading to bleeding (which can be catastrophic) and interruption of blood flow to the fetus.

### What are the signs and symptoms of a placental abruption?

Patients typically report severe abdominal pain and minimal or no vaginal bleeding. They often present with reduced fetal movements. The abdomen is described as feeling 'woody'.

## How is a placental abruption diagnosed?

It is a clinical diagnosis, and if suspected and fetal distress is present, the baby should be delivered, usually by caesarean section. At surgery, a retroplacental clot will be found.

## What complications can the mother have from placental abruption?

It can result in a massive obstetric haemorrhage, disseminated intravascular coagulation and death.

## How common is stillbirth?

The rate varies greatly across the world, but the latest UK rate is 3.7 babies per 1000 births.

## What chronic medical problems can increase the risk of stillbirth?

Diseases affecting vasculature and perfusion; for example, diabetes mellitus, renal disease, thrombophilia and systemic lupus erythematosus.

## What is assessed at a fetal growth scan?

The basic measurements are fetal head circumference, abdominal circumference and femur length. The amniotic fluid volume will also be assessed, and Doppler measurements of the umbilical artery and middle cerebral artery may be taken.

## Station 7.3    History: Anxious Pregnant Woman

### Doctor Briefing

You are a junior doctor in the antenatal clinic, and your next patient is Georgina Gordon, a 32-year-old woman who has been referred with increasing anxiety. She is 30 weeks pregnant and this is her first pregnancy. Please take a history from Miss Gordon and formulate an appropriate management plan.

### Patient Briefing

This is your first visit to the antenatal clinic. You are 32 years old and 30 weeks pregnant. This is your first pregnancy and it was planned.

You have been referred to clinic by your community midwife because you are reporting feeling incredibly anxious, mostly around the delivery of the baby. You are not sleeping well anymore, and you are struggling to concentrate at work. You are losing enjoyment in things and no longer feel excited about the pregnancy. You live with your partner, who is also very worried about you and has never seen you like this.

You have no history of mental health problems and are generally fit and well. Your sister has bipolar disorder.

You are mostly worried that something bad will happen at the delivery, and scared of not knowing what to expect.

### Mark Scheme for Examiner

#### Introduction

| | | | | | |
|---|---|---|---|---|---|
| Cleans hands, introduces self, confirms patient identity and gains consent for history taking | | | | | |
| Establishes current patient knowledge and concerns | | | | | |

#### History of Presenting Complaint

| Question | Justification | Answer | Thoughts | | | |
|---|---|---|---|---|---|---|
| When did you notice that you were starting to feel anxious? | To build up a picture of episode | 'I first noticed it after my 20-week scan and it has been getting worse since then' | Concerning, as has now been going on for nearly 3 months | | | |
| Have you ever experienced this type of feeling before? | While the patient may not have had a mental health diagnosis, may have had episodes of anxiety before | 'No, I have never felt like this' | Good to clarify the mental health history | | | |
| What do you feel anxious about? | To assess if anxiety is about pregnancy-related issues, and if the concerns are 'reasonable' | 'I am really scared of the birth, and that something terrible will happen to my baby. I have heard so many scary stories' | Reassuring, as no psychotic concerns offered at this stage | | | |
| How is this anxiety affecting you? | To assess effect illness is having on life | 'I can't concentrate at work, and I'm finding that I can't get to sleep, and that I wake up very early in the morning' | Concerning as starting to interfere with daily life and may impact on pregnancy | | | |
| How are you feeling about the pregnancy? | Important to see how illness is affecting this | 'I can't enjoy it any more. I was so excited at the start but now I just feel terrified' | | | | |

## History of Presenting Complaint

| Question | Justification | Answer | Thoughts | | | | | |
|---|---|---|---|---|---|---|---|---|
| Has anyone around you said that they are worried? | Useful to have opinions of people who know the patient well outside of illness | 'My partner is very worried; he says that he has never seen me like this' | Concerning that others are noticing a change; this should be taken seriously | | | | | |
| Have you tried anything to help? | To assess effects of treatment | 'No, I don't know where to start' | General idea obtained of the patient's previous attempts with getting help | | | | | |
| Sometimes when people are' anxious, they can start to feel like life isn't worth living. Have you felt like this at all? | Important to assess any risk of suicide | 'No, I don't feel like that' | Reassuring that there appears to be no risk | | | | | |

## Past Medical and Obstetrics History

| Question | Justification | Answer | Thoughts | | | | | |
|---|---|---|---|---|---|---|---|---|
| Do you have any chronic medical conditions? | Comorbidities have implications for both diagnosis and management | 'No' | No additional concerns | | | | | |
| Have you had a baby before? | Pre-eclampsia is more likely if it has occurred in a previous pregnancy | 'No' | No additional concerns | | | | | |

## Drug History

| Question | Justification | Answer | Thoughts | | | | | |
|---|---|---|---|---|---|---|---|---|
| Are you on any medication at the moment, or have any allergies? | Important to check in case of starting treatments. You must always check for allergies | 'No medications and no allergies' | No additional concerns | | | | | |
| Have you had all your immunisations? | Important to check pregnant women have had relevant vaccinations; for example, influenza and whooping cough | 'Yes' | No additional concerns | | | | | |

## Family History

| Question | Justification | Answer | Thoughts | | | | | |
|---|---|---|---|---|---|---|---|---|
| Are there any diseases that run in the family, including any mental health problems? | Bipolar disorder in a first-degree relative can increase the risk of puerperal psychosis | 'My sister has bipolar disorder but is well' | Possible concern as may increase risk of illness in this patient | | | | | |

## Social History

| Question | Justification | Answer | Thoughts | | | | | |
|---|---|---|---|---|---|---|---|---|
| Who is currently at home? Are you working? | Find out if there are any social concerns or if wider support is needed | 'I live with my partner and work full-time as a teacher' | No social concerns at present | | | | | |
| Do you feel supported and safe with your partner? | Important to consider domestic violence in pregnant women | 'We are happy and have no problems' | | | | | | |

**Social History**

| Question | Justification | Answer | Thoughts | | | | |
|---|---|---|---|---|---|---|---|
| Do you smoke? | Find out wider risk factors | 'No, I have never smoked' | No additional concerns at present | | | | |
| What is your average weekly alcohol consumption? | Find out wider risk factors as well as exploring causes for symptom changes | 'I don't drink alcohol at all; I never have' | Patient not disclosing any further concerns at present | | | | |
| Do you use any illegal drugs? | Many drugs can cause anxiety while taking them or withdrawing | 'No, I have never taken illegal drugs' | | | | | |

**Systems Review**

| Question | Justification | Answer | Thoughts | | | | |
|---|---|---|---|---|---|---|---|
| Just to check, have you had any problems with bladder or bowel function? | Both can be affected by feelings of anxiety | 'No, they have been normal' | No further concerns at present | | | | |
| Have you had any recent night sweats, fever, weight loss or fatigue? | It is essential to ask about B symptoms to rule out certain causes, such as infection | 'No' | No additional concerns | | | | |
| Have you experienced palpitations or feelings of breathlessness? | Can be caused by anxiety | 'Yes, I have felt palpitations at night when I have been trying to get to sleep' | This may need further investigation, and should not just be put down to anxiety | | | | |

**Finishing the Consultation**

| Question | Justification | Answer | Thoughts | | | | |
|---|---|---|---|---|---|---|---|
| Is there anything that you would like to tell me about? | May identify useful information that has been missed and helps to build rapport with the patient | 'I just want to feel better. I want some reassurance and to start to enjoy my pregnancy again' | Take the time to explain what will happen from here | | | | |
| Do you have any questions? | Allows any final concerns to be addressed | | | | | | |

**Present Your Findings**

Miss Gordon is a 32-year-old primiparous woman who presents to the antenatal clinic today with feelings of anxiety. She is 30 weeks pregnant, and her pregnancy has been uncomplicated to date. She first started feeling anxious after her anomaly scan, and feels it is getting worse. She is mostly concerned about the birth, and that something bad may happen to her baby. She is unable to concentrate at work, her sleep is affected, and she is unable to enjoy her pregnancy any more. She is experiencing palpitations at night. She has no suicidal ideation. Her partner has noticed a change in her and is concerned. She has no medical or drug history of note. Her sister has bipolar disorder.

My main differential is an acute anxiety disorder related to pregnancy. I would like to arrange cognitive behavioural therapy for her, and put her in touch with some local support groups. I will also arrange an electrocardiogram (ECG) to investigate her palpitations.

I plan to see her again in 2 weeks, and have explained that I may recommend pharmacological treatment at that stage and refer her to the perinatal mental health team

| General Points | | | |
|---|---|---|---|
| Polite to patient | | | |
| Maintains good eye contact | | | |
| Appropriate use of open and closed questions | | | |
| Assesses risk of suicide sensitively and appropriately | | | |

## ❓ QUESTIONS FROM THE EXAMINER

### How common is anxiety in pregnancy?
Around 13% of pregnant women experience anxiety. This increases to 20% in the first year after childbirth.

### How is anxiety assessed in pregnancy?
If a woman reports feelings of anxiety, then the GAD-7 scoring method should be used to assess her severity, and referral to an obstetrician should take place. Input may be needed from mental health professionals for further assessments.

### What is cognitive behavioural therapy?
It is a psychosocial intervention that works by challenging and aiming to change harmful thoughts.

### Which medications are safe to use for the management of anxiety in pregnancy?
In general, the rule is 'healthy mum, healthy baby', and most antianxiolytic medications are acceptable in pregnancy. It is important that women are fully informed when starting medications, as they may result in a small increase in the risk of birth defects or cause neonatal withdrawal. Sodium valproate should never be used in women of child-bearing capacity, as it is linked with significant birth defects.

### What psychotropic medications should not be used if breastfeeding?
Valproate should not be used (as above). The others that should not be used while breastfeeding are clozapine, carbamazepine and lithium.

### What is the rate of puerperal psychosis?
This affects 1–2 women per 1000.

### What increases the risk of puerperal psychosis?
Bipolar disorder (particularly bipolar I) is associated with a 50% risk of psychosis developing. A first-degree relative with bipolar disorder or puerperal psychosis also increases the risk.

### What are the options for tokophobia (fear of childbirth)?
Women should be referred to psychology services, with professionals who have experience in managing women during pregnancy. They should also have regular, empathetic input from a team of midwives and obstetricians, ideally with continuity of care in a perinatal mental health team.

### What considerations should be taken if a woman is on lithium in pregnancy?
Levels should be taken every 4 weeks, until 36 weeks' gestation, then increased to weekly until delivery at the recommendation of a psychiatrist. Recommend that the woman give birth on an obstetric unit. The medication should be stopped in labour, with levels checked 12 h after the last dose. Ensure the woman is well hydrated in labour due to risk of lithium toxicity.

### How common is anxiety in partners?
Ten per centof partners disclose feelings of anxiety in pregnancy and the postnatal period.

## Station 7.4 History: Antepartum Haemorrhage

### Doctor Briefing

You are a junior doctor on labour ward and have been asked to see Priya Patel, a 28-year-old woman, who has presented with vaginal bleeding. She is 30 weeks pregnant. Please take a history from Mrs Patel and then establish a differential diagnosis.

### Patient Briefing

You are 28 years old and 30 weeks pregnant. This was a planned pregnancy, and you and your husband have been very excited about this baby.

You started bleeding vaginally 3 h ago. You first noticed it on wiping after going to the toilet, and it has been getting heavier since that time. You have passed a few walnut-sized clots and had to change your pad a few times. In this time you haven't felt your baby move. You have no pain.

You have had an uncomplicated pregnancy before this, and are up to date with scans. You are due another scan at 32 weeks because your placenta is low-lying. You are rhesus-positive. You have no medical problems and are not taking any regular medications.

You are scared because you know that bleeding in pregnancy is abnormal, and worried for the safety of you and your baby.

### Mark Scheme for Examiner

**Introduction**

| | | |
|---|---|---|
| Cleans hands, introduces self, confirms patient identity and gains consent for history taking | | |
| Establishes current patient knowledge and concerns | | |

**History of Presenting Complaint**

| Question | Justification | Answer | Thoughts | | | |
|---|---|---|---|---|---|---|
| When did you first notice the bleeding? | Allows you to begin to assess the degree and severity of blood loss | 'It started 3 h ago' | She may have lost a significant amount of blood | | | |
| How heavy do you think the blood loss is in relation to a normal period? Have you had to change your pad? | | 'I have changed two pads since it started, and I have passed a few clots' | | | | |
| Do you have any photos of the blood loss? | Often patients will take pictures on camera phones, which helps to assess loss | 'No, I was too panicked to take a photo, but have the pads' | Having pictures often helps quantify the bleeding | | | |
| Have you had bleeding in the pregnancy before? | Will help to build a picture of acute or chronic problem | 'No, this is the first time' | Reassuring this is not a recurring issue | | | |
| Do you have any abdominal pain? | Bleeding from a placental abruption will be painful. Loss from a placenta praevia will be painless | 'No, I have no pain at all' | Fits more with a placenta praevia, less concerned about abruption | | | |
| What are your baby's movements like at the moment? | Lack of fetal movements is concerning for fetal well-being, particularly in acute blood loss | 'I haven't felt the baby move since this started' | Concerning for fetal well-being; fits with placental abruption or vasa praevia | | | |

## History of Presenting Complaint

| Question | Justification | Answer | Thoughts | | | | |
|---|---|---|---|---|---|---|---|
| Can you think of anything you were doing before the bleeding started? | A postcoital bleed would fit less with placental pathology | 'I was sitting at my desk working and then went to the toilet when I first noticed it' | Less likely to be cervical pathology or trauma | | | | |
| Are you up to date with your smear tests? | Important in assessing vaginal bleeding to consider cervical cancer | 'Yes, I had one before I got pregnant' | Unlikely to be cervical cancer | | | | |

## Drug History

| Question | Justification | Answer | Thoughts | | | | |
|---|---|---|---|---|---|---|---|
| Are you on any medication at the moment, or have any allergies? | Important to check not on any drugs that increase bleeding potential. You must always check for allergies | 'No medications and no allergies' | No additional concerns | | | | |
| Have you had all your immunisations? | Important to check pregnant women have had relevant vaccinations; for example, influenza and whooping cough | 'Yes' | No additional concerns | | | | |

## Family History

| Question | Justification | Answer | Thoughts | | | | |
|---|---|---|---|---|---|---|---|
| Does anyone in the family have any conditions that make them more prone to bleeding? | Important always to check for relevant heritable conditions | 'My family are all fit and well' | No additional concerns | | | | |

## Social History

| Question | Justification | Answer | Thoughts | | | | |
|---|---|---|---|---|---|---|---|
| Who is currently at home? Are you working? | Find out if there are any social concerns or if wider support is needed | 'I live with my husband and work part-time as a solicitor' | No social concerns at present | | | | |
| Do you feel supported and safe with your husband? | Important to consider domestic violence in pregnant women, especially with vaginal bleeding | 'We are happy and have no problems' | | | | | |
| Do you smoke? | Find out a patient's wider risk factors | 'No, I have never smoked' | No additional concerns | | | | |
| What is your average weekly alcohol consumption? | | 'I only have occasional alcohol outside of pregnancy' | | | | | |
| Do you take any drugs? | Cocaine can increase the risk of placental abruption | 'No, I have never taken drugs' | | | | | |

## Past Medical and Obstetrics History

| Question | Justification | Answer | Thoughts | | | | | |
|---|---|---|---|---|---|---|---|---|
| Have you had any problems in this pregnancy so far? | Find out more about the pregnancy | 'It has been straight-forward so far; mostly I have been seen by the midwife' | No additional concerns | | | | | |
| Are you rhesus-positive or negative? | Will need anti-D if rhesus-negative and fetus is positive or unknown | 'I am rhesus-positive' | Will not need anti-D. Rhesus status can always be checked in the patient notes if the patient is unsure | | | | | |

## Systems Review

| Question | Justification | Answer | Thoughts | | | | | |
|---|---|---|---|---|---|---|---|---|
| Just to check, have you had any problems with bladder or bowel function? | Find out if there are any wider concerns that have not arisen yet | 'No, they have been normal' | No additional concerns | | | | | |
| Have you had any recent night sweats, fever, weight loss or fatigue? | It is essential to ask about B symptoms to rule out certain causes, such as infection | 'No' | No additional concerns | | | | | |

## Finishing the Consultation

| Question | Justification | Answer | Thoughts | | | | | |
|---|---|---|---|---|---|---|---|---|
| Is there anything that you would like to tell me? | May identify useful information that has been missed and helps to build rapport with the patient. | 'I'm just really scared and I want to know if my baby and I are safe' | Take the time to explain what will happen from here | | | | | |
| Do you have any questions? | Allows any final concerns to be addressed | | | | | | | |

## Present Your Findings

Mrs Patel is a 28-year-old woman who presents today with vaginal bleeding. She is 30 weeks pregnant and this is her first pregnancy. The bleeding started 3 h ago, and is heavier than a period. She has passed clots and has had to change her pads several times. She has no abdominal pain and has not felt any fetal movements in that time. She has had an uncomplicated pregnancy to date and is otherwise fit and well. She takes no regular medications and has no allergies.

I am concerned that Mrs Patel may be having bleeding from a placenta or vasa praevia.

I would like to obtain intravenous access with two wide-bore cannulae, and send bloods for a full blood count, renal function, clotting screen and cross-match for 4 units of blood. I would like to check a fetal heart is present, and if so, perform a cardiotocograph to assess fetal well-being. I will involve the senior obstetrician and midwife in case of the need for emergency delivery

## General Points

| | | | | | |
|---|---|---|---|---|---|
| Polite to patient | | | | | |
| Maintains good eye contact | | | | | |
| Appropriate use of open and closed questions | | | | | |
| Acknowledges patient's fears and concerns | | | | | |

## ❓ QUESTIONS FROM THE EXAMINER

### What is a placental abruption?

When the placenta separates from the uterine wall before birth, leading to bleeding within the uterus and disruption of blood flow to the fetus.

### How do you tell the difference between a placental abruption and other causes of vaginal bleeding?

With vaginal bleeding and abdominal pain in the second or third trimester, an abruption should be the primary diagnosis. Most other causes of bleeding are painless.

### What is placenta praevia?

Implantation of the placenta in the lower segment of the uterus, which may or may not be covering the cervical os.

### What is vasa praevia?

Blood vessels within membranes, usually between two lobes of placenta, covering the cervical os.

### How do you tell the difference between a bleed from placenta and vasa praevia?

Although both will be painless, a bleed from vasa praevia will have signs of significant fetal distress or stillbirth, as fetal blood is being lost, whereas placenta praevia results in maternal blood loss.

### What is the priority in the management of antepartum haemorrhage?

The safety of the mother is the main priority, and an ABCDE approach should be used. When she is stable and safe, fetal concerns can be managed. In the care of a placental abruption, both are at risk from massive haemorrhage and emergency caesarean section is likely to be required.

### What does a CTG assess?

A transducer placed on the maternal abdomen detects the fetal heart rate and a trace is produced with the rate and variations within it. Another transducer on the abdomen detects the presence of uterine activity.

### How is a small antepartum haemorrhage managed?

Admit to hospital for observation and assess fetal growth by ultrasound once bleeding has settled, administer anti-D if the woman is rhesus-negative and fetus is rhesus-positive or status is unknown.

### What is anti-D?

The most common red cell alloantibody. Women can become sensitised if they are rhesus-negative and carrying a rhesus-positive fetus and have a sensitising event, leading to the production of anti-red cell immunoglobulin G (IgG) antibodies that cross the placenta. If this happens, this fetus and subsequent rhesus-positive fetuses are at risk of haemolytic disease of the fetus and newborn (HDFN), which can be fatal, due to fetal anaemia. To prevent this, rhesus-negative women are given routine antenatal anti-D prophylaxis (RAADP) to prevent HDFN. RAADP is commonly referred to as 'anti-D'.

### How is anti-D administered?

As an intramuscular injection at 28 weeks (1500 IU) or at 28 weeks and 34 weeks (if 500 IU used). Further doses should be given following a sensitising event (such as an antepartum haemorrhage). At delivery, fetal blood is tested from the umbilical cord. If the fetus is found to be rhesus-positive then further anti-D should be given to prevent HDFN in subsequent pregnancies.

## Station 7.5 History: Vaginal Discharge

### Doctor Briefing

You are a junior doctor in the gynaecology outpatient clinic and have been asked to see Diane Bruce, a 39-year-old woman, who is complaining of vaginal discharge. Please take a history from Mrs Bruce, present your findings and formulate an appropriate management plan.

### Patient Briefing

This is the first time you have been to the gynaecology department; your primary care physician made the referral. You have had vaginal discharge for about 3 months. It is yellowy-green, and present most days. It does not smell. You have never had anything like this before.

You split up with your husband a year ago, and have been seeing a new partner for about 6 months. You have a contraceptive implant and have not been using condoms. You have been having some spotting after sexual intercourse, and occasionally have deep pelvic pain during sex.

You are concerned that you may have a sexually transmitted infection (STI) and are worried about what this will mean for your health.

### Mark Scheme for Examiner

#### Introduction

| | | | | |
|---|---|---|---|---|
| Cleans hands, introduces self, confirms patient identity and gains consent for history taking | | | | |
| Establishes current patient knowledge and concerns | | | | |

#### History of Presenting Complaint

| Question | Justification | Answer | Thoughts | | | | |
|---|---|---|---|---|---|---|---|
| When did you first notice the discharge? | Build up a picture of an acute or chronic disease process | 'I think it has been there for about 3 months' | Relatively long time; however, it may have taken that time for referral | | | | |
| What does it look like? | Help with differential diagnosis | 'It is yellowy-green and quite thick' | Sounds like gonorrhoea or chlamydia | | | | |
| Does the discharge have a noticeable smell? | | 'Not that I have noticed' | | | | | |
| What have you tried for it already? | Assess previous treatment success | 'Nothing, the doctor said I should attend here first' | The patient has not yet received any medical treatment for this condition | | | | |
| Have you had any change in sexual partner in the last 12 months? | Assess risk of STI | 'Yes, my husband and I split up a year ago and I have a new partner' | More likely to be an STI | | | | |
| What contraception are you using? | | 'I have an implant in my arm' | Lack of barrier contraception increases the likelihood of an STI | | | | |

## History of Presenting Complaint

| Question | Justification | Answer | Thoughts | | | | | |
|---|---|---|---|---|---|---|---|---|
| In order for me to work out where to take tests from, it's important to know what type of sex you have been having. Have you had vaginal, oral or anal sex, or all three? | Swabs may need to be taken from the rectum or throat as well as vagina, but it is important to ask this question sensitively and in a non-judgemental way | 'I have had vaginal and oral sex' | Need to consider swabs in the throat as well as vagina | | | | | |
| Have you had any new symptoms during sex? | Assess risk of STI and complications such as pelvic inflammatory disease (PID) | 'I have had some bleeding after sex, and it sometimes hurts deep inside during sex' | Consider cervical pathology as well as an STI | | | | | |

## Past Medical and Gynaecological History

| Question | Justification | Answer | Thoughts | | | | | |
|---|---|---|---|---|---|---|---|---|
| Do you have any chronic medical conditions? | Comorbidities have implications for both diagnosis and management | 'No' | No additional concerns | | | | | |
| When was your last smear test, and what was the result? | Assess risk of underlying cervical pathology | 'I had a smear last year which was normal' | Less likely cervical pathology but important to examine thoroughly | | | | | |

## Drug History

| Question | Justification | Answer | Thoughts | | | | | |
|---|---|---|---|---|---|---|---|---|
| Are you on any medication at the moment, or have any allergies? | Unlikely to be on any medication, but important to check as people may not disclose their whole medical history. You must always check for allergies | 'No medications and no allergies' | No additional concerns | | | | | |
| Have you had all your immunisations? | Important to check pregnant women have had relevant vaccinations; for example, influenza and whooping cough | 'Yes' | No additional concerns | | | | | |

## Family History

| Question | Justification | Answer | Thoughts | | | | | |
|---|---|---|---|---|---|---|---|---|
| Are there any diseases that run in the family, including any cancers? | Important always to check for relevant heritable conditions | 'None that I am aware of' | No additional concerns | | | | | |

### Social History

| Question | Justification | Answer | Thoughts | | | | | |
|---|---|---|---|---|---|---|---|---|
| Who is currently at home? Are you working? | Find out if there are any social concerns or if wider support is needed | 'I live alone, and work full-time as a teacher' | No social concerns at present | | | | | |
| | Important to consider domestic violence in pregnant women | 'We are happy and have no problems' | | | | | | |
| Do you smoke? | Find out a patient's wider risk factors | 'No, I have never smoked' | No additional concerns | | | | | |
| What is your average weekly alcohol consumption? | | 'I don't drink alcohol' | | | | | | |
| Have you recently travelled abroad? | Ensure no tropical infections as a cause of the patient's symptoms and be aware of resistant organisms in other parts of the world | 'Not within the last few years' | No travel concerns at present | | | | | |

### Systems Review

| Question | Justification | Answer | Thoughts | | | | | |
|---|---|---|---|---|---|---|---|---|
| Just to check, have you had any problems with bladder or bowel function? | Find out if there are any wider concerns that have not arisen yet | 'No, they have been normal' | No additional concerns | | | | | |
| Have you had any recent night sweats, fever, weight loss or fatigue? | It is essential to ask about B symptoms to rule out certain causes, such as infection | 'No' | No additional concerns | | | | | |

### Finishing the Consultation

| Question | Justification | Answer | Thoughts | | | | | |
|---|---|---|---|---|---|---|---|---|
| Is there anything that you would like to tell me? | May identify useful information that has been missed and helps to build rapport with the patient | 'I'm really worried that I might have picked up an infection, and about how I will tell my new partner if I have' | Take the time to explain what will happen from here | | | | | |
| Do you have any questions? | Allows any final concerns to be addressed | | | | | | | |

### Present Your Findings

Mrs Bruce is a 39-year-old woman who presents with a history of vaginal discharge for 3 months. This discharge is yellowy-green and non-offensive. She has not yet tried anything for it. She has a new sexual partner and is not using barrier contraception. She has had episodes of postcoital bleeding and deep dyspareunia. Her smears are normal and up to date.

My main differential diagnosis is an STI such as chlamydia or gonorrhoea, but I would like to rule of cervical pathology.

I would like to perform abdominal and speculum examinations and carry out swabs for STIs. If this comes back positive, then I will refer her to the local sexual health clinic to guide further treatment and help her with contact tracing. In the meantime I have advised her to use condoms until her swab results come back

| General Points | | | | |
|---|---|---|---|---|
| Polite to patient | | | | |
| Maintains good eye contact | | | | |
| Appropriate use of open and closed questions | | | | |
| Asks about sexual history sensitively and in a non-judgemental manner | | | | |

## ❓ QUESTIONS FROM THE EXAMINER

### What is the bacterium that causes chlamydia infection?

It is caused by *Chlamydia trachomatis*, which is an obligate intracellular organism.

### What are the risk factors for chlamydia infection?

Lack of barrier contraception, age under 25 years old, new sexual partner or more than one sexual partner in the last year.

### How common is chlamydia infection?

It is the most common STI in people under the age of 25, with prevalence rates of up to 10%. It is estimated that 131 million people are infected worldwide each year.

### What are the long-term consequences of untreated chlamydia infection?

PID can lead to infertility, endometritis, chronic pelvic pain and increased risk of ectopic pregnancy. Fitz-Hugh–Curtis syndrome (perihepatic adhesions) can lead to abdominal pain. Sero-negative arthritis can develop.

### How likely is chlamydia to be transferred between sexual partners?

Chlamydia is highly likely to be passed between partners, with concordance rates of 75% in studies.

### How should chlamydia infection be diagnosed?

The nucleic acid amplification test (NAAT) is the gold standard for diagnosis. The most accurate test in women is a vulvovaginal swab, but endocervical swabs and urine can also be used. In some patients it may also be necessary to do rectal or pharyngeal swabs for the NAAT.

### What is the recommended treatment for chlamydia infection?

In the UK the current treatment regimens are doxycycline 100 mg bd for 7 days, or azithromycin 1 g orally as a single dose, followed by 500 mg once daily for 2 days. Treatment should be led by national guidance.

### What treatment should be recommended if the patient is pregnant and why?

Doxycycline is not safe in pregnancy, and so the azithromycin regimen should be used. As chlamydia can lead to preterm labour, neonatal conjunctivitis and pneumonia, it is important to carry out a test of cure 3 weeks after treatment.

### What is contact tracing?

This is carried out in sexual health clinics by trained healthcare advisors, who will help patients to go through their sexual history to work out who may be at risk of having the infection. It is important that this is not viewed as a blaming exercise, but a notification programme. Healthcare advisors can either help the patient decide how to contact the other sexual partners or make the contact for them. This contact can remain anonymous.

### How often does chlamydia infection resolve spontaneously?

In around 50% of cases the infection resolves by 12 months, but the mechanism is unknown and long-term damage may already have been caused and be irreversible.

## Station 7.6 History: Postmenopausal Bleeding

### Doctor Briefing

You are a junior doctor in the gynaecology clinic and have been asked to see Bethany Bates, a 68-year-old woman, who has come in with postmenopausal bleeding. Please take a history from Mrs Bates, present your findings and formulate an appropriate management plan.

### Patient Briefing

This is your first visit to the hospital. You have been referred by your primary care physician as you have noticed some vaginal bleeding. This had occurred after an episode of sexual intercourse. It was spotting only, and lasted a couple of hours. You have had a few similar episodes since. You have also experienced some soreness in your vulva.

You are otherwise fit and well. You have had three babies, all born by normal vaginal deliveries. Your smear tests are normal and up to date.

You are worried that this could be cancer of the womb.

### Mark Scheme for Examiner

#### Introduction

| | | | | |
|---|---|---|---|---|
| Cleans hands, introduces self, confirms patient identity and gains consent for history taking | | | | |
| Establishes current patient knowledge and concerns | | | | |

#### History of Presenting Complaint

| Question | Justification | Answer | Thoughts | | | | |
|---|---|---|---|---|---|---|---|
| When did you first notice the bleeding? | To assess if this is an acute or chronic problem | 'It first happened a few months ago' | Not likely an acute issue | | | | |
| Were you doing anything beforehand, such as having sexual intercourse? | Was this a provoked or unprovoked bleed? | 'I had been having sex just beforehand' | More likely to be a contact issue; for example, atrophy or cervical pathology | | | | |
| How many times has this happened now? | To assess if ongoing pathology | 'I have had a few episodes now' | Likely ongoing cause | | | | |
| How much bleeding have you had each time? | Assess blood loss and to consider causes | 'I have only had spotting that lasts a couple of hours' | Reassuring that there is no heavy bleeding | | | | |
| Have you had a change in sexual partner in the last year? | Assess risk of STI causing symptoms | 'I have been with my husband for 40 years' | Unlikely to be an STI | | | | |

#### Past Medical, Gynaecological and Obstetric History

| | | | | | | | |
|---|---|---|---|---|---|---|---|
| Do you have any other health problems? | Any conditions making it more likely to have bleeding | 'No, I am very well' | No additional concerns | | | | |
| When was your last smear test, and was it normal? | Assess likelihood of cervical pathology | 'I last had one about 5 years ago and this was normal' | Unlikely to be cervical cancer | | | | |
| How many children have you had? | Nulliparity is a risk factor for endometrial cancer | 'I have had three children' | Doesn't rule it out but is a protective factor | | | | |

## Drug History

| Question | Justification | Answer | Thoughts | | | | |
|----------|---------------|--------|----------|--|--|--|--|
| Are you on any medication at the moment, or have any allergies? | Unlikely to be on any medication but important to check as people may not disclose their whole medical history. You must always check for allergies | 'No medications and no allergies' | No additional concerns | | | | |
| Have you ever been on a drug that could affect your bleeding, such as aspirin or warfarin? | If there is a specific drug you need to consider, always ask. The patient may have recently stopped taking it. These drugs can have an effect on bleeding | 'No. I have never taken those medications' | No additional concerns | | | | |

## Family History

| Question | Justification | Answer | Thoughts | | | | |
|----------|---------------|--------|----------|--|--|--|--|
| Are there any diseases that run in the family, including any bowel cancers? | Important always to check for relevant heritable conditions, e.g. hereditary non-polyposis colorectal cancer (HNPCC) | 'Not that I know of' | No additional concerns | | | | |

## Social History

| Question | Justification | Answer | Thoughts | | | | |
|----------|---------------|--------|----------|--|--|--|--|
| Who is currently at home? Are you working? | Find out if there are any social concerns or if wider support is needed | 'I am retired and I live with my husband' | No social concerns at present | | | | |
| Do you feel supported and safe with your husband? | Important to consider domestic violence | 'We are happy and have no problems' | | | | | |
| Do you smoke? | Find out a patient's wider risk factors | 'I have never smoked' | No additional concerns | | | | |
| What is your average weekly alcohol consumption? | | 'I only have a small drink on special occasions' | No additional concerns | | | | |

## Systems Review

| Question | Justification | Answer | Thoughts | | | | |
|----------|---------------|--------|----------|--|--|--|--|
| Just to check, have you had any problems with bladder or bowel function? | Find out if there are any wider concerns that have not arisen yet | 'No, I have not had any problems' | No additional concerns | | | | |
| Have you lost any weight without trying recently? | Assess symptoms of possible underlying malignancy | 'Not that I have noticed' | No additional concerns | | | | |
| Have you had any recent night sweats, fever or fatigue? | It is essential to ask about B symptoms to rule out certain causes, such as infection | 'No' | No additional concerns | | | | |

**Finishing the Consultation**

| Question | Justification | Answer | Thoughts | | | | | |
|---|---|---|---|---|---|---|---|---|
| Is there anything that you would like to tell me? | May identify useful information that has been missed and helps to build rapport with the patient | 'I would just like anything nasty ruled out, I have heard about cancer of the womb and I am scared' | Take the time to explain what will happen from here | | | | | |
| Do you have any questions? | Allows any final concerns to be addressed | | | | | | | |

**Present Your Findings**

Mrs Bates is a 68-year-old woman who presents with a history of postmenopausal bleeding. This has occurred after sexual intercourse, and has been spotting only. She is fit and well, takes no medication and has no significant family history. She has had three children by vaginal delivery.

My main differential is vaginal atrophy however, I would like to exclude endometrial cancer.

I would like to perform abdominal and speculum examinations, and carry out a transvaginal ultrasound scan to assess the endometrial thickness. If this is increased, then I will perform an endometrial biopsy

**General Points**

| | | | | |
|---|---|---|---|---|
| Polite to patient | | | | |
| Maintains good eye contact | | | | |
| Appropriate use of open and closed questions | | | | |

## ❓ QUESTIONS FROM THE EXAMINER

### What is vaginal atrophy?

This is the thinning of the vaginal epithelium that occurs in oestrogen-deficient states, such as postmenopausally or during breast-feeding.

### How can vaginal atrophy be treated?

Topical oestrogen preparations can be used, as well as recommending lubricants for use during sexual intercourse.

### List three causes of postmenopausal bleeding, other than endometrial cancer and vaginal atrophy.

Vulval causes (lichen sclerosus, lichen planus, vulval cancer or intraepithelial neoplasia, trauma), vaginal causes (trauma, vaginal cancer), cervical causes (cervical polyps, cervical cancer), endometrial causes (endometrial polyps), causes related to the fallopian tubes (fallopian tube malignancy) and ovaries (rare oestrogen-secreting tumours). Sometimes there is a systemic cause, such as anticoagulants.

### What is the most common histological type of vulval cancer?

Squamous carcinomas account for over 90% of vulval cancers.

### How is vulval cancer treated?

The main treatment is surgical excision, which may need to include excision of the lymph nodes. In women who have involved margins, radiotherapy may be recommended. These women should be managed in a tertiary gynaecology centre.

## List the common risk factors for endometrial cancer.

Advancing age, late menopause, early menarche, nulliparity, obesity, oestrogen-only hormone replacement therapy, family history of HNPCC, polycystic ovarian syndrome and diabetes.

## What is HNPCC and what is the overall risk for endometrial cancer?

HNPCC (or Lynch syndrome) is an inherited form of bowel cancer associated with a 40–60% lifetime risk of endometrial cancer. It is inherited in an autosomal-dominant fashion, and is also associated with multiple other malignancies.

## How is endometrial cancer managed?

Total hysterectomy (abdominal or laparoscopic) with bilateral salpingo-oophorectomy. Women with more advanced disease will require radiotherapy, either external-beam or brachytherapy.

## What is the prognosis for endometrial cancer?

This is dependent on the stage of the cancer at diagnosis. The 5-year survival rates are 90% at stage 1, 75% at stage 2, 50% at stage 3 and 15% at stage 4.

## How common is primary vaginal cancer?

This is very rare, with about 250 cases diagnosed in the UK each year. It is much more common to have a secondary tumour in the vagina from cervical, vulval or endometrial cancer.

## Station 7.7   History: Pain in Early Pregnancy

### Doctor Briefing

You are a junior doctor on the gynaecology ward and have been asked to see Alice Arden, a 24-year-old woman who has presented with abdominal pain and is 6 weeks pregnant. Her primary care doctor has referred her to the hospital. Please take a history from Miss Arden, present your findings and formulate an appropriate management plan.

### Patient Briefing

You have been referred by your primary care physician to the gynaecology ward, after going to see them with sudden-onset right-sided abdominal pain. This woke you up from sleep this morning, and is still present. The pain is sharp and low down in the right side of your abdomen. You have not tried any painkillers and have never experienced anything like this before. You have had no vaginal bleeding, and your last period was 6 weeks ago.

This is your second pregnancy; you have a 4-year-old son, who was born by normal delivery. That pregnancy was uncomplicated. This pregnancy was planned.

You are scared that you might have an ectopic pregnancy, and are keen to know what is going on.

### Mark Scheme for Examiner

#### Introduction

| | |
|---|---|
| Cleans hands, introduces self, confirms patient identity and gains consent for history taking | |
| Establishes current patient knowledge and concerns | |

#### History of Presenting Complaint

| Question | Justification | Answer | Thoughts | |
|---|---|---|---|---|
| When did you first notice the pain? | Assess acute or chronic cause | 'It woke me up around 7 o'clock this morning, and hasn't gone away since' | More worrying as clearly an acute cause and severe enough to wake her from sleep | |
| How severe in the pain, on a scale of 1 to 10? | Assess severity to aid differentials and plan analgesia | 'Now it is about 8 out of 10' | Worrying as clearly severe | |
| Where in your tummy do you feel it worst? | A unilateral pain is more likely to be an ectopic pregnancy or ovarian cyst accident | 'It is really bad down in my lower tummy on the right' | Suggests unilateral pathology | |
| Have you had any vaginal bleeding? | More likely to be associated with a miscarriage or ectopic pregnancy | 'Not since my period' | Unlikely to be a miscarriage | |

#### Past Medical, Obstetric and Gynaecological History

| | | | | |
|---|---|---|---|---|
| How many pregnancies have you had before? | Important to determine previous outcomes to assess risks | 'I have had one baby boy. He was a normal delivery' | No previous ectopics or miscarriages is reassuring but does not rule these out | |
| When was your last period? | To assess likelihood of ectopic pregnancy | 'Six weeks ago' | Within reasonable window of ectopic pregnancy | |

## Past Medical, Obstetric and Gynaecological History

| Question | Justification | Answer | Thoughts | | | | |
|---|---|---|---|---|---|---|---|
| Was this a planned pregnancy, and how are you feeling about it? | To guide counselling and gain insight to the woman's thoughts | 'Yes, we have been really excited about it' | Take this into account if you need to break bad news later | | | | |
| Do you have any chronic medical conditions? | Comorbidities have implications for both diagnosis and management | 'No' | No additional concerns | | | | |

## Drug History

| Question | Justification | Answer | Thoughts | | | | |
|---|---|---|---|---|---|---|---|
| Are you on any medication at the moment, or have any allergies? | Unlikely to be on any medication but important to check, as people may not disclose their whole medical history. You must always check for allergies | 'No medications and no allergies' | No additional concerns | | | | |
| Have you had all your immunisations? | Important to check pregnant women have had relevant vaccinations; for example, influenza and whooping cough | 'Yes' | No additional concerns | | | | |

## Family History

| Question | Justification | Answer | Thoughts | | | | |
|---|---|---|---|---|---|---|---|
| Are there any diseases that run in the family? | Important always to check for relevant heritable conditions | 'Not that I know of' | No additional concerns | | | | |

## Social History

| Question | Justification | Answer | Thoughts | | | | |
|---|---|---|---|---|---|---|---|
| Who is currently at home? Are you working? | Find out if there are any social concerns or if wider support is needed | 'I am not working at the moment. I live with my husband and son' | No social concerns at present | | | | |
| Do you feel supported and safe with your husband? | Important to consider domestic violence in pregnant women | 'We are happy and have no problems' | | | | | |
| Do you smoke? | Find out a patient's wider risk factors | 'No, I do not smoke' | No additional concerns | | | | |
| What is your average weekly alcohol consumption? | | 'I don't drink alcohol in pregnancy, but have about four glasses of wine a week outside of pregnancy' | No additional concerns | | | | |

**Systems Review**

| Question | Justification | Answer | Thoughts | | | | |
|---|---|---|---|---|---|---|---|
| Just to check, have you had any problems with bladder or bowel function? | Find out if there are any wider concerns that have not arisen yet | 'No, but I have felt quite sick for a couple of weeks' | Symptoms of early pregnancy elicited. No further concerns at present | | | | |
| Have you had any discomfort or burning when passing urine? | Need to consider a urinary tract infection (UTI) | 'No, but I have been passing urine more frequently' | Need to consider UTI | | | | |
| Have you had any shoulder tip pain or chest pain? | Symptoms of a ruptured ectopic pregnancy and diaphragmatic irritation | 'No, only the tummy pain' | No additional concerns | | | | |
| Have you had any recent night sweats, fever, weight loss or fatigue? | It is essential to ask about B symptoms to rule out certain causes, such as infection | 'No' | No additional concerns | | | | |

**Finishing the Consultation**

| | | | | | | | |
|---|---|---|---|---|---|---|---|
| Is there anything that you would like to tell me? | May identify useful information that has been missed and helps to build rapport with the patient | 'I am worried that I might have an ectopic pregnancy, I really want this baby to be OK' | Take the time to explain what will happen from here | | | | |
| Do you have any questions? | Allows any final concerns to be addressed | | | | | | |

**Present Your Findings**

Miss Arden is a 24-year-old woman who presents today with abdominal pain in early pregnancy. Her last menstrual period was 6 weeks ago. The pain woke her up from sleep this morning, and remains 8 out of 10 in severity. It is localised in the right iliac fossa. She has had no vaginal bleeding. She has had one pregnancy in the past, which was uncomplicated. This pregnancy was planned. She has no significant medical or family history, takes no medication and has no allergies.

My main differential is an ectopic pregnancy, but I would like to exclude an ovarian cyst accident and UTI.

I would like to perform an abdominal and pelvic examination, carry out a urine dipstick test and arrange a transvaginal ultrasound scan

**General Points**

Polite to patient

Maintains good eye contact

Appropriate use of open and closed questions

## ❓ QUESTIONS FROM THE EXAMINER

### List three common causes of pain in early pregnancy.

Ectopic pregnancy, miscarriage, ovarian cyst accident and UTI.

### What are the most common ovarian cyst accidents?

Cyst rupture, torsion and cyst haemorrhage.

### What is the commonest benign ovarian cyst in pregnancy?

The commonest benign ovarian cyst is a dermoid cyst.

### How are benign ovarian cysts monitored in pregnancy?

Serial pelvic ultrasound scans are performed to monitor the growth of any ovarian cysts in pregnancy.

### How is an ovarian cyst accident managed?

There are two main options: conservatively, which is suitable for a cyst rupture, as fluid will normally be reabsorbed. Alternatively, surgical management will be needed for an ongoing haemorrhage (rare) or an ovarian torsion.

### What analgesia is suitable for pain in early pregnancy?

The standard pain ladder should be followed, but if there is a viable intrauterine pregnancy then NSAIDs should be avoided. It is therefore sensible to avoid these until a scan has taken place, and use alternative analgesia.

### What blood tests should be ordered for pelvic pain in early pregnancy and why?

A full blood count to assess haemoglobin level in case of intra-abdominal bleeding. Human chorionic gonadotrophin, which will be used to guide treatment in the case of an ectopic pregnancy. Rhesus status, which will be required in an ectopic pregnancy if anti-D is required.

### What findings would be suggestive of a UTI on a urine dipstick test?

Nitrites strongly suggest a UTI, and leukocytes and blood are suggestive of an infection, although less reliably.

### If all tests are normal and an intrauterine pregnancy was found, what advice could you give this woman?

Reassure her that nothing sinister has been found, and that her baby is growing in the correct place. Discuss simple analgesia if required. Advise that she should book her pregnancy with a community midwife to plan ongoing antenatal care.

### If this is an ongoing pregnancy, what medications would you advise a woman to take in early pregnancy?

All women should be advised to take folic acid (400 mcg once daily) in pregnancy to reduce the risk of neural tube defects, and this gestation is a good time to check if women are taking it, and advise them to do so if not.

## Station 7.8    Examination: Obstetric Examination

### Doctor Briefing

You are a junior doctor in the antenatal clinic and have been asked to see Clare Pfannenstiel, a 28-year-old woman who is 30 weeks pregnant. Please perform an obstetric examination and present your findings.

### Patient Briefing

This is your first visit to the antenatal clinic. Your midwife has referred you because you are a heavy smoker and are at risk of having a small baby. You are 30 weeks pregnant and this is your first pregnancy.

You have no health problems and take no medication. You have no pain at the moment.

You are not clear why you have been brought to clinic today.

### Mark Scheme for Examiner

**Introduction**

| | | | |
|---|---|---|---|
| Washes hands, introduces self, confirms patient identity and gains consent for examination | | | |
| Ensures a chaperone is present | | | |
| Appropriately exposes the patient whilst keeping dignity at all times, and repositions into a suitable position for the examination | | | |
| Asks patient if the patient has any pain currently | | | |

**General Inspection**

| What are you looking for or examining? | Justification | Thoughts | |
|---|---|---|---|
| General well-being | On initial glance, does the patient look well/unwell/in pain? | The patient looks well | |
| Obvious signs of pathology | Gives you an indication of the patient's baseline health | The patient appears to have a normal body mass index, and has no other signs of pathology | |

**Obstetric Examination – Inspection**

| | | | |
|---|---|---|---|
| Look at the abdomen | Assess general size of uterus, look for scars from previous abdominal surgery, look for skin changes of pregnancy | Uterus looks to fit with third trimester, no previous surgery, striae gravidarum present | |

**Obstetric Examination – Palpation**

| | | | |
|---|---|---|---|
| Measure symphysial–fundal height (SFH) | To give gross assessment of fetal size | Measures 31 cm, appropriate for this gestation | |
| Assess fetal lie | To assess longitudinal, oblique or transverse | Longitudinal lie at present | |
| Assess fetal presentation | To see which part of the fetus is closest to maternal pelvis | Appears to be cephalic | |

## Obstetric Examination – Palpation

| What are you looking for or examining? | Justification | Thoughts | | | | | |
|---|---|---|---|---|---|---|---|
| Assess fetal engagement | To see how much of the presenting part is in the pelvis | Fetal head is free; five-fifths are palpable | | | | | |
| Assess liquor volume | To assess if appropriate volume present | Appears to be normal on palpation | | | | | |

## Obstetric Examination – Auscultation

| | | | | | | | |
|---|---|---|---|---|---|---|---|
| Listen for fetal heart with Doppler or Pinard stethoscope | Assess fetal viability and well-being | Fetal heart present at 140 bpm, with no decelerations heard | | | | | |

## Finishing

| | | | | | | | |
|---|---|---|---|---|---|---|---|
| Check patient is comfortable, offer to help reposition her and give the privacy to change | Keeps the patient's dignity | Treating the patient with respect is important | | | | | |
| Remove your gloves and wash hands | Complying with hand hygiene is vital | No additional concerns | | | | | |

## Present Your Findings

Mrs Pfannenstiel is a 28-year-old woman who is 30 weeks pregnant. She has been referred as she has risk factors for developing a growth-restricted fetus. On examination she has an SFH of 31 cm; the fetal lie is longitudinal with a cephalic presentation. The fetal head is not engaged. The fetal heart rate is 145 bpm, with no decelerations heard.

Because she has risk factors, I am going to arrange growth scans for her, and she will return to clinic with the results of these

## General Points

| | | | | | |
|---|---|---|---|---|---|
| Polite to patient | | | | | |
| Maintains good eye contact | | | | | |
| Clear instruction and explanation to patient | | | | | |

## ❓ QUESTIONS FROM THE EXAMINER

### What landmarks should you use to auscultate the fetal heart?

Listen with a Pinard stethoscope or Doppler over the anterior fetal shoulder.

### What additional tests should be done at a routine antenatal visit?

Measurement of blood pressure and urine dipstick (looking for proteinuria or signs of infection).

## What role does an SFH measurement have?

Can be used as a guide of fetal growth (should be 2 cm either side of gestational weeks, i.e. a 30-week uterus should measure between 28 and 32 cm). The measurement should be plotted each time on an SFH chart, and falling centiles should raise the suspicion of inadequate fetal growth.

## At what gestation would you expect to be able to feel the uterine fundus?

From around 12 weeks this can be felt, with the uterus reaching the level of the umbilicus by 20–24 weeks' gestation.

## What other factors may affect the SFH?

Multiple pregnancies, uterine fibroids, disorders of amniotic fluid volume (oligohydramnios or polyhydramnios) and raised body mass index.

## What investigation should be undertaken if there are factors that may affect the SFH?

In these cases, women should have growth scans, as using SFH measurements will not be accurate.

## What is the initial investigation you can perform if you are unsure of the lie of the baby?

If in any doubt as to the lie of the baby, then an ultrasound scan should be performed to confirm the lie of the baby.

## When should antenatal SFH measurements be taken?

At each and every interaction with medical professionals in the community and hospital, from 24 weeks' gestation.

## If there are concerns about the SFH, how quickly should a woman have a growth scan?

Ideally within 5 days of recognition; however, in practice it is usually within 48 h.

## Why should an ultrasound scan be performed if you have any concerns about the SFH being either too short or too long?

The SFH is a screening tool used by the maternity team; it is not diagnostic. If there are any concerns that the measurements are not as suspected, an ultrasound to measure the growth of the baby formally is indicated.

## Station 7.9   Examination: Gynaecology Examination (Bimanual and Speculum)

### Doctor Briefing

You are a junior doctor in gynaecology and have been asked to see Josephine Sapphire, a 28-year-old woman, who has presented with severe pelvic pain and vaginal discharge. She suddenly became unwell last night and has been referred in by her primary care doctor. Please examine Miss Sapphire and present your findings.

### Patient Briefing

This is your first visit to the doctor. You have had tummy pain for the last few weeks, but it has suddenly got a lot more severe. You feel hot and sweaty and cannot get comfortable. You saw your primary care physician who said you had a very high temperature and needed to go to hospital. You have had smelly discharge for the last few days.

You have never had this examination before. On questioning, you have had three sexual partners in the last 6 months and you cannot remember if you used condoms. You have never been tested for an STI.

You are concerned because you don't know why you are so ill. Your doctor mentioned an infection in your pelvis but you want to know what caused it.

### Mark Scheme for Examiner

#### Introduction

| | | | |
|---|---|---|---|
| Washes hands, introduces self, confirms patient identity and gains consent for examination | | | |
| Ensures a chaperone is present | | | |
| Appropriately exposes the patient whilst keeping dignity at all times, and repositions into a suitable position for the examination | | | |
| Asks patient if she has any pain currently | | | |

#### General Inspection

| What are you looking for or examining? | Justification | Thoughts | |
|---|---|---|---|
| General well-being | On initial glance, does the patient look well/unwell/in pain? | The patient looks sweaty and unwell, which is clinically concerning | |
| Obvious clues | Gives you an indication of the patient's baseline health | No other obvious signs on inspection | |
| Surroundings | Checks for obvious clues to aid diagnosis or equipment/observations to aid assessment | The patient has had observations by the nurse but has not been cannulated yet | |

#### Abdominal Examination – Inspection

| | | | |
|---|---|---|---|
| Look at the abdomen | Note the size and look for any scars, distension or masses | Currently no evidence that the patient has had previous surgery | |

#### Abdominal Examination – Palpation

| | | | |
|---|---|---|---|
| Feel for superficial pain | Assess for tenderness, masses, guarding and distension | Patient is very tender in the lower abdomen; no masses felt | |
| Feel for deep pain | Again, assess for tenderness (rebound?), masses and guarding | Patient is very tender; some voluntary guarding in the pelvic region | |

**Abdominal Examination – Percussion**

| What are you looking for or examining? | Justification | Thoughts | | | | |
|---|---|---|---|---|---|---|
| Percuss the abdomen | Checking for dullness, tympanic or tender | No percussion tenderness | | | | |

**Abdominal Examination – Auscultation**

| | | | | | | |
|---|---|---|---|---|---|---|
| Listen for bowel sounds | Checking there are no issues such as ileus | Bowel sounds heard and normal | | | | |

**Pelvic Examination – Preparation**

| | | | | | | |
|---|---|---|---|---|---|---|
| Gather equipment and prepare the patient | Ensure the patient has no underwear on and provide a sheet to cover her | No additional concerns | | | | |

**Pelvic Examination – Inspection**

| | | | | | | |
|---|---|---|---|---|---|---|
| Look at the external genitalia for any abnormality | Checking for skin changes, masses, lesions or bleeding | External genitalia appear normal | | | | |

**Speculum Examination**

| | | | | | | |
|---|---|---|---|---|---|---|
| Lubricate the Cusco's speculum | Makes the examination more comfortable for the patient | No additional concerns | | | | |
| Part the labia minora and insert the speculum | The patient shouldn't be too tender | No additional concerns | | | | |
| Open the blades to visualise the cervix | Important to look at the cervix in order to note important clinical features on inspection | The cervix appears normal however, there is profuse offensive discharge. High index of suspicion for PID | | | | |
| Perform vaginal and/or cervical swabs if necessary | Checking for both STIs and vaginal pathogens | These are taken in this case | | | | |
| Gradually withdraw the speculum | Checking the vaginal walls as this happens | Vagina appears normal | | | | |

**Bimanual Examination**

| | | | | | | |
|---|---|---|---|---|---|---|
| Lubricate your gloved fingers and check the patient is happy for you to proceed | Patients may be uncomfortable from the speculum and want a moment before the bimanual examination | The patient is happy for the rest of the examination | | | | |
| Feel for uterus size and tenderness | The uterus may feel bulky or be tender | This is mildly uncomfortable, in keeping with your working diagnosis | | | | |
| Feel in both adenexae | Tenderness and masses are both felt for | The patient is very tender in both adenexae | | | | |
| Feel for cervical motion tenderness | Patients with PID or an ectopic pregnancy may be very tender | No acute tenderness felt | | | | |

**Finishing**

| What are you looking for or examining? | Justification | Thoughts | | | | |
|---|---|---|---|---|---|---|
| Check patient is comfortable, offer to help reposition her and give the privacy to change | Keeps the patient's dignity | Treating the patient with respect is important | | | | |
| Remove your gloves and wash hands | Complying with hand hygiene is vital | No additional concerns | | | | |

**Present Your Findings**

Miss Sapphire is a 28-year-old woman who presented with severe abdominal pain and vaginal discharge. On examination she looks uncomfortable at rest with generalised lower abdominal pain with some guarding to deep palpation. External genitalia were normal with profuse discharge seen on speculum examination. On bimanual examination she was generally tender but no masses were felt.

I feel the most likely diagnosis is PID, with the differential being ovarian cyst accident.

I would like to fully examine and take bloods from Miss Sapphire. I would also organise an ultrasound of her pelvis and send off the vaginal swabs I have taken. It is likely we will start on antibiotics

**General Points**

Polite to patient

Maintains good eye contact

Clear instruction and explanation to patient

## ❓ QUESTIONS FROM THE EXAMINER

**What is an important initial bedside investigation to perform in any woman with lower abdominal pain and why?**

Pregnancy test. In a woman of child-bearing age it is vital to determine whether she is pregnant. It is likely to change the management and investigation of the woman.

**What other bedside test is of equal importance when investigating lower abdominal pain?**

Urinalysis. A common differential of pelvic pain is UTI. Women have shorter urethras than men and are more predisposed to this. It is vital to exclude diagnoses that do not involve invasive testing.

**What are the common differentials for lower abdominal pain in young women?**

Pregnancy or pregnancy-related problems, UTI, PID, appendicitis, ovarian cyst accident and constipation.

**What is the first-line modality of imaging used to examine the pelvic organs of a woman?**

Ultrasound scan, usually a combination of transabdominal and transvaginal scanning.

**If further imaging of the pelvis was required, which modality would you use?**

MRI: this is much better at examining the pelvis than CT.

## What is the difference between the common two types of speculum used in gynaecology?

Most routine examinations involve using a Cusco's speculum, which has two blades and is self-retaining. These include taking smears, assessing the cervix, taking swabs for infection. A Sims speculum has one blade and is more commonly used by gynaecologists to assess for prolapse or to dilate the vagina to provide better access and visualisation of the vaginal cavity during a procedure.

## If you thought there was an abnormality on the patient's cervix when visualising it, what would you do?

Call the on-call gynaecology team for advice to determine the best follow-up for the patient, depending on the abnormality seen.

## If a patient has pelvic pain and you know she has an intrauterine form of contraception, what is important to note on examination?

The coil threads. Both the intrauterine system (such as the Mirena coil) and the intrauterine device (the copper coil) have threads attached that travel through the cervix and into the vagina. These allow clinicians to check that the coil is in situ. If the coil threads are not seen, then there is a small risk that the coil may have moved and perhaps perforated the uterus. This is most common in the few weeks following insertion.

## Describe a situation where it may be difficult to perform a pelvic examination.

Pelvic examination can be more difficult in postmenopausal women. They can sometimes experience vaginal dryness and structural changes, including atrophy, that make the vaginal canal narrower and the introitus smaller. If you feel you cannot examine a patient properly, it is important to discuss this with the gynaecology team.

## If a patient had an ovarian mass, give three things you might expect to find on examination.

Abdominal distension, tenderness in one of the iliac fossae on abdominal examination and a palpable mass on bimanual examination.

## Station 7.10 Communication: Consent for Caesarean Section

### Doctor Briefing

You are a junior doctor in the antenatal clinic and have been asked to see Joanne Taylor, a 22-year-old woman, who is 39 weeks pregnant. This is her first pregnancy and the baby is in a frank breech presentation. She is considering an elective caesarean section. Please explain the risks and benefits of the procedure to her. She has already had counselling about external cephalic version (ECV) and vaginal breech birth.

### Patient Briefing

You are 22 years old and this is your first pregnancy. This baby has been found to be breech at 39 weeks. One of the midwives has told you that this may mean you need a caesarean section, and you want to know more about the procedure.

You have no medical problems and your pregnancy has been uncomplicated up to now.

You are quite cross because you feel that this should have been picked up before now, and want an explanation as to why it has not been.

### Mark Scheme for Examiner

#### Introduction

Cleans hands, introduces self, confirms patient identity

Checks the identity of others in the room and confirms that the patient is happy for them to be present

Establishes current patient knowledge and concerns

#### Explaining the Procedure

| Statement/Question | Justification | Answer | Thoughts | | | | |
|---|---|---|---|---|---|---|---|
| A caesarean section is an operation that allows us to deliver the baby through a cut on your tummy | Start with a general open phrase to guide the patient | 'OK' | You know the patient is listening | | | | |
| It is usually performed under a spinal anaesthetic, allowing you to be awake for the procedure. This is safest for you and your baby | Important to signpost, as many patients assume all operations are carried out under general anaesthetic | 'OK' | The patient has no questions about the spinal | | | | |
| It usually takes about 10 min to deliver the baby, and about 45 min to close up, but you will be in the operating theatre for about 2 h | To give clear information on the procedure and what to expect | 'That is quicker than I expected!' | The patient has no questions about the timing of the operation | | | | |
| You will have a cannula in your hand, to allow us to give you fluids during the operation, and a tube in your bladder called a catheter | | 'That's good to know. I would have wondered what that was for' | Clearly thinking through what the operation will mean for her. She is engaged and well informed | | | | |
| You will stay in hospital for at least 1 night, more likely 2 nights | | 'I assumed this; it is what friends have told me' | | | | | |

## Explaining the Procedure

| Statement/Question | Justification | Answer | Thoughts | | | | | |
|---|---|---|---|---|---|---|---|---|
| You may need injections to thin your blood afterwards, to reduce the risk of blood clots. We will teach you how to do these when you go home | | 'Thank you for warning me' | | | | | | |
| You will not be able to drive for 6 weeks after having your baby by caesarean section | Women need to know to be able to plan their postnatal period | 'OK. Thank you for letting me know' | | | | | | |

## Explaining Risks and Benefits

| Statement/Question | Justification | Answer | Thoughts | | | | | |
|---|---|---|---|---|---|---|---|---|
| The benefit to you is that you will know the date of your baby's delivery | Important that patients understand risks and benefits of surgery | 'That is good' | No additional concerns | | | | | |
| Another benefit is that for your baby, an elective caesarean section is probably safer than a vaginal delivery | | | | | | | | |
| The main risks to you are bleeding, infection, damage to structures such as the womb, bowel, bladder or blood vessels and of developing blood clots in your legs or lungs. Everything is also written in an information leaflet I have for you | | 'I will need to think about these. Do you have this as written information?' | Appears to be taking risk seriously. Remember to provide the patient with an information leaflet as she is requesting written communication | | | | | |
| It may also affect how you labour with any further babies | | | | | | | | |
| The risks to the baby are the risk of a cut and of the baby needing to go to the neonatal intensive care unit (NICU) with short-term breathing problems | | | | | | | | |

## Discussing the Options

| Statement/Question | Justification | Answer | Thoughts | | | | | |
|---|---|---|---|---|---|---|---|---|
| You have the option of us turning your baby before it is born. This is called an external cephalic version or ECV | Women have to know other options that are available to make an informed decision | 'I will go home and think about my options' | Taking the time to make an informed decision | | | | | |
| Your other option is a vaginal breech delivery | | | | | | | | |

**Finishing the Consultation**

| Question | Justification | Answer | Thoughts | | | | | | |
|---|---|---|---|---|---|---|---|---|---|
| I understand that you are cross that this has only been found now, and I apologise for that. Would you like to discuss this further? | Good practice to acknowledge concerns and address them | 'I understand now that babies can turn themselves until this point, thank you' | Patient has good understanding | | | | | | |
| To summarise, we have discussed what a caesarean section is, as well as the risks and benefits. We have also talked about the alternative options that you have. You would like some more time to consider this. In the meantime, I will provide you with a leaflet with more information and am happy to assist in any way possible | Summarising the consultation and offering written communication | 'You've been wonderful, thank you!' | Leaflets will help to refresh the patient's memory | | | | | | |
| Do you have any other questions? I know that we have discussed a lot of new things; please take some time to digest the information | Allows any final concerns to be addressed | 'No, thank you, I would like to go home to think about what to do and talk to my partner' | The patient does not have any further questions | | | | | | |

**Present Your Findings**

Mrs Taylor is a 22-year-old woman who is having her first baby. She is 39 weeks pregnant, and her baby has been found to be in the breech position today.

I have discussed a caesarean section with her today, and she is aware of the risks and benefits. We have had a brief discussion about her other options of an ECV or a vaginal breech delivery.

She was initially quite cross about this, just having been diagnosed now. I have explained that babies often turn until late pregnancy, and she is happy with this explanation.

She is going to go home with written information and consider her options, and let us know tomorrow what she has decided to do. If she wishes a caesarean section, I will carry out formal consent

**General Points**

Polite to patient

Maintains good eye contact

Appropriate use of open and closed questions

Acknowledges patient is angry

## ❓ QUESTIONS FROM THE EXAMINER

### How common is infection following a caesarean section?

Six in 100 women having a caesarean section will develop an infection.

### How likely is it that a baby will get a laceration during a caesarean section?

Two babies in every 100 caesarean sections will have a laceration, but these tend to be very small and very rarely need any treatment.

### How common is a haemorrhage at a caesarean section?

Five in 100 women will have a haemorrhage at a caesarean section. Seven in 1000 women will go on to need an emergency hysterectomy to control the bleeding.

### What medications should be avoided following a postpartum haemorrhage at caesarean section?

Women should not be given non-steroidal anti-inflammatory drugs (NSAIDs), as these may affect renal function. Low-molecular-weight heparin should also be reviewed before being given.

### What options would this woman have in her next pregnancy for delivery?

She could have a repeat elective caesarean section, or she could aim for a vaginal birth after caesarean (VBAC). The main risk with this is uterine rupture, which occurs in one in every 200 women attempting a VBAC.

### What are the types of breech presentation?

There are three main types: frank, which is when the fetal legs are extended at the knees, with the feet near the fetal head; this presentation accounts for 65% of breech babies. Flexed is when the knees are bent, with the feet near the fetal bottom and this presentation accounts for 5–10% of breech babies. Footling is when the feet are presenting, more likely with preterm babies.

### Who should take consent for a caesarean section?

Ideally this should be done by the operating surgeon, but it should be taken by someone competent to undertake the procedure.

### What venous thromboembolism (VTE) prophylaxis should women have after a caesarean section?

All women should have thrombus embolus deterrent stockings, and should be assessed for low-molecular-weight heparin, and prescribed if they have risk factors.

### What pre-op medications should be given?

All women should receive an antiemetic and gastric protection; for example, omeprazole. This is to minimise the risk of aspiration.

### What is the role of the World Health Organization (WHO) checklist?

This is designed to maximise patient safety, and to ensure all members of the surgical team are aware of any concerns or issues. There should be a 'sign-in' performed with the woman on arrival, to check her identity, allergies and the procedure. A 'time-out' should be carried out before starting, and a 'sign-out' should be carried out upon leaving theatre to ensure everyone is aware of the postoperative plan.

## Station 7.11   Communication: Group B Streptococcus

### Doctor Briefing

You are a junior doctor in the antenatal clinic and have been asked to see Victoria Jones, a 28-year-old woman, who has been diagnosed with group B streptococcus (GBS) infection in pregnancy. She is worried about what this means for her and her baby, and would like to know more. Please explore her concerns and explain the diagnosis to her.

### Patient Briefing

You are 28 years old, and this is your third baby. You are keen to deliver at home, as your two previous births have been straightforward. You have been asked to come to antenatal clinic to discuss your swab result, which has shown GBS.

You are worried about what this means for you, your baby and your birth plans.

### Mark Scheme for Examiner

**Introduction**

Cleans hands, introduces self, confirms patient identity

Checks the identity of others in the room and confirms that the patient is happy for them to be present

Establishes current patient knowledge and concerns

**Explaining the Diagnosis**

| Statement/Question | Justification | Answer | Thoughts | | | | | |
|---|---|---|---|---|---|---|---|---|
| Group B streptococcus, sometimes called GBS, is a bacteria which many women carry in the genital tract | Begin with an introduction to the topic | 'OK' | You know the patient is listening | | | | | |
| It can be present in the vagina or in urine, and in your case it was on a vaginal swab | Start to build up more background knowledge | 'Oh, I didn't realise this' | The patient appreciates the information you are sharing | | | | | |
| Outside of pregnancy, it does not cause any problems. You do not have to have it treated at the time of diagnosis, but we recommend antibiotic treatment in labour | To put it in context to patient. Explaining what will happen and why | 'I have never heard of it before' | No additional concerns | | | | | |
| This is because GBS is the most common cause of severe early-onset neonatal infection | | 'Why can't we treat it now then?' | Patient understandably wants to know more | | | | | |
| If we treat it now, it does not mean that you will be clear at the time of labour | Explaining to the patient the current guidance is important, with the reasons why | 'OK, I see' | The patient has demonstrated that she understands what you have told her | | | | | |

**Explaining the Management Plan and its Consequences**

| | | | | | | | | |
|---|---|---|---|---|---|---|---|---|
| The treatment for GBS is intravenous antibiotics, in a drip in your arm or hand, at the time of labour | Straight forward explanation of procedure | 'Can I have that at home? I'm planning a home birth' | May have to deal with an angry or upset patient | | | | | |
| Unfortunately, this will have to take place in hospital, as antibiotics cannot be given intravenously at home | Be clear that this is definitely the case | 'Can I have my dose then go home?' | Need to be clearer that she will have to deliver in hospital | | | | | |

## Explaining the Management Plan and its Consequences

| Question | Justification | Answer | Thoughts | | | | | |
|---|---|---|---|---|---|---|---|---|
| Because you will need a dose every few hours during your labour, and the baby will need to be checked by the paediatricians, we recommend you deliver in hospital | Be clear and thorough, but not forceful | 'That is annoying, but I understand' | The patient appreciates the impact on the baby | | | | | |
| If you do not manage to get the antibiotics in time, for example in a very quick labour, your baby will need to stay in hospital for observation | Explain other possible eventualities | 'OK, I shall call the unit when I go into labour' | Seems to be happy with the plan and understands the reasoning | | | | | |

## Finishing the Consultation

| | | | | | | | | |
|---|---|---|---|---|---|---|---|---|
| I understand that this has surprised you, and will lead to a different birth plan than you had hoped. Is there anything I can do to make this easier for you? | Kind to be thoughtful and recognise patient's disappointment | 'No, I shall just have to get my head around it and plan childcare for my other children' | Seems to be happy to follow recommended plan | | | | | |
| To summarise, we have discussed what GBS is, the treatment for it and its impact on your birth plan. I will provide you with a leaflet with more information and am happy to assist in any way possible | Summarising the consultation and offering written communication | 'That's great, thank you' | Leaflets will help to refresh the patient's memory | | | | | |
| Do you have any other questions? I know that we have discussed a lot of new things; please take some time to digest the information | Allows any final concerns to be addressed | 'No' | The patient does not have any further questions | | | | | |

## Present Your Findings

Miss Jones is a 28-year-old woman who attended antenatal clinic today to discuss her diagnosis of GBS infection. She has had two babies before and was very keen for a home birth.

I have explained that while GBS will cause her no problems, it is potentially a very serious infection for newborn babies, and the most effective way to treat it is with intravenous antibiotics in labour. She is now happy with this plan and will deliver in hospital.

I shall make sure the discussion is documented in her notes and her GBS carrier status is made clear to those looking after her in labour

## General Points

| | | | | |
|---|---|---|---|---|
| Polite to patient | | | | |
| Maintains good eye contact | | | | |
| Appropriate use of open and closed questions | | | | |
| Acknowledges patient's disappointment with change in birth plan | | | | |

# ❓ QUESTIONS FROM THE EXAMINER

## What type of bacteria is GBS?

A Gram-positive coccus, also known as *Streptococcus agalactiae*. It is a beta-haemolytic, catalase-negative facultative anaerobe.

## What proportion of women are carriers for GBS?

20–40% of women carry GBS as a commensal organism.

## How is early-onset neonatal infection classified?

Infection diagnosed at less than 7 days of age. GBS is the most common cause, affecting 0.5 per 1000 births in the UK.

## Is it possible to screen for GBS?

Women can be screened, and in the USA this is recommended practice. In the UK, guidance is not to because many women carry the infection and their babies are born with no complications; screening does not predict which babies will become unwell; no screening test is entirely accurate; and treating all carriers of GBS would mean many women would receive antibiotics without benefit and possibly with harm, and could lead to antibiotic resistance.

## What are the risk factors for severe early-onset GBS infection in neonates?

Having a previous baby with GBS disease, diagnosis of GBS carrier status in pregnancy, preterm birth, prolonged rupture of membranes and maternal pyrexia and infection in labour.

## What antibiotics should be used for intrapartum prophylaxis in women who carry GBS?

The main recommended treatment is benzylpencillin. In women who are penicillin-allergic, this will depend on local resistance profiles, but vancomycin is recommended in the UK.

## Do women need treatment if they are having a caesarean section?

If they are having an elective caesarean section then they do not require treatment. If their membranes have ruptured before a planned or emergency caesarean then they should have antibiotics.

## Although this woman was not recommended to deliver at home, could she have a pool birth?

There is no evidence that this increases the risk to the baby, and so most hospitals would offer a pool birth if the woman wished.

## What if the patient declines antibiotics in labour, or does not get them in time?

The baby should stay in hospital for at least 12 h for observation, and should be checked by a paediatrician before discharge home.

## What antibiotics should a baby be given if severe early-onset GBS infection is suspected?

These babies should be given penicillin and gentamicin intravenously.

## Station 7.12 Communication: Placenta Praevia

### Doctor Briefing

You are a junior doctor in the antenatal clinic and have been asked to see Clare Smith, a 26-year-old woman, who has been diagnosed with placenta praevia on her anomaly scan. She is 20 weeks pregnant. She is worried what this means for her and her baby, and would like to know more. Please explain the diagnosis to her as well as the plan for the rest of her pregnancy.

### Patient Briefing

This is your first pregnancy and you have been sent to the antenatal clinic after your anomaly scan, to discuss the findings about your placenta. Nobody has explained anything to you so far.

You are frightened that this means there is something wrong with the pregnancy and want to know what it means for you and your baby.

### Mark Scheme for Examiner

#### Introduction

| | |
|---|---|
| Cleans hands, introduces self, confirms patient identity | |
| Checks the identity of others in the room and confirms that the patient is happy for them to be present | |
| Establishes current patient knowledge and concerns | |

#### Explaining the Diagnosis

| Statement/Question | Justification | Answer | Thoughts | |
|---|---|---|---|---|
| The placenta is the organ that develops along with your baby, to give the baby oxygen, nutrients and a blood supply | Start with a basic explanation of the role of the placenta | 'OK' | You know the patient is listening | |
| In an ideal setting, it grows on the inside walls of the womb, away from the cervix, which is the entrance to the vagina | | | | |
| In your case, the placenta is growing lower down than normal in the womb, and covering the cervix completely. It will still work normally however | Clear explanation of what the issue is | 'I understand, but why has this happened?' | Patient following explanation | |
| In most cases this has just happened by chance. Can I just check, have you had any surgery on your womb before? | Assessing risk of abnormally adherent placenta | 'No, I have never had surgery' | Likely to be an uncomplicated placenta praevia | |
| In the majority of cases, a low-lying placenta at 20 weeks will have moved out of the way by your delivery date, as the bottom half of the womb gets bigger | Be clear that this does not necessarily mean a complicated pregnancy | 'That's good to know. What happens now?' | Patient seems to understand the explanation | |

## Explaining the Plan for Pregnancy

| Question | Justification | Answer | Thoughts | | | | |
|---|---|---|---|---|---|---|---|
| To check if the placenta has moved away, we will arrange an ultrasound scan at 32 weeks to look at it | Being clear about ongoing management | 'OK' | The patient has no new questions | | | | |
| In the meantime, we would recommend that you do not have sexual intercourse, because of the risk of causing heavy bleeding | | 'Do you think that's likely?' | Important to acknowledge and answer her question | | | | |
| It is possible for women with a placenta praevia to have bleeding, although many do not. If you do have any bleeding it is important you contact Delivery Suite immediately | Patient safety must be of utmost importance during these consultations | 'That sounds scary. Will my baby be OK?' | Patient seems to understand potential seriousness of situation | | | | |
| In these cases, it is not the baby losing blood, but you. If you bleed very heavily then we would have to carry out an emergency caesarean section to keep you safe | Be clear the risk is to mum rather than baby | 'OK, I understand' | | | | | |
| If the placenta has not moved out of the way by 32 weeks, then it is more likely that it will not do so by the end of your pregnancy, and we would recommend a caesarean section for your delivery | Clearly explaining ongoing plan | 'That sounds fine' | No new concerns from the patient | | | | |
| This would potentially be riskier than a caesarean where the placenta was in the correct place, and you would have an increased chance of a serious haemorrhage, leading to a blood transfusion | | 'I'm happy to have blood if I need it' | This is good to know when planning surgery in complicated cases | | | | |
| Because of this increased risk of bleeding it is important you know that there is an increased chance of a hysterectomy to save your life | | 'That sounds awful … but I do understand' | The patient has taken on board what you are saying | | | | |

## Finishing the Consultation

| | | | | | | | |
|---|---|---|---|---|---|---|---|
| I understand that this is a lot to discuss today. Is there anything that I've missed, or anything that you are particularly concerned about? | Useful to acknowledge this may be quite unexpected and overwhelming. Also gives the opportunity for questions | 'No, thank you, you have been very helpful' | Seems to be clear on the plan | | | | |

**Finishing the Consultation**

| Question | Justification | Answer | Thoughts | | | | |
|---|---|---|---|---|---|---|---|
| To summarise, we have discussed what a low-lying placenta is and its implications for your pregnancy. I will provide you with a leaflet with more information and am happy to assist in any way possible | Summarising the consultation and offering written communication | 'That's great, thank you' | Leaflets will help to refresh the patient's memory | | | | |
| Do you have any other questions? I know that we have discussed a lot of new things; please take some time to digest the information | Allows any final concerns to be addressed | 'No' | The patient does not have any further questions | | | | |
| We will see you next at 32 weeks for that scan, but if you have any bleeding in the meantime, please contact Delivery Suite immediately. Do you have the telephone number? | Signposting for the patient | 'Yes, I have it, thank you' | Happy to end the consultation | | | | |

**Present Your Findings**

Miss Smith is a 26-year-old woman who presented to the antenatal clinic today following the diagnosis of a placenta praevia made at her anomaly scan. This is her first pregnancy and she has had no previous uterine surgery.

I have explained the diagnosis and the ongoing plan to her. She is aware to avoid sexual intercourse and to contact Delivery Suite immediately if she has any vaginal bleeding.

We will see her next at 32 weeks with an ultrasound scan to assess the placental site. If it remains covering the os or less than 20 mm clear, we will arrange a caesarean section for 39 weeks

**General Points**

Polite to patient

Maintains good eye contact

Appropriate use of open and closed questions

## ❓ QUESTIONS FROM THE EXAMINER

**How far away from the cervix does the placenta have to be to plan a vaginal delivery?**

It should be at least 20 mm clear of the internal os for a vaginal delivery to be planned.

**What are the types of placenta praevia?**

There are two main types: major, where the placenta is completely covering the internal os of the cervix; and minor, where the placenta is within the lower segment of the uterus but not covering the os.

**What types of surgery can increase the risk of an abnormally invasive placenta?**

Caesarean section, myomectomy, division of uterine septum.

## What types of abnormally invasive placenta are there?

There are three main types. Placenta accreta is when the placenta is abnormally adherent to the uterine wall. Placenta increta is when the placenta has abnormally invaded into the myometrium. Placenta percreta is when the placenta has gone through the myometrium and into the serosa; this type can involve neighbouring organs.

## How is an abnormally invasive placenta diagnosed?

It should be thought of in all women with a placenta praevia and previous uterine surgery. On ultrasound, you should look for abnormal colour Doppler flow. Magnetic resonance imaging (MRI) can also be useful in diagnosis.

## How should a woman be managed if she has a placenta praevia and attends with vaginal bleeding?

ABCDE assessment, intravenous access, bloods – full blood count, group and save, cross-match for 4 units of red blood cells if bleeding heavily, assess fetal well-being with CTG, consider delivery if bleeding is heavy and there is evidence of maternal compromise.

## What management should take place if the bleeding settles?

At least 48 h of observation in hospital. If women have had a large haemorrhage or repeated episodes, they may be recommended to stay in hospital until delivery.

## How should a caesarean section be planned in women with a placenta praevia?

The timing should be at 39 weeks unless there is heavy bleeding leading to emergency delivery. It should be done in a unit with access to facilities for high-volume blood transfusion, and with a senior obstetrician and anaesthetist present. There should also be at least 2 units of red blood cells cross-matched and available, and consider if cell salvage is available as well.

## What if the patient declines blood products?

This should be documented in the patient's notes, with most hospitals requiring the patient to sign an agreement before surgery. Cell salvage should be used, and women should be warned of the increased risk of hysterectomy at the time of surgery if heavy bleeding occurs.

## How should women be counselled for their next pregnancy?

If the placenta has moved after 32 weeks, they are not at increased risk in their next pregnancy.
If they have a caesarean, then they have an increased risk of another placenta praevia or of an abnormally invasive placenta.

## Station 7.13    Communication: Breech Presentation

### Doctor Briefing

You are a junior doctor in the antenatal assessment unit and have been asked to see Rachel Rae, a 26-year-old woman, who is 37 weeks pregnant and has been diagnosed as having a frank breech presentation during her first pregnancy. Please explain the diagnosis, then discuss the possibility of ECV, as well as other options if this fails to turn her baby.

### Patient Briefing

This is your first pregnancy and it has been uncomplicated so far. You are 37 weeks pregnant. You are very keen to have a vaginal delivery.

You are surprised to find out that your baby is breech, and want to know what this will mean for the delivery of your baby.

### Mark Scheme for Examiner

#### Introduction

| | | | | |
|---|---|---|---|---|
| Cleans hands, introduces self, confirms patient identity | | | | |
| Checks the identity of others in the room and confirms that the patient is happy for them to be present | | | | |
| Establishes current patient knowledge and concerns | | | | |

#### Explaining the Diagnosis

| Statement/Question | Justification | Answer | Thoughts | | | |
|---|---|---|---|---|---|---|
| I understand you have been told today your baby is breech. Do you understand what this means? | Clarify the level of knowledge the patient has and give information | 'I think it means my baby is bum down instead of head down?' | Clearly has some understanding | | | |
| Yes, your baby is bum down. Breech babies can also present with their feet | | 'OK' | Patient happy with this so far | | | |
| Some babies are breech because of the shape of the womb, or growths within it such as fibroids. Do you have any of these problems? | Building a picture of any contraindications to ECV, which must be done before offering it to women | 'Not that I know of' | No obvious contraindications, so can counsel about ECV | | | |
| Have you had any recent vaginal bleeding? | | 'No' | | | | |
| Have you had any signs that your waters have broken? | | 'No' | | | | |
| Has your midwife or obstetrician had any concerns about your baby's growth? | | 'No' | | | | |

**Discussing the Options**

| Question | Justification | Answer | Thoughts | | | | | |
|---|---|---|---|---|---|---|---|---|
| There are three main options to discuss for your delivery – vaginal breech, external cephalic version or ECV, which means turning your baby, and caesarean section. Would you like to discuss these now? | Signposting the conversation and establishing patient's wishes | 'I don't want a caesarean at all, so I would rather discuss the other two options please' | Can leave out caesarean section counselling with this woman at present | | | | | |
| With a planned vaginal breech delivery, we recommend you deliver in a consultant unit, as you may need help to have your baby, and these babies are more likely to need to see the neonatologists. A planned vaginal breech is riskier for the baby than a planned cephalic birth | Be clear about where delivery would take place and what may happen | 'That's helpful to know. I would rather there not be loads of people but I guess I understand why' | Patient clearly taking on board information | | | | | |
| If we were worried about the progress of the labour or thought that your baby was becoming distressed, we would recommend a caesarean section, just as we would for a cephalic baby. However it is more likely with a breech baby | | | It is always important to share all information about a procedure with a patient | | | | | |
| We can try to turn your baby with an ECV before labour. This involves you lying on the bed while an obstetrician tries to get your baby to turn around by pressing on the outside of your tummy | Explain ECV and its safety | 'Is it risky for my baby?' | Patient is engaged and asking appropriate questions | | | | | |
| We monitor your baby before and after the procedure, as well as carrying out a scan before we start. In a small proportion of babies, about 1 in 200, an emergency caesarean section is needed because the baby's heart beat shows signs of distress | Answer questions directly | 'Does it carry any risks for me?' | The patient seems to accept the small risk of caesarean section | | | | | |
| It is safe for you, but will feel uncomfortable. If you are too sore then we will stop trying immediately | Make sure you reassure the patient that she is in control at all times and has the right to remove consent | 'What will this mean for my labour?' | The patient has no questions about what you have just said. She is engaged and asking appropriate and expected questions | | | | | |

### Discussing the Options

| Question | Justification | Answer | Thoughts | | | | |
|---|---|---|---|---|---|---|---|
| Babies turned by ECV are more likely to have a vaginal birth than breech babies. When you go into labour you will have a slightly increased chance of an assisted vaginal birth or caesarean birth | Make sure the patient is aware of the increased labour risks associated with ECV | 'Is my baby likely to turn around again?' | The patient has picked up the fact that her baby could turn back around | | | | |
| About 5 in 1000 babies will turn back around by themselves | Reassurance is often needed here | 'That would be annoying!' | Yes! It can happen but is very unlikely | | | | |

### Finishing the Consultation

| | | | | | | | |
|---|---|---|---|---|---|---|---|
| To summarise, we have discussed what breech means and the various impacts on your birth plan. I will provide you with a leaflet with more information and am happy to assist in any way possible | Summarising the consultation and offering written communication | 'That's great, thank you' | Leaflets will help to refresh the patient's memory | | | | |
| Do you have any other questions? I know that we have discussed a lot of new things; please take some time to digest the information | Allows any final concerns to be addressed | 'No' | The patient does not have any further questions | | | | |

### Present Your Findings

Mrs Rae is 37 weeks pregnant and this is her first pregnancy. She has been found to have a baby in the breech position, and attended today to discuss her options. She has no contraindications to ECV. I have checked her notes and she is rhesus-positive.

I have discussed vaginal breech and ECV with her today. We did not cover caesarean section as she did not want to discuss this.

She is going to think about her options and attend the antenatal assessment unit tomorrow

### General Points

Polite to patient

Maintains good eye contact

Appropriate use of open and closed questions

## ❓ QUESTIONS FROM THE EXAMINER

### When would an ECV be carried out?

At 36–37 weeks, but it can be done up until delivery and during early labour.

### What are the contraindications to an ECV?

A confirmed need for a caesarean section, recent vaginal bleeding, abnormal CTG, rupture of membranes and multiple pregnancy.

## What should be done if the woman is rhesus-negative?

If the fetus is rhesus-positive or unknown, intramuscular anti-D should be given afterwards to minimise the risk of sensitisation. This should be done even if the procedure is unsuccessful.

## How successful is ECV?

About 50% of babies will turn, and this is more likely in multiparous women (60%).

## What can be done to make it more likely to be successful?

A medication (usually terbutaline) can be given to relax the woman, to make the baby easier to turn.

## Are there any natural methods of making babies turn from the breech position?

There is some evidence that a procedure called moxibustion can help, but this should only be carried out by somebody who is specially trained.

## What are the contraindications for a vaginal breech delivery?

Footling breech presentation, large-for-dates baby or significant growth restriction, hyperextension of the fetal neck, placenta praevia and fetal distress.

## What is the main cause for needing an emergency caesarean section after an ECV?

An abnormal CTG.

## Does a patient need to be starved before an ECV?

No. As the risk of requiring an emergency caesarean section is so low, guidelines state that women do not need to be starved before the procedure.

## Where should an ECV be carried out?

It is best practice to perform an ECV on central delivery suite, where there are the facilities to perform an emergency caesarean section if needed.

## Station 7.14    Communication: Miscarriage

### Doctor Briefing

You are a junior doctor working in the early pregnancy unit (EPU) and have been asked to see Emma Parker, a 32-year-old woman, who has had an ultrasound scan today and has been informed that she has had a miscarriage. She was referred to the clinic by her primary care doctor after some vaginal bleeding 2 days ago. Please explain the diagnosis and discuss her options with her.

### Patient Briefing

This is the first time you have been to the EPU. This was a planned pregnancy and you have been trying for this baby for about a year. You first had some vaginal bleeding 2 days ago. It started as spotting and then became much heavier, and lasted about 12 h. You had some tummy cramps at the same time. The bleeding has now completely stopped.

You have had two children before and these were uncomplicated pregnancies. You have no health problems, and are taking folic acid only.

You are worried that this means that you have lost the baby, and what this will mean for you in the future.

### Mark Scheme for Examiner

#### Introduction

Cleans hands, introduces self, confirms patient identity

Checks the identity of others in the room and confirms that the patient is happy for them to be present

Establishes current patient knowledge and concerns

#### Explaining the Diagnosis

| Statement/Question | Justification | Answer | Thoughts | | | |
|---|---|---|---|---|---|---|
| I'm afraid that I have some bad news. Do you have anyone here with you or would you like me to call someone for you? | Have a clear warning shot and check if the patient wants or needs support | 'No, thank you. My partner is at work' | Can continue with the consultation | | | |
| I'm sorry, but the scan you have had this morning has shown that you have had a miscarriage | Be very clear in plain language | 'Oh no … I was worried that this had happened' | Now aware that patient had wondered about this as a possibility | | | |
| This is not due to anything that you have done. Unfortunately around one in five pregnancies end in miscarriage, and in most cases we don't find out the reason why | Continue clear explanation | 'That is frustrating. What happens now?' | Seems to understand the diagnosis and wants to know what comes next | | | |

#### Explain the Management

| | | | | | | |
|---|---|---|---|---|---|---|
| There are three main options for what can happen next. Do you feel ready to discuss this or would you prefer to go over this another time? | This can be very overwhelming, and it is important to give the option of returning later to discuss options | 'I would like to hear the options today, then I can go home and discuss this with my partner' | The patient is happy for you to continue | | | |

**Explain the Management**

| Question | Justification | Answer | Thoughts |
|---|---|---|---|
| The first option is what is called conservative management, meaning that we allow what is there to pass naturally. This will mean that you will have a bit more bleeding, but should not require any drugs or operations | Give clear, concise information. You should highlight what the woman should expect in each procedure and also the risks | 'How likely is it that this will work?' | Clearly considering options carefully |
| Most miscarriages will complete within 7–14 days, and we would get you to take a pregnancy test after this time. If this is positive, or you change your mind at any time, you can contact us and we will see you again | | 'OK. What are my other options?' | |
| Another option is medical management, where a tablet is given, which is either swallowed or placed in the vagina, and this causes the cervix to open and the womb to contract, and then the products are passed | | 'Are there any risks with this?' | |
| You will have more bleeding, and there is a chance you may feel quite sick and experience diarrhoea or vomiting or abdominal pain | | 'OK. What is the third option?' | |
| The third option is surgical management. This involves passing a small suction tube through the cervix and into the womb, to remove the tissue that is still there | | 'Would I be awake for that?' | |
| It can either be done under a general anaesthetic, or with you awake in the outpatient clinic | | 'And what are the risks with this?' | |
| There are risks of bleeding and infection, and of damage to the womb needing keyhole or open surgery to repair. While these are rare risks, they are serious and have to be considered carefully | | 'OK. Thank you.' | |

**Finishing the Consultation**

| Question | Justification | Answer | Thoughts |
|---|---|---|---|
| Are there any questions that you have for me at this stage? | Acknowledge that this can be quite an overwhelming time and check if you have covered anything that she wishes to discuss | 'Will this affect me having more children?' | Able to establish patient's concern at this stage and can discuss further as appropriate |

**Finishing the Consultation**

| Question | Justification | Answer | Thoughts | | | | | |
|---|---|---|---|---|---|---|---|---|
| No. A miscarriage does not affect you having. I can provide you with written information about everything we have discussed so you can talk it all through with your partner | Important to reassure the patient and to answer her questions. Also vital to provide written information | 'Thank you' | You have addressed the patient's concerns | | | | | |
| To summarise, we have discussed the options to manage your miscarriage. I will provide you with a leaflet with more information and am happy to assist in any way possible | Summarising the consultation and offering written communication | 'Thank you' | Leaflets will help to refresh the patient's memory | | | | | |
| Do you have any other questions? I know that we have discussed a lot of new things; please take some time to digest the information | Allows any final concerns to be addressed | 'No' | The patient does not have any further questions | | | | | |

**Present Your Findings**

Miss Parker is a 32-year-old woman who presents today with an incomplete miscarriage which has been diagnosed on ultrasound scan. She presented originally to her general practitioner with vaginal bleeding, which has since stopped. She is fit and well, and has had two children before. These were uncomplicated pregnancies.

I have discussed the options for conservative, medical and surgical management with Miss Parker today, and she is going to go home to discuss these further with her partner. She will telephone the clinic to let us know if she has any questions and what she would like to do next

**General Points**

| | | | |
|---|---|---|---|
| Polite to patient, asks questions sensitively | | | |
| Maintains good eye contact | | | |
| Appropriate use of open and closed questions | | | |

## ❓ QUESTIONS FROM THE EXAMINER

### What is the role of an EPU?

To offer clinical care and emotional support to women with problems in early pregnancy, such as ectopic pregnancy or miscarriage. Women may be referred with pain or vaginal bleeding, and there will be the capacity for ultrasound scanning (usually on the same day) and blood tests if needed. EPUs may be staffed by specialist nurses, midwives or doctors.

### What setting should you use to break bad news?

A quiet room, with a clear notice outside that you should not be disturbed. The patient should be offered to have someone else with her to hear any bad news.

### What is a miscarriage?

According to World Health Organization (WHO), this is the expulsion of a fetus or embryo weighing less than 500 g, at less than 22 completed weeks' gestation. In the UK, a miscarriage is the loss of an intrauterine pregnancy before 24 weeks' gestation.

## What is the main cause of miscarriage?

Chromosomal abnormalities are the most common cause, attributed to 50% of miscarriages.

## What is the rate of uterine perforation in the surgical management of miscarriage?

Five in 1000 cases.

## Who should receive anti-D?

If the rhesus status of the fetus is unknown, then all rhesus-negative women undergoing medical or surgical management should receive anti-D, and all rhesus-negative women with a miscarriage after 12 weeks' gestation.

## Is it a problem if a woman does not make a decision about miscarriage management on the day she is seen?

No. Unless she is unstable or bleeding heavily, it better to give women time to make an informed decision and to discuss with relatives.

## Is everyone scanned in the EPU?

It is unlikely that an EPU will scan someone who is <5 weeks pregnant. This is because it is very unlikely that a fetal pole will be seen on scan.

## Can a miscarriage be confirmed on just one scan?

Yes. There are strict parameters on how a miscarriage is diagnosed. If a scan meets these criteria, then as long as two professionals agree it can be diagnosed on one scan.

## What if a scan does not meet the criteria for miscarriage diagnosis, but it is suspected?

In this case, the patient should have a repeat scan in 7 days' time.

## Station 7.15 Communication: Combined Oral Contraceptive Pill

### Doctor Briefing

You are a junior doctor in primary care and your next patient is Lauren Field, a 28-year-old woman, who wishes to start the combined oral contraceptive pill (COCP). She has a regular sexual partner, and they have been using condoms up to this point. Please explain how the COCP works and how to take it, as well as the risks and benefits of this form of contraception.

### Patient Briefing

This is the first time you have been to see the doctor for contraception advice, having previously only used condoms. You are looking to change to something different, and both you and your partner have been tested for STIs in the past 3 months.

You have no health problems, and no allergies or family history of note.

You want to know how the pill works, how effective it is and if there is anything else you should know while taking it.

### Mark Scheme for Examiner

#### Introduction

| | | | |
|---|---|---|---|
| Cleans hands, introduces self, confirms patient identity | | | |
| Checks the identity of others in the room and confirms that the patient is happy for them to be present | | | |
| Establishes current patient knowledge and concerns | | | |

#### Explaining How the COCP Works

| Statement/Question | Justification | Answer | Thoughts | | | |
|---|---|---|---|---|---|---|
| The COCP is a tablet containing a combination of two hormones, oestrogen and progestogen. The combination of these is what acts as a contraceptive | Start with a general explanation | 'OK' | You now know the patient is engaged and listening | | | |
| This is achieved by stopping you ovulating, which means releasing an egg each month | Be careful to explain things in clear language. Don't assume patients understand things the way doctors do | 'I understand' | Chunking here makes sure that the patient is following you | | | |
| It can be started at any time in your cycle, but it is easiest to start it on the first day of your period, then you will not need to use additional contraception | | 'What if I start it later?' | Patient is obviously thinking through process | | | |
| If you start it later than day 5 of your cycle (the fifth day of your period) then you should use extra contraception (such as condoms) for at least 7 days | | 'What happens with my period?' | A sensible question | | | |
| After taking the pill for 21 days, you have a pill-free week, and your period will start. Some pills have dummy pills instead of a pill-free week, and it is important to know which one you have | | 'What if I miss a pill?' | Really good for the patient to bring up something that should be discussed with all tablet contraceptives | | | |

## Explaining How the COCP Works

| Statement/Question | Justification | Answer | Thoughts | | | | | |
|---|---|---|---|---|---|---|---|---|
| If the missed pill is more than 24 h but less than 48 h late, you should take the missed pill immediately, and the rest of the packet should be taken as normal | Be careful to give very clear information here as it can be very confusing | 'What if I miss two pills?' | Sometimes important to not get too bogged down in detail. Remember, you can always signpost patients to resources | | | | | |
| If this is in the first 7 days of the packet, you should consider emergency contraception (EC) if you have had unprotected sex in the pill-free week or first week. Do you understand? | | 'Yes. What if it isn't in the first week?' | The patient is unlikely to remember these details seems keen to hear them | | | | | |
| If it is in the second week, you can carry on as normal as long as you have not missed any pills in the first week also. Does that make sense? | | 'Yes … and the third week?' | Answer her question | | | | | |
| If it is in the third week, you should miss out the pill-free week, and start the next packet when this one finishes. If you have a packet with dummy pills you should put these in the bin and start the next packet | | 'I see' | The patient seems happy you have covered this with her | | | | | |
| If you can't remember all of this today then you can find this information in the leaflet in your pill packet | Important to give written information in these situations | 'Thank you. That is useful to know' | The patient hasn't asked any further questions, so you can move on | | | | | |

## Explain the Risks and Benefits

| Statement/Question | Justification | Answer | Thoughts | | | | | |
|---|---|---|---|---|---|---|---|---|
| The benefits of taking the COCP include that you will not need to take any other contraception to stop you getting pregnant, and that it is non-invasive | Really important to cover the benefits and risks for all contraceptives | 'What is the chance of me getting pregnant while taking the pill?' | The patient is understandably keen to know the efficacy of these medications | | | | | |
| With perfect use, 3 per 1000 women using the COCP will get pregnant per year. In reality, this number is around 90 per 1000 | Be clear on how important it is to take it properly | 'OK, I understand' | Patient appears to be following the discussion | | | | | |
| The COCP will not protect you from STIs, so you may want to consider using condoms if you could be at risk | Remember to cover all safety aspects in consultations | 'My partner and I have both been tested for STIs, but that is useful to know' | The patient is following safe-sex standards. No further concerns here at the moment | | | | | |

**Explain the Risks and Benefits**

| Question | Justification | Answer | Thoughts | | | | | |
|---|---|---|---|---|---|---|---|---|
| Around one in five women find they have irregular bleeding while taking the COCP, and some women report mood changes | Be clear on side effects and serious things to watch out for | 'Thank you, that is helpful. I don't have any family members with breast cancer' | Seems to have taken in what you have said | | | | | |
| There is an increased chance of developing a clot in your leg or lung, called a venous thromboembolism or VTE. The risk of this is about double that of women not taking the COCP. You should see a doctor if you develop a hot, swollen calf or experience shortness of breath or chest pain | | | | | | | | |
| There is also a small increased chance of a stroke compared to women who are not taking the COCP | | | | | | | | |
| The COCP also puts you at an increased chance of breast cancer and cervical cancer; however these risks return to normal within 10 years of stopping. Although these risks are very small, you should not take the COCP if you have had breast cancer, and consider something else if you have a family history of it | | | | | | | | |

**Finishing the Consultation**

| Question | Justification | Answer | Thoughts | | | | | |
|---|---|---|---|---|---|---|---|---|
| To summarise, we have discussed the COCP, how it works and how to take it, as well as its risks and benefits. I will provide you with a leaflet with more information and am happy to assist in any way possible | Summarising the consultation and offering written communication | 'Thank you' | Leaflets will help to refresh the patient's memory | | | | | |
| Do you have any other questions? I know that we have discussed a lot of new things; please take some time to digest the information | Allows any final concerns to be addressed | 'No' | The patient does not have any further questions | | | | | |

**Present Your Findings**

Miss Field is a 28-year-old woman who has presented today to discuss the COCP. We have covered how it works, how to take it, its efficacy and risks and benefits.

I have checked her medical records and taken a thorough history and she has no contraindications.

I have given her a prescription today, and shall see her for a check-up in 6 months' time

| General Points | | | | | |
|---|---|---|---|---|---|
| Polite to patient | | | | | |
| Maintains good eye contact | | | | | |
| Appropriate use of open and closed questions | | | | | |

## ❓ QUESTIONS FROM THE EXAMINER

### How common is COCP use?

This varies across the world, but 20% of women in the UK aged 16–49 use it for contraception.

### Apart from inhibiting ovulation, what other effects does the COCP have?

It thickens cervical mucus to prevent sperm passage and thins the endometrium, making implantation less likely.

### What other types of combined contraceptive are available?

Transdermal patch or vaginal ring.

### When can the COCP be started after pregnancy?

Because of the risk of VTE, women should wait 6 weeks after having their baby to start the COCP.

### The COCP reduces the risk of which cancers?

Endometrial, colorectal and ovarian cancer. After 15 years of use, the risk of ovarian cancer is half that of women who have never taken the COCP.

### What is the risk of VTE when taking the COCP?

In healthy, non-pregnant women, the risk is two per 10,000. Use of COCP including ethinyloestradiol and levonorgestrel, norgestimate or norethisterone, it is 5–7 per 10,000. Use of COCP including ethinyloestradiol and gestodene, desogestrel or drospirenone, it is 9/12 per 10,000.

### What are the differences in monophasic and phasic pills?

Monophasic pills contain doses of oestrogen and progestogen that are the same throughout the cycle. Phasic pills may be biphasic, triphasic or quadriphasic (two, three or four different doses), and the amount of oestrogen and progestogen can vary throughout the cycle.

### What medications may interfere with the COCP?

Enyzme-inducing drugs; for example, rifampicin, St John's wort and some anticonvulsants.

### What specific advice should be given to women taking lamotrigine?

They have an increased risk of seizure, and a risk of toxicity when in their pill-free week, and so alternative contraception should be used when possible.

### What would you advise a woman taking the COCP to do if she develops diarrhoea or vomiting?

If she vomits within 2 h of taking it, she should take another pill. If she has symptoms for over 24 h, she should follow the same rules as for missed pills.

## Station 7.16    Communication: Emergency Contraception

### Doctor Briefing

You are a junior doctor in the sexual health clinic and have been asked to see Chloe Martin, a 16-year-old woman, who has presented to request emergency contraception (EC). Please discuss her options with her, as well as the risks and benefits of each.

### Patient Briefing

You have come to see the doctor, as you had sexual intercourse last night with your boyfriend, and the condom split. He is your only sexual partner, and you have been together for a year. You feel safe in the relationship. You are using only condoms for contraception, and have had no previous unprotected sex.

You have no medical problems and no allergies.

You are scared of getting pregnant and want to know more about EC.

### Mark Scheme for Examiner

#### Introduction

| | |
|---|---|
| Cleans hands, introduces self, confirms patient identity | |
| Checks the identity of others in the room and confirms that the patient is happy for them to be present | |
| Establishes current patient knowledge and concerns | |

#### Check History and Patient Safety

| Statement/Question | Justification | Answer | Thoughts | |
|---|---|---|---|---|
| If it's OK, can I just ask you a few questions so I know what options are best for you? | Start with an open phrase to let her know why you are asking the coming questions | 'Yes, that's fine' | The patient understands a history needs to be taken | |
| When did you have the unprotected sex that you are worried about? | Check the time frame to ensure the right options are offered | 'Last night. We were using a condom and it burst' | This means all options are available for EC | |
| Are you using any other contraception? | May not need it if using something else too | 'No, we only use condoms' | Definitely need to consider EC | |
| Have you had any other episodes of unprotected sex since your last period? | May not be able to offer anything if there were previous episodes in this cycle | 'No, only last night' | Leaves options open | |
| When was your last period, and are your periods regular? | Can offer copper coil within 5 days of ovulation | 'It was 2 weeks ago, and they happen about every 4 weeks' | No change in plan | |
| Did you feel forced into having sex with this partner? | Important to check patient safety | 'No, we have been together for a year, and I am happy with him. I didn't feel forced' | No additional concerns | |

## Check History and Patient Safety

| Statement/Question | Justification | Answer | Thoughts | | | | |
|---|---|---|---|---|---|---|---|
| I can offer you EC today, but this won't protect you from STIs. Would you like to arrange for tests to be done? | Important to think of issues other than pregnancy | 'Yes, please. I would like that' | Can arrange follow-up testing | | | | |
| Do you have any health problems, take any medicines or have any allergies? | In case of contraindications | 'No, nothing' | No additional concerns | | | | |

## Explain Options Available, Risks and Benefits

| Statement/Question | Justification | Answer | Thoughts | | | | |
|---|---|---|---|---|---|---|---|
| There are three options I can offer you today. Is it OK to talk through them now? | Check patient is ready to discuss options and signpost the discussion | 'Yes, please' | The patient is happy for you to proceed | | | | |
| The first is the copper coil. You can use this up to 5 days after unprotected sex. It is inserted through the neck of the womb, and can stay in place for up to 10 years as contraception | Explain clearly and in concise pieces | 'Does it hurt when it is put in?' | The patient is sharing her worry with you; it is vital you acknowledge and address this | | | | |
| It can be a bit uncomfortable, and you may have pain like period pain afterwards, which is usually helped by paracetamol | Making sure you answer the question the patient has asked | 'Are there any risks?' | Appears to be following what you are saying | | | | |
| There is a very small risk of the coil making a hole in the womb, or of the coil falling out after it is fitted | You must always go through the risks and benefits | 'What are the main benefits then?' | Chunking up your information helps the patient to understand and follow what you are saying | | | | |
| It can provide ongoing contraception, and is the most effective form of EC | Make sure you highlight the long-acting nature of the copper coil | 'That's good to know. What are my other options?' | The patient is keen to hear alternatives | | | | |
| The next options are tablets: ulipristal or levonorgestrel. Their main side effect is that they can cause vomiting | Most medications have common mild side effects, such as gastrointestinal disruption | 'What are my time limits on those?' | Patient is asking questions that you should be able to answer easily | | | | |
| Levonorgestrel can be used up to 72 h (3 days) after sex and ulipristal can be used up to 120 h (5 days) afterwards | It is vital to establish the timing of medication for EC | 'Which is better?' | Patient wanting to have the most effective contraception | | | | |
| Ulipristal is more effective, although it is less effective than the coil | Answer the questions directly | 'What if I am sick after taking it?' | She has picked up on the main side effect of vomiting | | | | |
| If you are sick less than 3 h after taking the tablet then you would need to take another dose | | 'OK, thank you, that's helpful' | No additional concerns | | | | |

**Finishing the Consultation**

| Question | Justification | Answer | Thoughts | | | | | |
|---|---|---|---|---|---|---|---|---|
| To summarise, we have discussed the various forms of EC. I will provide you with a leaflet with more information and am happy to assist in any way possible | Summarising the consultation and offering written communication | 'Yes, it'll be useful to take some information away for reference' | Leaflets will help to refresh the patient's memory | | | | | |
| Do you have any other questions? I know that we have discussed a lot of new things; please take some time to digest the information | Allows any final concerns to be addressed | 'No, thank you, that was helpful. I would like to have the coil fitted please' | The patient does not have any further questions | | | | | |

**Present Your Findings**

Miss Martin is a 16-year-old woman who has attended today requesting EC. She had unprotected sexual intercourse last night. I have no concerns regarding safeguarding today.

We have discussed her options, and she wishes to have a copper coil fitted.

I shall arrange for this to happen today, as well as relevant sexual health screening

**General Points**

Polite to patient

Maintains good eye contact

Appropriate use of open and closed questions

Uses non-judgemental language throughout

## ❓ QUESTIONS FROM THE EXAMINER

### How does the copper coil work to prevent pregnancy?

It has a direct toxic effect on sperm (reducing motility) and ova (affecting viability and transport). It also has a direct inflammatory effect on the endometrium, preventing implantation.

### How do the oral EC medications work?

Ulipristal is a selective progesterone receptor modulator, and delays ovulation by 5 days until sperm are no longer active. Levonorgestrel is a progestogen which inhibits ovulation by delaying or preventing follicular rupture.

### How effective is each method?

The copper coil has a 1 in 1000 pregnancy rate. Ulipristal has a 1–2 in 100 pregnancy rate. Levonorgestrel has a 2–3 in 100 pregnancy rate.

### What happens if a woman becomes pregnant after taking EC?

A copper coil should be removed, but the woman should be warned of the small risk of miscarriage. There is no increased risk of fetal abnormality or adverse pregnancy outcome if oral EC is taken.

## What should you do if you have concerns about the patient's safety or feel she was coerced?

Ensure discussion is well documented; make sure patient is going home somewhere safe and advise on refuge if needed; contact local safeguarding team for further advice.

## Can you take oral contraception more than once in a cycle?

You can take levonorgestrel more than once in a cycle but you can only take ulipristal once. That is why it is important to find out if the patient has used any other EC recently.

## Can you breastfeed and use EC?

You can breastfeed safely with the copper coil and levonorgestrel; however guidance is that you should avoid breastfeeding for 5–7 days if you take ulipristal.

## Is there a form of EC for men?

No.

## Where can you get EC?

Pharmacies, the emergency department, sexual health clinics and gynaecology units are the most accessible places to get EC.

## What STI screen should you offer women who accept it?

As a minimum, women should have a swab for chlamydia and gonorrhoea. They should also be risk-assessed for human immunodeficiency virus (HIV) and hepatitis B.

## Station 7.17    Communication: Cervical Smear Counselling

### Doctor Briefing

You are a junior doctor in a primary care practice and have been asked to see Miss Kerr, a 26-year-old woman, who is worried about her first cervical smear result. It has shown mild dyskaryosis and human papillomavirus (HPV), and she has an appointment for colposcopy. Please explain the diagnosis to her as well as what will happen at her colposcopy appointment.

### Patient Briefing

You have attended today to discuss the results of your first smear test, which you have received through the post. You are unsure what the results mean and are worried that it also means that you have an STI.

You want to know more about the diagnosis and what it means, what to expect when you go to the colposcopy clinic and what it could mean for your future.

### Mark Scheme for Examiner

#### Introduction

| | |
|---|---|
| Cleans hands, introduces self, confirms patient identity | |
| Checks the identity of others in the room and confirms that the patient is happy for them to be present | |
| Establishes current patient knowledge and concerns | |

#### Explaining the Diagnosis

| Statement/Question | Justification | Answer | Thoughts | |
|---|---|---|---|---|
| The cervical smear test is designed to pick up precancerous changes in the cervix | Start with an open statement | 'Yes, I am aware' | You know the patient is listening | |
| There are several different diagnoses that can come from a smear, and yours is one of these. Mild dyskaryosis is the medical term for mild changes in the cells of the cervix | Be clear and direct when explaining. It is useful to chunk things up into small sections | 'Does that mean I have cancer?' | Opens up one of patient's concerns | |
| It is very unlikely that you have cervical cancer with this result. Mild dyskaryosis usually means the cells are only beginning to become abnormal. | | 'Is the virus it mentioned bad? Have I caught an infection during sex?' | Leads into further concerns. HPV is often misunderstood and patients feel a lot of stigma around it. Have to make sure you are honest and clear | |
| Human papillomavirus or HPV is an incredibly common virus that is spread through sexual contact. However it can be inactive for a long time, and have no symptoms, so it is difficult to tell when you would have picked it up | | 'Why did they check for it during the smear test?' | | |

## Explaining the Diagnosis

| Statement/Question | Justification | Answer | Thoughts | | | | |
|---|---|---|---|---|---|---|---|
| It is important to screen for HPV because, although it can be asymptomatic, certain types can cause cervical cancer, and so if it is present, then you need closer surveillance to be safe | | 'Can I have treatment for it?' | | | | | |
| Some women will need treatment in the colposcopy clinic because of the changes associated with it, but most people will clear it within 2 years | | 'Can I do anything to help clear it?' | | | | | |
| Women who smoke are less likely to be able to clear the virus, so if you smoke then you should try to stop as soon as possible | | 'OK. Can you explain more about the colposcopy clinic please?' | | | | | |

## Explain the Colposcopy Clinic Visit

| Statement/Question | Justification | Answer | Thoughts | | | | |
|---|---|---|---|---|---|---|---|
| The colposcopy clinic takes place in the hospital outpatient department. You will be seen by a doctor or nurse who will ask you some questions and then examine your cervix with a special camera | Use plain language | 'Does it hurt?' | The patient is highlighting to you one of her anxieties | | | | |
| It is very similar to your smear test, and can be uncomfortable, but the test should not be painful | Always be open and honest with the patient | 'Will I need treatment?' | Sensible question; make sure you respond | | | | |
| If they find more concerning cells when they look with the camera, then you may need a biopsy or small sample of tissue. This is done with local anaesthetic and again can be uncomfortable | Remember to use lay terms throughout | 'Should I do anything special before or take anything with me?' | The patient is thinking about how to minimise her discomfort | | | | |
| It is a good idea to take paracetamol or ibuprofen before you go, and you can take someone with you if you would like support. Otherwise, you don't need to do anything else. You will receive written information about this | Clarify with the patient if she will receive written information | 'OK, thank you.' | The patient has no further questions, it appears | | | | |

## Finishing the Consultation

| Statement/Question | Justification | Answer | Thoughts | | | | |
|---|---|---|---|---|---|---|---|
| Do you have any other questions for me today? | Should help to uncover any further concerns not already addressed. Really important to check this | 'If I have to have treatment, will this stop me having children in the future?' | The patient has just shared a further anxiety | | | | |

### Finishing the Consultation

| Statement/Question | Justification | Answer | Thoughts | | |
|---|---|---|---|---|---|
| There is nothing that occurs at the colposcopy clinic that would stop you from having a baby. There is a type of treatment called a large-loop excision of the transformation zone, or LLETZ, which can be associated with preterm labour. This depends on the size of biopsy needed, and the team at the colposcopy clinic will be able to explain this to you if it is needed | Try to not get into too much detail but it is important to address her concerns | 'OK. Thank you, doctor' | The patient seems reassured | | |
| To summarise, we have discussed your results from the cervical smear and what to expect at your colposcopy visit. I will provide you with a leaflet with more information and am happy to assist in any way possible | Summarising the consultation and offering written communication | 'Thank you' | Leaflets will help to refresh the patient's memory | | |
| Do you have any other questions? I know that we have discussed a lot of new things; please take some time to digest the information | Allows any final concerns to be addressed | 'No' | The patient does not have any further questions | | |

### Present Your Findings

Miss Kerr is a 26-year-old woman who has attended today to discuss her first cervical smear test result. She has mild dyskaryosis and HPV infection.

I have explained the diagnosis and what to expect from her visit to the colposcopy clinic. I have also provided her with written information

### General Points

Polite to patient

Maintains good eye contact

Appropriate use of open and closed questions

Check for additional concerns

## ❓ QUESTIONS FROM THE EXAMINER

### What type of virus is HPV?

A DNA virus.

### What cancers are associated with HPV infection?

Cervical, vulval, vaginal, mouth, throat, penis and anal cancer.

## What are the two main subtypes of HPV associated with cervical cancer?

HPV subtypes 16 and 18, which cause around 70% of cervical cancers.

## What proportion of people become infected with HPV?

80% of sexually active people become infected with HPV in their lifetime.

## What subtypes of HPV are covered in the vaccination?

This depends on the country and vaccination programme. The vaccine currently used in the UK is Gardasil, which protects against subtypes 6, 11, 16 and 18. The two other licensed vaccines are Cervarix (subtypes 16 and 18 only) and Gardasil 9 (subtypes 6, 11, 16, 18, 31, 33, 45, 52 and 58).

## How is the HPV vaccine currently offered in the UK?

Girls and boys aged 12–13 years (11–12 years in Scotland) are covered in the screening programme. If it is missed, you can have it for free up until the age of 25 on the National Health Service.

## What is the rationale for starting cervical screening at **25 and not earlier?**

Screening in earlier age groups has not been shown to reduce cervical cancer in these groups. Many women under 25 may be exposed to HPV but clear it in this time, and so screening earlier could lead to unnecessary treatment, which can have consequences such as preterm labour in the future.

## What are the main histological subtypes of cervical cancer?

Squamous cell carcinoma accounts for 80% whereas adenocarcinoma accounts for 15–20%. Rarer tumours, including sarcomas, lymphomas, clear cell and small-cell neuroendocrine tumours, also exist.

## What are the presenting symptoms of cervical cancer?

Postcoital bleeding, intermenstrual bleeding, blood-stained vaginal discharge, postmenopausal bleeding and symptoms of advanced disease; for example, back or leg pain, bowel habit change, haematuria, malaise.

## How should the screening take place if the patient is pregnant?

Cervical screening should take place 3–4 months after delivery, if the woman has been invited to take part during her pregnancy. If she has symptoms then these should be investigated with urgency in the colposcopy clinic, and any lesions that are suggestive of invasion should be biopsied.

# Psychiatry

**8**

## Outline

---

| Station 8.1 | History: Alcohol |
|---|---|

### Doctor Briefing

You are a junior doctor in primary care and have been asked to see Mr Chang, a 58-year-old man, who has presented with an elevated gamma-glutamyl transpeptidase (GGT). His wife is concerned about how much he is drinking. Please take a detailed alcohol history from Mr Chang, present your findings and formulate an appropriate management plan.

### Patient Briefing

You are a 58-year-old solicitor. Two years ago, you became a partner at the solicitors, and your job has become more stressful since. You began drinking two beers after coming home from work but, in the last 2 months, this has increased to four beers every day. If you have had a particularly bad day, you can binge drink up to eight pints at one time.

You are aware that you have a drinking problem. You have not tried to quit drinking on your own but would like some help with this and to gain some control back over your life, such as a detox programme. When your wife has brought up your drinking before, you have become very defensive. You do not need an eye opener. You started drinking aged 17 and had been a social drinker until recently. You have no health conditions, take no medications and have not taken any illicit drugs. Your brother suffered with alcohol addiction and died 5 years ago.

You are concerned that if you don't get help, you will suffer from bad health associated with drinking too much alcohol, such as liver damage, which you've heard about.

### Mark Scheme for Examiner

#### Introduction

| | | | | | |
|---|---|---|---|---|---|
| Cleans hands, introduces self, confirms patient identity and gains consent for history taking | | | | | |

#### History of Presenting Complaint

| Question | Justification | Answer | Thoughts | | | | |
|---|---|---|---|---|---|---|---|
| What's brought you in today? | This question is general and open, so is a good way to start the consultation. It also helps to screen for insight as if the patient has attended voluntarily, this can show he may have some insight into the help needed | 'I've been told that one of my blood results is a bit high. I don't really know which one or why this is a problem' | This gives you some context and tells you that the patient isn't really sure what the problem is | | | | |

## History of Presenting Complaint

| Question | Justification | Answer | Thoughts | | | | | |
|---|---|---|---|---|---|---|---|---|
| One of the proteins that is raised is related to your liver. Sometimes, this can happen if there is a high alcohol consumption. Can I ask a few questions regarding your alcohol intake? | Always signpost the patient regarding where the consultation is going, especially if you are going to delve into personal questions that at times may come across as offensive | 'Go ahead' | The patient is expecting you to ask questions about his alcohol consumption | | | | | |
| How much alcohol do you drink in a typical week? | This question is important, as you need to establish current alcohol intake and to see whether this is above recommended limits | 'I drink about four beers a day, maybe more if it's a difficult day' | This patient is drinking 8 units a day, which is far above the recommended maximum 14 units a week. Follow-up questions need to include how often the patient is drinking, what alcohol he is drinking, whether he engages in binge drinking and what time he starts drinking | | | | | |
| What makes you start drinking? | This question can be used to screen for factors in the patient's life that might exacerbate drinking, such as stress or alcohol availability | 'I drink if I've had a particularly stressful day at work' | Stress is a common factor that leads to drinking. It may make stopping alcohol difficult if the stress continues or proper stress-coping techniques are not included within the management | | | | | |
| Have you ever felt that you should cut down on your drinking? | This is the first question in the CAGE tool, which is a widely used screening tool to assess alcohol use or dependence | 'I have felt for a while that I should cut down. I just wasn't sure how to go about it' | This patient has thought about cutting down before, so this adds 1 point to the CAGE screening tool | | | | | |
| Have other people annoyed you by criticising the amount you drink? | This is the second question in the CAGE tool | 'My wife. My wife thinks I drink too much and when she brings it up, it frustrates me a lot' | This patient responded yes to this question so this is +1 to the CAGE screening tool | | | | | |
| Have you ever felt guilty about your drinking? | This is the third question in the CAGE tool | 'I don't think I ever feel guilty about my drinking' | Patient does not show guilt about drinking, which doesn't add a further point to the CAGE screening tool | | | | | |
| Do you ever need a drink first thing in the morning? | This is the final question in the CAGE tool, to screen if the patient requires an eye opener | 'No' | This patient does not use an eye opener, which doesn't add a further point to the CAGE screening tool. Adding points from all the CAGE questions together, you get a score of 2. A score of 2 or above suggests alcohol misuse or dependence | | | | | |

## History of Presenting Complaint

| Question | Justification | Answer | Thoughts | | | | | |
|---|---|---|---|---|---|---|---|---|
| At what age did you start drinking? | This question should be used with other questions to establish past alcohol history and past drinking habits | 'I started drinking at 17 but have only drunk socially up until now' | This should ask you to prompt further on binge habits, triggers for drinking (such as socialising) and longest period of abstinence | | | | | |
| Is there a family history of alcoholism? | Alcoholism and drug addiction display strong family history, whether this a genetic or environmental connection | 'My brother was an alcohol addict and died about 5 years ago' | The patient has a positive family history of alcoholism | | | | | |
| Have you ever experienced any health problems associated with alcohol? | There are many health conditions linked to alcohol misuse, including gastrointestinal (GI) conditions, cardiovascular effects and psychiatric conditions | 'No, I don't think so' | No additional concerns | | | | | |
| Have you ever had any help from services in the past regarding your drinking? | In this question, you are looking for previous treatments and their outcomes, such as detoxification programmes, counselling, attending Alcoholics Anonymous | 'No, I haven't' | No prior contact with services | | | | | |
| Do you want to change your drinking habits? | This question assesses motivation to change. Success in changing drinking behaviour depends heavily on the individual's willingness to change | 'Definitely, I know I drink too much' | A positive step in changing drinking habits. This should be followed up with what help he thinks would be useful and a further discussion about options | | | | | |

## Past Psychiatric and Medical History

| | | | | | | | | |
|---|---|---|---|---|---|---|---|---|
| Have you ever struggled with your mental health? | Mental health conditions such as depression can exacerbate drinking | 'No' | No additional concerns | | | | | |
| Do you have any long-term health problems? | Alcohol abuse can lead to a variety of long-term conditions. The relationship between chronic illness and mental health conditions is also well established | 'No' | No additional concerns | | | | | |

### Drug History

| Question | Justification | Answer | Thoughts | | | | | |
|----------|---------------|--------|----------|--|--|--|--|--|
| Are you on any prescription medication at the moment or use anything over the counter? | It is important to find out in detail what medication the patient is taking regularly | 'No medications' | No additional concerns | | | | | |
| Do you have any drug allergies? | You must always check for allergies | 'No allergies' | No additional concerns | | | | | |

### Family History

| Question | Justification | Answer | Thoughts | | | | | |
|----------|---------------|--------|----------|--|--|--|--|--|
| Are there any diseases that run in the family, including any cancers? | Important always to check for relevant heritable conditions | 'Not that I'm aware of' | No additional concerns | | | | | |
| Does anyone in your family struggle with their mental health, specifically addiction? | Important to screen for family history of mental health disorders | 'Apart from my brother, whom I've mentioned' | Presence of mental illness within the family | | | | | |

### Social and Travel History

| Question | Justification | Answer | Thoughts | | | | | |
|----------|---------------|--------|----------|--|--|--|--|--|
| Who is currently at home? Are you working at the moment? | Find out if there are any social concerns or if wider support is needed. Alcoholism can be associated with absenteeism and loss of job. Alcoholism is also associated with divorce and lack of social support | 'I live with my wife. I am working as a partner at a solicitor's' | Partners can provide support, especially with ongoing treatment or management if required. Stress from work can be a trigger for drinking, and this should be covered in further detail | | | | | |
| Have you got any stress in your life at the moment? | Stressful circumstances can initiate or exacerbate psychiatric disorders and may be a trigger for drinking | 'I have a lot of stress from work, and I've noticed that I seem to drink more if I've had a bad day at work' | External stressors present, which seem to be a trigger for drinking | | | | | |
| Do you smoke tobacco or use any recreational drugs? | Find out a patient's wider risk factors | 'I used to smoke as a teenager but haven't smoked since. I haven't used drugs' | No additional concerns | | | | | |
| Any problems in getting along with people close to you? | Alcohol can put strain on family relationships and cause separation or divorce | 'My wife has been worried about the drinking and it has put some strain on our marriage' | Alcoholism seems to be affecting his personal life and relationships | | | | | |

## Social and Travel History

| Question | Justification | Answer | Thoughts | | | | | |
|---|---|---|---|---|---|---|---|---|
| Have you ever been in trouble with the police? | This question looks for unsociable behaviour and driving convictions that may have been caused by drinking | 'No' | No additional concerns | | | | | |

## Systems Review

| Question | Justification | Answer | Thoughts | | | | | |
|---|---|---|---|---|---|---|---|---|
| I'm just going to ask you some general questions about your health. Have you had any change in appetite/weight/bowel habits/water works/sleep? Do you find yourself sweating more or getting palpitations? Have you had any fevers? | A quick systems review of somatic symptoms that present with psychiatric disorders is important | 'No, I haven't noticed any of those' | No additional concerns | | | | | |

## Finishing the Consultation

| Question | Justification | Answer | Thoughts | | | | | |
|---|---|---|---|---|---|---|---|---|
| To summarise, your wife has been concerned about the amount of alcohol you've been drinking and you agree that your drinking has increased recently due to stress at work. Is that correct? | When summarising and finishing a consultation, it's important to recap the important information so far, the patient's key concerns and the plan moving forward | 'Yes, that's correct. I really do think I need some help to get the drinking under control' | Happy that the information that you have gathered is accurate | | | | | |
| Do you have any other questions or things to add? I know that we have discussed a lot of new things; please take some time to digest the information | May identify useful information that has been missed. Will also allow you to address any questions or concerns | 'No, I don't have any questions' | Take the time to explain what will happen from here | | | | | |

**Present Your Findings**

Mr Chang is a 58-year-old man who presented with an increased GGT, and we've discussed his increased alcohol intake. Before this, he said he was a social drinker, but now, due to increased stress at work, he drinks 56 units a week, usually beer. There are no features for a diagnosis of alcohol dependence syndrome. He has no other health problems and no psychiatric problems but has a family history of alcoholism. He has good insight and is aware that he drinks too much and is hoping to get help to reach abstinence.

I would like to examine Mr Chang fully and take a collateral history. I would also like to repeat his blood tests and organise a liver ultrasound scan. I will also refer to local drug and alcohol services so that he can receive appropriate support with reducing his alcohol intake

**General Points**

Polite to patient

Maintains good eye contact

Appropriate use of open and closed questions

## ❓ QUESTIONS FROM THE EXAMINER

### What is the treatment to prevent alcohol withdrawal syndrome?

Long-acting benzodiazepines; for example, diazepam.

### What is the role of disulfiram in the maintenance of abstinence?

Disulfiram can be used for those who have difficulty resisting alcohol. It blocks metabolism of alcohol, causing increased levels of acetaldehyde. Therefore, when alcohol is consumed, it causes headaches, flushing and nausea. It should never be used as a monotherapy and should be used in conjunction with supportive psychotherapy.

### What is the pathophysiology of Korsakoff's syndrome?

An organic brain disorder caused by a deficiency in vitamin $B_1$ (thiamine) resulting from long-term heavy drinking, resulting in short-term memory loss and confabulation.

### If someone presents with nystagmus, ataxia and delirium, what are you worried about and how should the patient be treated?

Wernicke's encephalopathy, which is treated with vitamin B and C infusions (e.g. Pabrinex intravenously).

### What is the recommended maximum weekly consumption of alcohol for an adult in the UK?

14 units.

### What are the cardinal symptoms of alcohol dependence?

Strong desire or compulsion to drink, difficulty controlling intake of substance, physiological withdrawal symptoms, tolerance, neglect of other responsibilities and persistence despite evidence of harmful consequences.

### What are the GI complications of alcohol abuse?

Liver cirrhosis, pancreatitis, gastritis, gastro-oesophageal reflux disease, peptic ulcer disease, hepatic encephalopathy, Mallory–Weiss tear and oesophageal varices.

**What would you expect to see on the full blood count of someone with alcohol dependence?**

Typically, alcohol dependence is associated with macrocytic anaemia.

**What are the clinical features on the hands that can indicate hepatic cirrhosis?**

Palmar erythema, Dupuytren's contracture, clubbing, pigmentation, jaundice, bruises and cyanosis.

**One year after a successful detox, what percentage of people in the UK stay abstinent and how does this change with engagement in specialist alcohol services?**

20%, increasing to 30% with engagement in specialist alcohol services.

## Station 8.2    History: Depression

### Doctor Briefing

You are a junior doctor in primary care and have been asked to see Mr Wood, a 50-year-old man, who has presented with difficulties sleeping. He has recently been made redundant and his wife has noticed that he is not enjoying things like he used to. She is worried about his mood. Please take a history from Mr Wood, present your findings and formulate an appropriate management plan.

### Patient Briefing

You have been struggling with your sleep recently, finding it difficult to fall asleep and often waking up at 4 a.m. and unable to fall back to sleep.

You lost your job as an accountant a month ago and have been feeling low ever since. You have been losing weight as you don't want to eat and aren't doing normal day-to-day activities, like showering or getting out of bed. You used to enjoy hiking but have since found no joy in this and have been unmotivated to go.

You have been drinking 20 units of alcohol a week, which is more than normal for you. You've not had any thoughts of self-harm, suicide or harming others.

You have no significant medical history and no family history of psychiatric illness. You have felt low before and had some talking therapy which helped. About a year ago, you had a period of very high mood, spent a lot of money on luxury items and gambled excessively.

Your wife and friends are worried about you as you haven't been your normal outgoing self, which you have noticed but put it down to your poor sleep.

### Mark Scheme for Examiner

**Introduction**

| Cleans hands, introduces self, confirms patient identity and gains consent for history taking | | | | |
|---|---|---|---|---|

**History of Presenting Complaint**

| Question | Justification | Answer | Thoughts | | | | | |
|---|---|---|---|---|---|---|---|---|
| What's brought you in today? | This question is general and open, so is a good way to start the consultation. It also helps to screen for insight as if the patient has presented voluntarily, this can show he may have some insight into the help he needs | 'My wife has encouraged me to come in today. I've been struggling with my sleep and I've not been feeling myself' | Clear worry from partner but also shows that the patient may have some insight | | | | | |
| How do you feel within yourself? Does this vary throughout the day? | This allows you to get a better idea of the patient's mood and allows you to screen for high and low moods | 'I'm feeling very low at the moment' | Low mood is one of the core depressive symptoms so needs to be explored further to establish a timeline and whether it has changed. A low mood present for over 2 weeks would suggest depression | | | | | |
| Do you still enjoy things that you used to? | This question screens for anhedonia, which is loss of interest | 'Yes, I used to hike every weekend. However I haven't felt like going for the last few weeks' | This patient displays evidence of anhedonia, which is one of the core symptoms of depression | | | | | |

**History of Presenting Complaint**

| Question | Justification | Answer | Thoughts |
|---|---|---|---|
| Do you find that you tire more easily? | Looking for fatigue, which is one of the core depressive symptoms | 'Yes, I don't have any energy recently, but I can't tell whether this is from the sleep problems' | This patient demonstrates some fatigue, which could be indicative of depression |
| How is your sleep? | Sleep disturbance is one of the biological/somatic symptoms of depression | 'Terrible! I can't seem to fall asleep and then when I do, I wake up very early and can't get back to sleep' | This patient is showing insomnia and early-morning wakening, which are both evidence of sleep disturbance, potentially secondary to depression. Other somatic symptoms such as reduced appetite, weight loss, constipation and loss of libido should all be screened for as well |
| How do you see yourself compared to other people? How do you feel about yourself? | These questions are used to assess feelings of worthlessness and current self-esteem | 'I'm just not good at anything. My wife deserves so much better than me' | Patient shows signs of worthlessness and low self-esteem. Alongside these cognitive symptoms of depression, other symptoms, including poor memory, poor concentration, guilt, tearfulness and agitation, need to be assessed |
| Have you ever heard things said when there is no one round and nothing can explain it? | This is one of the questions that can be used to help screen for abnormal perceptions | 'No' | No evidence suggesting hallucinations and, therefore, psychotic depression. However, more questions should be asked to screen more thoroughly |
| Do you ever have episodes where your mood is very elevated or you do things that you later regret? | These questions can be used to check for bipolar affective disorder which is a differential diagnosis of a depressive episode | 'Yes, I had an episode last year when I felt great! I bought lots of designer clothes and gambled a fair bit' | Suggestive of episode of previous mania and previous depression; implies this could be bipolar affective disorder |
| How would you describe yourself growing up? How do you think others would describe you? | Establishing a premorbid personality is an important step in a psychiatric history. It allows you to screen for potential personality disorders, such as avoidant personality disorder | 'I have always been happy and sociable' | The patient's premorbid personality does not suggest a personality disorder, but it would be good to check this in a collateral history |

## History of Presenting Complaint

| Question | Justification | Answer | Thoughts | | | | | | |
|----------|---------------|--------|----------|---|---|---|---|---|---|
| Have you ever had thoughts of harming yourself or others? Have you ever had thoughts of ending your life? | Risk assessments are essential in psychiatry, so never miss this. They are even more vital with patients presenting with low mood as they are at an increased risk of suicide | 'No, never' | Risk assessment is complete and there is no further concerns at this time | | | | | | |
| What do you think is going on? Do you think you would benefit from any help? | Establishing whether the patient has insight into his condition | 'I was thinking it could be depression. I just feel so low all the time. I think I would benefit from some help, yes' | This patient has insight into his mental health | | | | | | |

## Past Psychiatric and Medical History

| Question | Justification | Answer | Thoughts | | | | | | |
|----------|---------------|--------|----------|---|---|---|---|---|---|
| Have you ever struggled with your mental health? | Screening for previous psychiatric diagnosis or mood disorder | 'I felt low a few years ago and had some cognitive behavioural therapy (CBT)' | Suggestive of some prior mental health issues; could be a history of depression | | | | | | |
| Do you have any long-term health problems? | The relationship between chronic illness and mental health conditions is well established. Physical illness such as cancer, hypothyroidism and Cushing's syndrome can present like depression | 'No' | No additional concerns | | | | | | |
| Have you recently had any illnesses or hospital visits? | | 'No' | No additional concerns | | | | | | |

## Drug History

| Question | Justification | Answer | Thoughts | | | | | | |
|----------|---------------|--------|----------|---|---|---|---|---|---|
| Are you on any prescription medication at the moment or use anything over the counter? | Prescription medications strongly associated with depressive symptoms are oral contraceptives, corticosteroids and some antihypertensive drugs | 'No medications' | No additional concerns | | | | | | |
| Do you have any drug allergies? | You must always check for allergies | 'No allergies' | No additional concerns | | | | | | |

## Family History

| Question | Justification | Answer | Thoughts | | | | | | |
|----------|---------------|--------|----------|---|---|---|---|---|---|
| Are there any diseases that run in the family, including any cancers? | Important always to check for relevant heritable conditions | 'Not that I'm aware of' | No additional concerns | | | | | | |
| Does anyone in your family struggle with their mental health? | Important to screen for family history of mental health disorders | 'Not that I'm aware of' | No additional concerns | | | | | | |

## Social and Travel History

| Question | Justification | Answer | Thoughts | | | | | |
|---|---|---|---|---|---|---|---|---|
| Who is currently at home? Are you working at the moment? | Find out if there are any social concerns or if wider support is needed | 'I live with my wife, Jenny, and my two sons. I am not working as I lost my job recently' | Partners can provide support, especially with ongoing treatment or management if required. Unemployment is a risk factor for the development of depression | | | | | |
| Have you got any stress in your life at the moment? | Stressful circumstances can initiate or exacerbate psychiatric disorders | 'I'm worried about how Jenny and I will pay the bills since I don't have a job' | External stressors present which can exacerbate feelings of inadequacy and anxiousness | | | | | |
| Do you smoke tobacco? | Find out a patient's wider risk factors, as well as exploring causes for symptom changes. Alcohol is also a mood suppressor so can contribute to symptoms of low mood | 'No, I have never smoked' | No additional concerns | | | | | |
| What is your average weekly alcohol consumption? | | 'I have around 10 pints a week now. I used to have only a few at the weekend but now I drink most nights' | Patient seems to have increased alcohol consumption recently, above the recommended limits. This could be the reason for the depressive symptoms or alternatively could be a result of them | | | | | |
| Have you ever taken any recreational drugs? | Drug withdrawal can present as low mood and irritability | 'No' | No additional concerns | | | | | |

## Systems Review

| Question | Justification | Answer | Thoughts | | | | | |
|---|---|---|---|---|---|---|---|---|
| I'm just going to ask you some general questions about your health. Have you had any change in appetite/weight/bowel habits/water works? Do you find yourself sweating more or getting palpitations? Have you had any fevers? | A quick systems review of somatic symptoms that present with psychiatric disorders is important | 'No, I haven't noticed any of those' | No additional concerns | | | | | |

**Finishing the Consultation**

| Question | Justification | Answer | Thoughts | | | | |
|---|---|---|---|---|---|---|---|
| To summarise, you've been feeling quite low recently since losing your job and you have little motivation. You've also been struggling with your sleep and appetite. You would be open to receiving some help from us. Is this correct? | When summarising and finishing a consultation, it's important to recap the important information so far, the patient's key concerns and the plan moving forward | 'Yes, that's right' | Happy that the information that you have gathered is accurate | | | | |
| Do you have any other questions or things to add? I know that we have discussed a lot of new things; please take some time to digest the information. | May identify useful information that has been missed. Will also allow you to address any questions or concerns | 'No, I don't have any questions' | Take the time to explain what will happen from here | | | | |

**Present Your Findings**

Mr Wood is a 50-year-old man who presented with persistent low mood and poor sleep over the last month. He is also showing symptoms of fatigue, anhedonia and increased alcohol intake. He describes no thoughts of harm to himself or others. This is on the background of no medical or diagnosed psychiatric illness but with a history of what could be mania and depressive episodes.

I feel the most likely diagnosis is bipolar affective disorder, with the differentials of a moderate depressive episode.

I would like to get a collateral history to further my assessment, fully examine Mr Wood and organise a thorough set of bloods, as well as asking him to complete the CAGE questionnaire

**General Points**

| | | | |
|---|---|---|---|
| Polite to patient | | | |
| Maintains good eye contact | | | |
| Appropriate use of open and closed questions | | | |

## ❓ QUESTIONS FROM THE EXAMINER

### What are the three core depressive symptoms?

Low mood, anhedonia and low energy.

### What is Cotard's syndrome?

A type of psychotic depression where the patient believes that they are dead.

## What are the differences between primary and secondary mood disorders?

Primary mood disorders are not caused by a medical or psychiatric condition. Secondary mood disorders are caused by medical or psychiatric conditions, such as hypothyroidism or Cushing's syndrome.

## What factors in an older patient presenting with memory problems would make you think of a diagnosis of depression rather than dementia?

Short history of rapid-onset memory problems, biological symptoms (e.g. weight loss, sleep disturbance), patient concerned about poor memory, variable mini mental test score, global memory loss (dementia usually causes recent memory loss).

## What are the common side effects of selective serotonin reuptake inhibitors?

GI disturbance (either diarrhoea or constipation), feeling anxious, nausea and insomnia.

## What is seasonal affective disorder?

Depression that recurs in autumn and winter, associated with increased sleep.

## What is dysthymia?

Chronic low-grade depressive episode without other symptoms to give major depressive episode diagnosis.

## What endocrine disorders can present with low mood?

Hypothyroidism, hyperthyroidism, Cushing's syndrome, Addison's disease and hyperparathyroidism.

## When would electroconvulsive therapy (ECT) be an appropriate therapy for depression?

For severe depression that has not reacted to any drug therapy or for catatonic depression.

## What are the side effects of ECT treatment?

Nausea, confusion, headache and retrograde amnesia.

## Station 8.3    History: Mania

### Doctor Briefing

You are a junior doctor in primary care and have been asked to see Mrs Jones, a 28-year-old woman, who has presented with her husband. He reports that she has been acting strangely and has been on huge shopping sprees resulting in considerable debt. She has previously suffered from depression. Please take a history from Mrs Jones, present your findings and formulate an appropriate management plan.

### Patient Briefing

You have been in a great mood for the last few weeks. Your confidence is very high and your energy levels have never been better, meaning you haven't been having much sleep. You have been working on secret projects at night which have caused you to become rich. You are feeling very optimistic about your family and your financial standing. You have been going on huge shopping sprees, spending hundreds of pounds on clothes at a time. You are normally very responsible with money as you look after the family finances and budget.

You have not been seeing or hearing anything unusual. You have not had any thoughts of harming yourself or others. You do not smoke, drink alcohol or use recreational drugs.

You have no significant medical history and do not take any medication. You have had depressive episodes before, one aged 15, one at 21 and one after the birth of your son.

You don't feel unwell and you don't think you need any help. You get angry when your husband thinks there is a problem.

Instructions for patient: act very distractable and excited, change topics frequently and talk quickly.

### Mark Scheme for Examiner

#### Introduction

| Cleans hands, introduces self, confirms patient identity and gains consent for history taking | | | | | |
|---|---|---|---|---|---|

#### History of Presenting Complaint

| Question | Justification | Answer | Thoughts | | | | | |
|---|---|---|---|---|---|---|---|---|
| What's brought you in today? | This question is general and open, so is a good way to start the consultation. It also helps to screen for insight as if the patient has attended voluntarily, this can show she may have some insight into the help she needs | 'My husband brought me in today. I don't know why' | Clear worry from partner, but not from the patient | | | | | |
| How would you describe your mood? | This allows you to get a better idea of the patient's mood. For this history, we are screening for high mood, as the patient could be having a manic episode based on the briefing | 'I'm feeling fantastic, thank you! Everything's so wonderful. You're so beautiful too. Isn't the world just a great place to be? What a good time to be alive!' | An unusually elevated mood is one of the core features of mania. This patient does show an elevated mood so this should be followed up by establishing if there is a reason for the high mood or whether this is normal for the patient | | | | | |

**History of Presenting Complaint**

| Question | Justification | Answer | Thoughts | | | | | | | |
|---|---|---|---|---|---|---|---|---|---|---|
| How would you describe your energy levels? | Increased activity levels are associated with mania | 'I feel full of energy. I don't feel tired at all. I just keep going; I have so much to do anyway so I need to keep up. It's amazing!' | The patient demonstrates increased energy levels. Consider exploring further what she feels she needs to complete or keep up with | | | | | | | |
| Given that you've been so full of energy, how is your sleep? | Acknowledging what the patient has mentioned allows you to build a rapport. People with mania experience insomnia, as well as less sleep due to increased activity levels | 'I get a few minutes here and there but I don't need to sleep. I feel fabulous! Who needs to sleep when you have this much work to do?' | The patient demonstrates decreased levels of sleep and increased levels of activity at night, which is cohesive with a diagnosis of mania | | | | | | | |
| This question might be a bit personal, but has your interest in sex changed? | Warn the patient that a sensitive question is coming up. Increased libido can be a symptom of mania | 'Not that I've noticed. I don't have the time for that.' | No symptoms of increased libido | | | | | | | |
| Would you describe yourself as impulsive? | Assesses for disinhibition. This can take the form of overspending, gambling, illegal activity and other risk-taking behaviours | 'I mean, I've been treating myself lately with some shopping but we are rich, so why wouldn't I?' | This patient is demonstrating some disinhibition, and this should be followed up with further questions, such as: Do you feel that you've been taking more risks than you used to? Have you got into any trouble with the police lately or broken the law? | | | | | | | |
| How do you see yourself compared to other people? | Assesses self-worth. Mania can be associated with increased confidence, inflated self-esteem and grandiosity | 'Well, my family are extremely financially well off and we are very lucky. I don't want to sound spoilt but we are a bit better than everyone else … we're basically the royal family' | Consider exploring the patient's grandiose ideas and why she feels that she is comparable to high-profile people such as the royal family | | | | | | | |
| Do you have difficulties concentrating on things, such as reading a book or watching TV? | Assesses level of concentration. People experiencing mania often have reduced levels of concentration and increased activity levels | 'I can't just sit and watch TV or read a book! There's so much to do' | Signs of poor concentration | | | | | | | |

**History of Presenting Complaint**

| Question | Justification | Answer | Thoughts | | | | | |
|---|---|---|---|---|---|---|---|---|
| How do you think others would describe you? | Establishing a premorbid personality is an important step in a psychiatric history. It allows you to screen for potential personality disorders as well as establishing a baseline as to how the patient was prior to becoming unwell | 'I think others would describe me as quite sensible, but bubbly' | This should be followed up with: How would you describe yourself growing up? The patient's premorbid personality does not suggest a personality disorder, but it would be good to check this in a collateral history | | | | | |
| Have you ever had thoughts of harming yourself or others? Have you ever had thoughts of ending your life? | Risk assessments are essential in psychiatry, so never miss this for all patients | 'Of course not! Life's too wonderful, I could never give any of this up' | Risk assessment is complete and there are no further concerns at this time | | | | | |
| What do you think is causing your change in behaviour? Do you feel you need any help? | These questions can be used to assess whether the patient has insight into her condition | 'I don't think I need help at all. I feel amazing!' | This patient does not have insight into her symptoms | | | | | |

**Past Psychiatric and Medical History**

| Question | Justification | Answer | Thoughts | | | | | |
|---|---|---|---|---|---|---|---|---|
| Have you ever struggled with your mental health? | Screening for previous psychiatric diagnosis or mood disorder is important. If there is evidence of previous episodes of low mood, this could be indicative of bipolar disorder | 'I have had a few episodes of depression, quite a few years ago and then after the birth of my son' | Suggestive of some prior depressive episodes; combined with the manic episode, this could suggest bipolar disorder | | | | | |
| Do you have any long-term health problems? | The relationship between chronic illness and mental health conditions is well established. Brain tumours, hyperthyroidism and Cushing's can present similarly to manic episodes | 'No' | No additional concerns | | | | | |
| Have you recently had any illnesses or hospital visits? | Physical illness such as cancer, hypothyroidism and Cushing's syndrome can present like depression | 'No' | No additional concerns | | | | | |

**Drug History**

| Question | Justification | Answer | Thoughts | | | | |
|---|---|---|---|---|---|---|---|
| Are you on any prescription medication at the moment or use anything over the counter? | Withdrawal from antidepressants and steroid use can cause manic episodes | 'Nothing' | No additional concerns | | | | |
| Do you have any drug allergies? | You must always check for allergies | 'No allergies' | No additional concerns | | | | |

**Family History**

| Question | Justification | Answer | Thoughts | | | | |
|---|---|---|---|---|---|---|---|
| Are there any diseases that run in the family, including any cancers? | Important always to check for relevant heritable conditions | 'Not that I'm aware of' | No additional concerns | | | | |
| Does anyone in your family struggle with their mental health? | Important to screen for family history of mental health disorders | 'No' | No history of mental illness within family | | | | |

**Social and Travel History**

| Question | Justification | Answer | Thoughts | | | | |
|---|---|---|---|---|---|---|---|
| Who is currently at home? Are you working at the moment? | Find out if there are any social concerns or if wider support is needed | 'I live with my husband. I run my own business, which is doing so well' | Partners can provide support, especially with ongoing treatment or management if required. Depending on the patient's occupation, consider the impact this episode might have on others | | | | |
| Have you got any stress in your life at the moment? | Stressful circumstances can initiate or exacerbate psychiatric disorders. | 'No, I'm not worried about anything.' | No additional concerns | | | | |
| Do you smoke tobacco? | Find out a patient's wider risk factors as well as explore causes for symptom changes | 'No' | No additional concerns | | | | |
| What is your average weekly alcohol consumption? | | 'I might have a few glasses of wine at the weekend' | Patient does not display increased alcohol consumption | | | | |
| Have you ever taken any recreational drugs? | Manic episodes can increase risk-taking behaviours, such as recreational drug use | 'Never' | No additional concerns | | | | |

## Systems Review

| Question | Justification | Answer | Thoughts | | | | |
|---|---|---|---|---|---|---|---|
| I'm just going to ask you some general questions about your health.<br>Have you had any change in appetite/ weight/bowel habits/ water works?<br>Do you find yourself sweating more or getting palpitations?<br>Have you had any fevers? | A quick systems review of somatic symptoms that present with psychiatric disorders is important for mood disorders or anxiety disorders. This can be useful in screening for the differential diagnosis of hyperthyroidism | 'I've been eating more but my weight has stayed the same ... probably because I'm always rushed off my feet!" | No additional concerns | | | | |

## Finishing the Consultation

| | | | | | | | |
|---|---|---|---|---|---|---|---|
| To summarise, you've been feeling very well in yourself and have been very busy working on your secret projects, as well as spending more. You don't feel that you need any help from us today, despite your husband suggesting that you might benefit from some. Is that correct? | When summarising and finishing a consultation, it's important to recap the important information so far, the patient's key concerns and the plan moving forward | 'Exactly!' | Happy that the information you have gathered is accurate | | | | |
| Do you have any other questions or things to add?<br>I know that we have discussed a lot of new things; please take some time to digest the information | May identify useful information that has been missed. Will also allow you to address any questions or concerns | 'Nothing at all!' | Take the time to explain what will happen from here | | | | |

## Present Your Findings

Mrs Jones is a 28-year-old woman brought in by her husband. She presented with a 3-week history of elevated mood, increased energy and spending and reduced sleep. She has no thoughts of self-harm or harm to others and displays no features of psychosis. She has had previous depressive episodes.

I feel that the most likely diagnosis is a manic episode of a possible bipolar affective disorder, with a differential diagnosis of hyperthyroidism.

I would like to examine Mrs Jones fully and take bloods, and refer her urgently for a psychiatric assessment

| General Points | | |
|---|---|---|
| Polite to patient | | |
| Maintains good eye contact | | |
| Appropriate use of open and closed questions | | |

## ❓ QUESTIONS FROM THE EXAMINER

### What are the organic differential diagnoses for a manic episode?
Brain tumour, hyperthyroidism, Cushing's and head injury.

### What is the key difference between hypomania and mania?
Hypomania does not cause significant functional impairment, whereas mania does.

### What is the definition of a manic episode?
A period of elevated, expansive and irritable mood for over 1 week. Features include increased self-esteem, decreased need for sleep, increasingly talkative, flight of ideas or racing thoughts, distractibility, increased goal-directed activity and excessive involvement in pleasure activities.

### What conditions can present with mania?
Cushing's disease, thyrotoxicosis, encephalitis, syphilis.

### What are the risk factors for mania?
Family history, substance misuse, stress and antidepressant use in bipolar affective disorder.

### What is schizoaffective disorder?
The presence of psychotic features alongside a mood disorder, whether depression or mania.

### What is the first-line management for those with an acute manic episode?
Atypical antipsychotics such as olanzapine, quetiapine and risperidone.

### Which frequently prescribed class of drugs is a common cause for mania?
Glucocorticoids.

### What are the side effects of clozapine use?
Agranulocytosis, myocarditis, GI effects, neutropenia and arrhythmias.

### What is the mechanism of action of haloperidol and who is it contraindicated for?
Haloperidol is a typical antipsychotic, which is a dopamine $D_2$ receptor antagonist. It cannot be used in patients with Parkinson's disease.

## Station 8.4    History: Postnatal Depression (PND)

### Doctor Briefing

You are a junior doctor in primary care and have been asked to see Mrs Roberts, a 24-year-old woman, who has presented after giving birth to her first child. Her partner is concerned because she does not appear to be coping well. Her mood has been persistently low and she has been very tearful. Please take a history from Mrs Roberts, present your findings and formulate an appropriate management plan.

### Patient Briefing

You gave birth to your first child, Josh, 1 month ago. Your partner has encouraged you to come to the surgery today, as he doesn't feel that you have been yourself since the birth.

You are very anxious about whether you are doing the right things for Josh. You have been struggling to cope, tearful and often short-tempered with your partner. You have been neglecting to take care of yourself and have not been eating regularly. You've been having difficulty sleeping, despite Josh sleeping well, and feel exhausted all of the time.

Your pregnancy was planned and uncomplicated, and Josh has been a healthy baby. Initially establishing breastfeeding with Josh was hard, and this is something you are still having problems with. You have never had any thoughts of self-harm, suicide or harming Josh. You have never suffered a psychiatric illness before. You think your mother may have had depression after the birth of your brother. Your partner is very supportive and has been helping at home.

You are worried that you'll never be a good-enough mother for Josh.

### Mark Scheme for Examiner

#### Introduction

| Cleans hands, introduces self, confirms patient identity and gains consent for history taking | | | | | |
|---|---|---|---|---|---|

#### History of Presenting Complaint

| Question | Justification | Answer | Thoughts | | | | | |
|---|---|---|---|---|---|---|---|---|
| What's brought you in today? | This question is general and open, so is a good way to start the consultation. It also helps to screen for insight as if the patient has presented voluntarily, this can show she may have some insight into the help she needs | 'My partner encouraged me to come in today because I have been struggling since the birth of Josh' | Clear worry from partner; establishes a support network and shows that the patient may have some insight | | | | | |
| How do you feel within yourself? | This allows you to get a better idea of the patient's mood. For this history, we are screening for low mood, as the patient could have postnatal depression (PND) | 'I'm not feeling great at the moment. I'm feeling very low in myself. I think it's been a lot to cope with since the birth' | Low mood is one of the core depressive symptoms so needs to be explored further to establish a timeline and whether it has changed. In PND, an inability to cope is one of the clinical features | | | | | |
| Do you still enjoy things that you used to? | This question screens for anhedonia, loss of interest | 'Not really, I don't have time to do anything. I don't have time even to look after myself' | This patient is showing some signs of anhedonia but also self-neglect, which is common in PND | | | | | |

**History of Presenting Complaint**

| Question | Justification | Answer | Thoughts | | | | | | |
|---|---|---|---|---|---|---|---|---|---|
| Do you find that you tire more easily? | Screening for low energy, which is one of the core depressive symptoms | 'Yes, I've been very tired recently. I'm just so busy with Josh all the time' | This patient demonstrates fatigue, which could be indicative of depression | | | | | | |
| Do you find yourself getting anxious or worried for no apparent reason? | This is a common clinical feature of PND | 'Yes, I'm just worried all the time, but I think I'm mostly worried that I'm not looking after him well enough' | This patient seems to be very anxious and concerned that she is an inadequate mother | | | | | | |
| How is your sleep? | Sleep disturbance is one of the biological/somatic symptoms of depression. In new mothers, it is important to establish whether this is due to the baby's sleeping schedule or the mother's | 'I just can't seem to fall asleep, even though Josh is sleeping well' | This patient is showing insomnia, which can indicate a somatic symptom of depression. Other somatic symptoms, such as reduced appetite, weight loss, constipation and loss of libido, should all be screened for as well | | | | | | |
| How do you see yourself compared to other people? | Assesses for feelings of worthlessness and current self-esteem. In new mothers, this can present as inadequacy as a mother and feelings of guilt | 'I don't think I'm a good mother. I'm trying my best but I just feel that Josh would be better off without me' | Patient shows signs of inadequacy towards the baby. Alongside these cognitive symptoms of depression, other symptoms – poor memory, lack of concentration, tearfulness and agitation – need to be assessed | | | | | | |
| Have you ever heard things said when there is no one round and nothing can explain it? | This is one of the questions that can be used to help screen for puerperal psychosis, which can present with psychotic symptoms or thoughts of harming the baby | 'No' | No evidence suggesting auditory hallucinations. However, further questions should be asked to establish that this is not psychotic depression | | | | | | |
| Did you plan to have Josh? How was the pregnancy? How was the birth? How has breastfeeding been going? | Unplanned or unwanted pregnancy and difficulties with breastfeeding can be risk factors for developing PND | 'We had planned to have Josh and the pregnancy was good. The birth was OK too. I did struggle to establish breastfeeding and it is still a problem to this day but luckily we are closer to weaning now' | Breastfeeding difficulty is a risk factor for PND | | | | | | |

## History of Presenting Complaint

| Question | Justification | Answer | Thoughts | | | | |
|---|---|---|---|---|---|---|---|
| How would you describe yourself before the birth of Josh? | Establishing a premorbid personality is an important step in a psychiatric history. This can help you establish whether the symptoms had been ongoing before birth or since the birth | 'I have always been so bubbly and I was so excited for Josh but now I just feel so terrible' | The patient's premorbid personality suggests this is PND rather than an ongoing untreated depression | | | | |
| Have you ever had thoughts of harming yourself?  Have you ever had thoughts of ending your life?  Have you ever had any thoughts of harming Josh? | Risk assessments are essential in psychiatry, so never miss this. They are even more vital with patients presenting with low mood, as they are at an increased risk of suicide.  In suspected PND, it is important to ask about harm to the baby, as this can indicate severe PND or puerperal psychosis.  It is also essential to cover for safeguarding purposes | 'No, never. I would never harm myself or Josh' | Risk assessment is complete and there is no further concerns at this time | | | | |
| Would you say this might be depression?  Do you think you would benefit from any help? | Establishing whether the patient has insight into her condition | 'I was thinking I could be depressed and so does my partner. I do think some help might be beneficial for me' | This patient has insight into her mental health | | | | |

## Past Psychiatric and Medical History

| Question | Justification | Answer | Thoughts | | | | |
|---|---|---|---|---|---|---|---|
| Have you ever struggled with your mental health? | Screening for previous psychiatric diagnosis or previous mood disorder | 'No, never' | No additional concerns | | | | |
| Do you have any long-term health problems? | The relationship between chronic illness and mental health conditions is well established | 'No' | No additional concerns | | | | |
| Have you recently had any illnesses or hospital visits? | Acute psychotic reaction to a recent illness | 'No' | No additional concerns | | | | |

## Drug History

| Question | Justification | Answer | Thoughts | | | | |
|---|---|---|---|---|---|---|---|
| Are you on any prescription medication at the moment or use anything over the counter? | Prescription medications strongly associated with drug-induced psychosis include corticosteroids and antihistamines | 'No medications' | No additional concerns | | | | |
| Do you have any drug allergies? | You must always check for allergies | 'No allergies' | No additional concerns | | | | |

## Family History

| Question | Justification | Answer | Thoughts | | | | |
|---|---|---|---|---|---|---|---|
| Are there any diseases that run in the family, including cancers? | Important always to check for relevant heritable conditions | 'Not that I'm aware of' | No additional concerns | | | | |
| Does anyone in your family struggle with their mental health? | Important to screen for family history of mental health disorders | 'I think my mother had some depression after the birth of my brother' | History of mental illness within family, specifically PND, raises your suspicion | | | | |

## Social and Travel History

| Question | Justification | Answer | Thoughts | | | | |
|---|---|---|---|---|---|---|---|
| Who is currently at home? Are you working? | Find out if there are any social concerns or if wider support is needed | 'I live with my partner and my son Josh. I have been on maternity leave since Josh's birth' | Partners can provide support, especially with ongoing treatment or management if required | | | | |
| Do you have a good support network around you? | Poor social support can be a risk factor for PND | 'My partner has been really supportive and I have some close friends' | This patient seems to have some support at home, so encouraging her to talk to those around her might help | | | | |
| Have you got any stress in your life at the moment? | Stressful circumstances can initiate or exacerbate psychiatric disorders | 'Looking after the baby is causing me the most stress at the moment' | The baby seems to be the main reason behind the patient's anxiety | | | | |
| Do you smoke tobacco? | Find out a patient's wider risk factors as well as exploring causes for symptom changes. Alcohol is a mood suppressor so can contribute to symptoms of low mood | 'No' | No additional concerns | | | | |
| What is your average weekly alcohol consumption? | | 'The last time I drank alcohol was before I was pregnant' | No additional concerns | | | | |
| Have you ever taken any recreational drugs? | Drug withdrawal can present with low mood | 'No, never' | No additional concerns | | | | |

## Systems Review

| Question | Justification | Answer | Thoughts | | | | | |
|---|---|---|---|---|---|---|---|---|
| I'm just going to ask you some general questions about your health. Have you had any change in appetite/weight/ bowel habits/ water works? Do you find yourself sweating more or getting palpitations? Have you had any fevers? | A quick systems review of somatic symptoms that present with psychiatric disorders is important | 'No weight change but I haven't been eating very much' | No additional concerns | | | | | |

## Finishing the Consultation

| | | | | | | | | |
|---|---|---|---|---|---|---|---|---|
| To summarise, since Josh was born, you've been feeling quite low and have been struggling to cope. You have a good support network at home and would be open to receiving some help from us. Is that correct? | When summarising and finishing a consultation, it's important to recap the important information so far, the patient's key concerns and the plan moving forward | 'Definitely' | Happy that the information that you have gathered is accurate | | | | | |
| Do you have any other questions or things to add? I know that we have discussed a lot of new things; please take some time to digest the information. | May identify useful information that has been missed. Will also allow you to address any questions or concerns | 'No, thank you' | Take the time to explain what will happen from here | | | | | |

## Present Your Findings

Mrs Roberts is a 24-year-old woman who is mum to Josh, a 1-month-old baby. Since giving birth, she has felt low and is tearful and having trouble sleeping. She feels inadequate as a mother. She has no prior psychiatric history but a potential family history of PND. She has no thoughts of self-harm, suicide or of harming Josh.

This is consistent with a diagnosis of PND.

I would like to organise a thorough set of bloods to exclude an organic cause for low mood. Suggested management would be CBT and introduction of an antidepressant, as well as increased visits by the health visitor to allow for safety checks

| General Points | | | | |
|---|---|---|---|---|
| Polite to patient | | | | |
| Maintains good eye contact | | | | |
| Appropriate use of open and closed questions | | | | |

## ❓ QUESTIONS FROM THE EXAMINER

### What are the cardinal symptoms of PND?

Depressive symptoms, anxiety, concerns about baby's health, feeling of inadequacy and inability to cope and lack of bonding with baby.

### What are the risk factors for PND?

Family or personal history of PND or depression, adverse life events (for example, family death), difficulties with breastfeeding, unplanned/unwanted pregnancy and poor social support.

### When is the most likely time to develop 'baby blues'?

3–4 days post delivery.

### How should PND be managed?

Most cases can be managed at home supportively with information and reassurance, talking therapies and liaising with primary care physicians and local health visitors. Most cases will resolve with this management within a few weeks. If the PND is moderate or severe, it may require antidepressants as well.

### How should postnatal psychosis be managed?

Often it requires hospitalisation to a mother and baby unit. Antidepressants, antipsychotics and ECT may also be used.

### During pregnancy, what drugs should be avoided and why?

Lithium and valproate should be avoided if possible due to the risk of congenital defects.

### If antidepressants are to be used in the management of PND, which ones are considered safe for breastfeeding mothers?

Sertraline and paroxetine.

### How might a patient with 'baby blues' present?

Tearful, anxious about being a bad mother and feeling overwhelmed.

### What scoring system can be used to assess severity of PND in the UK?

The Edinburgh Postnatal Depression Scale.

### How can a patient with postnatal psychosis present?

Acute change in mood, auditory hallucinations, altered perceptions, thoughts of harming the baby, suicidal thoughts and other psychotic features.

## Station 8.5    History: Suicide Risk Assessment

### Doctor Briefing

You are a junior doctor in the emergency department (ED) and have been asked to see Mr Smith, a 45-year-old man, who has presented after attempting to hang himself. He has recently separated from his wife and has been struggling with low mood. He is now medically fit. Please take a history from Mr Smith, present your findings and formulate an appropriate management plan.

### Patient Briefing

You are a 45-year-old plumber and you have recently separated from your wife, Julie. Julie left you a month ago and took your daughter Rebecca (5 years old) with her. She left you after you had started drinking more, as you have been struggling to find work. You haven't been able to cope without them and feel that your life is no longer worth living. You feel very alone, as you have no close friends.

Ever since Julie left, you have been contemplating suicide, but in the last 3 days you came up with a firm plan. You had bought a rope, updated your will to leave everything to your daughter and wrote a note to your wife and daughter explaining why you had to do this. You attempted to hang yourself; however, the rope gave way. Your neighbour was alerted by the noise and came round to see what was wrong. He then brought you here today.

You have not attempted to commit suicide before and have no prior history of suffering with a mental health condition.

You don't want any help and would attempt suicide again.

### Mark Scheme for Examiner

#### Introduction

| | | | | | |
|---|---|---|---|---|---|
| Cleans hands, introduces self, confirms patient identity and gains consent for history taking | | | | | |

#### History of Presenting Complaint

| Question | Justification | Answer | Thoughts | | | | | |
|---|---|---|---|---|---|---|---|---|
| What's brought you in today? | This question is general and open, so is a good way to start the consultation. It also helps to screen for insight as if the patient has attended voluntarily, this can show he may have some insight into the help he needs | 'My neighbour found me trying to kill myself' | Patient has openly mentioned the suicide attempt, so this can be explored further. You want to aim your questioning to gather enough information for a timeline about 24 h before the attempt | | | | | |
| What was the method? | You need to establish the method as this might alter the management. For example, if it was a medication overdose, you need to establish what medication was taken and whether it was taken with alcohol as this might require urgent medical management | 'I tried to hang myself earlier today, but the rope broke' | The method of suicide varies between different demographics. Stereotypically, men are more likely to choose violent means and women are more likely to choose medication overdose | | | | | |
| How long have you been planning to do this? | This question helps to give you a timeline of events. It also allows you to see if there was much planning in the process or whether it was impulsive | 'I have been thinking about it for a while now but in the last few days, I decided to do it' | This patient shows a history of suicidal thoughts and there is some planning for the recent attempt | | | | | |

## History of Presenting Complaint

| Question | Justification | Answer | Thoughts | | | | | |
|---|---|---|---|---|---|---|---|---|
| Did you try not to be found? | Trying not to be found is a risk factor for complete suicide | 'I live at home alone so I didn't think I'd be found' | Risk factor for completed suicide present | | | | | |
| Did you think this would be lethal? | To assess whether the patient thought the attempt would be final or whether it was a cry for help, rather than finite | 'Yes, I thought it would work' | Evidence the patient thought the attempt was lethal | | | | | |
| How were you found? | This can be used to assess whether the patient sought help or whether he was 'discovered' | 'My neighbour heard some noise so came round to see if I was OK' | This patient was discovered rather than seeking help himself | | | | | |
| Did you write a note? Have you made a will? | Writing a suicide note or a will can show part of the planning process and is a risk factor for suicide | 'Yes, I wrote a letter to my wife and daughter, and I left everything to my daughter in the will' | The note writing and will show preplanning for the suicide attempt | | | | | |
| How do you feel about the suicide attempt? | This question helps to assess whether this is something the patient regrets or something he would attempt again | 'I wish I'd been successful' | The patient has persistent suicidal ideations and poses a risk to himself if discharged without further assessment | | | | | |
| How do you feel about the future? | Need to assess any thoughts, intentions or plans for suicide in the future. This is an open question which can start this conversation off | 'I mean, I don't really want a future. I just don't want to be alive' | The patient shows persistent suicidal ideations which would impact his management | | | | | |
| Do you think this is something you need help for? | Establish whether the patient has insight into his condition | 'I don't really want any help, I'd just like to be left alone' | This suggests recommendations to the patient may be refused and he may require admission under the Mental Health Act | | | | | |

## Past Psychiatric and Medical History

| Question | Justification | Answer | Thoughts | | | | | |
|---|---|---|---|---|---|---|---|---|
| Have you ever struggled with your mental health? | Screening for previous psychiatric diagnosis or previous mood disorder | 'Not really, only recently while I have been feeling pretty low since Julie left' | No past psychiatric history but continuous low mood triggered by a recent event | | | | | |
| Have you attempted suicide before? Do you self-harm? | Previous suicide attempt is a risk factor for suicide | 'No, I haven't' | No additional concerns | | | | | |

### Past Psychiatric and Medical History

| Question | Justification | Answer | Thoughts | | | | |
|---|---|---|---|---|---|---|---|
| Do you have any long-term health problems? | The relationship between chronic illness and mental health conditions is well established | 'No' | No additional concerns | | | | |

### Family History

| Question | Justification | Answer | Thoughts | | | | |
|---|---|---|---|---|---|---|---|
| Does anyone in your family struggle with their mental health? | Important to screen for family history of mental health disorders | 'No' | No history of mental illness within the family | | | | |

### Social and Travel History

| Question | Justification | Answer | Thoughts | | | | |
|---|---|---|---|---|---|---|---|
| Who is currently at home? Is there someone that you can talk to? | Establishing the patient's support network and whether wider social support might be required | 'I live alone, after my wife left me. I don't really have any close friends, no' | Social isolation and a change in life circumstance, such as a separation, are both risk factors for suicide | | | | |

### Systems Review

| Question | Justification | Answer | Thoughts | | | | |
|---|---|---|---|---|---|---|---|
| I'm just going to ask you some general questions about your health. Have you had any change in appetite/weight/bowel habits/water works/sleep? Do you find yourself sweating more or getting palpitations? Have you had any fevers? | A quick systems review of somatic symptoms that present with psychiatric disorders is important | 'My sleep has been poor. I've been really struggling to get to sleep so I've been quite tired recently' | Suggestive of some of the somatic symptoms associated with depression. Consider asking a more detailed depression history later on during the patient's assessment | | | | |

### Finishing the Consultation

| Question | Justification | Answer | Thoughts | | | | |
|---|---|---|---|---|---|---|---|
| To summarise, you've been having a tough time recently with your wife and your job, which led to you attempting to end your life earlier, when your neighbour found you. You feel that this is something you would attempt again and you don't want any help from us today. Is that correct? | When summarising and finishing a consultation, it's important to recap the important information so far, the patient's key concerns and the plan moving forward | 'Yes' | Happy that the information that you have gathered is accurate | | | | |

## Finishing the Consultation

| Question | Justification | Answer | Thoughts | | | | | |
|---|---|---|---|---|---|---|---|---|
| Do you have any other questions or things to add? I know that we have discussed a lot of new things; please take some time to digest the information | May identify useful information that has been missed. Will also allow you to address any questions or concerns | 'No' | Take the time to explain what will happen from here | | | | | |

## Present Your Findings

Mr Smith is a 45-year-old man who presented after being brought in by a neighbour who found him attempting suicide. He is at an increased risk of completed suicide with risk factors of planned intent, sex, age, social isolation and recent change of circumstances. He believed and intended that this attempt would take his life and he didn't think that he would be found. Mr Smith preplanned this attempt and made a will and wrote letters to his family.

This patient is probably suffering from untreated depression following separation from his wife.

In view that this patient has poor social support and still intends to kill himself, ideally I would like him to be assessed for potential inpatient admission (informal if possible) to keep him safe

## General Points

Polite to patient

Maintains good eye contact

Appropriate use of open and closed questions

## ❓ QUESTIONS FROM THE EXAMINER

### For this patient, what would indicate the need for further stay in hospital?
Poor social support and continued suicidal ideation.

### What jobs can put someone at a higher risk of suicide?
Doctors, dentists, farmers and lawyers.

### What are the demographics for a competed suicide?
Late-middle-aged male.

### How would you manage self-cutting?
Thorough psychiatric and social assessment to establish short-term risk of suicide. These patients may benefit from personal support and practical advice from a general practitioner (GP), social worker or community psychiatric nurse.

### How would you manage a suicide attempt?
Psychiatric assessment to assess future risk of suicide or self-harm, support network and insight into their condition. Any underlying disease should be treated, e.g. depression. The person could be offered psychological therapy through specialised groups, stress management and CBT.

**What is the purpose of Mental Health Act Section 2 in the UK?**

To allow for assessment for a suspected psychiatric illness by healthcare professionals.

**What is the purpose of Mental Health Act 4 in the UK?**

Emergency detainment of a patient for assessment, for up to 72 h.

**What are the social risk factors for suicide?**

Living alone, unemployment, recent bereavement, divorce or separation, drug or alcohol misuse and lower socioeconomic status.

**What are some protective factors for suicide?**

Family support, having children and strong religious belief.

**What risk factors increase the risk of a suicide attempt being successful?**

Efforts to avoid discovery, planning, leaving a written note, final acts such as sorting out finances and violent method.

## Station 8.6   History: Schizophrenia

### Doctor Briefing

You are a junior doctor in primary care and have been asked to see Mr Brown, a 19-year-old student, who has presented after hearing voices. He believes that his friends are out to get him, and his parents are worried that he has been acting strangely. Please take a history from Mr Brown, present your findings and formulate an appropriate management plan.

### Patient Briefing

You are a 19-year-old university student living at home with your parents. Your parents have brought you because they think you've been acting strangely recently.

For a month, you've been hearing your friends whispering that they hate you and want to hurt you. You constantly feel unsafe. The voices never tell you to harm yourself or others. You are defensive if someone tells you that the voices are not real. You feel that you can't control the voices and this means you've stayed in your room so your friends can't hurt you. You are feeling a little bit down as the voices have knocked your confidence, but you don't have fatigue or lack of pleasure.

Your thoughts feel chaotic – as if you don't have control over them, but you cannot elaborate any further.

You don't have any health problems and are not on any regular medications. You have smoked cannabis regularly since the age of 15. You used to drink 8 units of alcohol a week whilst socialising with friends. You do not use any other recreational drugs.

You have no thoughts of ending your life or harming others.

You don't understand why your parents seem so concerned but you know that haven't been feeling yourself recently.

### Mark Scheme for Examiner

| Introduction | | | | | | | | | |
|---|---|---|---|---|---|---|---|---|---|
| Cleans hands, introduces self, confirms patient identity and gains consent for history taking | | | | | | | | | |

**History of Presenting Complaint**

| Question | Justification | Answer | Thoughts | | | | |
|---|---|---|---|---|---|---|---|
| What's brought you in today? | This question is general and open, so is a good way to start the consultation. It also helps to screen for insight as if the patient has attended voluntarily, this can show he may have some insight into the help he needs | 'My parents think I've been acting strangely so they made me come. I don't really know why they think this' | Clear worry from parents; establishes a support network and signs of lack of insight into condition | | | | |
| Is there anything you are worried about? | This can allow for screening of persecutory delusions as well as being a good open question to ask at the beginning to guide the conversation | 'I'm worried that my friends are going to hurt me' | This answer needs further exploring, as it could demonstrate a persecutory delusion or a genuine concern for safety | | | | |
| Do you feel like anyone's out to get you? | Use this question to assess for persecutory delusions | 'My friends ... I just told you! They hate me and are going to hurt me' | This patient displays evidence of persecutory delusions that would require further exploration to understand why the patient believes people are going to hurt him and what they are going to do | | | | |

## History of Presenting Complaint

| Question | Justification | Answer | Thoughts | | | | | |
|---|---|---|---|---|---|---|---|---|
| Are there ever messages in the newspaper or on the TV just for you? Would you say you see things in the same way as others? | These two questions can be used to assess for delusions of reference and delusions of perception | 'No, I don't think so. I think I see things the same as others' | No delusions of reference or perception identified in this answer so other questions must be used to assess delusions further | | | | | |
| Do you have any special powers? Are you in a position of importance or power? | This question can assess for delusions of grandeur | 'No' | This patient does not show evidence for delusions of grandeur | | | | | |
| Have you ever heard things when there is nothing to explain it? | This question can be used to screen for auditory hallucinations | 'I hear my friends all the time. They say such horrible things' | Need to ask follow-up questions, including number of voices, what they say, whether they have told the patient to hurt himself | | | | | |
| Have you ever seen, smelled or tasted anything that you could not explain? | These questions are to screen for visual, olfactory or gustatory hallucinations | 'No' | No evidence for other types of hallucinations | | | | | |
| Do you ever feel like ideas are being deliberately inserted into your head?<br><br>Do you ever feel your thoughts have been taken away?<br><br>Can others hear your thoughts without you saying them out loud? | These questions can be used to screen for thought interference, which is a first-rank symptom of schizophrenia | 'My thoughts are … strange. It's all very chaotic, I feel like I don't have control over them, but no one can hear what I'm thinking, no' | Some suggestion of potential thought insertion/withdrawal, but nothing to suggest thought broadcast | | | | | |
| How would you describe yourself growing up? How do you think others would describe you? | Establishing a premorbid personality is an important part of a psychiatric history. Schizoid personality disorder can present as schizophrenia | 'I have always been happy and sociable' | The patient's premorbid personality does not suggest a diagnosis of a schizoid or schizotypal personality disorder. It would be a good idea to double-check this in a collateral history | | | | | |
| Have you had any periods of particularly low or high mood? | Screening for mood disorders or negative symptoms of schizophrenia | 'I have been feeling a bit down recently because of my friends, but not very low or very high' | Does not suggest a mood disorder such as depression with psychotic features or schizoaffective disorder | | | | | |

## History of Presenting Complaint

| Question | Justification | Answer | Thoughts | | | | |
|---|---|---|---|---|---|---|---|
| Have you ever had thoughts of harming yourself or others? Have you ever had thoughts of ending your life? | Risk assessments are essential in psychiatry so never miss this | 'No, never' | Risk assessment is complete and there are no further concerns at this time | | | | |
| What do you think is going on? Do you think you would benefit from any help? | Establishing whether the patient has insight into his condition | 'No, I don't think anything is wrong. I just want my friends to leave me alone' | This patient does not have insight into his current mental state | | | | |

## Past Psychiatric and Medical History

| Question | Justification | Answer | Thoughts | | | | |
|---|---|---|---|---|---|---|---|
| Have you ever struggled with your mental health? | Screening for previous psychiatric diagnosis or previous mood disorder | 'No, never' | No additional concerns | | | | |
| Do you have any long-term health problems? | The relationship between chronic illness and mental health conditions is well established | 'No' | No additional concerns | | | | |
| Have you recently had any illnesses or hospital visits? | Consider possible acute psychotic reaction to a recent illness | 'No' | No additional concerns | | | | |

## Drug History

| Question | Justification | Answer | Thoughts | | | | |
|---|---|---|---|---|---|---|---|
| Are you on any prescription medication at the moment or use anything over the counter? | Prescription medications strongly associated with drug-induced psychosis are corticosteroids and antihistamines | 'No medications' | No additional concerns | | | | |
| Do you have any drug allergies? | You must always check for allergies | 'No allergies' | No additional concerns | | | | |

## Family History

| Question | Justification | Answer | Thoughts | | | | |
|---|---|---|---|---|---|---|---|
| Are there any diseases that run in the family, including any cancers? | Important always to check for relevant heritable conditions | 'Not that I'm aware of' | No additional concerns | | | | |
| Does anyone in your family struggle with their mental health? | Important to screen for family history of mental health disorders | 'I think my mum had depression but she's fine now' | History of mental illness within family | | | | |

## Social and Travel History

| Question | Justification | Answer | Thoughts | | | | |
|---|---|---|---|---|---|---|---|
| Who is currently at home? Are you working? | Find out if there are any social concerns or if wider support is needed | 'I live with my parents and I'm a maths student at the local university' | Parents can provide support, especially with ongoing treatment or management if required. University students are a particularly vulnerable group to mental illness | | | | |
| Have you got any stress in your life at the moment apart from your friends? | Stressful circumstances can initiate or exacerbate psychiatric disorders | 'I'm approaching my end-of-year exams at university' | External stressors present and should be noted | | | | |
| Do you smoke tobacco? | Find out a patient's wider risk factors as well as exploring causes for symptom changes. Alcohol is also a mood suppressor so can contribute to symptoms of low mood | 'No, I have never smoked' | No additional concerns | | | | |
| What is your average weekly alcohol consumption? | | 'I have around four pints a week but haven't had any alcohol for a while' | No additional concerns | | | | |
| Have you ever taken any recreational drugs? | There is evidence to suggest a correlation between adolescent cannabis use and schizophrenia | 'I smoked cannabis when I was 15' | Cannabis is a risk factor for development of schizophrenia | | | | |

## Systems Review

| Question | Justification | Answer | Thoughts | | | | |
|---|---|---|---|---|---|---|---|
| I'm just going to ask you some general questions about your health. Have you had any change in appetite/weight/bowel habits/water works? Do you find yourself sweating more or getting palpitations? Have you had any fevers? | A quick systems review of somatic symptoms that present with psychiatric disorders is important for mood or anxiety disorders. This can be useful in screening for the differential diagnosis of hyperthyroidism | 'No, they have been normal' | No additional concerns | | | | |

## Finishing the Consultation

| Question | Justification | Answer | Thoughts | | | | | | |
|----------|---------------|--------|----------|---|---|---|---|---|---|
| To summarise, your parents brought you in today because they don't think that you've been feeling yourself recently. You've been hearing friends saying some unkind things and you feel that they are going to hurt you. You also feel that your thoughts have been chaotic and busy, but you don't think you need any help from us today. Is this correct? | When summarising and finishing a consultation, it's important to recap the important information so far, the patient's key concerns and the plan moving forward | 'Yes. Can I leave now?' | Happy that the information that you have gathered is accurate | | | | | | |
| Do you have any other questions or things to add? I know that we have discussed a lot of new things; please take some time to digest the information. | May identify useful information that has been missed. Will also allow you to address any questions or concerns | 'Can I leave now?' | Take the time to explain what will happen from here | | | | | | |

## Present Your Findings

Mr Brown is a 19-year-old student who presented with a persecutory delusion of his friends wishing to harm him with associated auditory hallucinations. He feels that his thoughts are chaotic, though he was not able to elaborate any further. He describes no thoughts of harm to himself or others. This is on the background of being normally fit and well but with a history of cannabis use.

I feel the most likely diagnosis is schizophrenia, with the differentials of a schizoaffective disorder.

I would like to get a collateral history to further my assessment, fully examine Mr Brown and organise a thorough set of bloods

## General Points

Polite to patient

Maintains good eye contact

Appropriate use of open and closed questions

**❓ QUESTIONS FROM THE EXAMINER**

**Name some risk factors for psychosis.**

Family history, perinatal complications, substance misuse, urbanisation at birth, stress.

**Name some organic syndromes can present as psychosis.**

Dementia, brain tumours, temporal-lobe epilepsy.

**What are the signs of a schizoid personality disorder?**

Lack of interest in relationships. Solitary lifestyle, emotional detachment.

**What drugs can cause drug-induced psychosis and how can we test for these?**

Drug-induced psychosis can be precipitated by amphetamines, Lysergic acid diethylamide (LSD and cocaine, which can all be tested for using a urine drug screen.

**What are the negative symptoms of schizophrenia?**

Social withdrawal, underactivity, emotionally flat, speech reduced, monosyllabic and slowness of movement.

**Name the first-rank symptoms of schizophrenia.**

Auditory hallucinations, thought broadcasting, thought insertion, thought withdrawal, delusions of control and delusional perceptions.

**What are the first-line medications for schizophrenia?**

Atypical antipsychotics such as olanzapine or risperidone.

**What are delusions of perception?**

When someone attributes false meaning to normal perceptions. It's a two-stage process; for example, in the above case, Mr Brown might have noticed that the road signs changed, which meant that he is king of the world.

**What is neuroleptic malignant syndrome?**

A life-threatening reaction to antipsychotic medications, with symptoms of fever, tremor, rigidity, autonomic dysfunction and delirium.

**What is acute dystonia and how can it be treated?**

Involuntary contractions of face, neck, arms and other muscles, caused by imbalance of dopaminergic and cholinergic neurotransmission. This can be managed with procyclidine.

## Station 8.7   Examination: Mental State

### Doctor Briefing

You are a junior doctor in a primary care practice and have been asked to see Mrs Bradley, a 58-year-old woman, who has recently separated from her husband and lost her job. There is a concern that she is very depressed. Please perform an MSE, present your findings and formulate an appropriate management plan.

### Patient Briefing

You have been feeling very low and hopeless for the last month. Three months ago, your 35-year marriage broke down and you and your husband are now separated. In the last few weeks, you have been made redundant from your job as a cleaner.

- *Appearance and behaviour*: You look poorly kempt, with signs that you have neglected all self-care. You are able to engage with the doctor but become tearful when asked about your husband and job. You maintain eye contact intermittently.
- *Mood*: Your mood is very low and this varies throughout the day, being worse in the morning.
- *Speech*: You sound depressed in tone and speak slowly with a low volume. When answering questions, you give short answers most of the time.
- *Thoughts*: You have overwhelming feelings of inadequacy and low self-esteem. You husband felt you were no longer compatible but you think your husband left you because he was having an affair. You have had fleeting thoughts of self-harm but have no intentions to act on these and have no thoughts of suicide.
- *Perceptions*: You have not had any unusual perceptions.
- *Cognition*: You are orientated to time, place and person and are able to count backwards in sevens.
- *Insight*: You have good insight into your current mental state and are aware that you need help.

### Mark Scheme for Examiner

#### Introduction

| Cleans hands, introduces self, confirms patient identity and gains consent for history taking | | | | | | |
|---|---|---|---|---|---|---|

#### History of Presenting Complaint

| Question | Justification | Answer | Thoughts | | | | | |
|---|---|---|---|---|---|---|---|---|
| What's brought you in today? | This question is general and open, so is a good way to start the consultation. It also helps to screen for insight as if the patient has attended voluntarily, this can show she may have some insight into the help she needs | 'I came here today because I've been feeling really low this last month and I think I need help' | Establishes why the patient has come in and helps to steer the conversation. Also implies that the patient has insight into her condition and would be willing to receive help | | | | | |
| Appearance | When initially interacting with the patient, you should assess appearance specifically: how she is dressed. Looking poorly kempt can be a sign of self-neglect, which could be associated with depression or dementia. Dressing inappropriately, such as wearing sunglasses while being indoors, can be associated with psychosis. Also note if there is evidence of self-harm or self-neglect | Patient looks poorly kempt, in baggy clothing with matted hair, and appears to be neglecting self-care | This patient is poorly kept and is neglecting self-care. Consider what could have led her to this and try to discuss it with her to have insight into this aspect of her life | | | | | |

**History of Presenting Complaint**

| Question | Justification | Answer | Thoughts | | | | | |
|---|---|---|---|---|---|---|---|---|
| Behaviour | Throughout the whole interaction with the patient, pay attention to the way she behaves and interacts with you.<br>Does she maintain eye contact? Is she tearful, visibly anxious or suspicious? | The patient engages well with the conversation, with infrequent eye contact. At times she becomes tearful, especially if asked about husband or job | The patient is tearful but has engaged with the conversation | | | | | |
| Speech | Throughout the conversation, pay attention to the way the patient speaks. Listen to the tone, rhythm, rate and volume. Manic patients can speak quickly and loudly whereas depressed patients may speak more slowly and quietly | The patient speaks at a low volume and slow pace. She occasionally gives one-word answers | The patient speaks slowly and quietly but engages well with the conversation and answers questions appropriately | | | | | |
| Mood:<br>How do you feel within yourself?<br>Does this vary throughout the day?<br>Have you ever felt on top of the world, like you could do anything?<br>Does your mood vary?<br>Do you find yourself getting tearful? | This allows you to assess the subjective mood of the patient. You should also give your objective impression of the patient's mood. The mood element of the MSE is mostly assessed in the history of presenting complaint part of the consultation. This should cover both ends of the mood spectrum | 'I'm feeling very low at the moment and it's worse in the morning. I just don't want to get out of bed any more. I do find myself getting tearful. I can't think of my husband without crying' | Low mood is one of the core depressive symptoms so needs to be explored further to establish a timeline and whether it has changed. A low mood present for over 2 weeks would indicate depression. Further questioning should cover anhedonia and fatigue. You should also screen for any manic moods, whether recently or in the past | | | | | |
| Thought:<br>What is worrying you at the moment? | These questions are used to assess thought.<br>Thought form can be assessed through the coherence of the conversation; however, thought content is assessed through the questions you ask, such as delusions or obsessions.<br>Thoughts of self-harm and suicidal thoughts will also need to be covered, if not done so earlier | 'I'm worried about where I'm going to live. My husband and I have split up and I've just lost my job so I don't have an income' | This patient appears to have normal thought form and no delusions, obsessions or thought possession. She has some anxious thoughts regarding her upcoming living circumstances | | | | | |
| Thought:<br>Have you ever felt people were against you? | | 'No, I'm not paranoid ... just worried' | | | | | | |
| Thought:<br>Have there been times when you've felt something strange was going on? | | 'Nothing strange' | | | | | | |

## History of Presenting Complaint

| Question | Justification | Answer | Thoughts | | | | | |
|---|---|---|---|---|---|---|---|---|
| Thought: Have you ever felt as though your thoughts have been removed or that you have thoughts that aren't yours? Or that your thoughts can be heard by everyone else? | It is important to assess for thought insertion, withdrawal and broadcast which, if positive, could point towards schizophrenia | 'No' | No additional concerns | | | | | |
| Thought: Have you ever had any thoughts to harm or kill yourself? | A risk assessment is essential to any psychiatric history and is also essential in a MSE. Suicidal thoughts and thoughts of self-harm come into both the mood and thought elements of an MSE, and are important to elicit so that you can manage the patient appropriately | 'I have had thoughts of self-harm but I haven't acted on them. I have never had any thoughts of killing myself' | This patient has had thoughts of self-harm but no suicidal thoughts. It is important to explore the protective factors that have stopped her from acting on her thoughts so far | | | | | |
| Perception: Have you ever heard or seen things when nothing can explain them? | This question can be used to help screen for psychotic depression presenting with hallucinations | 'No' | No evidence suggesting auditory hallucinations and therefore psychotic depression. More questions should be asked to screen for this more thoroughly | | | | | |
| Cognition | Vital to establish whether the patient is cognitively aware. You should note if the patient is orientated to time, place and person. If required, you can carry out other tests, such as Mini-Mental State Examination (MMSE) | Patient is orientated to time, place and person and would complete an MMSE to no concerns if requested | This patient is orientated to time, place and person and can engage in the conversation. There is no concern regarding cognitive impairment | | | | | |
| Insight | Vital to establish the patient's level of insight which can be assessed using the questions below:<br>• Do you think there has been a change in your mental health?<br>• What do you think might be causing it?<br>• Do you think you need any treatment? | 'My mental health has got much worse in the last month and I think this is down to my marriage breaking down and me losing my job. I think I need some help' | This patient has insight into her mental health and is keen for support | | | | | |

**Finishing the Consultation**

| Question | Justification | Answer | Thoughts | | | | | |
|---|---|---|---|---|---|---|---|---|
| Do you have anything to add? | May identify useful information that has been missed. Will also allow you to address any questions or concerns | 'No' | Take the time to explain what will happen from here | | | | | |

**Present Your Findings**

Mrs Bradley is a 56-year-old woman who presented with low mood. She was wearing appropriate clothes but was poorly kempt with matted hair. Eye contact was intermittently maintained. She engaged well throughout the interview but was tearful at times. Her mood was subjectively and objectively very low, with a reactive affect. Her thought form is normal but with feelings of inadequacy and low self-esteem, following the recent separation from her husband. She has had thoughts of suicide but has no intention of acting on them, and there are no thoughts of self-harm. She displays no evidence of abnormal perceptions. I assess Mrs Bradley to be of reasonable intelligence and she is orientated to time, place and person. She has good insight into her condition and is aware that she needs treatment.

I would like to organise a thorough set of bloods and will signpost her to relevant support groups for psychological therapy. Then I would arrange for a follow-up in 1 week's time to review her

**General Points**

| Polite to patient | | | | |
|---|---|---|---|---|
| Maintains good eye contact | | | | |
| Appropriate use of open and closed questions | | | | |

## ❓ QUESTIONS FROM THE EXAMINER

**How might the speech of a patient indicate schizophrenia?**

Flight of ideas, pressure of speech, excessive amounts of speech.

**How could you describe the affect of a patient with mania?**

Heightened.

**What are neologisms?**

Words a patient is using but where the meaning is unintelligible to another person.

**What is thought blocking?**

A sudden cessation of thought, usually mid-sentence, with the patient unable to remember what was previously said.

**What is a pseudohallucination?**

A hallucination (sensory perception without any relevant external stimulation) where the patient is aware that it is not real.

**What should be assessed in the cognition element of the MSE?**

Orientation to time/place/person, concentration levels, short-term memory.

## What is echolalia?

Repetition of another person's words.

## Describe the difference between objective and subjective mood.

Objective mood is how we observe and describe the patient's mood. Subjective mood is how the patient describes and reports their mood.

## What is meant by the phrase 'word salad'?

Speech/thinking that is unintelligible to others because it consists of words or phrases that are joined together with no meaningful connection.

## What is the passivity phenomenon?

The belief that your actions, feelings or impulses are controlled by an external force.

## Station 8.8    Examination: Cognitive

### Doctor Briefing

You are a junior doctor in primary care and have been asked to see Mr Ahmed, a 68-year-old man, who has been referred because his son has noticed his increasing forgetfulness. The son is worried that his father may have some memory problems. Please perform a cognitive assessment on Mr Ahmed, present your findings and formulate an appropriate management plan.

### Patient Briefing

You are Mr Ahmed, a 68-year-old retired accountant. Your son has brought you in today because he thinks your memory is getting worse. You think the memory decline is just getting old and don't think your memory is a problem

- *Orientation*: You are orientated to year/month/season (3/5), orientated to country/county/time (3/5)
- *Registration*: You can register all three items (lemon, key, ball) (3/3)
- *Attention and calculation*: when asked to spell WORLD backwards or count from 100, you say that you are not good with numbers, and spell DRLOW (3/5)
- *Recall*: You manage to recall one object mentioned previously (lemon) (1/3)
- *Language*: You can follow the instructions and close your eyes (1/1)
- *Language*: You are able to name pen and watch. You can repeat the sentence (3/3)
- *Reading and writing*: You can read and follow commands on the paper and construct a sentence (2/2)
- *Three-stage command*: You take the paper, forget to fold it in half, then put it on the floor (2/3)
- *Construction*: You copy the diagram successfully (1/1)

### Mark Scheme for Examiner

#### Introduction

| | | | | |
|---|---|---|---|---|
| Cleans hands, introduces self, confirms patient identity and gains consent for history taking/cognitive assessment | | | | |

#### Performing a Cognitive Assessment

| Question | Justification | Answer | Thoughts | | | | | |
|---|---|---|---|---|---|---|---|---|
| I'd like to perform a memory test today. This will involve some questions and tasks. Some of the questions sound a bit strange but they are part of the routine test. Please try your best and don't worry if you don't know the answers. Is that OK? Do you have any questions? | It is important to explain the assessment to gain consent. It also helps to alleviate any concerns the patient may have | 'That's fine. I have no questions' | Proceed with the examination | | | | | |
| What is the date? The day? The month? The year? The season? | These questions are used to assess orientation to time. This gives you a score out of 5 which forms part of the MMSE score | 'I don't know the day or date, but it's October 2022, which means that it is autumn' | The patient is orientated to the month, year and season, which gives you a score of 3/5 | | | | | |
| What country are we in? Which county? What town/city? What is the name of the building? On what floor are we? | These questions are used to assess orientation to place. This gives you a score out of 5 which forms part of the MMSE score | 'England. Kent. Tunbridge Wells. I don't know the building or the floor though' | The patient is orientated to the country, county and town, which gives you a score of 3/5 | | | | | |

## Performing a Cognitive Assessment

| Question | Justification | Answer | Thoughts | | | | | |
|---|---|---|---|---|---|---|---|---|
| I am going to say three objects. Please repeat the words after me now, and I will also ask you for them again later. The objects are: lemon, key and ball. Can you repeat the words I said? | This tests registration and is one point per correct word | 'Lemon, key, ball' | This patient recalled all three words, which gives a score of 3/3 | | | | | |
| Spell the word 'world' backwards or Keep subtracting 7 from 100 and stop after five answers | These questions are used to assess attention and calculation. You should give the patient the choice of these options by asking whether they prefer tasks with numbers or letters | 'D R L O W.' | This gives a score of 3/5 | | | | | |
| What were the three objects I told you earlier? | This question assesses recall and scores 1 point per correct object | 'Lemon ... I don't remember the others, sorry.' | The patient recalled one word correctly, so scores 1 point | | | | | |
| Can you tell me the name of the following? [point to watch and then to pencil] | This is one of the tasks used to assess language | 'Watch and pencil' | This patient names the two items correctly, which scores 2 points | | | | | |
| Can you repeat the following: 'No ifs, ands or buts.' | This is one of the tasks used to assess language, and if correctly repeated scores 1 point | 'No ifs, ands or buts' | This patient correctly recalled the sentence and scores 1 point | | | | | |
| [Show a card that says 'Close your eyes'] Can you read what is written and complete the task? | This is used to assess reading and scores 1 point | Patient closes his eyes | This patient scores 1 point as he completed the task correctly | | | | | |
| Can you write down a short sentence for me? It can be about anything | This can be used to assess writing and if done correctly scores the patient 1 point | Patient writes: 'Yesterday I walked the dog to the local park' | The patient completed this task correctly so scores 1 point | | | | | |
| Take this paper in your right hand, fold it in half and place it on the floor | This is a three-stage command and scores a point for each step completed correctly | The patient takes the paper, doesn't fold it in half and places it on the floor | This patient completed two steps correctly, which scores 2 points | | | | | |
| Try to copy this drawing for me | The drawing is a picture of interlocking pentagons. If correctly copied, this scores 1 point | The patient correctly copies the diagram | The patient correctly copied the diagram, which scores 1 point | | | | | |

**Present Your Findings**

Mr Ahmed is a 68-year-old man who has presented with a gradual decline of memory since the death of his wife. He scored 21/30 on his MMS with poor performance in orientation and recall. This decline of memory could be consistent with a diagnosis of early-onset dementia, grief or depression. From this assessment alone, it cannot be determined which of these it is.

I would like to obtain a collateral history, particularly looking at long-term cognitive impairment, as well as taking a focused depression history

**General Points**

Polite to patient

Maintains good eye contact

Appropriate use of open and closed questions

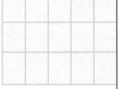

## ❓ QUESTIONS FROM THE EXAMINER

### How do you differentiate between delirium and dementia?

Delirium is a sudden, reversible state of confusion which fluctuates in severity and can be attributed to a physical illness or drug toxicity. Dementia has an insidious onset and is more constant in its level of confusion.

### What are the treatment options for moderate Alzheimer's dementia?

Acetyl cholinesterase inhibitors; for example, donepezil, galantamine, rivastigmine.

### What different electrolyte imbalances can cause delirium?

Hyperthyroidism, hypothyroidism, hypoparathyroidism, hyperparathyroidism, hyponatraemia, hypernatraemia, hypercalcaemia, Cushing's syndrome, hypoglycaemia and hyperglycaemia.

### After completing the MMSE, what further tests could be completed to test executive function?

Frontal Assessment Battery and/or Addenbrooke's Cognitive Examination Revised.

### What are the symptoms of Lewy body dementia?

Hallucinations, parkinsonism (rigidity, bradykinesia, tremor), memory loss.

### What are the symptoms of frontotemporal dementia?

Changes in personality, changes in behaviour, aphasia, trouble recognising objects, hyperorality.

### What common cardiovascular drugs cause delirium?

Beta-blockers, calcium channel blockers, digoxin.

### What are the three symptoms of normal-pressure hydrocephalus?

'Wet' – incontinent; 'wobbly' – difficulty walking; 'wacky' – cognitive impairment or short-term memory loss.

### Vitamin deficiencies can cause delirium and cognitive decline. Which vitamins?

Thiamine and vitamin $B_{12}$.

### What is the difference between how hypoactive and hyperactive delirium present?

Hypoactive presents as withdrawn, feeling lethargic, drowsy, very sleepy. Hyperactive patients are restless, agitated, hallucinating.

## Station 8.9 Communication: Assessing Capacity

### Doctor Briefing

You are a doctor in the later-life liaison psychiatry team and have been asked to see Mr Webber, an 80-year-old man with vascular dementia, who was admitted following a fall. There is concern about how Mr Webber is coping at home, but he is refusing a package of care at discharge. Please assess his capacity to make the decision to refuse care at home and present your findings.

### Patient Briefing

You have been newly diagnosed with vascular dementia. A week ago, you fell in your bathroom and fractured your wrist. This was your third fall. You insist that you have always coped well at home, been able to feed yourself, managed medications, cooked and performed other tasks independently.

You are refusing care at home because you feel that you do not need it. You feel that you are able to look after yourself in the long run, and are willing to accept help from family initially until you have fully recovered from the fracture. You acknowledge the benefit of having a care package but are adamant that you do not need it.

You are able to understand the information relevant to the decision and to repeat this information back. You can retain the information given. You can weigh up the information in making a reasoned decision. You can communicate the decision that you have made.

### Mark Scheme for Examiner

#### Introduction

| | | | |
|---|---|---|---|
| Cleans hands, introduces self, confirms patient identity. Have a colleague with you to document and witness the interaction if needed | | | |

#### Discussion

| Question | Justification | Answer | Thoughts | | | |
|---|---|---|---|---|---|---|
| There have been some concerns about how you will manage at home after we discharge you and this is what I'd like to explore with you today | This opening introduces the conversation and describes the conversation's direction | 'Go ahead' | The patient knows what to expect of the conversation | | | |
| Do you mind explaining to me why you have come into hospital? | This question can be used to assess awareness level and establish a rapport with the patient | 'I broke my wrist. I think I fell over' | This shows that Mr Webber is aware of his circumstances | | | |
| How are you feeling now? | This question is used to gauge the patient's current well-being | 'I'm feeling much better now' | This patient has awareness of his condition | | | |
| Consider if there is an impairment of, or disturbance in, the functioning of the person's mind or brain. | | | | | | |
| If the answer is yes, continue with the assessment. | | | | | | |
| If the answer is no, the assessment should not be completed and the patient is presumed to have capacity | | | | | | |
| Consider the timeframe for the decision and whether capacity may be regained if the decision is delayed | | | | | | |

**Discussion**

| Question | Justification | Answer | Thoughts | | | | |
|---|---|---|---|---|---|---|---|
| Explain how some patients benefit from a package of care upon leaving the hospital to help them in their recovery. Explore the benefits of receiving care. Ask the patient to repeat this back to you | It is important to give the patient information and the reasoning behind your decisions. Throughout this part of the conversation, you need to use jargon-free language. You need to be assessing whether the patient can understand the information and whether he can repeat it back to you. You need to assess whether the patient can retain the information | Repeats information back correctly | The patient understands what the care package can provide. He has correctly repeated it back and shows that he can retain the information long enough to make a decision | | | | |
| So we were considering that you may need some care after leaving hospital. What do you think about that? | This is an open question to explore the patient's thoughts on the topic and establishes his current understanding | 'I don't think I need it. I can look after myself; I've not had any trouble before. I don't want to waste anybody's time' | Patient is adamant he does not need care. He has demonstrated that he understands the purpose of the care package | | | | |
| Can you see the benefit of receiving some care? | This can help assess whether the patient has addressed the risks and benefits of his decision, therefore weighing up the information in a reasoned decision | 'I can see that it would help around the house but I feel that I will be able to cope OK alone. My family can help with the cooking and cleaning if I do struggle until I'm fully recovered' | Evidence that the patient understands the benefit of care and can weigh up the benefits and risks | | | | |
| Just so we're clear, you don't want any care at home? | The last element of full capacity is being able to communicate the decision the person has made. This can be in any form of communication – verbally, using an interpreter, written or other | 'No, I would not like care at home' | This patient is able to communicate his decision | | | | |

**Finishing the Consultation**

| Question | Justification | Answer | Thoughts | | | | |
|---|---|---|---|---|---|---|---|
| To summarise, you wouldn't like a care package on discharge and would prefer for your family to look after you in the short term. You feel that you can look after yourself well at home after that. Is that correct? | When summarising and finishing a consultation, it's important to recap the important information so far, the patient's key concerns and the plan moving forward | 'Yes, that's correct' | Happy that the information that you have gathered is accurate | | | | |

## Finishing the Consultation

| Question | Justification | Answer | Thoughts | | | | |
|---|---|---|---|---|---|---|---|
| Do you have any other questions or things to add?<br><br>I know that we have discussed a lot of new things; please take some time to digest the information | May identify useful information that has been missed. Will also allow you to address any questions or concerns | 'No, thank you' | Take the time to explain what will happen from here | | | | |

## Present Your Findings

Mr Webber is an 80-year-old man who presented following a fall. He has a diagnosis of vascular dementia and lives alone. He is refusing a package of care on discharge. Upon discussion with Mr Webber, he believes that he is able to cope at home, despite two previous falls.

I have had a detailed discussion today regarding his support at home and in my opinion, I feel that Mr Webber had the capacity to make such a decision. Therefore we should respect his wish to refuse care at home

## General Points

Polite to patient

Maintains good eye contact

Appropriate use of open and closed questions

## ❓ QUESTIONS FROM THE EXAMINER

### Define consent.

An informed, freely given decision from a patient with capacity to do so.

### What legislation is valid for capacity in England and Wales?

Mental Capacity Act 2005.

### What is the role of a medical proxy in the UK?

Allows another person to be appointed to make healthcare decisions on your behalf if you are no longer able to do so.

### Under what conditions is consent considered to be valid?

Consent is valid when it is voluntary, informed and the patient has capacity.

### What is the use of Gillick competency?

To determine whether a patient under the age of 16 is able to consent to their own medical treatment.

### What does the role of the Mental Health Act in the UK play with consent?

Allows a patient with a mental disorder to be detained if they are at risk of harm to themselves or others. This allows you to treat their mental illness without their consent.

**What are the principles of Deprivation of Liberty Safeguarding as enforced in the UK?**

It's a formal application to the local authority which assesses if a treatment/management option which might deprive a patient of their liberty (e.g. mittens or bed rails) are in the best interest of the patient. Legal authorisation is required for this restrictive practice to continue.

**By what means can advance decisions be made in the UK?**

They can be made verbally unless they are specifically refusing life-sustaining treatment, which then are required to be written and witnessed.

**What is the role of Section 4 of the Mental Health Act in the UK?**

Admission for emergency treatment which is valid for 72 h. Needs to be signed by a doctor and an approved social worker. Cannot treat without the patient's consent under this section. This can then be converted to Section 2 to allow for further assessment.

**What is the process for appeal of a Section 2 or 3 of the Mental Health Act in the UK?**

They need to be appealed at a mental health review tribunal. For a Section 2, appeal must be within 14 days and for Section 3, it must be within 6 months.

## Station 8.10   Communication: Commencing Lithium Treatment

### Doctor Briefing

You are a junior doctor working on a psychiatry ward and you have been asked to see Mr Wallace, a 36-year-old man, after his ward round where your consultant discussed the option of starting lithium. Please counsel Mr Wallace about starting lithium treatment for his bipolar affective disorder.

### Patient Briefing

You have been in the hospital for some time now after being treated for a period of mania. You have a diagnosis of bipolar disorder type 1, for which you do not take any medication. You do not have any existing medical problems.

The consultant has talked about starting you on a drug called lithium. You are happy to discuss starting this drug, but do not know much about it.

You have some questions: you've read on the internet that you will need regular blood tests and would like to know why these are necessary. You would also like some more information about the side effects of lithium.

You are able to understand and repeat the information given. You are unsure whether you would like to start lithium but will discuss this with your wife.

### Mark Scheme for Examiner

#### Introduction

| | |
|---|---|
| Cleans hands, introduces self, confirms patient identity and gains consent for history taking | |

#### History of Presenting Complaint

| Question | Justification | Answer | Thoughts | | | | | |
|---|---|---|---|---|---|---|---|---|
| I understand you discussed a change in medication with one of the doctors earlier. Is that correct? | It is important to establish the patient's understanding of the situation so far. From this, you can then discuss the purpose of the conversation | 'He did, yes. I think it was called lithium?' | This patient is aware that the medication is changing which means that he will be expecting some information about this | | | | | |
| I plan to talk to you about the possibility of starting lithium therapy and this will involve discussing the side effects, monitoring and lithium toxicity. | | 'That would be useful' | The patient is ready to receive information about the medication | | | | | |
| Lithium is a mood stabiliser and its aim is to maintain your mood at a constant level | Background information on lithium. Ensure that you use jargon-free language and regularly check the patient's understanding | 'OK' | Splitting information into chunks helps aid understanding when information giving | | | | | |
| If lithium isn't taken as prescribed or if there is a rapid reduction in the dose, this can result in the relapse of the symptoms of bipolar. | Discussion of compliance should be done in a non-judgemental way with pathways for support explained | 'I understand' | Make sure to check patient's understanding after each section of information given | | | | | |

**History of Presenting Complaint**

| Question | Justification | Answer | Thoughts | | | | | |
|---|---|---|---|---|---|---|---|---|
| Lithium has a variety of different side effects, like increased urinary frequency, weight gain, tiredness and concentration problems. Most of the side effects are dose-dependent so will improve with a dose adjustment | Lithium has many side effects, so knowing some of the common ones is vital to allow the patient to be aware of them as well | 'Are there any more side effects?' | If asked for side effects, then it's important to give a few examples. It is important to mention these to the patient, whether this be unprompted or prompted by questions | | | | | |
| Lithium can also have some long-term lasting effects on the kidneys and the thyroid gland, such as diabetes insipidus | | 'I see' | The patient appears to have understood; you can move on to the next section | | | | | |
| Lithium is a potentially toxic substance and if the lithium levels are increased, patients can experience some symptoms of toxicity. Early symptoms of lithium toxicity include a tremor, poor appetite, nausea and vomiting and lethargy. If the levels of lithium in the plasma continue to rise, it can cause seizures and potentially death | Provide the patient with information about lithium toxicity. It is important that patients know the symptoms of lithium toxicity and how to avoid it; for example, fluid intake in hot weather and maintaining salt intake | 'Oh gosh, that sounds so serious' | You should continue to warn the patient about other problems with lithium, but do so in an unbiased way | | | | | |
| It is important to inform your doctor that you have started lithium as it interacts with many other medications, and to avoid use of non-steroidal anti-inflammatory drugs (NSAIDs) such as ibuprofen as these also interact with lithium | Give the patients information about drug interactions | 'That's fine' | Move on to inform the patient about monitoring | | | | | |
| It is important whilst you are on lithium to have regular blood tests, which become less frequent as the dose is established. Once the dose is stable, blood tests are every 3 months for the first year and can then be measured every 6 months | Give the patient information about the monitoring of lithium so that he knows what to expect after commencement | 'Why are these blood tests necessary?' | Address any concerns or queries that the patient may have throughout | | | | | |

### History of Presenting Complaint

| Question | Justification | Answer | Thoughts | | | | |
|---|---|---|---|---|---|---|---|
| With the initial blood tests, we look at your red and white blood cells and kidney and thyroid function. In the regular blood tests, we also look at the lithium level. We need to make sure the level is high enough to be an effective treatment, but not high enough to cause problems | Explain in lay terms the details of the blood tests and the significance of the narrow therapeutic window | 'I see' | Ensure that you have covered everything that you were planning to | | | | |

### Finishing the Consultation

| | | | | | | | |
|---|---|---|---|---|---|---|---|
| In summary, we have discussed the benefit of starting lithium to help stabilise your mood. We've also talked about its side effects and monitoring needs. How do you feel about starting the medication? | When summarising and finishing a consultation, it's important to recap the important information so far, the patient's key concerns and the plan moving forward | 'I'd like to discuss with my family first as I'll definitely need their support with the monitoring' | Patient has appraised how lithium therapy might affect his life. Time to discuss with family is a good step in ensuring the monitoring is achievable for him | | | | |
| Do you have any other questions or things to add? I know that we have discussed a lot of new things; please take some time to digest the information | May identify useful information that has been missed. Will also allow you to address any questions or concerns | 'No, thank you' | Take the time to explain what will happen from here | | | | |

### Present Your Findings

Mr Wallace is a 36-year-old man who has a diagnosis of bipolar affective disorder type 1. He has recently recovered from an episode of mania and would like to try a mood stabiliser.

Today I have discussed the side effects, longer-term complications, toxicity risks and monitoring of lithium with Mr Wallace. He was able to understand the information discussed and repeat it back to me. I have given him some written information so that he can discuss this with his family. If Mr Wallace agrees, then we will complete work-up for the commencement of lithium

### General Points

| | | | |
|---|---|---|---|
| Polite to patient | | | |
| Maintains good eye contact | | | |
| Appropriate use of open and closed questions | | | |

## ❓ QUESTIONS FROM THE EXAMINER

### How long after the last dose of lithium should the plasma levels be checked?

12 h.

### Once the lithium dose is stable, how often should the blood tests be repeated?

Every 3 months for the first year and then measured every 6 months in people without comorbidities, interacting drugs or compliance issues.

### Before starting treatment on lithium, what tests are required?

Full blood count, urea and electrolytes renal function, thyroid function tests, baseline electrocardiogram, baseline weight.

### Why is it important to monitor lithium levels closely?

It has a very narrow therapeutic index. If it exceeds 1.5 mmol/L, most patients will experience some symptoms of toxicity and if it exceeds 2.0 mmol/L, it can be life-threatening.

### What are the long-term effects of lithium treatment?

Nephrogenic diabetes insipidus, hypothyroidism, interstitial nephritis and reduced glomerular filtration rate.

### What are the common side effects of lithium treatment?

Polyuria, polydipsia, weight gain, impaired memory, fine tremor and GI disturbances.

### What is Ebstein's anomaly?

A congenital malformation of the tricuspid valve in the heart. Its risk is increased by the use of lithium in the first trimester of pregnancy.

### How may a patient with lithium toxicity present?

Diarrhoea, vomiting, agitation. poor coordination and coarse tremors.

### How does lithium cause hypercalcaemia?

Lithium alters the set point for parathyroid hormone release, resulting in hyperparathyroidism. This is resolved upon lithium cessation.

### What drugs can increase the risk of lithium toxicity, due to their ability to impair lithium excretion by the kidneys?

Diuretics (particularly bendroflumethiazide), angiotensin II receptor blockers, angiotensin-converting enzyme inhibitors, NSAIDs and metronidazole.

# Paediatrics

9

## Outline

## Station 9.1    History: Paediatric History Taking

### Doctor Briefing

You are a junior doctor in primary care and have been asked to see Summer, a 3-year-old girl. Her mother, Mrs Howard, has brought her in because she has noticed a rash and Summer has been more agitated than normal. Please take a history from Mrs Howard and Summer, then present your findings and formulate an appropriate management plan.

### Patient Briefing

Summer is your first child. She currently attends nursery, where you note a couple of children have been unwell. Today you've noticed a rash over her hands. The lesions are raised and grey-white and some of them are filled with pus. She has also been crying a lot and it's getting difficult to put her to sleep. She's not been feeding well.

She has no past medical history, and your pregnancy was uneventful. She is up to date with all her vaccinations and has no known allergies. She is growing and developing well.

You think she may have chickenpox and you were wondering if there was anything that could help.

### Mark Scheme for Examiner

#### Introduction

| | |
|---|---|
| Washes hands, introduces self, confirms patient identity and gains consent for examination | |
| Enquires about parental ideas and concerns | |

#### History of Presenting Complaint

| Question | Justification | Answer | Thoughts | |
|---|---|---|---|---|
| Please can you tell me about what's been happening with Summer? | Open question to allow mother to provide the essential features and guide the rest of the history | 'She has a rash on her hands which appeared yesterday and she's been more agitated lately' | Rash could be dermatological or an infective disease issue. Onset was recent | |

## History of Presenting Complaint

| Question | Justification | Answer | Thoughts | | | | | |
|---|---|---|---|---|---|---|---|---|
| Is the rash itchy? Has she been scratching it? | Itchy lesions indicate possible allergy or certain infections (e.g. chickenpox) | 'No, it's not itchy but it is pretty sore' | Less likely to be allergic | | | | | |
| Do the areas affected feel warm to touch? Or has Summer felt warm to you? Have you taken her temperature? | A temperature points to possible infection, and local heat to an inflammatory process | 'Yes, she does, I recorded her temperature yesterday as 38°C. And the spots are warm' | Infection is a possible cause | | | | | |
| Whereabouts is the rash? Has this changed over time? | Identify the affected sites and consider distribution pattern (e.g. dermatomal) | 'I can see them on her hands mostly, but I think there are some around her mouth and on the bottom of her feet. They have not changed since I first noticed them' | Distribution is classic of hand, foot and mouth disease (HFMD) but could still be chickenpox. In chickenpox, the lesions tend to appear centrally (on the face and stomach) before spreading to the limbs | | | | | |
| What do the spots look like? | Obtain a detailed description of the rash. This can help differentiate between eczematous rashes, allergic reactions and infection | 'They are slightly raised, look grey-white and also some have pus in them. I think it might be chickenpox' | Description of a vesicular rash consistent with HFMD | | | | | |
| Does the rash disappear when you apply pressure to it? | Assess whether the rash is non-blanching, particularly when considering meningococcal disease | 'Yes, it does' | Less worrying as blanching | | | | | |
| Does the rash look the same throughout or do some of the spots look different to you? | Older HFMD lesions crust and become punched-out ulcers | 'No, I think they're all the same' | Patient is most likely still in early stages of the disease | | | | | |
| Have you given Summer anything for the rash? | Identify the impact of any interventions to help with diagnosis and assessing severity | 'I've given her some Calpol which settles her down for a couple of hours. Antihistamines have not helped' | Unlikely to be allergic | | | | | |
| Is anyone at nursery or home unwell? Has anyone had any similar problems recently? | Viral causes spread quickly throughout a household | 'Yes, some kids in her nursery have been unwell. I am not sure what this was for' | HFMD can spread through contact with vesicle fluid | | | | | |

## Birth History

| Question | Justification | Answer | Thoughts | | | | | |
|---|---|---|---|---|---|---|---|---|
| Can you please tell me a bit about your pregnancy? At how many weeks was Summer born? What type of delivery did you have? Were there any complications or stays in hospital following birth? How much did she weigh? | Preterm children and those with a complex neonatal course may be more susceptible to illness | 'She was born at 39 weeks. Uncomplicated vaginal delivery. 3.2 kg at birth. No stays in hospital following birth' | No additional concerns | | | | | |

## Past Medical and Surgical History

| | | | | | | | | |
|---|---|---|---|---|---|---|---|---|
| Has Summer ever been hospitalised? Does she have any known medical conditions or has she ever had surgery? | Identify any pre-existing conditions that would suggest immunodeficiency, such as cancer | 'No' | No additional concerns | | | | | |

## Feeding History

| | | | | | | | | |
|---|---|---|---|---|---|---|---|---|
| How has she been feeding? Is she eating and drinking as normal for her? Have there been any issues with regard to gaining weight? | Determine the impact on child's well-being. Identify any loss of appetite or any introduction of new foodstuffs that could cause an allergic reaction | 'Yes, she is drinking normally, but she is not feeding very well. There have been no problems with weight gain' | Patient is generally unwell, as expected in a viral illness | | | | | |

## Developmental History

| | | | | | | | | |
|---|---|---|---|---|---|---|---|---|
| Are there any concerns regarding Summer's development? How is she doing at nursery? | Identify any developmental concerns | 'No. Nursery is going well' | Patient seems to be developing as expected | | | | | |

## Drug History

| | | | | | | | | |
|---|---|---|---|---|---|---|---|---|
| Is Summer on any medications? | Identify possible drug reactions | 'No' | No additional concerns | | | | | |
| Is she up to date with all her vaccinations? | Rashes might relate to vaccine-preventable diseases | 'Yes' | No additional concerns | | | | | |
| Does she have any allergies? | Identify possible triggers of skin outbreaks | 'No' | No additional concerns | | | | | |

## Family History

| | | | | | | | | |
|---|---|---|---|---|---|---|---|---|
| Are there any conditions that run in the family? Do you have any other children? | Identify any family history of conditions that may affect the skin | 'No, everyone's fit and well. Summer is an only child' | No additional concerns | | | | | |

## Social and Travel History

| Question | Justification | Answer | Thoughts | | | | |
|---|---|---|---|---|---|---|---|
| Who is normally at home with Summer? | Identify main carers and home support | 'Myself and Summer's father' | No additional concerns | | | | |
| Does anyone in the household smoke? | Identify exposure to second-hand smoke | 'No' | No additional concerns | | | | |
| Has Summer or anyone in the household recently travelled abroad? | Screen for tropical diseases with dermatological presentations | 'No, we've all been at home for the last few months' | Not likely to be a tropical skin disease | | | | |
| Has a social worker ever been formally involved in Sarah's care? | Identify any potential risk of harm to the child that could result in injuries easily mistaken for rash, such as burns | 'No' | No social concerns | | | | |

## Systems Review

| Question | Justification | Answer | Thoughts | | | | |
|---|---|---|---|---|---|---|---|
| Any headaches, drowsy episodes or fits? Any chest pain or dizzy episodes? Any vomiting, diarrhoea or tummy pain? Any wheeze, cough or breathlessness? Any joint or bone pain? Any problems passing urine? Any bruising or bleeding? | Rash can be part of a systemic disease | 'No' | No additional concerns | | | | |

## Finishing the Consultation

| Question | Justification | Answer | Thoughts | | | | |
|---|---|---|---|---|---|---|---|
| Is there anything else that you would like to tell me about? | May identify useful information that has been missed and help to build rapport with the parent. Provides the opportunity to assure the mother that she has done the right thing by bringing her child in and that all the appropriate investigations will be done to determine the cause | 'I am worried that she is not eating as normal for her. However I am able to persuade her to eat a little when she is more settled throughout the day' | Take the time to explain what will happen from here, and reassure further about it being OK to eat less when ill | | | | |
| Do you have any questions? | Allows any final concerns to be addressed | | | | | | |

**Present Your Findings**

Summer is a 3-year-old child who has been a close contact of children who have been unwell at her nursery. She has presented today with a new rash over her hands and feet and around her mouth, which her mother has described as grey-white, and some of the lesions are pus-filled. She has not been feeding as normal and appears agitated. Calpol tends to help settle her for a couple of hours. There are no other concerning features.

I would like to examine Summer fully, but my main differentials would be HFMD or chickenpox.

Following an examination, if it was HFMD, I would reassure the mother that it is likely to be self-limiting and give the mother a patient information leaflet and safety net for any potential worrying features

**General Points**

Polite to patient/parent

Appropriate use of open and closed questions

## ? QUESTIONS FROM THE EXAMINER

**What is the causative organism in HFMD?**

It is a viral infection, commonly caused by coxsackievirus (A-16 most commonly) and enterovirus (although this presents more severely).

**What would the management be for HFMD?**

Supportive management (particularly adequate fluid and food intake) and reassurance as the disease is self-limiting and resolves within a week. Calpol or ibuprofen may be used to support with painful lesions.

**What are potential complications of HFMD?**

Aseptic meningitis, encephalitis, pulmonary oedema and myocarditis (especially with enterovirus infection).

**What is the typical presentation of chickenpox?**

An itchy, rapidly progressive maculopapular rash which then forms fluid-filled lesions (vesicles) that eventually crust over or form blisters.

**What is the causative organism of chickenpox?**

Varicella-zoster virus (herpesvirus type 3).

**What are some of the red-flag symptoms of sepsis in a child under 5 years old?**

Unresponsive, drowsy, weak/high-pitched/continuous cry, severe tachycardia or tachypnoea, bradycardia, non-blanching rash, mottled, ashen, cyanotic, hypothermia or looks very unwell to a healthcare professional.

**How can human immunodeficiency virus (HIV) be transmitted from mother to child?**

Vertical transmission antenatally through the placenta, perinatally due to exposure to maternal blood during childbirth or postnatally via breast milk.

**How would you describe the dermatological presentation of Lyme disease?**

Target lesion (erythema migrans).

**When are children with varicella-zoster virus (chickenpox) infectious?**

From 48 h before the onset of rash until all the lesions have crusted over.

**What is characteristic of the distribution of vesicles due to shingles infection?**

They follow a dermatomal distribution, commonly along the V1 division of the trigeminal nerve.

## Station 9.2  History: Crying Baby

### Doctor Briefing

You are a junior doctor in primary care and have been asked to see Mabel, a 4-month-old girl. Mabel's mother, Mrs Jackson, has brought her in because she will not stop crying. Please take a history from Mrs Jackson regarding Mabel, present your findings and formulate an appropriate management plan.

### Patient Briefing

Mabel is your 4-month-old daughter and your only child. You noticed Mabel has been crying on and off for the past day and there is nothing you can do to settle her. You've also noticed that sometimes when she's lying in her cot, she pulls her legs up towards her body and curls up before she starts crying. Her tummy has started to look a bit bigger than normal, despite her not feeding very well over the last couple of days. She has vomited a small amount of greenish liquid this morning, immediately after her feed.

If questioned specifically, Mabel had some red jelly-like stools this morning, which worried you as it looked like it could be blood. She does not have a fever, and no one in the household is unwell at present or has similar symptoms. There has not been any recent travel and she is exclusively breastfed. She is up to date with all her vaccinations.

You are concerned about the red stools and vomiting. You are both very tired following a sleepless night due to Mabel's distress.

### Mark Scheme for Examiner

#### Introduction

| | | | | | |
|---|---|---|---|---|---|
| Washes hands, introduces self, confirms patient identity and gains consent for examination | | | | | |
| Enquires about parental concerns | | | | | |

#### History of Presenting Complaint

| Question | Justification | Answer | Thoughts | | | | |
|---|---|---|---|---|---|---|---|
| What's been happening with Mabel? | Open question to allow mother to provide the essential features and guide the rest of the history | 'She's been crying a lot since yesterday and she just doesn't look right to me' | Mother is very concerned. Onset is recent | | | | |
| Have you noticed whether there is a pattern to when she cries? | Establish a time course and identify any triggers | 'Not really. She just cries on and off throughout the day. Although it tends to be worse following feeding' | No obvious trigger, although it might be related to reflux | | | | |
| How does it compare to her normal cry? | Distinguish level of discomfort and identify distinctive cries | 'It's just her normal cry but there are times when it sounds like she's screaming' | Patient appears to be in fluctuating discomfort | | | | |
| Is there anything that you can do to settle her? | Identify possible relieving factors | 'Nothing at all. I have tried Calpol; however it didn't provide any relief' | Concerning that there seems to be no relief | | | | |
| Has anything made her crying worse? | Identify possible exacerbating factors | 'Sometimes I feel like she is worse after she feeds' | Indicates potential gastrointestinal (GI) cause | | | | |
| Does she seem more tired than usual? | Indicates fatigue, potentially dehydration | 'Yes' | Indicates that she may be unwell with it and feeding less | | | | |

## History of Presenting Complaint

| Question | Justification | Answer | Thoughts | | | | |
|---|---|---|---|---|---|---|---|
| Has she been feeding less? | Determine the impact on baby's well-being | 'I feed her more frequently now as she always seems to be hungry but I'm not sure how much she has been taking' | At risk of becoming dehydrated | | | | |
| Has she vomited or had diarrhoea? | Vomiting may indicate a cause, e.g. gastroenteritis or bowel obstruction | 'Yes, a little just this morning. It was green. Her stool was red and jelly-like in consistency' | Bilious vomiting present; suggests obstruction in lower GI tract. Stool suggestive of intussusception | | | | |
| Does she ever look floppy to you since all this started? | Could be a feature of sepsis or a neurological condition | 'No' | No additional concerns | | | | |
| Is there any possibility she may have hit her head recently? | Excludes any intracranial injuries | 'No' | No additional concerns | | | | |
| Has she been passing urine and stools? | Identifies dehydration, potential urinary tract infection and features of GI upset. Ask about each feature extensively if positive | 'Yes, I have to change her nappies regularly' | No concerning urinary symptoms | | | | |
| Does her tummy look any bigger to you? | Identifies noticeable abdominal distension; could be sign of a mass or constipation | 'Yes, actually it does. I hadn't noticed this before' | Potential mass in abdomen, suggestive of obstruction | | | | |
| Does she feel warmer than usual? | Identifies general features of infection/sepsis | 'No' | No additional concerns | | | | |
| Has this ever happened before? | Previous or recurrent episodes may indicate a more chronic problem | 'No' | Either the first presentation of a chronic problem or, more likely, an acute problem | | | | |

## Birth History

| | | | | | | | |
|---|---|---|---|---|---|---|---|
| Can you please tell me a bit about your pregnancy? At how many weeks was Mabel born? What type of delivery did you have? Were there any complications or stays in hospital following birth? How much did she weigh? | There may be underlying conditions or risk factors from pregnancy that are important | 'No, normal pregnancy and scans, normal vaginal delivery, on time, weighing 3.6 kg' | No identifiable risk factor for neonatal infections | | | | |

## Past Medical and Surgical History

| Question | Justification | Answer | Thoughts | | | | | |
|---|---|---|---|---|---|---|---|---|
| Has Mabel ever been hospitalised? Does she have any known medical conditions or has she ever had surgery? | Identify any pre-existing conditions that may predispose to illness | 'No' | No additional concerns | | | | | |

## Drug History

| Question | Justification | Answer | Thoughts | | | | | |
|---|---|---|---|---|---|---|---|---|
| Is Mabel on any medications? Or has she taken any over-the-counter medication recently? | May be a potential side effect of medication | 'I gave Mabel some Calpol to try and settle her last night; however it didn't seem to work' | No additional concerns | | | | | |
| Is she up to date with all her vaccinations? | Identify potential risk of vaccine-preventable illness | 'Yes' | No additional concerns | | | | | |
| Does she have any allergies? | Identify allergens that could cause GI upset | 'No' | No identifiable trigger | | | | | |

## Family History

| Question | Justification | Answer | Thoughts | | | | | |
|---|---|---|---|---|---|---|---|---|
| Are there any conditions that run in the family? Do you have any other children? | Identify any family history or conditions that may affect the skin | 'No, everyone's been fit and well. Mabel is an only child' | No additional concerns | | | | | |

## Social and Travel History

| Question | Justification | Answer | Thoughts | | | | | |
|---|---|---|---|---|---|---|---|---|
| Who's normally at home with Mabel? | Identify main carers and family dynamics | 'Myself, my partner and my mum' | No additional concerns | | | | | |
| Is anyone at home unwell or have any similar problems recently? | Viral causes spread quickly throughout a household | 'No' | Unlikely to be infective | | | | | |
| And how about you? How have you been? And how has your mood been? | Screen for postnatal depression as maternal complaints can in reality be a sign of poor mood or difficulty coping | 'I have been coping well until recently, as I haven't been able to sleep and I am very worried about Mabel' | Some concerns regarding maternal well-being | | | | | |
| Has Mabel or anyone around her recently travelled abroad? | Remember that children are vulnerable to infections potentially carried by family members | 'No, we've all been at home for the last few months' | Lower chance of an infectious cause | | | | | |
| Does anyone in the household smoke? | Indicates exposure to second-hand smoke | 'No' | No additional concerns | | | | | |

## Social and Travel History

| Question | Justification | Answer | Thoughts | | | | |
|---|---|---|---|---|---|---|---|
| Has a social worker ever been formally involved in Mabel's care? | Children are also vulnerable to neglect and abuse. Asking about social work helps identify any potential risk of harm to the child that could result in injuries | 'No' | Reassured that Mabel is well looked after | | | | |

## Systems Review

| Question | Justification | Answer | Thoughts | | | | |
|---|---|---|---|---|---|---|---|
| Any headaches, drowsy episodes or fits? Any vomiting, diarrhoea or tummy pain? Any wheeze, cough or breathlessness? Any joint or bone pain? Any problems passing urine? Any bruising or bleeding? | Crying can be part of a systemic disease | 'No' | No additional concerns | | | | |

## Finishing the Consultation

| Question | Justification | Answer | Thoughts | | | | |
|---|---|---|---|---|---|---|---|
| Is there anything else that you would like to tell me about? | May identify useful information that has been missed and help to build rapport with the parent. Provides the opportunity to assure the mother that she has done the right thing by bringing her child in and that all the appropriate investigations will be done to determine the cause | 'No, I'm just very worried because of the red stool. Plus, I'm not getting much sleep' | Take the time to explain what will happen from here | | | | |
| Do you have any questions? | Allows any final concerns to be addressed | | | | | | |

## Present Your Findings

Mabel is a 4-month-old girl who has presented with abdominal distension, red jelly-like stools and bilious vomiting. She has been noted to pull her legs up towards her body and has been crying inconsolably. She is up to date with all of her vaccinations.

My main differentials would be intussusception, volvulus, an incarcerated or strangulated hernia and GI inflammation due to allergy or infection.

I would like to check her FBC, U&Es and C-reactive protein (CRP), dip her urine and order an abdominal ultrasound. I would also like to admit her to hospital, give her some fluids if dehydrated and monitor for any worsening features. Depending on the results of the tests, I would then like to discuss the case with a paediatric surgeon for a definitive management plan

| General Points | | | | |
| --- | --- | --- | --- | --- |
| Polite to patient/parent | | | | |
| Appropriate use of open and closed questions | | | | |

## ❓ QUESTIONS FROM THE EXAMINER

### How does a volvulus differ from an intussusception?

A volvulus is a malrotation of the GI tract where the loop of bowel twists on itself, whereas an intussusception is an invagination of one part of the GI tract into another.

### What radiological feature would you look for to differentiate between an intussusception and a volvulus?

An intussusception can be seen on ultrasound scan as a target/doughnut sign (mostly commonly in the ileocaecal region) whereas a volvulus can be seen on an abdominal X-ray, showing a characteristic coffeebean sign (most commonly in the sigmoid region).

### Where is the most common site for intussusception to occur and what anatomical anomaly could cause this?

It usually occurs in the ileocaecal area.

### What might happen with untreated intussusception?

Blood vessels can be drawn into the site of intussusception, resulting in ischaemic injury, leading to inflammation, oedema and bleeding. This will eventually become necrotic, increasing the risk of perforation, pneumoperitoneum and peritonitis.

### What is the anatomical landmark that separates the upper and lower GI tract?

The ligament of Treitz or the suspensory muscle of the duodenum located at the duodenojejunal flexure.

### What features could you elicit in the history that would raise concerns of non-accidental injuries?

Features may include: history inconsistent with presentation, inconsistent histories from various family members/carers, injury to non-bony prominences, uncertain time of onset, unexplained injuries, abnormal sites of injuries inconsistent with expected milestones, parental drug and alcohol abuse and multiple attendances to primary/secondary care.

### If a non-accidental injury is suspected, how would you escalate your concerns as a junior doctor?

Firstly, communicate to the parents that you would like the child to stay in hospital, then discuss your concerns with a senior immediately. Consider further blood tests, radiological imaging and other appropriate investigations depending on presenting clinical features. Notifying social workers, safeguarding on-call consultant and the relevant authorities is also important.

### How would you differentiate between gastro-oesophageal reflux and obstruction?

Simple reflux occurs after feeding. It usually only contains milk or recently ingested fluids and can be managed conservatively in most cases. Obstructive causes would result in projectile bilious vomiting, constipation and failure to pass flatus; positional changes do not usually make a difference.

### What is the genetic abnormality in cri-du-chat syndrome?

It is a chromosomal deletion of the p arm of chromosome 5.

### What would a high-pitched cry make you worry about?

Cerebral irritation from, for example, a head injury or meningitis.

## Station 9.3   History: Febrile Convulsions

### Doctor Briefing

You are a junior doctor in the emergency department (ED) and have been asked to see Fred, a 2-year-old boy who has been brought in by his mother. He has presented with a temperature and a fit. You examined the patient and found signs consistent with acute otitis media. Take a history from the mother and arrive at a likely diagnosis.

### Patient Briefing

Feng is your second child. You are worried because he had a seizure that lasted for approximately 2 min. This is the first time that this has happened. He has had a temperature for the past 2 days with a runny nose and cough. You have been giving him paracetamol as per your general practitioner's advice, which has helped a bit. You thought this was a simple cold as his older brother has similar symptoms.

Feng was born at term. There were no antenatal concerns and his delivery was uncomplicated. He currently attends nursery, but you don't know if anyone else has been unwell. He has missed some of his routine childhood vaccinations, as you've been unable to attend clinic due to a busy work schedule, but you cannot recall which ones.

You are concerned that there is something seriously wrong and want to know if there will be any long-term complications for his health.

### Mark Scheme for Examiner

#### Introduction

| | | | | |
|---|---|---|---|---|
| Washes hands, introduces self, confirms patient identity and gains consent for examination | | | | |
| Enquires about parental concerns | | | | |

#### History of Presenting Complaint

| Question | Justification | Answer | Thoughts | | | | |
|---|---|---|---|---|---|---|---|
| What's been happening with Feng? How has Feng's health been before today? | Establishes a possible preceding risk factor for developing seizures, such as infection or diagnosed neurological disorder | 'He's been having fevers for the past 2 days and has had a fit today' | Likely infection; need to narrow down the source | | | | |
| Who witnessed the episode? Did anyone manage to record or time the episode? | Identifies a witness who can give an accurate description of what happened. Establishes the duration of seizure activity | 'Yes, myself and his older brother. We didn't get a video, but it was about 2 min long' | Witnessed seizure means history likely to be more accurate | | | | |
| Could you describe what happened just before the episode? | Detailed description to narrow down trigger of the seizure and to screen for any potential injuries. Enquire in more detail for signs of infection, history of head injuries or behavioural problems | 'He was complaining of discomfort; he kept tugging at his ears. Next thing I know, he's fallen to the floor and is shaking his arms and legs' | Potentially triggered by ear infection | | | | |
| What height did he fall from and which part of his body hit the floor first? | Identifies risk of head injury | 'He fell from standing. I think it was his shoulder that hit the floor first' | Reassured that head injury is less likely | | | | |

## History of Presenting Complaint

| Question | Justification | Answer | Thoughts | | | | | |
|---|---|---|---|---|---|---|---|---|
| Could you describe what he was doing during the episode? | A detailed description of the episodes helps confirm a seizure occurred, and if it was atypical | 'His arms and legs were jerking a lot and it looked like his jaw was clenched' | Likely to be generalised tonic-clonic seizure | | | | | |
| Did he wet or soil himself during this time? | Often occurs during a seizure | 'No' | No additional concerns | | | | | |
| Did he sustain any injuries during the episode? | Identify potential injuries that require attention soon | 'I don't think so. We put a pillow under his head just in case' | No additional concerns | | | | | |
| What did you do when he had the episode? | Understand interventions that were employed to help or to terminate seizure | 'I immediately phoned the ambulance. They took maybe 7 min to arrive, but the seizure stopped after 2 min' | Length of seizure consistent with febrile convulsion | | | | | |
| What did the ambulance crew do? | Establish whether medications were given and when | 'They observed him briefly, checked his pulse and temperature, then brought him to hospital. He was very sleepy' | Self-limiting seizure with postictal period | | | | | |
| And what happened after the episode? | A full recovery is characteristic of seizures. If there is a new neurological deficit, other neurological conditions need to be considered | 'He was tired and sleepy whilst we were in the ambulance but he's starting to look brighter now and returning to his normal self' | Full recovery. Likely to be febrile convulsion | | | | | |
| Has anyone in the household or at nursery been unwell recently? | Ill contacts may explain source of infection | 'No' | No additional concerns | | | | | |

## Birth History

| | | | | | | | | |
|---|---|---|---|---|---|---|---|---|
| Can you please tell me a bit about the pregnancy? At how many weeks was Feng born? What type of delivery was there? Were there any complications or stays in hospital following birth? How much did he weigh? | Preterm children and those with a complex neonatal course may be more susceptible illness | 'He was born at 39 weeks. Vaginal delivery. No complications. 3 kg at birth' | No additional concerns | | | | | |

## Past Medical and Surgical History

| Question | Justification | Answer | Thoughts | | | | | |
|---|---|---|---|---|---|---|---|---|
| Has Feng had these episodes before? | Establishes diagnosis of epilepsy or previous febrile convulsion | 'No' | No evidence for underlying condition | | | | | |
| Has Feng ever been hospitalised? Does he have any known medical conditions, like epilepsy? | Important to elicit any other underlying conditions that the patient may have | 'No' | No additional concerns | | | | | |

## Developmental History

| Question | Justification | Answer | Thoughts | | | | | |
|---|---|---|---|---|---|---|---|---|
| How has his development been? How is he finding nursery? | Elicit developmental concerns if there are any | 'Things are fine at nursery, and both myself and nursery are happy with his development' | No additional concerns | | | | | |
| Is he able to communicate with two words strung together? | Identify any specific developmental delay using milestones appropriate to age | 'Yes' | No additional concerns | | | | | |
| Can he scribble in circular pattern? | | 'Yes' | No additional concerns | | | | | |
| Is he able to walk, run and jump? | | 'Yes to all of those' | No additional concerns | | | | | |
| How does he eat and drink? What does he do when he plays? | | 'He eats with a fork and a spoon. He is happy playing alongside other children and has a great imagination' | No additional concerns | | | | | |
| Have you noticed if he's stopped doing things he previously could do? | Identify developmental regression, particularly in neurological presentations, as it could suggest more serious and evolving pathology | 'No' | No additional concerns | | | | | |

## Drug History

| Question | Justification | Answer | Thoughts | | | | | |
|---|---|---|---|---|---|---|---|---|
| Is he on any medications at the moment, or does he have any allergies? Has he taken any medications over the counter recently? | It is good practice to check the patient's full drug history and allergy status | 'I've given him some paracetamol as my doctor suggested. He doesn't have any allergies' | No additional concerns | | | | | |

## Drug History

| Question | Justification | Answer | Thoughts | | | | | |
|---|---|---|---|---|---|---|---|---|
| Is he up to date with his childhood vaccinations? | Ensure preventable diseases are not causing an infection | 'I think he might have missed some of the more recent ones as I've not been able to take him to them yet' | Consider checking his records to clarify which ones the patient has received | | | | | |

## Family History

| | | | | | | | | |
|---|---|---|---|---|---|---|---|---|
| Are there any conditions that run in the family, particularly related to seizures? Do you have any other children? | Identify potential genetic link to febrile convulsions or epilepsy | 'No. Feng has one adopted brother who is well' | No additional concerns | | | | | |

## Social History

| | | | | | | | | |
|---|---|---|---|---|---|---|---|---|
| Who is normally at home with Feng? | Identifies main carers and home support | 'Me, my husband, and his older brother' | No additional concerns | | | | | |
| Does anyone in the household smoke? | Exposure to second-hand smoke | 'No' | No additional concerns | | | | | |
| Has Feng or anyone around him recently travelled abroad? | Screen for tropical infection | 'No, we've all been at home for the last few months' | Not likely to be an unusual infection | | | | | |
| Have any social workers ever been involved in Feng's care? | Identify any risk of non-accidental injuries or abuse/neglect that could lead to head injuries | 'No' | No additional concerns | | | | | |
| Do you feel well supported at home? | Provides an opportunity to empathise with father but also identifies any risk that patient may not be well cared for | 'Not really. My partner and I work long hours to scrape enough money to pay for Feng and his brother' | Father is struggling to cope. Could signpost to additional support services | | | | | |

## Systems Review

| | | | | | | | | |
|---|---|---|---|---|---|---|---|---|
| Any headache, drowsy episodes or fits? Any chest pain or dizzy episodes? Any vomiting, diarrhoea, tummy pain or weight loss? Any wheeze, cough or breathlessness? Any joint or bone pain? Any problems passing urine? Any bruising or bleeding? | Helps identify focus of any infection, and any underlying condition that may predispose to seizures | 'No' | No additional concerns | | | | | |

## Finishing the Consultation

| Question | Justification | Answer | Thoughts | | | | | |
|---|---|---|---|---|---|---|---|---|
| Is there anything else that you would like to tell me about? | May identify useful information that has been missed and help to build rapport with the parent. Provides the opportunity to assure the father that he has done the right thing by bringing his child in and that all the appropriate investigations will be done to determine the cause | 'I'm just so worried something might be really wrong. Are there any long-term complications from having a fit?' | Take the time to explain what will happen from here | | | | | |
| Do you have any questions? | Allows any final concerns to be addressed | | | | | | | |

## Present Your Findings

Feng is a 2-year-old boy who has presented with a 2-min, self-terminating seizure, and a 2-day history of fever, sore ears and coryzal symptoms. He has fully recovered and is otherwise well.

My main differential diagnosis is a simple febrile seizure. However, I would also consider other causes of transient loss of consciousness such as epilepsy, breath-holding attacks and vasovagal syncope.

I would like to investigate this patient further by checking a blood glucose and a urine dipstick. I would want to observe Feng in hospital, and at discharge, ensure the parents know what to do if it happens again, including first aid for seizures. I would also explore reasons behind missing previous vaccinations and encourage uptake

## General Points

| Polite to patient/parent | | | |
|---|---|---|---|
| Appropriate use of open and closed questions | | | |

## ❓ QUESTIONS FROM THE EXAMINER

### What is the typical age range for febrile convulsions?

6 months to 6 years.

### What is the difference between a generalised and a focal seizure?

Generalised seizures affect both cerebral hemispheres and are accompanied by a loss of consciousness, whereas focal seizures begin in one region of the brain and do not always cause loss of consciousness.

### What would you take into consideration when deciding what kind of antiepileptic medication to prescribe long-term?

I would like to determine the type of seizures experienced, the tolerability of the side effects of indicated medications, medications already trialled, the gender of the patient and any plans for pregnancy. Febrile seizures, in general, do not need antiepileptic medications to be prescribed.

### What is the mechanism of action of benzodiazepines?

They increase the effectiveness of gamma-aminobutyric acid (GABA) by increasing chloride ion influx through GABA receptors. This causes hyperpolarisation of the neuronal cell membrane, preventing conduction of action potentials across the neuron.

## If a generalised tonic-clonic seizure did not terminate with one dose of buccal midazolam, what would you do next?

Wait 10 min for the first dose to take effect. If the seizure has not terminated at this point, give one further dose of benzodiazepine and call for immediate senior help. Observe for any signs of relief, monitor the airway and gain IV access if the seizure has not terminated. Following the Advanced Paediatric Life Support (APLS) algorithm, consider another antiseizure medication, e.g. phenytoin or levetiracetam, if the seizure still has not terminated.

## How would you differentiate between a seizure and a vasovagal syncope?

Vasovagal syncope typically has obvious triggers, such as hot climate, pain or anxiety, comes on within minutes and resolves within a minute with prompt full recovery. Seizures are less likely to have identifiable triggers and take longer to recover from. There may also be tongue biting and incontinence.

## What is the risk of developing epilepsy from one episode of febrile convulsions?

Most cases of febrile convulsions are not associated with epilepsy, although the risk is slightly increased. However, there is an increased risk if there are underlying neurodevelopmental conditions, a strong family history of epilepsy or prolonged, recurrent or focal febrile convulsions.

## When would you consider admitting a child with a first febrile seizure?

Admission should be considered if: it's a first seizure, lasts more than 15 min, is focal, happens twice in 24 h, has incomplete recovery after 1 h, in children under 18 months old, suspected serious cause for infection (e.g. pneumonia), no apparent focus of infection or significant parental anxiety.

## How would the lumbar puncture results differ between viral and bacterial meningitis?

Viral meningitis would typically have elevated lymphocytes rather than neutrophils. Glucose is typically reduced in bacterial but not viral causes.

## What ophthalmological signs would you look for if you suspect a raised intracranial pressure?

The main ophthalmological signs would be papilloedema and the sunset sign (paralysis of the upwards gaze).

## Station 9.4   History: Wheeze

### Doctor Briefing

You are a junior doctor in the ED and have been asked to see Tommy, a 3-year-old boy who has presented with a wheeze. Please take a history from Mrs Shire, his mother present your findings and formulate an appropriate management plan.

### Patient Briefing

Tommy is your third child, and both his two older siblings suffer from eczema. You first noticed him wheezing after he had been playing in the garden with the dog a few weeks ago. His wheeze lasts for several minutes following exercise and is relieved by resting. However, since then, his wheezing episodes have been getting worse and he's developed a dry cough at night. He has otherwise been fit and well.

He does not have any significant past medical history and is up to date with his immunisations. There are no developmental concerns. No one in the household has travelled abroad recently or been unwell.

You think this may be asthma as you had it as a child and his older siblings presented in the same way. However, you would like a formal assessment and possibly some inhalers to help him.

### Mark Scheme for Examiner

#### Introduction

| | | | |
|---|---|---|---|
| Washes hands, introduces self, confirms patient identity and gains consent for examination | | | |
| Enquires about parental concerns | | | |

#### History of Presenting Complaint

| Question | Justification | Answer | Thoughts | | | | |
|---|---|---|---|---|---|---|---|
| What's been going on with Tommy? Could you describe the wheeze for me? Would you be able to demonstrate the sound he makes? | Gain a clear idea of how loud and where the wheeze is | 'Yes, I have noticed that he is very wheezy when he is playing sport or running around in the garden. It's a high-pitched whistling sound' | It's an expiratory sound consistent with a wheeze. Rule out a stridor (upper-airway sound) | | | | |
| When did you first notice it? | Identify trigger and onset to guide diagnosis | 'A few weeks back after Tommy had been running around in the garden with our dog' | Two possible triggers identified: exercise and allergies to dog | | | | |
| Is Tommy known to be allergic to anything? | Identify any potential triggers | 'I don't think so' | Does not rule out allergic response, but parents may need counselling on common allergens | | | | |
| Has the wheeze changed since then? | Identify patterns, timings and worsening features | 'Yes, it seems to be getting worse following exercise and in the mornings. I have also noted that he is coughing at night' | Diurnal pattern characteristic of asthma | | | | |
| Has anything made it better? | Identify relieving factors | 'It seems to improve a bit with rest' | Potentially relieved by rest and change of environment | | | | |

## History of Presenting Complaint

| Question | Justification | Answer | Thoughts | | | | |
|---|---|---|---|---|---|---|---|
| Does the wheeze cause any problems for him day to day? | Identify features that could indicate severity | 'Not really' | May only be experiencing mild to moderate asthma | | | | |
| How is his breathing when he is wheezing? | Identifies severity of respiratory distress | 'He really struggles to breathe but it settles quickly when he rests' | May be exercise-related. Being relieved without medication at present | | | | |
| Does he go blue or stop breathing with the wheeze? Does he make any funny sounds on breathing in? | Indicates a severe picture of airway obstruction | 'No' | No additional concerns | | | | |
| Does he have a cough? If so, does he bring up anything? | Could indicate asthma or infection | 'Only at night, and no, he doesn't bring anything up' | Less likely to have concurrent chest infection. Nocturnal cough classic of asthma | | | | |
| Does he have a fever? | Identify possible infection from elsewhere | 'No' | No additional concerns | | | | |
| Is anyone in the household unwell or have similar problems recently? | Viral causes spread quickly throughout a household | 'No' | Less likely to be an infective exacerbation | | | | |

## Birth History

| | | | | | | | |
|---|---|---|---|---|---|---|---|
| Can you please tell me a bit about the pregnancy? At how many weeks was Tommy born? What type of delivery did your partner have? Were there any complications or stays in hospital following birth? How much did he weigh? | Prematurity is a risk factor for atopy. Complications and neonatal infections could cause chronic lung diseases | 'Tommy was born at 36 weeks by normal vaginal delivery. There were no complications or stays in hospital following the birth. He was a good weight; I can't remember the figure' | Prematurity may contribute to atopy risk | | | | |

## Past Medical and Surgical History

| | | | | | | | |
|---|---|---|---|---|---|---|---|
| Does he have asthma, food allergies, eczema or hayfever? | Asthma commonly exists with other atopic syndromes | 'No' | No additional concerns | | | | |
| Does he have any other medical conditions? | Identify diseases that could predispose patient to chest infections and difficulty breathing, such as cystic fibrosis | 'No' | No additional concerns | | | | |

## Past Medical and Surgical History

| Question | Justification | Answer | Thoughts | | | | |
|---|---|---|---|---|---|---|---|
| Has he ever been hospitalised due to difficulty breathing? Or for anything else? | Number and nature of admissions due to asthma indicate severity | 'No' | No additional concerns | | | | |

## Feeding History

| Question | Justification | Answer | Thoughts | | | | |
|---|---|---|---|---|---|---|---|
| Is he eating and drinking as normal for him? | Determine overall illness and hydration | 'Yes, he is drinking and eating normally' | No additional concerns | | | | |

## Developmental History

| Question | Justification | Answer | Thoughts | | | | |
|---|---|---|---|---|---|---|---|
| Do you have any concerns about his development? How is nursery? | Premature children may have slower development. Severe asthma can have an impact on development due to medication used and hindrance to daily activities | 'No, he's been hitting all of his milestones' | No additional concerns | | | | |

## Drug History

| Question | Justification | Answer | Thoughts | | | | |
|---|---|---|---|---|---|---|---|
| Is he on any medications? Has he taken any over-the-counter medications recently? | Important to note effectiveness of current asthma treatment, if any | 'None' | Treatment for asthma follows a stepwise approach. A trial of salbutamol may be beneficial | | | | |
| Does he have any allergies? | Allergens could be a trigger for asthma | 'Not that I'm aware of' | No obvious allergies identified by father. This does not completely exclude the possibility of allergies | | | | |

## Family History

| Question | Justification | Answer | Thoughts | | | | |
|---|---|---|---|---|---|---|---|
| Are there any conditions that run in the family? Do you have any other children? | Ask specifically for atopic conditions | 'Yes, both his siblings have eczema and I used to have asthma as a child' | Strong family history of atopy suggestive of asthma as main diagnosis | | | | |

## Social and Travel History

| Question | Justification | Answer | Thoughts | | | | |
|---|---|---|---|---|---|---|---|
| Who is normally at home with Tommy? | Identify main carers | 'Me, my partner, his siblings and my parents' | No additional concerns | | | | |
| Do you have any pets at home? | Pets can trigger allergies | 'Yes, we have one dog, which actually he may be allergic to, but I'm not sure' | Potential allergen. Consider testing or advise to avoid allergen | | | | |

## Social and Travel History

| Question | Justification | Answer | Thoughts | | | | |
|---|---|---|---|---|---|---|---|
| Does anyone smoke around Tommy? | Second-hand smoke can exacerbate asthma | 'Yes, his grandfather' | Another potential trigger | | | | |
| Is anyone in the household unwell or have similar problems recently? | Viral causes spread quickly throughout a household | 'No' | Less likely to be an infective exacerbation | | | | |
| Has Tommy or anyone around him been abroad recently? | Recent travel, depending on destination, would warrant thinking about infectious diseases common to other climates | 'No' | No additional concerns | | | | |
| Have any social workers ever been involved in Tommy's or his sibling's care? | Identify if there are any social issues that could impact the children's health | 'No' | No additional concerns | | | | |

## Systems Review

| | | | | | | | |
|---|---|---|---|---|---|---|---|
| Any headache, drowsy episodes or fits? Any chest pain or dizzy episodes? Any vomiting, diarrhoea, tummy pain or weight loss? Any night sweats? Any joint or bone pain? Any problems passing urine? Any bruising or bleeding? | Wheeze can be part of other conditions, e.g. reflux or heart failure | 'No' | No additional concerns | | | | |

## Finishing the Consultation

| | | | | | | | |
|---|---|---|---|---|---|---|---|
| Is there anything else that you would like to tell me about? | May identify useful information that has been missed and help to build rapport with the parent. Provides the opportunity to assure the father that he has done the right thing by bringing his child in and that all the appropriate investigations will be done to determine the cause | 'No. I'm quite certain this is asthma as I used to have it. I'm just hoping to get some inhalers' | Take the time to explain what will happen from here | | | | |
| Do you have any questions? | Allows any final concerns to be addressed | | | | | | |

## Present Your Findings

Tommy is a 5-year-old boy who has presented with a wheeze over the past few weeks that follows a diurnal pattern and is associated with dry cough at night. His siblings have eczema and his father had childhood asthma. His grandfather is a smoker.

My main differential is asthma, but I would also consider viral-induced wheeze or a chest infection.

To investigate further I would like to do a respiratory and cardiovascular examination. I would consider doing allergen testing, fractional exhaled nitric oxide (FeNO) testing, spirometry and peak flow monitoring. If a diagnosis of asthma was confirmed, I would prescribe a salbutamol inhaler, an inhaled corticosteroid and a spacer. I would then follow the British Thoracic Society (BTS)/Scottish Intercollegiate Guidelines Network (SIGN) Guidelines and step up treatment as appropriate. It would also be appropriate to discuss smoking cessation with the family, particularly if the grandfather lives in the same household

## General Points

Polite to patient/parent

Appropriate use of open and closed questions

## ❓ QUESTIONS FROM THE EXAMINER

### What is the pathophysiology of asthma?

The main features that give rise to the asthmatic phenotype are airway hyperresponsiveness, bronchial inflammation and airflow limitation.

### What are some causes of asthma exacerbations in children?

Animal hair, pollen, infection, exercise and smoke.

### Describe the difference between a wheeze and stridor.

A wheeze is a polyphonic sound produced by partially obstructed airway (bronchospasms) and is more commonly heard during expiration. A stridor is a harsh, monophonic sound caused by partially obstructed airway, in or just above the larynx, and is more commonly heard during inspiration.

### When started treatment for asthma, what might the treatment goals be?

To manage the condition with the minimum amount of medication and side effects to eliminate daytime symptoms, nighttime waking due to asthma and asthma attacks and to reduce limitations on daily activities.

### What are the side effects of salbutamol?

It can cause tachycardia, shakiness and headaches. It may also cause low potassium and raised lactate.

### What are the risks of regular high-dose steroids for long-term asthma management?

It can cause adrenal suppression, which can lead to stunted growth and weight gain.

### How does heart failure lead to wheezing?

It reduces right ventricular output and leads to congestion of fluid in the pulmonary vasculature. The fluid causes pulmonary oedema and turbulent air flow within the lungs.

**What features make a murmur more likely to be pathological rather than innocent?**

Harsh, loud, diastolic murmurs that may radiate or have an associated thrill or symptoms such as cyanosis. However, this is not always the case.

**How is the severity of heart failure staged in children?**

Using the modified Ross criteria to identify typical symptoms of each stage.

**How would you describe a murmur caused by a patent ductus arteriosus?**

It is a classically a continuous 'machinery-like' murmur, best heard below the left clavicle, or an early systolic murmur in the left eternal edge.

## Station 9.5   History: Neonatal Jaundice

### Doctor Briefing

You are a junior doctor seeing Mrs Jones and her daughter Sarah, a 1-week-old baby. Mrs Jones has noticed a yellow tinge to her daughter's skin and is quite concerned. Please take a history from Mrs Jones, present your findings and formulate an appropriate management plan.

### Patient Briefing

Sarah is your first child; you gave birth to her a week ago. You first noticed a mild yellow tinge in the whites of Sarah's eyes 2 days ago and it now looks like her skin is yellowing too. You did not have any antenatal or postnatal complications and you had a normal vaginal delivery. On questioning, you reveal that Sarah is exclusively breastfed and feeds every 2 h. After feeding, you've noticed that she possets occasionally, but doesn't vomit.

On specific questioning regarding her stools and urine, you reveal that her stool is pigmented and her urine looks normal.

On specific questioning about Sarah's development, when the community midwife last visited you, she noted that Sarah had not grown much since the last visit. Sarah is not on any regular medications.

There is no past family history of note and everyone in the family is currently well. You live with your partner and you feel well supported.

You are concerned about Sarah's yellow skin because you are aware that jaundice means something is wrong with the liver.

### Mark Scheme for Examiner

#### Introduction

| | | | |
|---|---|---|---|
| Washes hands, introduces self, confirms patient identity and gains consent for examination | | | |
| Enquires about parental concerns | | | |

#### History of Presenting Complaint

| Question | Justification | Answer | Thoughts | | | | |
|---|---|---|---|---|---|---|---|
| Can you tell me what's been happening with Sarah? | Open question to allow mother to provide the essential features and guide the rest of the history | 'She's becoming more yellow and not feeding as well. I am very concerned' | Jaundice may be made worse by poor feeding, or perhaps there is an underlying cause for both (e.g. sepsis) | | | | |
| When did you first notice your baby turning yellow? | Serious pathology is more likely with onset in first 24 h | 'I first noticed her eyes turning yellow 2 days ago but now her skin is also looking yellow' | Onset is around 72 h after birth, which reduces the risk of it being sepsis or blood group incompatibility | | | | |
| Is she more lethargic or floppy? Any changes in her activity level? | Asking about general well-being can help to screen for possible infection and anaemia | 'No, she is acting the same' | No additional concerns | | | | |
| Does she appear paler to you? | May have associated anaemia | 'No' | No additional concerns | | | | |
| Has she been ill or had a fever recently? | Neonatal infection is a possible cause of jaundice | 'No' | No additional concerns | | | | |

## History of Presenting Complaint

| Question | Justification | Answer | Thoughts | | | | | |
|---|---|---|---|---|---|---|---|---|
| Are there any liver or blood disorders in your family or your partner's family? | Neonatal jaundice may be caused by an underlying pathological disease, most commonly affecting the liver or haematological system | 'No' | No additional concerns | | | | | |

## Birth History

| Question | Justification | Answer | Thoughts | | | | | |
|---|---|---|---|---|---|---|---|---|
| At what gestational age was Sarah born? What type of delivery? Were there any complications? How much did she weigh? How long did you stay in hospital? | Preterm children are at greater risk of jaundice | 'She was born at 39 weeks. I delivered normally, and there weren't any complications. We were sent home after 24 h. She weighed 3.4 kg' | No additional concerns | | | | | |
| Did you have a temperature during labour? Did you have group B streptococcal infection during pregnancy? Were antibiotics given during labour? Did your waters break for a particularly long time? | Risk factors for infection that might cause jaundice | 'I didn't have any temperature, infection or antibiotics. Sarah was born 6 h after my waters broke' | No risk factors for infection identified | | | | | |
| What is your blood type? Do you know Sarah's blood type? | Risk factors for haemolytic disease | 'I am AB-positive, but Sarah has never been checked' | Risk of blood group incompatibility low | | | | | |

## Past Medical and Surgical History

| Question | Justification | Answer | Thoughts | | | | | |
|---|---|---|---|---|---|---|---|---|
| Has Sarah ever been hospitalised? Does she have any known medical conditions? | There may have been a previous admission for jaundice or a related condition | 'No' | No additional concerns | | | | | |

## Feeding History

| Question | Justification | Answer | Thoughts | | | | | |
|---|---|---|---|---|---|---|---|---|
| How is Sarah being fed? How is it going? | Breastfeeding is a potential cause of physiological jaundice | 'She's exclusively breastfed and has been feeding every 2 h or so. She feeds for around 15 min a time, but I'm worried she is not taking enough' | Feeding but may have only picked up recently | | | | | |

## Feeding History

| Question | Justification | Answer | Thoughts | | | | | |
|----------|--------------|--------|----------|---|---|---|---|---|
| Has Sarah been growing well? | To establish how well the patient has been gaining weight compared to others within the same cohort | 'She's on the 50th centile and doing well. However, her health visitor mentioned that she hadn't gained any weight since her last visit' | Growing well | | | | | |
| How often do you have to change her nappies? Can you describe the appearance of her stools and urine? | Pale stools, dark urine and cholestasis are signs suggestive of cholestasis | 'I change her every few hours, which is normal for her. Her urine and stools look normal to me' | There is no evidence of significant dehydration, or concerns about biliary atresia | | | | | |

## Drug History

| Question | Justification | Answer | Thoughts | | | | | |
|----------|--------------|--------|----------|---|---|---|---|---|
| Is Sarah on any medications? Have you given Sarah any over-the-counter medications recently? | Unlikely, but this needs to be explicitly stated, as certain medications could trigger haemolytic anaemia, such as nitrofurantoin. Some medications may cause liver failure, and jaundice, in large quantities | 'No' | Unlikely to be an iatrogenic event | | | | | |
| Does Sarah have any allergies that you are aware of? | Increasing metabolism due to acute allergic response may cause jaundice | 'No' | No additional concerns | | | | | |

## Family History

| Question | Justification | Answer | Thoughts | | | | | |
|----------|--------------|--------|----------|---|---|---|---|---|
| Does Sarah have any siblings? Did they have jaundice at this age? | Jaundice can be caused by diseases characterised by haemolytic anaemia or increased bilirubin production. They may be hereditary | 'No, Sarah is our first child' | Less concerned about congenital disorders | | | | | |
| Are there any blood disorders or liver conditions that run in the family? | | 'No' | | | | | | |

## Social History

| Question | Justification | Answer | Thoughts | | | | | |
|----------|--------------|--------|----------|---|---|---|---|---|
| Who lives at home with Sarah? | Identify main carers and home support | 'My partner and I' | No additional concerns | | | | | |
| Has Sarah or anyone in the household recently travelled abroad? | Children are vulnerable to infections potentially carried by family members | 'No, we've all been at home for the last few months' | No additional concerns | | | | | |

## Social History

| Question | Justification | Answer | Thoughts | | | | |
|---|---|---|---|---|---|---|---|
| Does anyone in the household smoke? | Identify if there is exposure to second-hand smoke | 'No' | No additional concerns | | | | |
| Has a social worker ever been formally involved in Sarah's care? | Children are also vulnerable to neglect and abuse. Asking about social work helps identify any potential risk of harm to the child that could lead to jaundice, such as physical abuse and possible malnourishment | 'No' | Reassured that Sarah is well looked after | | | | |

## Systems Review

| Question | Justification | Answer | Thoughts | | | | |
|---|---|---|---|---|---|---|---|
| Any fits or funny movements? Any vomiting or diarrhoea? Any wheeze, cough or breathlessness? Any bruising or bleeding? | To look for complications of jaundice, e.g. kernicterus, and wider possible causes | 'No, everything else has been fine' | No additional concerns | | | | |

## Finishing the Consultation

| Question | Justification | Answer | Thoughts | | | | |
|---|---|---|---|---|---|---|---|
| Is there anything else that you would like to tell me about? | May identify useful information that has been missed and help to build rapport with the parent. Provides the opportunity to assure the mother that she has done the right thing by bringing her child in and that all the appropriate investigations will be done to determine the cause | 'I am so worried there is something seriously wrong with Sarah. I've heard that yellowing of the skin can affect her brain' | Take the time to explain what will happen from here | | | | |
| Do you have any questions? | Allows any final concerns to be addressed | | | | | | |

## Present Your Findings

Sarah is a 1-week-old breastfed baby who has presented with a 2-day history of jaundice but is otherwise well. There is no significant birth, family or social history.

This is most likely a physiological jaundice, following breastfeeding. However, I would also consider Gilbert syndrome, birth trauma (e.g. cephalohaematoma), polycythaemia and sepsis.

I would like to check a bilirubin and plot the value on a jaundice chart. This may require phototherapy or a repeat bilirubin measurement. I will check to ensure feeding is going well, and if bilirubin levels are significantly below the treatment threshold, discharge home, with advice to come back in if the jaundice worsens, or there are any concerns. I would also offer the mother support from a breastfeeding specialist

| General Points | | | |
|---|---|---|---|
| Polite to patient/parent | | | |
| Appropriate use of open and closed questions | | | |

## ❓ QUESTIONS FROM THE EXAMINER

### How long can breast milk jaundice last?

Up to 12 weeks.

### What is the difference between conjugated and unconjugated bilirubin?

Conjugated bilirubin is water-soluble, cannot cross the blood–brain barrier and is freely excreted in the urine. Unconjugated bilirubin is insoluble in water, binds tightly to albumin and can cross the blood–brain barrier.

### How is conjugated bilirubin produced in the body?

It is an end-product of haemoglobin breakdown in the liver via the enzyme uridine 5'-diphospho-glucuronosyltransferase (UDP-glucuronosyltransferase).

### What is kernicterus?

It is a rare complication of hyperbilirubinaemia where bilirubin binds irreversibly to neuroreceptors in the basal ganglia of the brain, resulting in permanent neurological effects. Symptoms may include fatigue, drowsiness, hypotonia, diminished primitive reflexes and respiratory distress.

### What autosomal-dominant condition might lead to a haemolytic jaundice?

Hereditary spherocytosis.

### What is the significance of pale stools in patients with biliary atresia?

Pale stools are caused by a lack of the brown-pigmented stercobilin. In biliary atresia, flow of bile from the gallbladder is obstructed, causing less bile to be available in the gut for conversion to stercobilin.

### How would you identify a dehydrated neonate/infant during examination?

Clinical signs suggestive of dehydration in a neonate include: sunken fontanelles and/or eyes, reduced skin turgor, increased capillary refill time, increased heart rate, lethargy, poor tone and decreased urine output.

### How does the onset of physiological jaundice differ from pathological jaundice?

Physiological jaundice usually appears after 24 h, whereas pathological jaundice is more likely to appear in the first 24 h of life.

### What investigations would you request to measure bilirubin levels non-invasively?

Transcutaneous bilirubinometer.

### What is the surgical treatment for congenital biliary atresia?

Kasai procedure, and if that fails, a liver transplant.

## Station 9.6    History: Faltering Growth

### Doctor Briefing

You are a junior doctor attached to the paediatric team. The primary care physician has referred 9-month-old, James because of poor weight gain. You are asked to take a history from his mother, Lucy, present your findings and formulate an appropriate management plan.

### Patient Briefing

Abishek is your 9-month-old son. He is your first child. You've noticed that he is very small and does not seem to have grown much since his birth. His health visitor has also expressed concerns regarding his growth and has recommended you visit the doctor. You have also noticed that he frequently gets a continuous cough which has been on and off for a couple of months. He's been having some foul-smelling, pale stools. Recently he has not been feeding as normal and has only been managing half of his bottle.

When he was born, he weighed 3.6 kg (50th centile). Currently, he weighs approximately 7 kg, which lies between the second and ninth centile. He was born via vaginal delivery at term, and it took 24 h for him to pass meconium. You did not want any antenatal screening tests whilst you were pregnant. You were discharged after 24 h.

You wonder if he is allergic to something or whether he has asthma like his brother. You're worried as he looks more poorly today.

### Mark Scheme for Examiner

#### Introduction

| | | | | |
|---|---|---|---|---|
| Washes hands, introduces self, confirms patient identity and gains consent for examination | | | | |
| Enquires about parental concerns | | | | |

#### History of Presenting Complaint

| Question | Justification | Answer | Thoughts | | | | |
|---|---|---|---|---|---|---|---|
| What's been happening with Abishek? | Open question to allow mother to provide the essential features and guide the rest of the history | 'I'm worried as he hasn't been growing. His health visitor recommended that I organise a visit due to his poor growth' | Need to focus on chronic issue of growth | | | | |
| When did you start having concerns about Abishek's growth? | Establishing a timeline helps identify if there is an acute change or if the problem is more long-term, suggestive of a congenital/genetic disorder | 'The health visitor mentioned that he had not gained weight for a couple of months. We weighed him at the doctors when he was 6 months old, and he was quite small. He has not seemed to improve or gain weight since' | Suggests an overall chronic problem, possibly respiratory in nature | | | | |
| Were there any issues before that? Do you have any other concerns? | Identify further and pre-existing concerns and what may have been considered at the time | 'He's always been on the smaller side as my husband and I are also quite small, but recently I'm not sure if he has gained any weight at all' | Constitutional delay may be a factor, but this seems to be more than that | | | | |

## History of Presenting Complaint

| Question | Justification | Answer | Thoughts | | | | |
|----------|---------------|--------|----------|---|---|---|---|
| Are there any problems with his bowels? Has he had any vomiting or diarrhoea? | Establishes any concerning features indicative of a GI problem | 'Yes, I've noticed some pale, smelly stools in his nappy since a few days ago. No vomiting or diarrhoea' | Steatorrhoea noted; could be a pancreatic or GI cause | | | | |
| Have you noticed any other symptoms, e.g. a cough, recurrent infections or shortness of breath? | Identifies a source of infection | 'He's been coughing a lot' | Suggests a respiratory tract infection | | | | |
| Is anyone in the household unwell? | Children may be vulnerable around others with infectious diseases | 'No' | No additional concerns | | | | |
| Does he bring anything up when he coughs? Does he have any difficulty breathing? Does he have a fever? | Acute or long-term infection | 'Yes – often thick green sputum. He often has a temperature but his breathing is OK otherwise' | Possible chronic chest infection | | | | |
| Have you tried anything to make it better? | Knowing what may have worked helps with diagnosis | 'He has had two courses of antibiotics, which haven't really helped' | May have resistant or chronic infection | | | | |

## Birth History

| Question | Justification | Answer | Thoughts | | | | |
|----------|---------------|--------|----------|---|---|---|---|
| Can you please tell me a bit about your pregnancy? At how many weeks was Abishek born? What type of delivery did you have? Were there any complications or stays in hospital following birth? What was his birth weight? How long was it before he pooed? | Preterm children are more susceptible to infections and poor growth | 'Abishek was born on time, and I had a vaginal delivery that went well. He was 3.6 kg. He pooed after a day' | No additional concerns | | | | |

## Past Medical and Surgical History

| Question | Justification | Answer | Thoughts | | | | |
|----------|---------------|--------|----------|---|---|---|---|
| Has Abishek ever been hospitalised? Does he have any known medical conditions or has he ever had surgery? | Identify any pre-existing conditions that are associated with slower growth | 'No' | No additional concerns | | | | |

## Past Medical and Surgical History

| Question | Justification | Answer | Thoughts | | | | | |
|---|---|---|---|---|---|---|---|---|
| Is he unwell often? How many times would you say he has been unwell in the last year? | Screen for recurrent infections | 'Yes. I find that he coughs quite a lot and it only settles for a few days and the comes back again. It hasn't been bad enough to be admitted to hospital' | Recurrent chest infections are a feature of cystic fibrosis | | | | | |

## Feeding History

| Question | Justification | Answer | Thoughts | | | | | |
|---|---|---|---|---|---|---|---|---|
| How has he been feeding? When did you start weaning Abishek? Is he eating and drinking as normal for him? | Identify any nutritional problems | 'He's drinking formula milk and taking it well. He started solids at 6 months, has a balanced diet, but is fussy' | There is not an obvious issue with poor intake, although there could still be malabsorption | | | | | |
| How has his weight changed over time? | Look at pattern of growth to identify possible cause of small size | 'He was born a good size, but has gradually been dropping down the centile line, from the 50th to between the second and ninth centile' | Short and small for age, with gradual decline, suggesting chronic condition | | | | | |

## Developmental History

| Question | Justification | Answer | Thoughts | | | | | |
|---|---|---|---|---|---|---|---|---|
| Is he able to sit? | Elicit stage of gross motor development appropriate for age | 'Yes, he can sit with a nice straight back' | No developmental concerns | | | | | |
| Does he pick things up with his hands? How does he do this? | Elicit stage of fine motor development appropriate for age | 'Yes, he uses the tips of his fingers and thumb to do it' | No developmental concerns | | | | | |
| Has he been able to make any sounds? What kind of sounds does he make? | Elicit stage of language and speech appropriate for age | 'Yes, he occasionally says dada' | No developmental concerns | | | | | |
| How is he around strangers? What kind of things does he do when playing? | Establish if the child has reached social developmental milestone appropriate for age | 'He gets a little anxious with strangers but settles if we stay with him. He likes peek-a-boo' | No developmental concerns | | | | | |
| Have you noticed if he's stopped doing things he previously could do? | Identify developmental regression | 'No' | No additional concerns | | | | | |

## Drug History

| Question | Justification | Answer | Thoughts | | | | | |
|---|---|---|---|---|---|---|---|---|
| Does Abishek take any regular medications? Have you given him any over-the-counter medications recently? | Take note of corticosteroid use as can affect growth, particularly in known asthmatics. Due to recurrent infections, take note of antibiotic use as well | 'No' | No additional concerns | | | | | |
| Is Abishek allergic to anything? | Ensure no allergic cause for condition, and to help with any possible medication choice | 'Not that I know of, but I am worried he might be' | No additional concerns | | | | | |
| Are his vaccinations up to date? | Ensure preventable diseases are not causing an infection | 'Yes, all of them' | No additional concerns | | | | | |

## Family History

| Question | Justification | Answer | Thoughts | | | | | |
|---|---|---|---|---|---|---|---|---|
| Are there any conditions that run in the family? Do you have any other children? Does anyone in the family have bowel conditions, or lung conditions, like cystic fibrosis or primary ciliary dyskinesia? | Screen for possible inherited disease | 'No. Abishek is an only child' | No additional concerns | | | | | |

## Social and Travel History

| Question | Justification | Answer | Thoughts | | | | | |
|---|---|---|---|---|---|---|---|---|
| Who lives at home with Abishek? | Identify main carers and home support | 'My partner and I live at home with Abishek' | No additional concerns | | | | | |
| Does anyone in the household smoke? | Elicit possibility of exposure to second-hand smoke | 'No' | No additional concerns | | | | | |
| Has Abishek or anyone in the household recently travelled abroad? | Screen for tropical diseases with respiratory presentations | 'No, we've all been at home for the last few months' | Not likely to be a tropical disease | | | | | |
| Have any social workers ever been involved in Abishek's care? | Identify risk of neglect that could lead to poor growth | 'No' | No additional concerns | | | | | |

## Systems Review

| Question | Justification | Answer | Thoughts | | | | |
|---|---|---|---|---|---|---|---|
| Any drowsy episodes or fits? Any sweating? Any joint or bone pain? Any problems passing urine? Any bruising or bleeding? | Screen for any systemic disease | 'No' | No additional concerns | | | | |

## Finishing the Consultation

| | | | | | | | |
|---|---|---|---|---|---|---|---|
| Is there anything else that you would like to tell me about? | May identify useful information that has been missed and help to build rapport with the parent. Provides the opportunity to assure the mother that she has done the right thing by bringing her child in and that all the appropriate investigations will be done to determine the cause | 'I'm just really worried that he's not gaining weight as normal. I am trying to feed him as much as possible. Is there anything I can do to support him? | Take the time to explain what will happen from here | | | | |
| Do you have any questions? | Allows any final concerns to be addressed | | | | | | |

## Present Your Findings

Abishek is a 9-month-old boy who has been referred due to poor weight gain. He also has an associated cough and foul-smelling pale stools. He has been struggling to gain weight over the last few months.

My main differential diagnosis is cystic fibrosis, but I would also consider primary ciliary dyskinesia, GI conditions (e.g. coeliac disease or inflammatory bowel disease) and non-organic causes for poor growth.

I would like to investigate further by performing an abdominal and chest examination. I will review his growth chart. I would also like to order an FBC, U&Es, LFTs, CRP, erythrocyte sedimentation rate, coeliac screen, chest X-ray, sweat test and immune-reactive trypsinogen test. I would then review again with the results

## General Points

| | | | | |
|---|---|---|---|---|
| Polite to patient/parent | | | | |
| Appropriate use of open and closed questions | | | | |

## ❓ QUESTIONS FROM THE EXAMINER

### How would you determine mid-parental height?

Take the combined height of the mother and father. Add 13 for a boy; subtract 13 for a girl. Divide the total by 2.

### What worrying features would you look for when plotting weight on a growth chart?

A worrying feature is either being persistently very low, especially if disproportionate to the mid-parental height, or if weight is dropping through centile lines.

## How would you identify constitutional delay of growth and puberty and faltering growth?

Children with constitutional delay of growth and puberty are of short stature with delayed bone maturation and puberty, despite adequate nutrition, and are otherwise well. It is often familial.

## Aside from cystic fibrosis, name three other conditions screened for using the newborn blood spot screening test in the UK.

Screening tests include: sickle cell disease, congenital hypothyroidism and inherited metabolic diseases (such as phenylketonuria, medium-chain acyl-CoA dehydrogenase deficiency, maple syrup urine disease, isovaleric acidaemia, glutamic aciduria type 1 and homocystinuria.

## How is cystic fibrosis inherited?

It is an autosomal-recessive condition.

## What is the pathophysiology of cystic fibrosis?

It is a genetic defect in the cystic fibrosis transmembrane conductance regulator (CFTR) gene which results in chloride ions remaining intracellularly, leading to high osmolality within the cells. This then causes water to move into cells via osmosis, leading to thick, dehydrated secretions. The most common mutation is F508del.

## Why is genetic testing important in the planning of management in cystic fibrosis?

Depending on the type of genetic defect affecting the CFTR gene, small-molecule therapy may be effective for certain mutations, potentially curing the chloride channel defect.

## What are the histopathological differences between Crohn's disease and ulcerative colitis?

Crohn's disease has characteristic non-caseating granulomas and transmural inflammation with normal glands, but ulcerative colitis will show polymorphonuclear cell aggregates with mucosal and submucosal inflammation and distorted glands, but no granulomas.

## How could you determine the severity of an acute presentation of colitis?

Using the Paediatric Ulcerative Colitis Activity Index, which takes into account abdominal pain, rectal bleeding, stool consistency, number of stools in 24 h, nocturnal stools and activity level.

## Why must anti-TTG and other immunological assay testing be carried out while gluten is still included in the diet?

Gluten is required to produce the antibodies and therefore if it is excluded pre-emptively, there is a risk of a false-negative test.

## Station 9.7    History: Non-Accidental Injury

### Doctor Briefing

You are a junior doctor in the ED and have been asked to see Fred, a 3-month-old boy. Fred was brought in by his mother, Mrs Williams, after he 'rolled off the sofa'. He has broken his right humerus; which has been confirmed on X-ray. Please take a history from Mrs Williams about Fred, present your findings and formulate an appropriate management plan.

### Patient Briefing

Fred is your fifth child from an unexpected pregnancy. He is now 3 months old. You live alone with your five children and you are not supported by any other family members or friends.

Fred rolled off the couch this morning, but you did not witness this. You were not made aware until lunch time when your eldest child, who is 15, told you what happened, as you've been exhausted and in bed all morning. You are unable to recall the events accurately and feel irritated when pressed for more information. You feel like you are being judged for being a single mum.

This is Fred's third attendance in the ED in 2 months. The previous two attendances were for similar problems, again not witnessed by yourself. He does not have any other significant past medical history.

You are not concerned as Fred seems fine to you. You want to take your kids home and rest.

### Mark Scheme for Examiner

#### Introduction

| | | | | | |
|---|---|---|---|---|---|
| Washes hands, introduces self and confirms patient identity and gains consent for examination | | | | | |
| Enquires about parental concerns | | | | | |

#### History of Presenting Complaint

| Question | Justification | Answer | Thoughts | | | | | |
|---|---|---|---|---|---|---|---|---|
| What's been happening with Fred? | Open question to allow mother to provide the essential features and guide the rest of the history | 'He had a fall, but seems to be OK now' | No obvious parental concern, despite a fracture | | | | | |
| What was Fred doing just before the incident? | Establish who Fred was with, what he was doing and form a clear image of how the incident could feasibly and potentially happen | 'I don't know. I think he was playing with his brother' | Mother is not a main witness; probably would need another collateral history for full picture | | | | | |
| Who witnessed the fall? | Asking for specifics helps identify key people with relevant information. Also, if mechanism of injury is suspicious, the witness may have more information or may be a suspect | 'Finn, his older brother' | Ideally will need to speak to Finn to get more information. Also need to know whether it is appropriate for Finn to be supervising the baby | | | | | |
| How did he fall? | Correlate the story with the child's development/physical capabilities and think whether it is feasible for the child to have injured himself in this way | 'He rolled off the sofa. I don't know exactly how. I wasn't there' | Not consistent with developmental ability of 3-month-old | | | | | |

## History of Presenting Complaint

| Question | Justification | Answer | Thoughts | | | | | |
|---|---|---|---|---|---|---|---|---|
| When did he fall? | Note the time between incident and attendance, to assess appropriate speed of care seeking | 'Last night. I'm not sure of the exact time. His brother only told me this morning and I only had the time to bring him in now' | Child's health needs not met appropriately – unnoticed fracture from evening before | | | | | |
| How high did he fall from? | Note if height correlates with the injury sustained | 'Just about the height of the couch on to the floor' | Height may be consistent with a fracture, but there may also have been a more significant injury | | | | | |
| How was he immediately after the incident? Did anything help, like any medications? | Assess severity of initial injury | 'He cried a lot. There was a lot of noise, but it settled by the end of the evening. I thought it was bad colic. He didn't sleep well, and I eventually realised from my other son that he had fallen. It all made sense then. Sorry I didn't think to give any medications at the time' | Likely was in a lot of pain from the untreated fracture. Unclear why pain medication not given | | | | | |
| Did he hit his head, or injure any other part of his body do you think? Are there any bumps or bruises on him? | Important to assess any head injury, or injuries elsewhere | 'No, I don't think so' | Appears to be an isolated fracture | | | | | |
| Has he vomited? Has he been drowsy? Has he had any fits or funny turns since the fall? Has there been any change in behaviour? | Even if head injury not reported, important to screen for it | 'He's vomited once but is now back to his normal self' | No major concern around a serious head injury | | | | | |
| Has he been feeding normally? | Poor feeding is a red flag for any paediatric condition | 'Yes. I am not sure how much though' | May be an issue with feeding, perhaps related to untreated pain | | | | | |

## Birth History

| | | | | | | | | |
|---|---|---|---|---|---|---|---|---|
| Can you please tell me a bit about your pregnancy? At how many weeks was Fred born? What type of delivery did you have? Were there any complications or stays in hospital following birth? What was his birth weight? | Preterm children may be at higher risk of fractures | 'He was born at term via a vaginal delivery, and everything was fine. His birth weight was 3.5 kg' | No additional concerns | | | | | |

## Past Medical and Surgical History

| Question | Justification | Answer | Thoughts | | | | | |
|---|---|---|---|---|---|---|---|---|
| Has he had any previous hospital admissions or ED attendances? | Repeated ED attendance, especially at different hospitals, and within a short timeframe is likely a red flag | 'Yes. This is the third time he's been brought into hospital' | Multiple ED attendances and injuries raise concerns about possible neglect | | | | | |
| Has he had any metabolic bone diseases or bleeding disorders? | May predispose to fractures/injuries | 'No' | No additional concerns | | | | | |
| Does he have any known medical conditions? Has he ever had surgery? | Other conditions may also be of importance | 'No' | No additional concerns | | | | | |

## Developmental History

| Question | Justification | Answer | Thoughts | | | | | |
|---|---|---|---|---|---|---|---|---|
| Is he able to lift his head and raise his chest when lying on his front? | Elicit stage of gross motor development appropriate for age | 'Yes' | No additional concerns | | | | | |
| Does he reach for objects, and hold objects placed in his hand? | Elicit stage of fine motor development appropriate for age | 'Yes' | No additional concerns | | | | | |
| Does he follow objects with his eyes? | Elicit stage of development of vision | 'Yes' | No additional concerns | | | | | |
| What kind of noises does he normally make? Does he recognise your voice? | Elicit stage of speech and language development appropriate for age | 'He's always been really quiet but he makes occasional noises. He dditions me"' | No additional concerns | | | | | |
| Does he smile or laugh? | Establish social milestones appropriate for age | 'Yes, both' | No additional concerns | | | | | |
| Have you noticed if he's stopped doing things he previously could do? | Identify developmental regression | 'No' | No additional concerns | | | | | |

## Drug History

| Question | Justification | Answer | Thoughts | | | | | |
|---|---|---|---|---|---|---|---|---|
| Is he on any medications at the moment, or does he have any allergies? Any over-the-counter medications given? | It is good practice to check the patient's full drug history and allergy status | 'No' | No additional concerns | | | | | |

## Drug History

| Question | Justification | Answer | Thoughts | | | | | |
|---|---|---|---|---|---|---|---|---|
| Are his vaccinations up to date? | Ensure preventable diseases are not causing an infection | 'Yes, he has had them all' | No additional concerns | | | | | |

## Family History

| Question | Justification | Answer | Thoughts | | | | | |
|---|---|---|---|---|---|---|---|---|
| Do any conditions run in the family? | Screen for conditions that may predispose to injuries | 'No' | No additional concerns | | | | | |
| Does anyone in the family have mental health issues or chronic illnesses? | Vulnerable adults may need extra support as new parents | 'I've got depression and I've been seeing a community psychologist' | Mother may be needing additional support in the context of a new child | | | | | |

## Social History

| Question | Justification | Answer | Thoughts | | | | | |
|---|---|---|---|---|---|---|---|---|
| Who normally lives at home with Fred? | Knowing who is involved in Fred's care will help identify if there are safeguarding issues | 'Me and my other children' | Ensure mum has appropriate support at home | | | | | |
| Have any social workers ever been involved in your household, whether with you, Fred or his siblings? What was it for? | Identify risk of neglect that could lead to poor growth | 'Yes, they've visited sometimes. I can't remember why, but it's all fine now' | Important to understand why they were involved, and if additional support is needed | | | | | |
| Is Fred's father in the picture? Are there other children? Where do they stay? What are their names and ages? Does anyone else look after the children? | Complicated family dynamics could lead to an unstable environment for a young child. Also gives an indication of how well supported mother is | 'No. I have four other children with the same father, all boys. They are Finn, 15, George, 11, Steve, 7 and Daphney, 4. We all live together in a flat in Peckham. Dad lives in Barcelona and never sees them' | No close familial support. Suspicion of basic needs not met | | | | | |
| Does anyone else see any of your children? Who else have they been with in the last 48 h? Do you have a current partner or any other children? | Important to ensure safety of other children, and check who has been around at the time of the injury | 'No one else has seen them since the injury. The older kids all go to Canterbury School. My brother Jamie has the kids sometimes; he's with the others now' | No obvious additional source of risk, and children appear safe with a relative. Need to get all names and addresses of family members/contacts | | | | | |
| Are you having any difficulties supporting your family (financially or otherwise)? | Explore all the familial stressors and whether the mother needs additional help | 'Sometimes. I'm working when I can but sometimes I just can't cope and I get too tired' | Financial and social stresses are present in the family, which may also require support | | | | | |

**Finishing the Consultation**

| Question | Justification | Answer | Thoughts | | | | | |
|---|---|---|---|---|---|---|---|---|
| Is there anything else that you would like to tell me about?<br>Do you have any questions? | May identify useful information that has been missed and help to build rapport with the parent. Provides the opportunity to assure the mother that she has done the right thing by bringing her child in and that all the appropriate investigations will be done to determine the cause<br>Allows any final concerns to be addressed | 'I don't really know. I think he is OK' | Reluctance to stay in hospital – needs support and communication of need for medical intervention | | | | | |

**Present Your Findings**

Fred is a 3-month-old boy who has presented with a broken right humerus due to a fall last night, witnessed only by his older brother, Finn. There have been multiple recent attendances for unwitnessed injuries, and the presentation of this fracture is late. There are also challenges in the home environment, making me concerned that Fred may be suffering from neglect and a possible non-accidental injury.

I would like to raise concerns with a senior doctor and the safeguarding team. I would draw a body map with any injuries, and record details of all carers, including full names and addresses. I would like to investigate Fred's injuries with bloods, including FBC, U&Es, LFTs and clotting. Further investigations may include a full skeletal survey, computed tomography (CT) head and ophthalmological examination. I would like to admit the child to hospital for further investigations and treatment, whilst also discussing this case with our safeguarding lead and social services

**General Points**

| | | | | | |
|---|---|---|---|---|---|
| Polite to patient/parent | | | | | |
| Appropriate use of open and closed questions | | | | | |

## ❓ QUESTIONS FROM THE EXAMINER

### What are the four categories of child abuse?

Physical, sexual, emotional and neglect.

### What is a 'child protection medical'?

It is an extensive history and examination carried out by a senior doctor on children for whom there are safeguarding concerns, in order to put in place a plan to ensure safeguarding of the child.

### Which areas on the body would be typical sites for non-accidental injuries to occur?

Areas include: non-bony aspects such as inner aspects of arms, soles of feet, back and side of trunk (not including spine), chest and abdomen, soft tissue of cheeks, ears and intraoral injury.

## What is the pathophysiology of osteogenesis imperfecta?

It is a genetic disorder that results in the synthesis of defective collagen type 1, which causes bone, teeth, ligament, sclera and skin fragility.

## What factors might make you classify a burn as being accidental?

Splash marks and irregular burn margins are consistent with accidental injury. Uncommon burn areas (e.g. genitals, face, soles of feet), history not matching up with injuries or burns with a well-demarcated area (e.g. a sock distribution indicates that the child was held down in hot fluid) are likely to be non-accidental.

## What actions might social services take to support a vulnerable child?

They might remove a child from their home, put them on a child protection plan or a child in need plan.

## Why is an ophthalmological review important in safeguarding cases with babies?

The most common pattern of injury is retinal haemorrhages. However, depending on the type of trauma that occurred there may also be evidence of periocular bruising, subconjunctival haemorrhages and retinal detachment.

## What is the definition of emotional abuse?

This is the persistent emotional maltreatment of a child, causing severe and persistent adverse effects to their well-being and emotional development.

## What is the 'triangle of safety' in relation to non-accidental injury?

This is between the ear, side of the face and the shoulder – injuries in this area are suspicious for non-accidental injury.

## What is an ossification centre and what is its relevance in the context of fractures?

It is the site of osteoblast accumulation in connective tissue which results in the formation of bone. It can be confused with a fracture.

## Station 9.8    Examination: Newborn Baby Check

### Doctor Briefing

You are a junior doctor covering the postnatal ward. You routinely perform a baby check on baby Barton, who is 12 h old. He is the first child of a 36-year-old woman and was born by normal vaginal birth. Combined antenatal screening was not undertaken. Before you see the baby, the midwife has called your attention to the baby's facial features.

### Patient Briefing

This is your first child, Wilfrid. You had a spontaneous vaginal delivery 12 h ago. You delivered at 38 weeks' gestation. You have noticed that Wilfrid has a large dark red lesion on his face. He has otherwise been well; you have not noticed any fits or seizures, fever or increased work of breathing.

You have not had any antenatal screening tests for genetic disorders as the results wouldn't have changed the outcome for you. There is no family history of congenital disorders. He passed meconium a few minutes following birth and has successfully latched on to feed twice already.

You are worried what this skin lesion on his face might be.

### Mark Scheme for Examiner

#### Introduction

| | | | | | | |
|---|---|---|---|---|---|---|
| Washes hands, introduces self, confirms patient identity and gains consent for examination | | | | | | |
| Enquires about parental concerns | | | | | | |
| Appropriately exposes the patient and positions comfortably for the examination | | | | | | |

#### General Inspection

| What are you looking for or examining? | Justification | Thoughts | | | | |
|---|---|---|---|---|---|---|
| Tone, posture and movements. Assess tone by gently moving the newborn's limbs | Identify gross neurological abnormalities | Baby moving well and flexes arms. No additional concerns | | | | |
| Note any birthmarks, rash, abnormal skin colour or discoloration | Important to document these as some can look like bruises or may be associated with eye problems, neural tube defects and vascular problems | Area of a large dark red lesion, not raised, on left cheek under the eye and at the border of the left nostril. Position could indicate associated eye or cerebral vasculature associations | | | | |
| Comment on cry or general behaviour | Note if very irritable or if lack of movement | Cries appropriately when roused but settles quickly | | | | |
| Offer to weigh and measure height | Track growth development | No concerns. Growth is following a centile line | | | | |

#### Head Examination (Inspection, Palpation)

| | | | | | | |
|---|---|---|---|---|---|---|
| Comment on shape of the head | Note if symmetrical, abnormally large or small | Normal head shape and circumference for patient's age | | | | |
| Measure and plot the head of circumference | Track growth development | | | | | |

## Head Examination (Inspection, Palpation)

| What are you looking for or examining? | Justification | Thoughts | | | | |
|---|---|---|---|---|---|---|
| Palpate for both anterior and posterior fontanelles and comment on size. Check for extra fontanelles. Inspect the cranial sutures | Check for sunken fontanelles indicating dehydration or swellings that are contained within or have crossed suture lines. Look for fusion of sutures | No additional concerns | | | | |
| Look for any possible dysmorphic facial features. Note appearance and asymmetry and document any marks | If present, may suggest possible genetic problem | No dysmorphic features noted | | | | |
| Inspect eyes. Check red reflex in both eyes with ophthalmoscope | Absence indicates possible congenital cataracts or retinoblastoma | Red reflex present in both eyes | | | | |
| Assess suck reflex | Ensure a good latch to finger; this reassures baby is capable of adequate feeds | Suck reflex present | | | | |
| Check for cleft palate, cleft lip and tongue tie | Early identification allows for early surgical intervention with good prognosis. Severe cleft palates can cause problems with feeding | No additional concerns | | | | |
| Check position of ears and overall appearance (including pinna, periaural bruising or deformity) | Low-set ears are a sign of dysmorphism. Skin tags near the ears can be normal but can also be associated with hearing loss | No additional concerns | | | | |

## Chest Examination (Inspection, Palpation, Auscultation)

| | | | | | | |
|---|---|---|---|---|---|---|
| Assess respiratory effort | Assess for respiratory distress | Normal respiratory effort | | | | |
| Auscultate for heart sounds and measure heart rate | May indicate congenital heart disease | Heart sounds and rate normal | | | | |
| Auscultate lung fields | Assess for respiratory pathology, e.g. congenital infection | Lung fields clear bilaterally | | | | |

## Abdominal Examination (Inspection, Palpation, Auscultation)

| | | | | | | |
|---|---|---|---|---|---|---|
| Inspect umbilical stump. Assess whether it is clean and dry | Ensure good hygiene and no sign of infection | No additional concerns | | | | |
| Check patency of anus | Anorectal malformations can be associated with urogenital malformations | Patent anus | | | | |
| Palpate for umbilical/inguinal hernias and organomegaly | Inguinal hernias may require surgery | No signs of umbilical/inguinal hernias | | | | |

## Abdominal Examination (Inspection, Palpation, Auscultation)

| What are you looking for or examining? | Justification | Thoughts | | | | |
|---|---|---|---|---|---|---|
| Palpate for femoral pulses on both sides | Weakened pulses or dysrhythmia could indicate cardiovascular problems | Femoral pulses normal bilaterally | | | | |
| Auscultate for bowel sounds | Change in bowel sounds could indicate obstruction | Bowel sounds present | | | | |

## External Genitalia Examination (Inspection, Palpation)

| | | | | | | |
|---|---|---|---|---|---|---|
| If male, inspect the tip of the penis. If female, inspect labia, clitoris and any discharge | Note presence of hypospadias in men and abnormal/excess discharge in women | No additional concerns | | | | |
| If male, palpate for the testes | Document undescended testes and at which level they can be felt | No additional concerns | | | | |

## Hip Examination

| | | | | | | |
|---|---|---|---|---|---|---|
| Perform Barlow and Ortolani manoeuvre | Screening test for hip dysplasia | No additional concerns | | | | |

## Limb Examination (Inspection)

| | | | | | | |
|---|---|---|---|---|---|---|
| Look at and count digits. Check for symmetry of limbs (in both size and length) | Note position of limbs (indications of nerve palsies), polydactyly and webbed digits | 10 digits on each hand and foot | | | | |
| Check palmar crease | Single palmar creases are associated with Down's syndrome | No additional concerns | | | | |
| Inspect feet and assess for any ankle deformities | Exclude talipes or other physical abnormality that may impede motor development | No additional concerns | | | | |

## Spine Examination (Inspection)

| | | | | | | |
|---|---|---|---|---|---|---|
| Check curvature of spine | Assess for scoliosis | Normal curvature of the spine | | | | |
| Look for sacral dimples or tufts of hair | Exclude presence of spina bifida | No evidence of sacral dimples or hair | | | | |

## Movement and Reflexes

| | | | | | | |
|---|---|---|---|---|---|---|
| Check Moro reflex | Absent or asymmetrical reflex could indicate developmental complications or birth injury. Commonly impaired in infants with kernicterus and potentially exaggerated in those with encephalopathy | Moro reflex present | | | | |

## Movement and Reflexes

| What are you looking for or examining? | Justification | Thoughts | | | | |
|---|---|---|---|---|---|---|
| Check head lag | Persistent or exaggerated head lag could suggest a neurological concern | No head lag | | | | |
| Check palmar grasp reflex | Indicates development of rudimentary fine motor skills | Grasp reflex present | | | | |

## Finishing

| | | | | | | |
|---|---|---|---|---|---|---|
| Check patient is comfortable, record basic observations and cover the patient up | Keeps the patient's dignity | Treating the patient with respect is important | | | | |
| Remove your gloves and wash hands | Complying with hand hygiene is vital | No additional concerns | | | | |

## Present Your Findings

Wilfrid is a 12-h-old baby who has been referred for a newborn baby check. On examination, there is a large dark red discoloration on the left side of his face and on his nose. The examination was otherwise unremarkable.

My top differential is a port-wine stain birthmark. However, other differentials I would like to consider are haemangioma, birth trauma and a salmon patch.

I would like to discuss this patient further with my seniors. If there is any concern about Sturge–Weber syndrome, a magnetic resonance imaging (MRI) head may be warranted. Given the proximity to the eye, referral to an ophthalmologist for glaucoma screening is also needed. The risks and benefits of laser treatment to the lesion may need to be discussed in due course

## General Points

| | | | |
|---|---|---|---|
| Performs examination safely and confidently | | | |
| Clear instruction and explanation to patient/parents | | | |

## ❓ QUESTIONS FROM THE EXAMINER

### What is the genetic abnormality in Down's syndrome?

Trisomy 21, i.e. there are three copies of genes from chromosome 21 present.

### What are the genetic variations that cause Down's syndrome?

Trisomy 21, robertsonian translocation of chromosome 21 and mosaic Down's syndrome.

### At what age would you expect the closure of the ductus arteriosus?

At 24–48 h for healthy, full-term newborns.

### What would the main differentials be for an absent red reflex?

Congenital cataracts and a retinoblastoma.

## How would you differentiate between an innocent murmur and a pathologic murmur in neonates?

Innocent murmurs are usually systolic, soft, vary with position and have no associated symptoms. Pathologic murmurs are more likely to be diastolic, harsh/loud and may cause symptoms. However, this may not always be the case.

## Describe the difference between the Barlow manoeuvre and the Ortolani manoeuvre.

Barlow's is a movement of adduction of the hips in an attempt to dislocate the femoral head posteriorly from the acetabulum, while Ortolani's is a gentle abduction of the hip in order to reduce a potentially dislocated femoral head back into the acetabulum.

## How would you reduce the risk of spina bifida during the antenatal period?

Prescribe folic acid supplements, advise against alcohol consumption and be aware of any medications that may potentially increase the risk of spina bifida, such as antiepileptics and antipsychotics. These mothers may be prescribed a higher dose of folic acid and will be monitored closely throughout pregnancy.

## What is the pathological defect in spina bifida?

It is a neural tube defect whereby the neural tube fails to close during the first month of embryonic development.

## What is the pathophysiological process of a congenital indirect inguinal hernia?

It is caused by the improper closure of the processus vaginalis, leading to protrusion of an abdominal viscus.

## What is the significance of a one-sided absent Moro reflex compared to a symmetrically absent Moro reflex?

One-sided absence indicates injury at or beyond the level of the brachial plexus, such as a fractured clavicle or Erb's palsy. Symmetrically absent Moro reflexes suggests injury within the central nervous system or bilateral brachial plexus (or beyond) injury.

## Station 9.9   Examination: Developmental Delay

### Doctor Briefing

You are a junior doctor in a neonatal outpatient clinic and have been asked to see Khalid, a 24-month-old boy who is attending with his mother Leila for a routine developmental follow-up. He was born at 26 weeks' gestation, and he left the neonatal intensive care unit (NICU) at 3 months of age, after overcoming numerous complications. Please examine Khalid, then present your findings and present your findings.

### Patient Briefing

Khalid is your second child. He was born premature at 26 weeks' gestation via caesarean section due to an infection you had, which made you very unwell. He had to be admitted to NICU for 3 months, due to his prematurity, and you were treated with intravenous (IV) antibiotics. You both recovered well and have had no issues since leaving the hospital.

His older sister is 3 years old. Today, you are concerned because Khalid has not started walking yet. You do not know of any family members with any genetic disorders. However, you recall that your uncle had difficulty walking when he was younger and is now wheelchair-bound. You are unsure of his diagnosis.

You are concerned that his developmental progress is much slower than his sister's. The health visitor has also expressed concerns regarding his development.

### Mark Scheme for Examiner

#### Introduction

| | | | | |
|---|---|---|---|---|
| Washes hands, introduces self, confirms patient identity and gains consent for examination | | | | |
| Enquires about parental concerns | | | | |
| Appropriately exposes the patient whilst keeping dignity at all times and repositions into a suitable position for the examination | | | | |

#### General Inspection

| What are you looking for or examining? | Justification | Thoughts | | | | |
|---|---|---|---|---|---|---|
| Assess gross appearance of child. Offer to measure weight and weight | Appearance allows rough estimation of age and visible conditions. Ensure good physical growth by plotting against the relevant charts | Looks appropriate for age, with no obvious pathology. Child is growing adequately | | | | |
| Note any dysmorphic features | Many syndromes can lead to cognitive impairment resulting in developmental delay | No dysmorphic features of note | | | | |
| Look around for hearing aids, a wheelchair and walking aids | Gives clues regarding mobility and developmental domain of concern | No obvious disability | | | | |
| Note if child is walking or talking, and how he is interacting. Assess interaction with yourself, other healthcare professionals and family/carers | Immediate and simple assessment of gross motor, speech and social development | Child is being carried by parent. There is some speech with poorly formed words | | | | |

## Gross Motor Development

| What are you looking for or examining? | Justification | Thoughts | | | | |
|---|---|---|---|---|---|---|
| Observe and comment on movement of all four limbs | Allows you to gauge the general tone of the child and whether there is a gross deformity characteristic of a nerve palsy | Child seems very stiff | | | | |
| Have the child sit unsupported and comment on posture | Postural instability or inability to sit may reflect a proximal muscle weakness or poor gross motor development | Able to sit up straight | | | | |
| Assess if child can stand from sitting and stay in a standing position | Helps to assess leg strength and balance | Child adopts a tripod stance and pushes on legs up to standing (Gower's sign positive). Unable to stand unaided | | | | |
| Assess if child can walk or run. Assess if the child can pick up objects from standing, walk up the stairs, cruise, jump and kick a ball | If walking has not occurred by 18 months, it is a developmental red flag and warrants further investigation | Unable to walk; prefers to sit and shuffle on bottom | | | | |

## Fine Motor Development

| | | | | | | |
|---|---|---|---|---|---|---|
| Observe child's play/interaction with toys and other individuals in the room | Important to observe how the child hold objects of interest. Note the strength used and the type of grasp (palmar or pincer) used | Reaches out for a toy or able to point and indicate desire for toy | | | | |
| Assess if child is able to pick up pencil | Helps to assess whether pincer grip is strong or effective | Able to hold a pencil but uses firm palmar grasp | | | | |
| Assess if child can scribble with a pencil | Assesses child's fine motor control | Able to draw lines and scribble, but not any shapes | | | | |
| Assess if child can build a tower with building blocks | Assesses child's fine motor control | Able to complete task with a lot of encouragement and build a tower of three blocks but no more | | | | |

## Speech, Language and Hearing Development

| | | | | | | |
|---|---|---|---|---|---|---|
| Determine the main spoken language of the family | Ensure there is no language barrier – the child can understand instructions given | The family speaks English | | | | |
| Ask if Khalid can follow any instructions. Assess if the child is able to pick up a toy or point to body parts | Appropriate responses indicate that the child is able to hear and understand the instruction and allows you to test whether the child has a level of language skills appropriate to his level | Able to point to three body parts. Able to follow simple instructions | | | | |
| Ask how many words are in the child's vocabulary | Assesses development of speech | '10–20 words' | | | | |

## Social/Self-Care Development

| What are you looking for or examining? | Justification | Thoughts | | | | | |
|---|---|---|---|---|---|---|---|
| Ask if child has imitated parents' actions at home | Common example to ask is if the child mimics doing housework | 'Sometimes' | | | | | |
| Ask about how the child prefers to eat | Assess ability to eat | 'He eats with a fork and spoon' | | | | | |
| Ask about how the child plays and with whom | Elicit social interaction and forms of play | 'He plays with his sister and other children. He likes dolls' | | | | | |
| Ask if child gets involved in dressing/undressing | Assess ability to self-care | 'Yes, he can take his socks/shoes off' | | | | | |

## Finishing

| | | | | | | | |
|---|---|---|---|---|---|---|---|
| Ask if there has been any regression in milestones, which the parent/carer may be aware of. Ask about whether the health visitor/nursery provider has raised any concerns | Regression is often a red flag and suggests that there may be a serious developing pathology that has caused developmental delay | No additional concerns | | | | | |
| Check patient is comfortable and help the parent/carer redress him | Keeps the patient's dignity | Treating the patient with respect is important | | | | | |
| Remove your gloves and wash hands | Complying with hand hygiene is vital | No additional concerns | | | | | |

## Present Your Findings

Khalid is a 24-month-old boy (19 months corrected) who presented for routine developmental assessment in neonatal clinic with his mother. On examination there are signs of spasticity in the lower limbs but no obvious signs of dysmorphism.

On gross motor assessment, he is able to sit up with a straight back but does so with spastic movements. He cannot stand unaided and is unable to walk (9 months).

On fine motor assessment, he can hold a pencil and build a tower of three blocks and is able to scribble (18 months).

On language assessment, he is able to point to body parts and has 10–20 words in his vocabulary (18 months).

On social assessment, he has imitative play, taking shoes/socks off and smiles (18 months).

I feel that the most likely diagnosis is gross motor developmental delay. Given his history, my differentials would include cerebral palsy, congenital myopathy and Duchenne's/Becker's muscular dystrophy.

To complete my examination, I would like to perform a full examination, including a neurological assessment. I would take bloods for full blood count (FBC), urea and electrolytes (U&Es), liver function tests (LFTs), ferritin, thyroid function tests (TFTs), bone profile and creatinine kinase. I would also like to discuss his case with a senior and get multidisciplinary team input for ongoing management

| General Points | | | | |
|---|---|---|---|---|
| Performs examination safely and confidently | | | | |
| Clear instruction and explanation to patient/parents | | | | |

## ❓ QUESTIONS FROM THE EXAMINER

### What does prematurity mean?

It refers to the birth of a child before 37 weeks of pregnancy.

### How would you correct the age of a premature baby?

Determine the gestational age when the baby was born. Work out the number of weeks left to term. Subtract this value from the chronological age.

### At what age would you stop correcting for prematurity?

Around 2 years of age, although there is variability in this practice.

### What is the difference between Duchenne and Becker muscular dystrophy?

Duchenne is the result of a nonsense mutation, while Becker is a missense mutation. This causes the dystrophin gene in Duchenne to be fully dysfunctional, whereas the dystrophin gene in Becker remains partially functional, resulting in longer life expectancy and milder symptoms in Becker.

### What is the mode of inheritance for Duchenne and Becker muscular dystrophy?

X-linked recessive.

### What is the meaning of the term 'global developmental delay'?

It is an umbrella term used to describe developmental delay in two or more developmental domains.

### What is autistic spectrum disorder?

Autistic spectrum disorder is a developmental disorder characterised by marked impairments in:
- Social interaction: lack of ability to have normal social interactions
- Communication: significant speech delay, with some never acquiring speech, and lack of non-verbal communication (e.g. eye contact, social smiling, facial expressions, gestures)
- Repetitive and stereotyped behavioural patterns

### What do you understand by the term 'intellectual disability'?

This is an umbrella term that encompasses a spectrum of difficulties, predominantly noticed in the developmental period, in:
- Understanding new or complicated information (cognitive)
- Ability to cope and communicate independently (social and language)
- Practical skills (motor)

### What is cerebral palsy?

It is a neurological disorder caused by non-progressive injury in the developing brain, acquired before the age of 2. Children with cerebral palsy tend to have difficulties with movement, tone and posture.

### What are the clinical subtypes of cerebral palsy and which areas of the brain do they affect?

The main subtypes of cerebral palsy are spastic, dyskinetic, ataxic and mixed. The areas of the brain affected are the cerebral cortex, basal ganglia and the cerebellum respectively. In mixed cerebral palsy, multiple areas of the brain may be affected.

## Station 9.10   Communication: Type 1 Diabetes Mellitus

### Doctor Briefing

Zac White is a 10-year-old boy who has been recently diagnosed with type 1 diabetes mellitus and is about to commence insulin therapy. Please explain the diagnosis and his insulin treatment to him. Address any concerns that he or his parent may have.

### Patient Briefing

Zac is your first child. You have noticed that he is not as active as his school friends. He often complains that he is tired and there are times when he looks very drowsy to you. You decided to bring him to the doctor to have him checked and they have informed you that Zac has type 1 diabetes mellitus.

You do not know much about the condition but have been told that he needs regular injections. You feel very nervous about this. You would like to know more about the disease, the treatments and how best to care for Zac.

### Mark Scheme for Examiner

#### Introduction

| | | |
|---|---|---|
| Cleans hands, introduces self and confirms patient identity | | |
| Checks the identity of others in the room and confirms that the patient/parent is happy for them to be present | | |
| Establishes current patient/parent knowledge and concerns | | |

#### Establishing the Patient's/Parent's Level of Understanding and Current Concerns

| Statement/Question | Justification | Answer | Thoughts | | | | |
|---|---|---|---|---|---|---|---|
| What's been going on with Zac? | Establish the presenting symptoms and obtain a summary of what has happened from the patient's/parent's perspective | 'He was getting tired a lot, and he needed the toilet a lot even in the middle of the night. The doctor before took some blood and told us that he has diabetes' | Symptoms are consistent with diagnosis | | | | |
| Has anyone explained what diabetes is to you? | Establish patient's/parent's level of understanding of the diagnosis and its implications | 'No' | Will need to start from beginning | | | | |
| Do you or Zac have anything specific you'd like to know about diabetes? | Establish what is the most worrying aspect of the diagnosis to the parent. This will guide how you structure your explanations and how much information you should provide | 'I was told that Zac needs to inject himself with insulin every day. So I would like to know how to do this, how it may affect his life and whether there are any side effects' | Make a note of the information the patient is specifically querying about and ensure you address this | | | | |

## Explaining the Diagnosis

| Statement/Question | Justification | Answer | Thoughts | | | | |
|---|---|---|---|---|---|---|---|
| Diabetes is a condition where the body has trouble taking up sugar to use as energy | State very simply what is the nature of the disease | 'Oh. That makes sense' | Patient seems to be understanding what you have covered so far | | | | |
| Zac have been diagnosed with type 1 diabetes, which means that his body does not have enough insulin, a hormone that helps him use up the sugars from your food as energy | Relating the diagnosis back to the relevant history helps put the symptoms in context and reinforces how the diagnosis was made | | | | | | |

## Insulin Treatment and Monitoring

| Statement/Question | Justification | Answer | Thoughts | | | | |
|---|---|---|---|---|---|---|---|
| To manage the condition, we need to replace the insulin | Explain the rationale behind the treatment | 'Will it hurt?' | Try to be reassuring and address the patient's concern. Involving the parent can improve compliance with medications | | | | |
| We can do this by injecting insulin into his belly or his arm. It may cause a little bit of discomfort but it is tolerated well by young patients | Explain how treatment is delivered | | | | | | |
| It can be tricky to work out the right amount of insulin he needs, as it depends on how much and what kind of food he eats so we need to monitor his blood sugars closely by using a special continuous glucose-monitoring device | Explain the importance of monitoring and highlight the potential challenges that will be faced in controlling blood glucose | 'OK' | No additional concerns | | | | |
| If he has low sugars, this test will show a level of 4 or less. If this happens, he must have some sugary food or drink. Sometimes he may feel dizzy or more tired and this is the first sign of low blood sugar and sometimes he may not even feel any different | Clearly states how to identify and treat hypoglycaemia | 'I understand' | Patient understands the signs and symptoms of hypoglycaemia | | | | |

## Insulin Treatment and Monitoring

| Statement/Question | Justification | Answer | Thoughts | | | | | |
|---|---|---|---|---|---|---|---|---|
| It is normal for blood sugars to increase after eating. But we should aim for it to be less than 10 after meals. Usually parents help to keep an eye on the sugar levels and to measure out the insulin | Involving parents will help share the responsibility and highlight to the patient that there will be help available | 'OK' | Patient seems to understand how to identify hyperglycaemia | | | | | |
| Sometimes in diabetes the body thinks it's starving, even though you have eaten, and starts using fat to make sugars but in doing this it also makes something called ketones. High levels of ketones in the body can make someone very unwell. They may feel very thirsty, sick, tired and confused, with difficulty breathing, tummy pain and vomiting. This is serious so if this happens, Zac must inform someone and he should be brought to the hospital immeidately. | Explain the life-threatening complications so that both patient and parents can look out for it | 'Oh gosh, we'll bear all of that in mind' | Remember to provide reassurance that there are steps that can be taken to prevent these outcomes and that help will be available if they feel they are unable to cope | | | | | |
| If he gets a fever or becomes unwell, he may need more energy to fight any infections, so he will need to increase his insulin and check his sugar levels more often | Explain the rationale behind sick-day rules | 'I see' | No additional concerns | | | | | |
| It's important that we take care of Zac's blood sugars because if they are left too high for too long they may start causing him problems in his body. This includes his eyes, nerves, feet, kidneys and heart. So it's also important that he continues to see doctors who can help you manage these | Identify the potential lasting effects if diabetic control is not obtained | 'OK' | Patient aware of the long-term complications | | | | | |

## Insulin Treatment and Monitoring

| Statement/Question | Justification | Answer | Thoughts | | | | |
|---|---|---|---|---|---|---|---|
| These doctors may need to see Zac regularly so that if there are any problems, we can treat them early. There will be lots of professionals involved to ensure we stay on top of things | Clearly state what to expect in terms of long-term care | I understand | Patient aware of the ongoing care required to manage this condition | | | | |

## Finishing the Consultation

| Statement/Question | Justification | Answer | Thoughts | | | | |
|---|---|---|---|---|---|---|---|
| To summarise, as I have given you a lot of information, we have discussed what diabetes is, as well as the complications and treatment options | Short summary of the key points discussed so far | 'Yes' | Summarising at the end or having the patient/parent summarise back to you helps reinforce understanding | | | | |
| I can give you some things for you to read to understand diabetes and blood sugars better. And you can always come back and ask me more questions if you would like | Leaflets and other resources will help to refresh the patient's memory | 'That'd be helpful, thank you so much' | | | | | |
| Do you have any other questions or things to add? I know that we have discussed a lot of new things; please take some time to digest the information | May identify useful information that has been missed. Will also allow you to address any questions or concerns | 'No, thank you' | | | | | |

## Present Your Findings

Zac is a 10-year-old boy who has presented with fatigue, polyuria and nocturia. He has recently been diagnosed with type 1 diabetes.

Today, he has attended with his parents and we have discussed the diagnosis, its treatment and complications. I have given them some leaflets and have safety-netted them for worrying complications and to come back if they feel they need more guidance

## General Points

| | | | | |
|---|---|---|---|---|
| Polite to patient/parent | | | | |
| Appropriate use of open and closed questions | | | | |

## ? QUESTIONS FROM THE EXAMINER

### What is the biochemical difference between carbohydrates, fats and proteins?

Carbohydrates are large molecules made from glucose and other simple sugars; fats are made from fatty acids and glycerol while proteins are made from amino acids.

### What is the Krebs cycle?

It is a process that makes up part of aerobic respiration where adenosine triphosphate is produced from acetyl coenzyme A.

### What are the exogenous and endogenous functions of the pancreas?

The pancreas functions as an exogenous gland as it produces digestive enzymes such as pancreatic amylase, trypsinogen and lipase. Its endogenous functions include secreting hormones such as insulin and glucagon in order to maintain homeostasis of blood glucose.

### How might diabetic retinopathy present?

It may be picked up on screening, but otherwise could present with eye pain/redness, blurred/patchy vision, floaters, poor night vision or gradual/sudden visual loss.

### What are the World Health Organization (WHO) criteria for diagnosing type 1 diabetes in symptomatic patients?

For symptomatic patients, a fasting plasma glucose of greater than 7.0 mmol/L or a random plasma glucose of 11.1 mmol/L is diagnostic of type 1 diabetes.

### What is the difference between type 1 and type 2 diabetes?

Type 1 is considered an autoimmune disease that develops rapidly and at a younger age, causing the body to have a reduced or complete lack of production of insulin. Type 2 is related to insulin resistance, and typically occurs in older people, particularly in the context of obesity, though it is increasingly being seen in younger people.

### What precautions should you take when before stopping insulin infusions following the resolution of diabetic ketoacidosis?

It is important to ensure that oral fluids are tolerated, ketosis is resolving and subcutaneous insulin is given well in advance of stopping the insulin infusion.

### How would you advise the patient to manage episodes of hypoglycaemia?

Have a glass of fruit juice or a glucose tablet and recheck glucose within 15 min. Repeat the process if necessary, then consider having a biscuit or slice of toast (long-acting carbohydrates) afterwards.

### What are the risk factors for developing hypoglycaemia in newborns?

Risk factors include: prematurity, low birth weight, gestational diabetes and babies that are large for gestational age.

### What healthcare professionals would be included in the long-term care of a patient with type 1 diabetes?

Type 1 diabetes requires a large multidisciplinary team. Specialists may include: a dietitian, psychologist, ophthalmologist, diabetologist, general practitioner, podiatrist and specialist diabetes nurse.

## Station 9.11 Communication: MMR Vaccine

### Doctor Briefing

You are a junior doctor working in primary care and have been asked to see Mr and Mrs Fletcher who have come to see you with their daughter, Sandy. They are keen to get the measles, mumps and rubella (MMR) vaccine for her but have some concerns about what they have heard on social media. Please explain the vaccination, discuss the risks and benefits and gain consent.

### Patient Briefing

Sandy is your first child and she has just turned 1. Both you and your partner have been vaccinated for MMR, and you are keen for her to be vaccinated as well. However, you have recently come across a research study that suggests this vaccine can cause autism. You are very worried about this. You also have friends who have advised against the vaccine, as their only child has been diagnosed with autism around the same time as obtaining the MMR vaccination.

Sandy doesn't have any allergies and she is up to date with all her other immunisations.

You would like to find out more about the benefits and risks of the MMR vaccination.

### Mark Scheme for Examiner

#### Introduction

| | | | | |
|---|---|---|---|---|
| Cleans hands, introduces self and confirms patient identity | | | | |
| Checks the identity of others in the room and confirms that the patient/parent is happy for them to be present | | | | |
| Establishes current parental knowledge and concerns | | | | |

#### Establishing the Parent's/Parent's Level of Understanding and Current Concerns

| Statement/Question | Justification | Answer | Thoughts | | | | |
|---|---|---|---|---|---|---|---|
| Could you tell me a bit about what's brought you in today? Is there anything in particular you'd like to discuss about the MMR vaccine? | Establish quickly the reason behind the visit and construct your consultation around the main concerns | 'We've heard some disturbing things about the vaccine. We've seen posts on Facebook that say that it causes autism. So we want to know what harm this vaccine could cause to our daughter' | Main concerns are development of autism and why vaccines are encouraged | | | | |
| Has anyone explained to you how this vaccine works? | Establish how much they know about the basic science behind vaccines | 'No. But we've done our own research and we know there's dangerous viruses in them, just in small doses' | There may be a misconception regarding how vaccines work | | | | |
| Have either you or Sandy experienced problems with vaccines before? | Establish whether there's a known allergic reaction to vaccines or their components | 'No' | No additional concerns | | | | |

## Establishing the Parent's/Parent's Level of Understanding and Current Concerns

| Statement/Question | Justification | Answer | Thoughts | | | | | |
|---|---|---|---|---|---|---|---|---|
| Has Sandy been diagnosed with any medical conditions before, including problems with her immune system? Does she have any allergies or previous anaphylactic reactions? | Establish whether there are any vaccine contraindications | 'No' | No additional concerns | | | | | |
| What was the last vaccination Sandy had and when was this? | Ensure that no other live vaccine was given up to 3 weeks before the MMR appointment | 'She had the meningitis B and 6-in-1 vaccine, almost 8 months ago' | No additional concerns | | | | | |
| Is your child currently unwell? | Establish an active febrile illness | 'No' | No additional concerns | | | | | |

## Explanation of the MMR Vaccine

| | | | | | | | | |
|---|---|---|---|---|---|---|---|---|
| The MMR vaccine is a live vaccine. So there are live viruses in it, but these viruses have been weakened so that they cannot cause a strong reaction or serious symptoms, but it is enough to give you immunity | Acknowledge that you have heard and taken in what the parents have said with regard to their understanding of how vaccines work but also gently correct any misconceptions you've identified | 'I see. So, there won't be any side effects?' | Potential new misconception regarding the effects of the vaccine | | | | | |
| Some children do experience some discomfort at the injection site, a rash and maybe a fever for a few days, but these symptoms can be managed with some paracetamol. Any major side effects are extremely rare, unless the child is allergic to a component of it or already has a weakened immune system | Sensitively address concerns or misunderstandings as they arise | 'I see' | No further questions at present | | | | | |
| I know that you are also concerned about the link between MMR vaccines and autism. I can assure you that this claim has been investigated extensively by the medical community and there is no link | Acknowledge the main concern and reassure parents further investigations have been done | 'But our friends' child was diagnosed with autism after having this vaccine' | Explore this correlation further and explain what autism is | | | | | |

## Explanation of the MMR Vaccine

| Statement/Question | Justification | Answer | Thoughts | | | | |
|---|---|---|---|---|---|---|---|
| I understand that the timing must have been suspicious, but there is no proven link between the MMR vaccination and autism. There are also other factors that may have increased the risk of the condition. Also, many children display the behavioural symptoms of autism spectrum disorder between 12 and 18 months of age, which is a similar timing to the MMR vaccination | Try to put it into context for Mr and Mrs Fletcher and offer them reassurance | 'We understand that. But how can the benefits of this vaccine possibly outweigh the possibility of developing autism, even if it's extremely unlikely?' | Explore the benefits of having the vaccine | | | | |
| There are many benefits to having the vaccine. There are personal benefits to your child and then there are benefits to other children if your child gets vaccinated as well | Break down the benefits of MMR vaccines in simple digestible concepts that won't overwhelm Mr and Mrs Fletcher | 'What are these benefits?' | No additional concerns | | | | |
| The personal benefit of this is that your child will have protection against three diseases: measles, mumps and rubella. They can cause very distressing symptoms and can lead to long-term complications that will affect their health and development | | 'Yes, I think that's why we both had it as a baby' | | | | | |
| The benefit to other children is that the more people who are vaccinated, the less disease there is in the population, and therefore you are protecting everyone else. This is particularly important for children who cannot be vaccinated, if for example they have severe allergies or immunodeficiencies. So the vaccinated children will be protected from disease but vulnerable children will also be protected | | 'I understand now' | | | | | |

## Finishing the Consultation

| Question | Justification | Answer | Thoughts | | | | | | |
|---|---|---|---|---|---|---|---|---|---|
| I appreciate I've given you a lot of information today; would you be able to summarise back to me what you've understood from today? | Short summary of the key points discussed so far | 'The MMR vaccine is a safe vaccine. Some people may experience some side effects but they are rarely very harmful. There is no evidence that MMR vaccines cause autism and there are many benefits of taking the vaccine for Sandy and the kids around her' | Clear understanding of conversation | | | | | | |
| I will provide you with a leaflet with more information and I am happy to meet you again if that would be useful, if you have further things you would like to go through | Leaflets and other resources will help to refresh the patient's memory | 'That'd be helpful, thank you so much' | | | | | | | |
| Do you have any other questions or things to add? I know that we have discussed a lot of new things; please take some time to digest the information | May identify useful information that has been missed. Will also allow you to address any questions or concerns | 'No, thank you. We'll go home and read the information before making a decision' | | | | | | | |

## Present Your Findings

Sandy is a 1-year-old child who is due to have her MMR vaccination. Her parents have attended today to discuss concerns regarding the vaccination.

The concerns raised were regarding the vaccine's link to autism and other potential side effects. I have reassured them that autism is not linked to the MMR vaccine. We have also discussed the risks and benefits of having the vaccine. They would like to take some time to consider the information before making an informed decision on the vaccination

## General Points

Polite to patient/parent

Appropriate use of open and closed questions

## ❓ QUESTIONS FROM THE EXAMINER

### What is the difference between live attenuated vaccines and inactivated vaccines?

Live attenuated vaccines contain a weakened form of the organism whereas inactivated vaccines contain components of the organism, which is killed or inactivated. Live vaccines create long-lasting antibodies, whereas inactivated vaccines stimulate a weaker immune response compared to live vaccines, meaning they may require several boosters throughout a lifetime.

## What are some contraindications of vaccinations?

Contraindications are vaccine-specific. They may include: active febrile illness, known anaphylaxis reaction from previous vaccines/biochemical components of a vaccine or immunosuppression.

## What is the difference between passive and active immunity?

Passive immunity is immunity acquired through vertical transmission (mother to child) or through immune serum medications (monoclonal antibodies). Active immunity is immunity developed after being exposed to an infection or from a vaccine.

## Which potential side effects of vaccines should be discussed before administration?

All major and common side effects need to be discussed. Common side effects include: swelling, redness and discomfort at injection site, fever, malaise and anaphylaxis.

## What diseases are being vaccinated against in the 6-in-1 vaccination, given at 2 months?

Diphtheria, pertussis, polio, tetanus, *Haemophilus influenzae* type B and hepatitis B.

## What is the difference between an epidemic and a pandemic?

An epidemic refers to a disease that spreads to many people within one population in a specific geographic area over a short period of time, e.g. measles outbreaks. A pandemic refers to a disease that spreads across different populations, across a wider geographical area, e.g. COVID-19.

## How do newborns have immunity against diseases within the first few months of life?

Newborns gain immunity through maternal antibodies during the antenatal period, whereby immunoglobulin G (IgG) from maternal blood is transferred across the placental to the fetus. Additionally, breastfed newborns gain maternal IgA from breastfeeding.

## Explain the pathophysiology of a secondary immune response.

A secondary immune response occurs in response to a subsequent exposure to the same antigen. Memory B cells would have been formed from the first exposure and will be circulating readily during the second exposure, causing the immune system to mount a faster and more aggressive response to the same antigen.

## Explain the pathophysiology of an anaphylactic reaction.

Anaphylaxis arises from an IgE-mediated response to a foreign antigen, leading to the release of a wide range of inflammatory mediators, released by mast cell and basophil degranulation. This can result in severe cardiorespiratory compromise.

## Are there any circumstances where children can be given vaccines without parental consent?

There is no compulsion in the UK to take vaccines, although this is not the case in all countries. Risks and benefits ought to be explained to the parent (and child, if appropriate), but in no circumstances should vaccines be given without parent/child consent.

## Station 9.12   Communication: Genetic Counselling – Cystic Fibrosis

### Doctor Briefing

Mr and Mr Taylor have been called to the rapid-access paediatric clinic as their 2-week-old baby, Matthew, has suspected cystic fibrosis (CF) from the newborn-screening blood (Guthrie) test.

### Patient Briefing

Matthew is your first child. He has not been gaining weight as expected. He has fallen across a centile line since his birth, and the doctors were concerned as he did not pass meconium until 72 h following birth. He had some blood taken from his heel, and you have been told that the results are suspicious of cystic fibrosis.

Neither you nor your partner have ever heard of cystic fibrosis. You would like to know what it is and whether Matthew has it for definite. You would also like to know the treatment, outcome and prognosis. You both are very anxious about it.

### Mark Scheme for Examiner

#### Introduction

| | | | |
|---|---|---|---|
| Cleans hands, introduces self and confirms patient identity | | | |
| Checks the identity of others in the room and confirms that the patient/parent is happy for them to be present | | | |
| Establishes parent's knowledge and concerns | | | |

#### Establishing the Parent's Level of Understanding and Current Concerns

| Statement/Question | Justification | Answer | Thoughts | | | | |
|---|---|---|---|---|---|---|---|
| Please can you tell me what's been going on? Were there any concerns when Matthew was born or during the pregnancy? | Establish the presenting symptoms and obtain a summary of what has happened from the parent's perspective | 'We have been really happy with Matthew, but his blood test came back positive for cystic fibrosis. Now that we've been thinking about it, the health visitor said he hasn't been putting on weight very well, and it took a couple of days for him to pass meconium. Everything else is fine' | Cystic fibrosis is consistent with the clinical picture | | | | |
| Has anyone explained the results to you? | Establish the parent's understanding of what's happening | 'No. But they said Matthew might have cystic fibrosis' | The parent is aware of the condition that is being suspected | | | | |
| Are there any concerns that you'd like to address in this discussion? | Establish any specific information the parent wants from this discussion | 'We don't really know what it is. Please could you explain the disease and how it's treated?' | Remember to address the parent's concerns during your discussion | | | | |
| Of course. Before I start, do you know of anyone who has this condition?' | Try to relate back to any personal experience to help with explanations | 'No' | The parents likely have little prior knowledge | | | | |

## Explanation of Cystic Fibrosis

| Statement/Question | Justification | Answer | Thoughts | | | | |
|---|---|---|---|---|---|---|---|
| Cystic fibrosis is a genetic condition that causes a build-up of mucus in the lungs and pancreas | Simple and short explanation of pathophysiology | 'OK. So one of us has this condition too?' | Misconception regarding mode of inheritance | | | | |
| Cystic fibrosis is a genetic condition. So, we can offer genetic testing for you both as well | Correct misconception and offer testing. Reassure that there is no one to blame for genetic conditions | 'That would be good. What are the chances that any children we have in the future will have this condition?' | Calculate risk of inheriting autosomal-recessive traits | | | | |
| There would be roughly a 25% chance for future children to develop this condition | 1 in 4 equates to 25%, which is the classic probability for a recessive trait | 'I see ... How does this disease affect Matthew?' | Try to approach the symptoms of cystic fibrosis systematically | | | | |
| The main organs affected are the lungs and the pancreas. Thick mucus within the lungs can be difficult to clear and this makes people more susceptible to multiple infections. In the pancreas, mucus may stop digestive enzymes from getting to the digestive system, causing malnutrition. The delayed passage of meconium may have been related to the condition, which can affect the gut | Cystic fibrosis can affect people in many ways. Stick to the main common concerns first and explore the rest if any concerns arise | 'That sounds awful. It seems like if Matthew has this, he'll be unwell for most of his life' | Empathise with how parents are feeling | | | | |
| There are some forms of cystic fibrosis that are less serious than others. It depends on the type of cystic fibrosis gene that a person has. But different specialists will work together to ensure the right balance of therapies and medications are provided to reduce the risk of malnutrition and other problems from arising | Reassure that it is a well-rounded care to ensure every chance is given to the cystic fibrosis patient to have a good quality of life | 'OK. So how old can people with cystic fibrosis live up to?' | Answer the parent's questions at this point | | | | |

## Explanation of Cystic Fibrosis

| Statement/Question | Justification | Answer | Thoughts | | | | | |
|---|---|---|---|---|---|---|---|---|
| People with cystic fibrosis can now be expected to live well into adulthood, and survival rates continue to improve as we understand the condition better, but it very much depends on the individual child | Reassure that childhood deaths are rare | 'I understand' | Acknowledge parental concerns and provide reassurance | | | | | |

## Making a Plan

| | | | | | | | | |
|---|---|---|---|---|---|---|---|---|
| I understand that this may be a lot of information to process; however, we will be monitoring your baby closely. Firstly, we need to confirm whether Matthew does indeed have cystic fibrosis | Draw parents' attention back to the next step in management | 'Is there still a chance that the test could be wrong then?' | Give objective answer. Do not 'sugarcoat' or provide certainty of diagnosis until further testing is done | | | | | |
| The initial test was a screening test, meaning that we aren't certain Matthew has the condition yet. We can find out by doing a sweat test and a genetic test | State the investigations used for diagnosis of cystic fibrosis | 'Yes, let's go ahead' | No additional concerns | | | | | |
| Once we know the diagnosis for sure we can schedule more discussions and explore how the disease will affect Matthew and how we can support him | Plan for future appointments and briefly outline what to expect | 'Yes, we'll see how it goes then' | No additional concerns | | | | | |

## Finishing the Consultation

| | | | | | | | | |
|---|---|---|---|---|---|---|---|---|
| I've given you quite a lot of information; could you please summarise what you've understood from today? | Short summary of the key points discussed so far | 'Yes, Matthew has been showing signs that he may have cystic fibrosis, which is an inherited disease. We need to do further testing to know for sure. If he does have it, then there are lots of treatment options and teams to support him' | Summarising at the end or having the parent summarise back to you helps reinforce understanding | | | | | |

### Finishing the Consultation

| Statement/Question | Justification | Answer | Thoughts | | | | |
|---|---|---|---|---|---|---|---|
| I will provide you with a leaflet with more information and am more than happy to see you again if that would be useful, if you have further things you would like to go through | Leaflets and other resources will help to refresh the patient's memory | 'That'd be helpful, thank you so much' | | | | | |
| Do you have any other questions or things to add? I know that we have discussed a lot of new things; please take some time to digest the information | May identify useful information that has been missed. Will also allow you to address any questions or concerns | 'No, thank you' | | | | | |

### Present Your Findings

Matthew is a 2-week-old boy with poor growth and delayed passage of meconium, whose newborn blood spot test results suggest he may have cystic fibrosis. His fathers have attended today to discuss this.

We have discussed cystic fibrosis, principles of management, the impact of the disease and the next steps necessary for a definitive diagnosis. I have signposted the parents to educational resources and organised a follow-up appointment for diagnostic results and further discussions

### General Points

| | | | | |
|---|---|---|---|---|
| Polite to patient/parent | | | | |
| Appropriate use of open and closed questions | | | | |

## ❓ QUESTIONS FROM THE EXAMINER

### What is a gene?

A sequence of nucleotides that carry hereditary genetic information that translates into physical/biochemical/functional traits.

### What is an allele?

A variation or alternate forms of a gene.

### What is ivacaftor?

Ivacaftor is a specific treatment for certain gene mutations in the *CFTR* gene (e.g. G551D mutation). It directly treats the underlying cause of cystic fibrosis, helping the defective cellular channel to open.

### What is the most common cystic fibrosis gene mutation in the UK?

F508del.

## What are trinucleotide repeat disorders?

They are genetic conditions caused by an increased number of repetitions of specific trinucleotide sequences, such as Huntington's chorea and fragile X syndrome.

## How and when is the newborn blood spot screening test done in newborns?

It is a heelprick blood test done on day 5 of life.

## What is the significance of a positive nuchal translucency sign?

Nuchal translucency may be a normal finding but is also associated with pathology, including genetic syndromes such as Down syndrome and Turner syndrome.

## Explain the difference between karyotyping and fluorescence in situ hybridisation (FISH).

Karyotyping enables the identification of structural abnormalities and numerical changes in chromosomes as it shows the chromosomes in pairs and in descending order according to size. FISH utilises florescent probes to bind to a specific part of a chromosome to detect either the presence or absence of specific DNA sequences.

## Explain the similarities and differences between the genetic abnormalities of Down's, Edward's and Patau syndromes.

These syndromes are caused by trisomy or an extra copy of a specific chromosome, but it is a different chromosome in each case. Down's is 21, Edward's 18 and Patau 13.

## What is gene therapy?

It is the therapeutic delivery of genetic material into a patient's cells.

## Station 9.13    Communication: Counselling For Down's Syndrome

### Doctor Briefing

Mr and Ms Bradley are pregnant with their fourth child. They are concerned about the possibility of Down's syndrome due to Mrs Bradley's age (35 years old). Please advise the couple as to what Down's syndrome is and what screening options are available.

### Patient Briefing

This is your fourth pregnancy, and you are 17 weeks pregnant. You did not plan for this pregnancy. Your first child was born when you were 21 years old. Your youngest is 12 years of age now.

Neither you nor your partner has a family history of Down's syndrome, but you work as a teaching assistant in a school that caters to children with special needs and have some understanding of the challenges of raising a child with Down's syndrome.

You have been told from your ultrasound and initial screening tests that this pregnancy is high-risk for Down syndrome. You would like to know more about the condition, and the options available for diagnostic testing.

### Mark Scheme for Examiner

#### Introduction

| | | | | |
|---|---|---|---|---|
| Cleans hands, introduces self and confirms patient identity | | | | |
| Checks the identity of others in the room and confirms that the patient is happy for them to be present | | | | |
| Establishes parent's current knowledge and concerns | | | | |

#### Establishing the Parent's Level of Understanding and Current Concerns

| Statement/Question | Justification | Answer | Thoughts | | | | |
|---|---|---|---|---|---|---|---|
| How is the pregnancy going? What has brought you in today? | Obtain a summary of what has happened from the parent's perspective | 'This is our fourth pregnancy. Everything has been going well so far, but I've been told that my screening test showed an increased risk of Down syndrome. My other kids have all been fine, but I was younger then' | Parent aware of Down syndrome possibility and probably age as a risk factor | | | | |
| How have your scans been? And your pregnancy otherwise? | Establish any additional risks | 'No, I don't have any other concerns. It was just the blood tests and the ultrasound that showed risk of Down syndrome was increased' | Has good understanding of test results | | | | |
| Do you have any personal experience with Down's syndrome? | Establish patient's understanding of the condition | 'Yes, I work as a teaching assistant with children with special needs' | Probably knowledgeable regarding children with Down's syndrome | | | | |
| Could you briefly summary what you know about the condition? | Quickest way to identify any misconceptions | 'I know that children with Down syndrome can have learning difficulties and certain health problems' | Some initial understanding present | | | | |

## Establishing the Parent's Level of Understanding and Current Concerns

| Statement/Question | Justification | Answer | Thoughts | | | | | |
|---|---|---|---|---|---|---|---|---|
| Are there any specific concerns you'd like to discuss? | Establish what the patient expects from this discussion | 'I'd like to know whether there are any other tests we can do to diagnosis whether this child has Down's syndrome or not' | Remember to discuss diagnostic antenatal tests | | | | | |

## Explanation of Down's Syndrome

| | | | | | | | | |
|---|---|---|---|---|---|---|---|---|
| Down's syndrome is a genetic condition that occurs when a baby has an extra set of genes from chromosome 21 | State clearly what is the underlying pathology | 'How does that happen?' | Use simple language to explain key concepts | | | | | |
| It spontaneously occurs. The chances of this happening increase with maternal age | State clearly the main risk factors. It is also good practice to acknowledge that you had heard what the patient had alluded to earlier | 'So, what does this extra set of genes do?' | Explore symptoms and possible complications | | | | | |
| Children with Down's syndrome tend to have distinctive physical features and may develop at a slower rate, as you may have noticed from your work. They may need more guidance and help with learning and social interactions | Explore the main features of the condition and the challenges that may be faced | 'Yes, I've seen that with the kids I teach' | Parent appears to be on the same page as you | | | | | |
| You may also have noticed that every child with Down's syndrome is different in terms of their capabilities. Some children can lead independent adult lives with minimal assistance whereas others may need full-time support | Discuss the variability of the condition | 'What about their general health?' | Explore associated conditions and how they are managed | | | | | |

**Explanation of Down's Syndrome**

| Statement/Question | Justification | Answer | Thoughts | | | | | |
|---|---|---|---|---|---|---|---|---|
| Down's syndrome can be associated with a number of health issues, such as problems with the eyes, heart, glands, gut and immune system. However, we monitor children closely and can manage these issues early if detected. A multiprofessional team is employed to care for the child's health needs. Children with Down's syndrome can lead full, happy and healthy lives | Discuss the known associated health issues and how they can be managed. Reassure that there will be an established multidisciplinary team | 'I didn't quite expect that. But of course, I'd like to prepare myself for all this. Is there a way we can be sure if this baby will have Down's syndrome?' | Explore antenatal tests that have been done and their results | | | | | |

**Making a Plan**

| Statement/Question | Justification | Answer | Thoughts | | | | | |
|---|---|---|---|---|---|---|---|---|
| The test that you did recently was an initial screening test to see how likely it is that you are carrying a child with Down's syndrome | Relate the clinical concerns back to the patient's experience to help reassure her that her concerns are being investigated | 'I see. So, the tests might be wrong?' | Need to clarify still high-risk, but cannot be certain until definitive testing | | | | | |
| I can understand that you'd like certainty. There are further tests we can do before delivery to give you clearer information | Empathise with the patient's worries and provide options to move forward. Provide realistic options and explore the risks and benefits | 'What are my options?' | As patient is past 14 weeks, chorionic villus sampling is inappropriate. At her gestational age, non-invasive prenatal testing (NIPT) or amniocentesis would be recommended | | | | | |
| Since you are now 17 weeks, we would have to do an amniocentesis, which means we would pop a needle into your tummy and take a sample of the amniotic fluid to test the baby's cells. However, as with all tests, it is not without risks. These risks include bleeding, infection and miscarriage | | 'That sounds painful. I'll need some time to consider. Can I not have a simple blood test or something?' | Allow the patient time to think it over. Reassure that decision does not have to be made immediately | | | | | |

## Making a Plan

| Statement/Question | Justification | Answer | Thoughts | | | | |
|---|---|---|---|---|---|---|---|
| So, there are blood tests available now called non-invasive prenatal testing or NIPT. However, they are not available in all centres across the UK. Unfortunately, we are not able to do them at our centre yet. Would a positive diagnostic test change anything for you? | Ensures impact of decision anticipated | 'I'm not sure. I think I'd still like to continue the pregnancy, but it would be helpful knowing what to expect' | Allow time to consider options | | | | |

## Finishing the Consultation

| Statement/Question | Justification | Answer | Thoughts | | | | |
|---|---|---|---|---|---|---|---|
| I've given you a lot of information today and it can be difficult to absorb. Would you like to summarise what you've understood from today's chat? | Short summary of the key points discussed so far | 'Yes, there are screening tests available to see if there is a chance that my baby has Down's syndrome. Following a high-risk screening test, there are further options available to diagnose Down's syndrome accurately. However, they do come with associated risks, such as miscarriage' | Summarising at the end or having the patient summarise back to you helps reinforce understanding | | | | |
| I will provide you with a leaflet with more information on the condition and on amniocentesis, so that you can read more about them. I am more than happy to see you again if that would be useful, if you have further things you would like to go through | Leaflets and other resources will help to refresh the patient's memory | 'Thank you' | | | | | |
| Do you have any other questions or things to add? I know that we have discussed a lot of new things; please take some time to digest the information | May identify useful information that has been missed. Will also allow you to address any questions or concerns | 'No' | | | | | |

**Present Your Findings**

Mrs Bradley is a 42-year-old woman who is 17 weeks pregnant. This is her fourth pregnancy. Her previous pregnancies were uncomplicated. She attended today with her husband following a screening test for Down's syndrome.

Today we've discussed the risk factors for Down's syndrome, screening tests and features/symptoms of Down's syndrome. We have also discussed further diagnostic testing, specifically amniocentesis. She has been signposted to some resources and was encouraged to reattend if she had further questions or concerns

**General Points**

Polite to patient

Appropriate use of open and closed questions

## ❓ QUESTIONS FROM THE EXAMINER

**What is brachycephaly?**

It is the flattening of the contour of the head due to early fusion of the coronal sutures.

**What are the structural abnormalities of the GI tract that are associated with Down's syndrome?**

Duodenal atresia and Hirschsprung's disease.

**What is the most common cardiac structural defect associated with Down's syndrome?**

Atrioventricular septal defect.

**How would you manage a patient with Down's syndrome complaining of loud snoring?**

Down's syndrome is associated with sleep apnoea due to enlarged tonsils and smaller upper airways. This may be investigated with a sleep study and pulse oximetry.

**Why is it important to monitor thyroid function in Down's syndrome?**

It is associated with hypothyroidism.

**Why are speech and language therapists (SALT) involved in the care of patients with Down's syndrome?**

Patients with Down's can be hypotonic and may have large protruding tongues and difficulty with communication. SALT can help assess for a safe swallow and with speech development.

**How are atrioventricular septal defects managed?**

Dependent on the size, management can be conservative, medical or surgical. Small ventricular septal defects close spontaneously. Diuretics (such as captopril) can be used to manage small defects. Surgical correction is reserved for larger defects.

**How would you ensure the growth of a patient with Down's syndrome is normal?**

Plot height and weight on a growth chart specifically for children with Down's syndrome. It is a different chart from the standard chart as children with Down's have a slower growth rate.

**What haematological malignancies are associated with trisomy 21?**

It is associated with leukaemia, especially acute lymphoblastic and myeloid types.

**What important spinal complication is associated with Down's syndrome?**

It is important to be aware of atlantoaxial instability, as this puts children at high risk of serious spinal injury if their neck is overextended. Healthcare professionals must be aware of this risk when performing emergency airway procedures.

## Station 9.14 Practical Skills: Inhaler Technique

### Doctor Briefing

Mrs Andrews has come to your clinic with her son James, an 8-year-old boy. He has recently been diagnosed with asthma and has commenced using regular inhalers. Please teach him how to use an inhaler with a spacer, explaining the steps to the examiner.

### Patient Briefing

You are James, an 8-year-old boy who was diagnosed with asthma a week ago. You have a good understanding of the disease and have been told that this condition affects your lungs sometimes. For example, when you play sports, your chest feels tight and you find it more difficult to breathe. As a result, you have been given two inhalers. However, you have never seen or used an inhaler before.

You would like a doctor to explain to you how to use an inhaler and spacer so that you can do it properly when you need it.

### Mark Scheme for Examiner

#### Introduction

| | | | | |
|---|---|---|---|---|
| Cleans hands, introduces self and confirms patient identity | | | | |
| Checks the identity of others in the room and confirms that the patient is happy for them to be present | | | | |
| Establishes current patient knowledge and concerns | | | | |

#### Explaining the Procedure

| Statement/Question | Justification | Answer | Thoughts | | | | |
|---|---|---|---|---|---|---|---|
| Do you know what an inhaler is? Have you ever seen one before? | Establish a baseline of patient's understanding | 'It is supposed to help me feel better with my asthma, especially when I am having an asthma attack' | Understands the need for medication and appropriate time to use it | | | | |
| This [blue] inhaler is a reliever and contains some medications that will help you breathe more easily when you are feeling wheezy or short of breath. You will also have a [brown] inhaler which is a preventer, and you will take this every day. Today I'm going to show you how to use the inhaler and it will hopefully help to improve your shortness of breath and wheezing | Clearly state what the inhaler is for and how it would help with the patient's symptoms | 'Yes, please' | The patient is ready to take on board what you say | ' | | | |
| If you find that after a couple of puffs you don't feel any better, you cannot speak in full sentences or your lips go blue, you need to tell someone you trust (your parents/teacher/carer) and call an ambulance immediately | Clearly state the red flags that would indicate the patient requires more medical intervention | 'Yes, I remember the other doctor told me that those were the most important things to remember' | The patient has already been given important safety-net information | | | | |

**Explaining the Procedure**

| Statement/Question | Justification | Answer | Thoughts | | | | | |
|---|---|---|---|---|---|---|---|---|
| Before you use it, you will need to check the expiry date | Ensure effective medication is being used | 'That makes sense, like with food, right?' | Be encouraging and praise the child as appropriate | | | | | |
| Yes, exactly! Make sure you are sitting up straight, then shake the inhaler and remove the cap | Highlight the importance of positioning in relation to the delivery of medications to the airways | 'Done!' | Patient able to carry out the steps up until now | | | | | |
| Now this is a spacer, and it is a tube which can help you get all the medication into your lungs. So you can insert the inhaler into the spacer. Then put your lips around the mouthpiece of the spacer | Use simple language. Make sure patient understands which is the inhaler and which is the spacer. Clearly identify the different parts of the spacer and demonstrate how to assemble the device | 'That makes sense' | | | | | | |
| Once you're all set up, then press the top of the inhaler and take five normal breaths | Once the patient is in a good position and everything has been set up properly, instruct the patient how to take the dose of the medication | 'No problem!' | | | | | | |
| 'Wait 30 s to see if you feel better. If you don't, you take another puff just like before' | Give clear instructions on how to manage a mild acute exacerbation | 'OK' | The patient comprehends your advice | | | | | |
| 'When you are done, remove the inhaler from the spacer and replace the cap on the inhaler. Remember to wash your spacer once a week with warm soapy water and let it drip dry. Every 3–6 months you should get a new spacer. Another thing to remember is if you are taking your preventer inhaler [brown/white/purple] you must remember to wash your mouth out after you have taken in the medication' | Ensure that it is stressed that the spacer needs to be washed and changed. You may need to redirect your attention to the parent at this point, as it is likely that the parents will be responsible for this step | 'Fine' | No additional concerns | | | | | |

## Check Patient Understanding

| Statement/Question | Justification | Answer | Thoughts | | | | | |
|---|---|---|---|---|---|---|---|---|
| Now that I've shown you how to do it, do you think you can have a try and show me how you'd use your inhaler and spacer? | Having patients demonstrate it back to you is the best way to check their understanding and highlight anything they may have forgotten. Correct any mistakes, remember to be patient and maintain a calm and encouraging manner | 'Yes, I will give it a go' | No additional concerns | | | | | |
| That was very good! Well done, James. Now do you or your mother have any questions you'd like to ask me? Do you need me to go through anything again? | Explore any concerns patient or his mother has. Provide them with adequate information that will ensure good compliance and good understanding of the condition | 'Nothing. That was very helpful, thank you!' | No additional concerns | | | | | |

## Finishing the Consultation

| Statement/Question | Justification | Answer | Thoughts | | | | | |
|---|---|---|---|---|---|---|---|---|
| To summarise, I have shown you how to use the inhaler, and you have also demonstrated it in front of me | Short summary of the key points discussed so far | 'Yes, I feel much more at ease with it now' | Summarising at the end or having the patient/parent summarise back to you helps reinforce understanding | | | | | |
| I will provide you with a leaflet with more information and video links so that you can rewatch what we have gone through today | Leaflets and other resources will help to refresh the patient's memory | 'That'd be great' | | | | | | |
| Do you have any other questions or things to add? Is there anything you are particularly worried about? | May identify useful information that has been missed. Will also allow you to address any questions or concerns | 'No, thank you' | | | | | | |

## Present Your Findings

James is an 8-year-old boy who has recently been diagnosed with asthma. He has attended today with his mother for a review of his inhaler technique. Today I have explained and demonstrated the correct technique of using an inhaler and spacer. I have also provided them with information leaflets and signposted them to their general practitioner and the asthma clinic if they have any further questions or concerns

| General Points | | | | |
|---|---|---|---|---|
| Polite to patient/parent | | | | |
| Appropriate use of open and closed questions | | | | |

## ❓ QUESTIONS FROM THE EXAMINER

### What is the mechanism of action of corticosteroids?

They have an anti-inflammatory effect that reduces mucosal oedema and vascular permeability by acting as glucocorticoid receptor agonists.

### Why should children with asthma have their oral hygiene checked regularly?

Regular use of inhalers can lead to dry oral mucosa. Use of steroids can cause immunosuppression, both of which lead to increased risk of development of oral thrush.

### What are some physical signs seen on patients with severe chronic asthma?

Pectus carinatum and Harrison's sulcus.

### What are some physical observations that may be identified in a baby suffering from respiratory distress?

Nasal flaring, grunting, head bobbling, wheezing, poor feeding, cyanosis, poor tone, lethargy and abdominal breathing.

### How does a spacer help in delivering medications?

Spacers ensure efficient delivery of medication into the lungs. Without them there is a risk that the medication may not reach the lower airways due to poor inhaler technique. This means spacers result in more effective treatment delivery, especially for those who have difficulty with coordinating between pressing the inhaler and taking a deep breath.

### Why must spacers be allowed to drip dry rather than towel dried?

Drip-drying allows the surface to maintain its antistatic property, which allows medications to flow optimally through optimally through the chamber into the patient's airways.

### How might nebulised ipratropium affect the eye?

Avoid the eyes as it can cause acute angle closure glaucoma. It may also cause a dilated pupil.

### How does a paediatric airway differ from an adult airway?

The airway is smaller in diameter and shorter in length. In addition, children have relatively larger tongues compared to the space in the oropharynx, and their larynx is more anterior and their adenoids tend to be bigger. They may also not have teeth, which affects intubation.

### How do you position a 9-month-old child's head if there is a concern about the airway?

Maintain the child's head in a neutral position (rather than in hyperextension).

### What are 'preschool wheezing disorders'?

These are conditions that occur before the age of 5 years old, where the patient does not have a diagnosis of asthma but has a wheeze, usually associated with viral infection. The lungs do not have the same changes as with asthma and there are no interval symptoms between flare-ups and no nocturnal cough.

## Station 9.15  Practical Skills: Peak Flow

### Doctor Briefing

You are the junior doctor in the clinic. Mrs Patel has come to your clinic with her 7-year-old son, Sandeep. He has recently been diagnosed with asthma and has been advised to keep a peak flow diary. Please teach him how to perform a peak flow, explaining the steps to the examiner.

### Patient Briefing

You are Sandeep, a 7-year-old boy. You were told that you have asthma a few months ago and were given a salbutamol inhaler to use when needed. You have been using it on and off since.

The doctor has previously explained that in order to know if the treatment is working and whether your asthma is well controlled, you need to keep a diary of your peak flow readings. You don't really know what this is, and neither does your foster mother. You also don't know how to use the tube that the doctor had given you to work out the peak flow.

Therefore, you would like a healthcare professional to show you how to do it properly so that you can fill in your diary correctly.

### Mark Scheme for Examiner

#### Introduction

| | | | |
|---|---|---|---|
| Cleans hands, introduces self and confirms patient identity | | | |
| Checks the identity of others in the room and confirms that the patient/parent is happy for them to be present | | | |
| Establishes current patient/parent knowledge and concerns | | | |

#### Explaining Peak Flow

| Statement/Question | Justification | Answer | Thoughts | | | |
|---|---|---|---|---|---|---|
| Sandeep, please could you tell me what you know about asthma? | Establish baseline understanding | 'It makes me wheezy sometimes, after I've been playing sport' | Patient has identified the trigger | | | |
| And has anyone explained to you how we check if it's getting worse? | Establish management plans that were previously relayed | 'Using a peak flow, I think. But I don't really know what that is' | Identify knowledge gaps that need to be explored | | | |
| Peak flow is a measurement of how well your lungs are working. In the middle of the tube, there is an arrow that can move. The harder you blow, the further it goes and the higher the peak flow number. The higher the number, the better your lungs are | Clearly state the purpose of this procedure | 'That makes so much more sense now! But what is it actually for?' | Ensure patient understands the importance of peak flow measurements | | | |
| This helps us know how well your lungs are normally functioning and whether your asthma is getting worse. It also helps us make sure you are on the correct inhalers that will help you control your asthma | Clearly state how you will use the information to highlight the importance of recording the measurements | 'I understand' | | | | |

## Explaining Peak Flow

| Statement/Question | Justification | Answer | Thoughts | | | | | |
|---|---|---|---|---|---|---|---|---|
| You will need to do this in the morning and in the evening every day. Please, may I show you how to measure it? | Clearly state when you'd like the patient to take his measurements. Obtain consent to explain and demonstrate the procedure | 'Yes, please' | The patient is ready to learn how to measure peak flow | | | | | |

## Explaining and Demonstrating a Peak Flow Measurement

| | | | | | | | | |
|---|---|---|---|---|---|---|---|---|
| Before you start you should wash your hands and take a clean mouthpiece. Attach the mouthpiece to the peak flow tube, make sure it's secured tightly and then move this arrow down to zero | Set the scene for the patient. Make sure he understands all the preparations required before taking a reading to ensure accuracy | 'Done' | Ensure that the patient is keeping up with each step of the procedure | | | | | |
| Stand up straight and hold the peak flow tube in your hand. Make sure your fingers don't block the scale otherwise the arrow can't move. Take a deep breath, as deep as you can. Hold it in. Put your lips around the mouthpiece tightly, but don't bite down. Then lift your chin slightly and blow as hard and as fast as you can | Give clear instructions on how to use the device to give the most accurate and best reading possible | 'OK' | | | | | | |
| Record the number that the arrow points at and move it back to zero. Try another two times and write down the highest number out of the three times on to this sheet with the date and the time | Ensure patient understands that it is the best number and overall trend that need to be reviewed | 'Fine' | | | | | | |

## Check Patient Understanding

| | | | | | | | | |
|---|---|---|---|---|---|---|---|---|
| Now that I've shown you how to do it, do you think you can have a try and show me how you'd take your peak flow measurement and record it? | Having patients demonstrate it back to you is the best way to check their understanding and highlight anything they may have forgotten. Correct any mistakes, remember to be patient and maintain a calm and encouraging manner | 'Yes, I think I can try' | No additional concerns | | | | | |

## Check Patient Understanding

| Statement/Question | Justification | Answer | Thoughts | | | | |
|---|---|---|---|---|---|---|---|
| That was very good! Well done, Sandeep. Now do you or your foster mother have any questions you'd like to ask me? | Explore any concerns patient or patient's mother have. Provide them with adequate information that will ensure good compliance and good understanding of the condition | 'Nothing. That was very helpful, thank you!' | No additional concerns | | | | |

## Finishing the Consultation

| | | | | | | | |
|---|---|---|---|---|---|---|---|
| I know I've given you a lot of information today. Would you be able to tell me one important point that you have learnt? | Short summary of the key points discussed so far | 'I need to check how good my breathing is by measuring my peak flow every morning and evening' | Summarising at the end or having the patient/parent summarise back to you helps reinforce understanding | | | | |
| I will provide you with a leaflet with more information and am more than happy to see you again if that would be useful, if you have further things you would like to go through | Leaflets and other resources will help to refresh the patient's memory | 'Thank you' | | | | | |
| Do you have any other questions or things to add? I know that we have discussed a lot of new things; please take some time to digest the information | May identify useful information that has been missed. Will also allow you to address any questions or concerns | 'No, thank you' | | | | | |

## Present Your Findings

Sandeep is a 7-year-old boy who has recently been diagnosed with asthma. He is currently on a salbutamol inhaler. He has attended the clinic with his foster mother for instructions on how to do a peak flow measurement and keep a peak flow diary.

Today, I have demonstrated the correct technique of measuring peak flow and provided them with useful resources if they have any further questions or concerns

## General Points

Polite to patient/parent

Appropriate use of open and closed questions

## ❓ QUESTIONS FROM THE EXAMINER

### How would you test lung function in a more definitive way?

FeNO and spirometry with bronchodilator reversibility.

### What is vital capacity?

The total volume of air exhaled after forced maximal inhalation.

### What is tidal volume?

The volume of air that is exhaled and inhaled during normal resting respiration.

### What is $FEV_1$?

The volume of air forcibly exhaled in 1 s after maximal inhalation.

### How do peak flow measurements affect the treatment of asthma?

They give a baseline value of what a patient's normal peak flow should be. If the readings remain greater than 80% of their best or predicted peak flow, this means the asthma is well controlled. If there is an acute exacerbation the peak flows would help grade the exacerbation and this guides management of asthma and in the acute clinical setting. However, peak flows are challenging to perform in acute exacerbations and the clinical picture alone should guide you towards the acute asthma severity.

### At what time of day are peak flow readings expected to be worse in asthmatic patients?

In the morning, asthma typically follows a diurnal pattern, showing improvement later in the day. A difference of approximately 15% between morning and evening measurements is consistent with a diagnosis of asthma.

### Where should acute exacerbations of asthma be managed?

Depending on the severity, exacerbations can be managed at home, by the primary care doctor or in hospital. Mild episodes, depending on the confidence of the family, ought to be managed at home, and recorded for the next asthma medication review. This will be treated with back-to-back inhalers and a spacer as per the child's treatment plan. Moderate asthma will require an increased inhaler use and possibly short courses of steroids. Again, metered-dose inhaler and spacer is the preferred management plan for moderate asthma; however, if the child is not improving following 10 puffs, then urgent medical advice is needed. Severe and life-threatening asthma should be managed in the secondary care setting as escalation to the high dependency unit/intensive therapy unit/intensive care unit may be needed.

### How is bronchodilator reversibility helpful in lung function testing?

In children a 12% or greater improvement in lung function or peak flow following bronchodilator administration is a positive test and diagnostic of asthma. However, this is only useful in children over 5 years old, when lung function can be measured.

### What are common triggers for asthma exacerbations?

Viral respiratory tract infections, changes in environment, e.g. moving from warm to cold, environmental allergens, e.g. pollen, exercise, smoke, and strong emotional triggers.

### What is the prognosis of childhood asthma?

For many children their asthma tends to disappear with age. However, a late diagnosis of childhood asthma is likely to continue into adulthood. There is still a significant mortality and morbidity associated with the condition.

# Ophthalmology

## Outline

---

### Station 10.1 History: Red Eye

#### Doctor Briefing

You are a junior doctor in the ED and have been asked to see Aaron James, a 62-year-old man who has presented with a red right eye associated with pain and photophobia. He has a past medical history of ankylosing spondylitis. Please take a history from Mr James, present your findings and formulate an appropriate management plan.

#### Patient Briefing

You have come to the ED today because you are experiencing severe pain in your right eye. This started this morning when you were woken up by the pain. You describe it as a deep, boring pain, confined to your right eye. It does not radiate, is constantly present, and you rate the pain as 10/10.

You also noticed that your right eye appears red, mainly the temporal half of the eye. Nothing really helps the pain, and you have become more sensitive when looking at bright lights. You have not had any neck stiffness, fever, nausea or vomiting.

The vision in your right eye is mildly reduced. Your left eye is completely normal. There has not been any discharge from your eyes. Your sinuses are non-tender. You have not had any trauma to the eyes.

On questioning about your past medical history, you reveal that you have a background of rheumatoid arthritis and ankylosing spondylitis. Regarding family background, your mother has systemic lupus erythematosus (SLE).

You are concerned because your eye is really painful and you are worried that you are going to become blind.

#### Mark Scheme for Examiner

##### Introduction

| | | | |
|---|---|---|---|
| Cleans hands, introduces self, confirms patient identity and gains consent for history taking | | | |

##### History of Presenting Complaint

| Question | Justification | Answer | Thoughts | | | |
|---|---|---|---|---|---|---|
| How long have you been experiencing pain in your eye? | Helps to determine if this is acute or chronic | 'Since this morning' | Given the sudden onset, it is important to rule out an acute pathology | | | |

## History of Presenting Complaint

| Question | Justification | Answer | Thoughts | | | | | |
|---|---|---|---|---|---|---|---|---|
| Which eye is affected, right, left or both? | Certain conditions are more likely to present bilaterally, and vice versa. If the presentation is bilateral, but one eye started before the other, consider conjunctivitis | 'It's only my right eye' | Consider unilateral causes of eye pain | | | | | |
| How would you describe the pain? | The character of the pain can give you an idea as to what is causing it | 'It is a deep, boring pain that's always there' | A deep pain is typically associated with scleritis and migraines | | | | | |
| Does the pain radiate? | Important to know if the pain radiates to the back of the eye or causes a headache to establish the cause | 'No' | No additional concerns | | | | | |
| On a scale of 0–10, with 10 being the worst pain ever, how would you rate it? | Gives you an idea as to how severe the pain is | '10/10' | This suggests very intense pain | | | | | |
| Are your eyes looking red? | Helps you to ascertain if you need to consider causes of a red eye | 'The right eye is really red all over. The left eye is normal' | This suggests a large area of diffuse injection of the right eye | | | | | |
| Have you noticed any skin changes or swelling around the eye? | Important to rule out orbital cellulitis and herpes zoster ophthalmicus | 'No' | No additional concerns | | | | | |
| Are you experiencing other symptoms, such as sensitivity to bright light or loss of vision? | These associated symptoms are important to enquire about to narrow your list of differential diagnoses | 'I have noticed that I'm a bit more sensitive to light and my right eye is slightly blurry' | The patient is experiencing photophobia and reduced vision, which could suggest AACG, scleritis, anterior uveitis or meningitis | | | | | |

## Past Medical History

| Question | Justification | Answer | Thoughts | | | | | |
|---|---|---|---|---|---|---|---|---|
| Have you ever had these symptoms before? | Check that these are not recurring symptoms | 'No' | No additional concerns | | | | | |
| Do you wear contact lenses? | Use of contact lenses is a risk factor for corneal ulcers | 'Yes, I've been using them for over 10 years without any problems' | Consider conditions commonly seen in contact lens wearers | | | | | |
| Have you had any recent procedures or surgeries to your eyes? | Vital to consider any potential complications from eye surgery or injections, such as endophthalmitis | 'No' | No additional concerns | | | | | |
| Have you ever been treated for any sexually transmitted infections (STIs)? | This question is important as gonorrhoea and chlamydia are known to be associated with eye infections | 'No, and my recent STI screen was clear' | No additional concerns | | | | | |

## Past Medical History

| Question | Justification | Answer | Thoughts | | | | |
|---|---|---|---|---|---|---|---|
| Do you suffer from any medical conditions, especially autoimmune diseases? | Certain eye conditions are associated with some systemic diseases | 'I have rheumatoid arthritis and ankylosing spondylitis' | This increases the suspicion of scleritis and anterior uveitis | | | | |

## Drug History

| Question | Justification | Answer | Thoughts | | | | |
|---|---|---|---|---|---|---|---|
| Are you on any medications at the moment, or have any allergies? | Good practice to check the patient's full drug history and allergy status | 'No medications and no allergies' | No additional concerns | | | | |
| Have you recently used any topical eye treatments? | Anything applied to the eyes topically can cause localised inflammation or infection | 'No' | No additional concerns | | | | |

## Family History

| Question | Justification | Answer | Thoughts | | | | |
|---|---|---|---|---|---|---|---|
| Are there any diseases that run in the family, specifically any systemic or ophthalmic diseases? | Important always to check for relevant heritable conditions, that could increase the patient's risk of eye problems | 'My mother has SLE' | This increases the suspicion of scleritis and anterior uveitis | | | | |

## Social History

| Question | Justification | Answer | Thoughts | | | | |
|---|---|---|---|---|---|---|---|
| Are you working? | Find out if the patient is in a job that is at high risk of eye injuries | 'No, I am retired' | No occupational concerns | | | | |
| Do you smoke? | Find out a patient's wider risk factors | 'No, I have never smoked' | No additional concerns | | | | |
| What is your average weekly alcohol consumption? | | 'I only drink a glass of wine once a week' | No additional concerns | | | | |

## Systems Review

| Question | Justification | Answer | Thoughts | | | | |
|---|---|---|---|---|---|---|---|
| Just to check, have you had any fever, headache, neck stiffness, nausea or vomiting? | These are important questions to ask about to rule out systemic infections, such as meningitis | 'No' | No additional concerns | | | | |
| Have you experienced any problems with your skin, joints or bowels? | Screening for systemic diseases | 'No more than usual' | No additional concerns | | | | |

**Finishing the Consultation**

| Question | Justification | Answer | Thoughts | | | | |
|----------|---------------|--------|----------|--|--|--|--|
| Is there anything that I've missed that you would like to tell me about? | May identify useful information that has been missed. Will also help to build rapport with the patient | 'No, I'm just really worried about it and want it to get better' | Take the time to explain what will happen from here | | | | |
| Do you have any questions? | Allows any final concerns to be addressed | | | | | | |

**Present Your Findings**

Mr James is a 62-year-old man who has presented with a red right eye associated with pain and photophobia. He woke up with a deep boring pain in his right eye that is non-radiating, and the severity is rated to be 10/10. There is also diffused injection of the right eye and right vision is reduced. He is experiencing photophobia. The patient suffers from rheumatoid arthritis, and his mother has SLE.

My main differential would be scleritis, with differential diagnosis of episcleritis and anterior uveitis.

I am going to refer Mr James immediately to ophthalmology and will consider prescribing systemic non-steroidal anti-inflammatory drugs to reduce the inflammation in the meantime

**General Points**

| | | | | |
|--|--|--|--|--|
| Polite to patient | | | | |
| Maintains good eye contact | | | | |
| Appropriate use of open and closed questions | | | | |

## ❓ QUESTIONS FROM THE EXAMINER

### What is the meaning of the term 'uvea'?

The uvea is a collective term for the iris, choroid and ciliary bodies.

### Give three examples of diseases that are associated with the HLA B-27 gene, which is associated with anterior uveitis.

These include psoriasis, ankylosing spondylitis, inflammatory bowel disease, reactive arthritis and Reiter's syndrome.

### If a patient presents with a red eye and the blood vessels blanch after the application of phenylephrine, what condition does this suggest?

This points towards a diagnosis of episcleritis.

### Which specific infection must you consider after recent eye – especially cataract – surgery?

Endophthalmitis is a complication to be aware of post-cataract surgery.

### Which systemic diseases are most commonly associated with dry eyes?

Autoimmune diseases; for example, Sjögren's syndrome, rheumatoid arthritis, SLE and diabetes.

### Name three risk factors that may increase your risk of AACG.

These include being female, aged 55–70 years old, hyperopia, family and personal history of AACG and recent use of pupil dilators.

## Name three common precipitants of subconjunctival haemorrhage.

Subconjunctival haemorrhage can occur during excessive straining; for example, coughing, sneezing and vomiting. It can also happen due to eye trauma (including infection) or by rubbing the eye too hard.

## Name three common causative organisms of orbital cellulitis.

*Staphylococcus aureus* and streptococci species are the most common bacterial organisms. Other pathogens include *Aeromonas hydrophila*, *Pseudomonas aeruginosa* and *Eikenella corrodens*.

## What is a known contraindication to the use of chloramphenicol?

Acute porphyrias.

## What is the most common problem associated with contact lens use?

Superficial punctate keratitis.

## Station 10.2    History: Sudden Loss of Vision

### Doctor Briefing

You are a junior doctor in the ED and have been asked to see Monica Goodfellow, a 62-year-old woman, who has presented today with sudden visual loss in her left eye. She has also been having terrible headaches and generally feels unwell. Please take a history from Mrs Goodfellow, present your findings and formulate an appropriate management plan.

### Patient Briefing

You have come to the ED today because a few hours ago, your left-eye vision reduced dramatically. You are now only able to see vague shapes such as the outline of fingers or people. At the time, you were watching television in a dark room. You are also experiencing severe pain in your left eye and left brow, rating its severity as 9/10. Your left eye also looks really red, and your partner said that your left eye appears hazy on the surface.

On specific questioning, you are experiencing pain around your left brow and eye. Since the onset of the loss of vision, you have felt a bit nauseous, but have not vomited. There have not been any skin changes, discharge or sensitivity to bright lights.

On specific questioning, you have never experienced this before. Apart from being long-sighted you have not had any problems with your eyes before. You have not had any eye trauma or surgery recently.

You are concerned that this visual loss is going to be permanent and that your right-eye vision is also going to be affected.

### Mark Scheme for Examiner

#### Introduction

| | | | | | |
|---|---|---|---|---|---|
| Cleans hands, introduces self, confirms patient identity and gains consent for history taking | | | | | |

#### History of Presenting Complaint

| Question | Justification | Answer | Thoughts | | | | |
|---|---|---|---|---|---|---|---|
| How long have you had visual loss? | Helps to determine if this is acute or chronic | 'Since this evening' | Given the sudden onset, it is important to rule out an acute pathology | | | | |
| What were you doing at the time? | Establish if there were any significant events at the time of onset – for example, head trauma – that could precipitate an intracranial bleed or lifting heavy weight that may induce a vitreous haemorrhage | 'I was watching TV in a dark room' | This environment would require the pupils to dilate; therefore, this should be considered when deciding the main diagnosis | | | | |
| Which eye is affected, right, left or both? | Certain conditions are more likely to present bilaterally, and some are more likely to be unilateral | 'It's only my left eye. My right seems fine' | Consider unilateral causes of vision loss | | | | |
| How much are you able to see compared to before? | Extent of the vision loss allows you to determine the patient's visual acuity and visual field | 'Everything was clear before, but now the left eye is blurry and I can only make out shapes, like number of fingers' | A significant sudden reduction in vision is concerning and you must rule out acute causes | | | | |

## History of Presenting Complaint

| Question | Justification | Answer | Thoughts | | | | |
|---|---|---|---|---|---|---|---|
| Have you got any pain in or around your eyes? | Painless loss of vision is classically associated with central retinal vein occlusion (CRVO) and central retinal artery occlusion (CRAO) | 'Yes, I have got really bad pain in my left eye and up to the left eyebrow' | Eye pain is a concerning factor that needs to be explored more | | | | |
| Are you having any headaches? | Headaches associated with vision loss can be a presentation of giant-cell arteritis (GCA) | 'Just the pain around my left eyebrow, which feels like a headache' | This kind of headache doesn't sound consistent with GCA but could allude to another diagnosis | | | | |
| Are you particularly sensitive to the light, or have you had any nausea or vomiting? | These symptoms combined with a headache are typical of meningitis but could be caused by other conditions | 'I feel a bit sick but haven't vomited. I don't seem to have a problem with the light' | With the combination of headache/eye pain and nausea, consider pathology related to raised intracranial or intraocular pressure (IOP) | | | | |
| Have you had any pain on brushing your hair, in the jaw or in your muscles and joints? | Scalp tenderness, jaw claudication and polymyalgia rheumatica (PMR) are typically associated with GCA | 'No' | This points away from GCA | | | | |
| Do your eyes look different, such as, any redness? | Helps you to build a better image of what the eye looks like | 'The left eye is really red and my partner said that it looks hazy' | Consider causes of a red eye and potential obstructions on the surface of the cornea | | | | |
| Do you have any eye discharge? | Discharge from the eye could suggest conjunctivitis, and excessive tears could be due to dry eyes | 'No' | No additional concerns | | | | |

## Past Medical History

| Question | Justification | Answer | Thoughts | | | | |
|---|---|---|---|---|---|---|---|
| Do you have any known eye problems, including prescriptions? | Specifically ask about spectacles as this tells us a lot about the shape of the eyeballs | 'I am long-sighted' | Hypermetropia increases the risk of AACG | | | | |
| Are you known to have a history of PMR, aortic aneurysms/dissection or large-artery stenosis? | PMR is a result of the same disease process as GCA, while the latter conditions are known complications of GCA | 'No' | No additional concerns | | | | |

## Drug History

| Question | Justification | Answer | Thoughts | | | | |
|---|---|---|---|---|---|---|---|
| Are you on any medications at the moment, or have any allergies? | It is good practice to check the patient's full drug history and allergy status | 'No medications and no allergies' | No additional concerns | | | | |

## Drug History

| Question | Justification | Answer | Thoughts | | | | |
|---|---|---|---|---|---|---|---|
| Have you recently used any steroids? | The use of steroids can mask symptoms of GCA | 'No' | No additional concerns | | | | |

## Family History

| Are there any diseases that run in the family, specifically PMR, GCA or migraines? | The presentation could be a manifestation of these conditions | 'My brother suffers from migraines a lot' | Could consider migraine as a differential diagnosis | | | | |
|---|---|---|---|---|---|---|---|

## Social History

| Are you working? | Find out if the patient is in a job that is very stressful, which could trigger migraines and tension headaches | 'No, I am retired' | No occupational concerns | | | | |
|---|---|---|---|---|---|---|---|
| Do you smoke? | Smoking increases the risk of various ophthalmic conditions | 'No, I don't smoke' | No additional concerns | | | | |
| What is your average weekly alcohol consumption? | Excessive alcohol intake can cause visual loss secondary to nutritional deficiencies | 'I rarely drink alcohol' | No additional concerns | | | | |

## Systems Review

| Have you had any back pain, abdominal pain, chest pain or symptoms of stroke? | Important to ask regarding possible systemic manifestations of GCA | 'No' | No additional concerns | | | | |
|---|---|---|---|---|---|---|---|
| Have you had any unexplained weight loss, fevers or night sweats? | Screening for vasculitis such as GCA | 'No' | No additional concerns | | | | |
| Have you felt particularly tired? | Malaise and fatigue could be suggestive of systemic diseases, such as lymphoma and hypothyroidism, which are risk factors for CRVO | 'Not really, no more than usual' | No additional concerns | | | | |
| Have you experienced any problems with your skin, joints or bowels? | Screening for systemic diseases | 'No more than usual' | No additional concerns | | | | |

## Finishing the Consultation

| Question | Justification | Answer | Thoughts | | | | | |
|---|---|---|---|---|---|---|---|---|
| Is there anything else that you would like to tell me about? | May identify useful information that has been missed and help to build rapport with the patient | 'No, I've told you everything' | Take the time to explain what will happen from here | | | | | |
| Do you have any questions? | Allows any final concerns to be addressed | | | | | | | |

## Present Your Findings

Mrs Goodfellow is a 62-year-old woman who has presented with sudden loss of vision in her left eye. She is only able to count fingers, and the vision loss is associated with severe eye pain, radiating to the left brow. It began when she was watching TV in a dark room this evening. She feels nauseous but is not photophobia. She is known to be hypermetropic.

My main differential would be AACG, with differential diagnosis of migraine and scleritis.

I would like to measure the patient's IOP and urgently refer her to ophthalmology for confirmation of diagnosis and commencement of IOP-lowering treatment

## General Points

Polite to patient

Maintains good eye contact

Appropriate use of open and closed questions

## ❓ QUESTIONS FROM THE EXAMINER

### Why may a patient experience jaw claudication if they have GCA?

Jaw claudication is highly predictive of GCA and it is a result of ischaemia of the maxillary artery, which supplies the masseter muscles.

### Name three risk factors for retinal detachment.

These include increased age, personal or family history of retinal detachment, extreme myopia (near-sightedness), previous eye surgery and eye injury.

### How many types of CRVO exist and what are they?

There are two main types of CRVO: non-ischaemic CRVO (milder) and ischaemic CRVO (more severe).

### Name three risk factors for CRAO.

These include arterial hypertension, diabetes, carotid artery disease, coronary artery disease, transient ischaemic attacks, strokes and smoking.

### What procedure can be performed to reduce the risk of a recurrent episode of AACG?

Laser or surgical iridectomy can be performed in the affected eye only, or in both eyes.

### Name two potential causes of vitreous haemorrhage.

These include proliferative diabetic retinopathy, posterior vitreous detachment and ocular trauma.

### What complications are associated with GCA?

These include blindness, aortic aneurysm, stroke, myocardial infarction and peripheral arterial disease.

### What are optic radiations?

Optic radiations are the axons from the neurones in the lateral geniculate nucleus to the primary visual cortex. There is one on each side of the brain and they carry information along the calcarine fissure.

### In terms of histopathology, what may be seen during a retinal examination in a patient presenting with amaurosis fugax?

You may notice a Hollenhorst plaque lodged within a retinal vessel; this appears as yellow, bright and refractile.

### Name the seven leading causes of vision impairment worldwide.

These include uncorrected refractive errors, cataract, age-related macular degeneration, glaucoma, diabetic retinopathy, corneal opacity and trachoma.

## Station 10.3  History: The Watery Eye

### Doctor Briefing

You are a junior doctor in the ED and have been asked to see Phyllis Jones, a 43-year-old woman who has presented with constantly watery eyes, which have felt increasingly sore. She is very anxious and thinks that her vision is slightly blurred. Please take a history from Mrs Jones, present your findings and formulate an appropriate management plan.

### Patient Briefing

You have come to the ED today because both of your eyes have been constantly watery and became much worse today. This has come on progressively over the last couple of weeks, with it being worst in the morning. They are also both really sore, which you describe as grittiness, and rate it as a 4/10 in severity. On inspection, both of your eyes are also mildly red. Your vision can be intermittently blurry for a few seconds. You deny any double vision, eye pain, change in appearance to the eyes or face.

On questioning, you have not had any procedures performed to your eyes nor any eye trauma. You have not been exposed to any fumes. You do not wear glasses or contact lenses. You do not suffer from allergies. You work as a writer and have been working from home this month. It seems to get worse when you are reading documents online.

On questioning, you reveal that you got a cat half a year ago. You deny experiencing a runny nose.

You are concerned that you've got something stuck in your eyes or that you've got an infection.

### Mark Scheme for Examiner

#### Introduction

| Cleans hands, introduces self, confirms patient identity and gains consent for history taking | | | | |
|---|---|---|---|---|

#### History of Presenting Complaint

| Question | Justification | Answer | Thoughts | | | | |
|---|---|---|---|---|---|---|---|
| How long have you had watery eyes? | Helps to determine if this is acute or chronic | 'It started 2 weeks ago, getting worse by the day' | Sounds relatively acute | | | | |
| Which eye is affected, right, left or both? | Certain conditions are more likely to present bilaterally, and some are more likely to be unilateral | 'Both' | Bilateral watery eyes could suggest dry-eye disease or environmental factors | | | | |
| Is it present all the time? | As well as establishing if the watery eyes are constant or intermittent, you should find out if there is any diurnal variation | 'It's worst when I wake up" | Dry-eye disease is often worse in the morning | | | | |
| Can you describe the discharge? | Differentiate betwen the various causes of eye discharge | 'It's just watery and clear. There's no gunk or anything' | Less likely to be bacterial conjunctivitis | | | | |
| Does anything make it worse? | Exacerbating factors are helpful clues to the diagnosis | 'It's worst when I've been working at the computer' | Dry-eye disease is often worsened by prolonged computer use, whereas if the watery eyes are worse when looking down, it could be due to an eyelid positional problem | | | | |

## History of Presenting Complaint

| Question | Justification | Answer | Thoughts | | | | | |
|---|---|---|---|---|---|---|---|---|
| Does anything make it better? | Alleviating factors are just as important clues | 'When I take a break from work' | Consistent with dry-eye disease | | | | | |
| Have you had any trauma to your eyes, including exposure to chemical fumes? | Eye trauma could injure the eyes directly | 'No' | Less likely to be foreign body or reaction to environmental factors | | | | | |
| How would you describe the soreness? | Character of the pain helps to differentiate between causes | 'Both eyes feel gritty, like something is stuck' | A typical description of dry-eye disease | | | | | |
| Have you had any visual change, including double vision? | Important to establish if vision is affected to avoid misdiagnosis | 'I have not had double vision but sometimes my vision appears blurry, which lasts for a few seconds' | Non-specific visual changes present, but no diplopia | | | | | |
| Have there been any changes to the appearance of the eyes, including skin changes and swelling? | Establish the likelihood of other causes, such as orbital cellulitis, thyroid eye disease, lid laxity | 'There's no swelling or skin changes, but both eyes look a bit red' | Redness could suggest inflammation or infection | | | | | |
| Has there been any asymmetry of your face? | Important to rule out facial nerve palsy or lid abnormalities | 'No' | No additional concerns | | | | | |
| Have you had this before? | Establish if this is a recurring problem | 'Only last summer when I had the air conditioner on all the time' | Dry-eye disease is often exacerbated by air-conditioned and heated rooms, as well as dusty and windy environments | | | | | |

## Past Medical History

| Question | Justification | Answer | Thoughts | | | | | |
|---|---|---|---|---|---|---|---|---|
| Do you have any known eye problems, especially recurrent eye infections or eyelid abnormalities? | Recurrent eye infections can lead to scarring, obstruction or eversion of the punctum | 'No' | No additional concerns | | | | | |
| Are you known to suffer from facial nerve palsy? | Facial nerve palsy is associated with a reduced blink reflex | 'No' | No additional concerns | | | | | |
| Do you suffer from any medical conditions, especially autoimmune diseases? | Certain conditions are associated with various eye problems (outlined in 'Family History', below) | 'I suffer from depression' | No additional concerns | | | | | |

## Drug History

| Question | Justification | Answer | Thoughts | | | | | |
|---|---|---|---|---|---|---|---|---|
| Are you on any medications at the moment, or have any allergies? | Good practice to check the patient's full drug history and allergy status | 'No medications and no allergies' | No additional concerns | | | | | |
| Have you recently used any eye drops, especially containing preservatives? | Lubrication drops with preservatives can cause your eyes to water | 'No' | No additional concerns | | | | | |

## Family History

| Question | Justification | Answer | Thoughts | | | | | |
|---|---|---|---|---|---|---|---|---|
| Are there any diseases that run in the family, especially any autoimmune diseases? | Thyroid disease, type 1 diabetes and vitiligo would increase suspicion for thyroid eye disease. Rheumatoid arthritis and Sjögren's syndrome are often associated with dry-eye disease | 'My dad has type 2 diabetes' | No additional concerns | | | | | |

## Social History

| Question | Justification | Answer | Thoughts | | | | | |
|---|---|---|---|---|---|---|---|---|
| Are you working? | Jobs at increased risk of exposure to chemical fumes, mental grinding or cement use can increase the risk of foreign bodies | 'I am a writer' | No occupational concerns | | | | | |
| Do you smoke? | Smoking relates to poor prognosis of thyroid eye disease and worsening severity | 'I rarely smoke' | No additional concerns | | | | | |

## Systems Review

| Question | Justification | Answer | Thoughts | | | | | |
|---|---|---|---|---|---|---|---|---|
| Have you experienced any problems with your skin, joints or bowels? | It is important to screen for rheumatoid arthritis, Sjögren's syndrome, psoriasis and Graves' disease | 'No more than usual' | No additional concerns | | | | | |
| Have you had any palpitations, diarrhoea, temperature intolerance or restlessness? | Screening for thyroid disease | 'No' | No additional concerns | | | | | |

## Finishing

| Question | Justification | Answer | Thoughts | | | | |
|---|---|---|---|---|---|---|---|
| Is there anything else that you would like to tell me about? | May identify useful information that has been missed and helps to build rapport with the patient | 'No, I've told you everything' | Take the time to explain what will happen from here | | | | |
| Do you have any questions? | Allows any final concerns to be addressed | | | | | | |

## Present Your Findings

Mrs Jones is a 43-year-old woman who has presented with constantly watery eyes, which have felt increasingly sore. This started 2 weeks ago and both of her eyes are affected. The epiphora is aggravated by prolonged computer use. They are also mildly injected and have a sense of grittiness to them. She experiences blurry vision intermittently but denies any diplopia or eye pain.

My main differential would be dysfunctional tear syndrome/dry-eye syndrome, with differential diagnoses of viral conjunctivitis or allergic eye disease.

I would like to examine the patient's eyes under a slit lamp and perform a tear film break-up time test and/or Schirmer test to confirm my main diagnosis. I would also advise trialling preservative-free artificial tears

## General Points

| | | | | |
|---|---|---|---|---|
| Polite to patient | | | | |
| Maintains good eye contact | | | | |
| Appropriate use of open and closed questions | | | | |

## ❓ QUESTIONS FROM THE EXAMINER

### In general, alkali eye burns usually lead to more severe injuries than acidic eye burns, with the exception of which acid?

Chemicals with a higher pH penetrate more layers of the eyes than chemicals with a lower pH, and therefore can lead to more extensive injuries. An exception to this is hydrofluoric acid burn, which is as dangerous as an alkali chemical burn.

### Name three common precipitants of dry eyes.

These include prolonged contact lens use, long periods of time looking at a digital screen, air-conditioned or heated environments and windy, cold or dusty air.

### What microorganism is responsible for the development of dendritic keratitis?

Herpes simplex virus (HSV).

### How many types of HSV are there and what are their primary sites of infection?

There are two main types of HSV: HSV-1 and HSV-2. Typically, HSV-1 causes infection in the face, lips and eyes; meanwhile HSV-2 infects the genitalia, although it may be transmitted through infected secretions either venereally or at birth.

### What structure within the eye is responsible for the secretion of oil and why does it do this?

Meibomian glands are small oil glands that line the margin of the eyelids, and their function is to secrete oil, which contributes to the tear film and stops tears from evaporating.

### How do tears normally flow?

Tears are produced by the lacrimal glands, which are situated at the upper lateral part of the eyes. When you blink, the inner eyelids spread the tears across the eyes to keep them lubricated. The tears then migrate into the lacrimal puncta, down the lacrimal canal and sac, and into the nasolacrimal ducts.

### What clinical test can be used to assess for lower-lid laxity?

The snap-back test can be performed, whereby gentle digital pressure is used to draw the lower eyelid down. If it remains in a frank ectropion position for longer than expected, then it is a positive test for lower-lid laxity.

### Which muscle elevates the upper eyelid?

Levator palpebrae superioris.

### What is the triad of symptoms of acute Horner's syndrome?

Anhidrosis, miosis and ptosis.

### For which three conjunctival syndromes is *Chlamydia trachomatis* known to be responsible?

Trachoma, adult and neonatal conjunctivitis and lymphogranuloma venereum can all be secondary to *Chlamydia trachomatis* infections.

## Station 10.4    History: Flashing Lights and Floaters

### Doctor Briefing

You are a junior doctor in the ED and have been asked to see Sheila Jameson, a 67-year-old woman who has presented with flashes and floaters, with a small black curtain in her right-eye vision. Please take a history from Mrs Jameson, present your findings and formulate an appropriate management plan.

### Patient Briefing

You have come to the ED today because you are seeing flashes and floaters in both of your eyes. This started 6 months ago. The flashing lights are worse when you move your head and they look like arcs of white light. The floaters are tiny black specks and have increased in number in your right eye over the last week. You have come to ED today because since this afternoon, you have also been seeing a small black shadow in the corner of your right eye, that you describe is 'like a curtain'.

On specific questioning, you are not experiencing any eye pain, headache, red eye or double vision. You have had diabetes for over 20 years, for which you take metformin and insulin, but you've never managed to get good control. You have recently been diagnosed with high blood pressure, that is currently managed by lifestyle adjustments.

On specific questioning, a year ago you had laser surgery performed on both of your eyes because of your diabetes.

You are concerned that you are going blind, as your ophthalmologist had warned you of this if you do not get your diabetes under control.

### Mark Scheme for Examiner

#### Introduction

| | | | | |
|---|---|---|---|---|
| Cleans hands, introduces self, confirms patient identity and gains consent for history taking | | | | |

#### History of Presenting Complaint

| Question | Justification | Answer | Thoughts | | | | |
|---|---|---|---|---|---|---|---|
| Which eye is affected, right, left or both? | It is important to determine which eye is affected, and if one preceded the other | 'I can see flashes and floaters in both eyes, but the right eye has a shadow' | Both eyes would generally suggest less sinister pathology, but consider an acute problem in the right eye | | | | |
| Did they come on gradually or suddenly? | Determine if this is acute or chronic and to understand the symptoms' progression | 'The flashes and floaters came on 6 months ago, but the shadow appeared today' | Consider an acute-on-chronic condition. Symptoms that come on suddenly are more concerning for a sinister pathology | | | | |
| Describe the flashing lights | Characteristics of the light help to determine the cause. For example, in migraines patients typically see colourful and/or zigzag lines | 'The flashes are like arcs of white light' | Typical description of flashes associated with vitreous traction on the retina | | | | |
| Does anything make the flashes worse or better? | Exacerbating and relieving factors are important to elicit | 'When I move my head, the flashes are worse' | Flashing lights brought on with head or eye movement suggest vitreous traction on the retina | | | | |
| Describe the floaters | To ascertain the extent of visual disturbance | 'They are like small black specks, but there are now more in the right eye' | Constant new floaters suggest a more sinister pathology | | | | |

## History of Presenting Complaint

| Question | Justification | Answer | Thoughts | | | | | |
|---|---|---|---|---|---|---|---|---|
| Are the flashes and floaters present intermittently or constantly? | Also note if it is worse at a specific time of the day | 'They are constantly there' | Floaters are present at all times | | | | | |
| Describe the shadow | To ascertain which area of the vision is affected | 'Just in the top corner of my right eye, there is a small black shadow, similar to a curtain' | A black curtain in the vision associated with flashes and floaters is a classical sign of retinal detachment | | | | | |
| Do you have any eye pain, headache, double vision or red eyes? | Important associated symptoms to enquire about to rule out other causes | 'No' | Must explore retinal detachment, which often presents with painless visual field loss | | | | | |

## Past Medical History

| | | | | | | | | |
|---|---|---|---|---|---|---|---|---|
| Do you have any known eye problems, including prescriptions? | Myopia and hyperopia increase the risk for various conditions | 'I am short-sighted' | Myopia is a risk factor for retinal tears and detachments | | | | | |
| Do you suffer from any medical conditions, especially diabetes or hypertension? | Important to consider chronic conditions and their effects on the eyes | 'I've had type 2 diabetes for over 20 years and have recently been diagnosed with high blood pressure' | Consider complications of diabetic retinopathy | | | | | |
| Have you ever had a retinal tear or detachment? | This would increase the risk of recurrence | 'No' | No additional concerns | | | | | |
| Have you had any procedures performed on your eyes? | If surgery has been performed, then you need to consider potential complications | 'A year ago, I had laser surgery done to both of my eyes because of diabetes' | Consider complications of eye surgery. The patient most likely had laser photocoagulation | | | | | |

## Drug History

| | | | | | | | | |
|---|---|---|---|---|---|---|---|---|
| Are you on any medications at the moment, or have any allergies? | Good practice to check the patient's full drug history and allergy status | 'I am on diabetic medications, including metformin and insulin. I do not have any allergies' | Insulin for type 2 diabetes implies that the condition has been difficult to control | | | | | |

## Family History

| | | | | | | | | |
|---|---|---|---|---|---|---|---|---|
| Has anyone in the family had migraines or retinal detachments? | Positive family history increases the risk of these conditions | 'No' | No additional concerns | | | | | |

## Social History

| Question | Justification | Answer | Thoughts | | | | | |
|---|---|---|---|---|---|---|---|---|
| Are you working? | Highly stressful jobs could increase the suspicion for migraines | 'I am retired' | No occupational concerns | | | | | |
| Do you smoke? | To elicit social risk factors | 'No' | No additional concerns | | | | | |
| Do you drink alcohol? | | 'No' | No additional concerns | | | | | |

## Systems Review

| Question | Justification | Answer | Thoughts | | | | | |
|---|---|---|---|---|---|---|---|---|
| Have you had any recent head or eye injuries? | Rule out traumatic causes | 'No' | No additional concerns | | | | | |
| Have you had any limb weakness, facial asymmetry, speech impairment or loss of sensation? | Rule out possible stroke | 'No' | No additional concerns | | | | | |
| Have you had any neck pain/stiffness, vomiting, headache, fever or sensitivity to light? | Rule out possible meningitis | 'No' | No additional concerns | | | | | |
| Have you experienced any problems with your skin, joints or bowels? | Screening for systemic diseases | 'No more than usual' | No additional concerns | | | | | |

## Finishing the Consultation

| Question | Justification | Answer | Thoughts | | | | | |
|---|---|---|---|---|---|---|---|---|
| Is there anything else that you would like to tell me about? | May identify useful information that has been missed and help to build rapport with the patient | 'No, I've told you everything' | Take the time to explain what will happen from here | | | | | |
| Do you have any questions? | Allows any final concerns to be addressed | | | | | | | |

## Present Your Findings

Mrs Jameson is a 67-year-old woman who has presented with bilateral flashes and floaters, associated with a small black curtain in her right eye. Flashes and floaters began 6 months ago, but the small black curtain was only noticed this afternoon. She does not have any eye pain, headache, red eye or diplopia. There is a background of poorly controlled diabetes for over 20 years, for which the patient is on metformin and insulin, and last year she had laser eye surgery. She also has hypertension that is conservatively managed.

My main differential would be a potential retinal detachment secondary to proliferative diabetic retinopathy with differential diagnoses being a retinal tear, vitreous traction and hypertensive retinopathy.

I would like to examine the patient using a fundoscope and slit lamp, then refer to ophthalmology. I would also provide the patient with information on improving diabetes and hypertension control

| General Points | | | | |
|---|---|---|---|---|
| Polite to patient | | | | |
| Maintains good eye contact | | | | |
| Appropriate use of open and closed questions | | | | |

## ❓ QUESTIONS FROM THE EXAMINER

### What is the blood supply to the retina?

The retina is supplied by the central retinal artery and the choroidal blood vessels, both of which originate from the ophthalmic artery.

### Name three risk factors for posterior vitreous detachment.

These include increased age, personal or family history, extreme myopia, previous eye surgery and eye trauma.

### What is the role of the vitreous humour?

The vitreous humour provides and preserves the eye in its intended shape and transmits light on to the retina.

### Which part of the eye is responsible for central vision?

The macula.

### How many types of surgeries can be used to treat retinal detachment and what are they?

There are three main types of surgery for retinal detachment: vitrectomy, scleral buckle surgery and pneumatic retinopexy.

### If you have had a pneumatic retinopexy, why are you recommended against flying?

During a pneumatic retinopexy, a gas bubble is inserted into the eye. The change in air pressure can expand the gas bubble and increase the pressure within your eye, which can be serious and sight-threatening.

### What procedure can be performed to visualise the blood flow to the back of the eyes?

Fundus fluorescein angiography can help to visualise the blood flow to the back of the eyes.

### Within the UK, approximately what proportion of diabetic patients develop diabetic retinopathy?

In the UK, within 20 years of diagnosis, nearly all people with type 1 diabetes, and almost two-thirds of people with type 2 diabetes, have some degree of retinopathy.

### How often is the diabetic eye screening in the UK?

Diabetic patients are advised to get their eyes checked annually to screen for diabetic retinopathy, and sooner if they experience any symptoms. There are separate screening rules if a patient with diabetes is pregnant.

### Why might a patient not be certified by a consultant ophthalmologist for being partially or severely sight-impaired?

If the patient does not meet the criteria for visual acuity or visual field, if the sight loss is only temporary or if the patient is currently receiving treatment that may improve the sight, then the consultant ophthalmologist may not issue the certificate at the moment.

## Station 10.5 History: Periocular Pain With Headache

### Doctor Briefing

You are a junior doctor in the ED and have been asked to see John Wright, a 77-year-old man who has presented with pain around his right eye, extending over his head. He also has a facial rash, which came up 2–3 days after the pain. Please take a history from Mr Wright, present your findings and formulate an appropriate management plan.

### Patient Briefing

You have come to the ED today because you have deep pain in your right eye and on the right eyelid, which radiates to the forehead on the right-hand side. You have noticed that the right eyelid is swollen, red and warm to touch. Your left eye is normal.

On specific questioning, you have noticed a rash on your face, that you describe as a 'red circle' around your right eye. The eye pain started 2 days ago, then the rash appeared today. There is no associated discharge, masses or pruritus.

On specific questioning, the vision from your right eye is mildly reduced (you describe it as being 'fuzzy') and there is pain with eye movements occasionally, such as when you look to either side.

On specific questioning, you have not had any procedures performed on your eyes recently. There is no history of trauma. Last week you were treated for acute sinusitis, and you are still experiencing a runny nose. You are still getting fevers intermittently, but you have put that down to your sinus infection. You have not had any neck stiffness or photophobia.

You are concerned that the swelling is going to increase.

### Mark Scheme for Examiner

#### Introduction

| | | | | | |
|---|---|---|---|---|---|
| Cleans hands, introduces self, confirms patient identity and gains consent for history taking | | | | | |

#### History of Presenting Complaint

| Question | Justification | Answer | Thoughts | | | | | |
|---|---|---|---|---|---|---|---|---|
| Where is the pain and does it radiate? | Periocular pain may originate from the eye, sinuses, orbit or intracranial space | 'It's behind my right eye and goes to the right eyelid and forehead' | Consider the deeper structures of the eye and causes of unilateral headache, such as migraines | | | | | |
| How would you describe the pain? | Character of the pain can be a clue; for example, sharp burning sensation indicates neuropathic pain which could be from trigeminal nerve inflammation | 'Like a sharp pressure' | Consider sinusitis or migraine | | | | | |
| When did the pain start? Did it all come together? | The chronological order of symptoms can give clues to the underlying cause | 'Yes, it gradually started worsening over the last 2 days' | The condition is progressively worsening | | | | | |
| Does anything make the pain worse? | Exacerbating and relieving factors can aid diagnosis. For example, worsening headache on standing could be secondary to cerebrospinal fluid leak, and being in a dark room might help with migraines | 'When I look from side to side the eyes hurt more' | Ophthalmoplegia is a concerning feature and could indicate orbital cellulitis | | | | | |
| Does anything make the pain better? | | 'No medication ... nothing seems to make it better' | Less likely to be migraines | | | | | |

## History of Presenting Complaint

| Question | Justification | Answer | Thoughts | | | | | |
|---|---|---|---|---|---|---|---|---|
| Is anywhere on your face tender to touch? | Rule out potential facial inflammation or infection | 'All around my right eye is really sore to touch' | Could be orbital cellulitis or sinusitis | | | | | |
| Have you had any visual change, including double vision? | Bleeding at the back of the eye may result in the patient seeing a brown spiral. 'Zigzag' visions are typically associated with migraines with aura | 'The vision in the right eye has been constantly blurry since yesterday' | Blurry vision could be secondary to compression of deeper structures or superficial/deep infections | | | | | |
| Have there been any new skin changes or swelling on the face? | A rapidly growing rash may suggest facial cellulitis or necrotising fasciitis. If it is within a dermatomal distribution, such as trigeminal nerve ophthalmic division, it could suggest herpes zoster ophthalmicus (HZO) | 'The skin around the right eye is really red, swollen and warm, and it's getting worse. The left eye is normal' | Need to rule out cellulitis (facial and orbital) and necrotising fasciitis | | | | | |
| Have you had any discharge? | Discharge can indicate infection | 'No' | No additional concerns | | | | | |
| Is your eye itchy or red? | Rule out causes of a red eye | 'No' | No additional concerns | | | | | |
| Have you had any nausea/vomiting/ neck stiffness/ photophobia? | Rule out meningism | 'No' | No additional concerns | | | | | |
| Have you had any slurred speech or limb weakness? | Rule out stroke | 'No' | No additional concerns | | | | | |

## Past Medical History

| Question | Justification | Answer | Thoughts | | | | | |
|---|---|---|---|---|---|---|---|---|
| Do you have any known eye problems, such as eye infection? | Recurrent eye infections can lead to scarring, obstruction or eversion of the punctum | 'I used to get conjunctivitis a lot' | Consider complications of conjunctivitis, such as orbital abscess | | | | | |
| Do you have diabetes or human immunodeficiency virus (HIV)? | Screening for immunosuppression which increases the risk of HZO | 'No' | No additional concerns | | | | | |

## Drug History

| Question | Justification | Answer | Thoughts | | | | | |
|---|---|---|---|---|---|---|---|---|
| Are you on any medications at the moment, or have any allergies? | Good practice to check the patient's full drug history and allergy status | 'No medications and no allergies' | No additional concerns | | | | | |

### Family History

| Question | Justification | Answer | Thoughts | | | | |
|---|---|---|---|---|---|---|---|
| Are there any problems that run in the family, such as headaches? | Positive family history for certain conditions may increase the patient's risk | 'My mum and sister suffer from migraines' | Blurry vision and headache could be secondary to migraine, but it doesn't explain the swelling | | | | |

### Social History

| Question | Justification | Answer | Thoughts | | | | |
|---|---|---|---|---|---|---|---|
| Have you had any recent travels? | Consider reaction to insect bites and transmissible infectious diseases | 'Not for 5 years' | No additional concerns | | | | |
| Do you work with chemicals? | Consider exposure to solvents and potential chemical eye injury | 'No, I am a receptionist' | No additional concerns | | | | |
| Do you smoke? | Smoking impairs the immune system which may become vulnerable to reactivation of viruses | 'I do not smoke' | No additional concerns | | | | |

### Systems Review

| Question | Justification | Answer | Thoughts | | | | |
|---|---|---|---|---|---|---|---|
| Have you had any recent infections? | Some infections increase the risk of eye problems | 'I've recently had sinusitis' | This could be a precipitant of orbital cellulitis | | | | |
| Have you been under a lot of stress? | Stress is a risk factor for HZO | 'No' | No additional concerns | | | | |
| Have you experienced any problems with your skin, joints or bowels? | Screening for systemic diseases | 'No more than usual' | No additional concerns | | | | |

### Finishing

| Question | Justification | Answer | Thoughts | | | | |
|---|---|---|---|---|---|---|---|
| Is there anything else that you would like to tell me about? | May identify useful information that has been missed and help to build rapport with the patient | 'No, I've told you everything' | Take the time to explain what will happen from here | | | | |
| Do you have any questions? | Allows any final concerns to be addressed | | | | | | |

### Present Your Findings

Mr Wright is a 77-year-old man who has presented with unilateral right-eye pain and a facial rash. The eye pain is located on the right eyelid, that is also red, warm and swollen. Two days after the onset of right-eye pain, the patient developed a red circular rash around the right eye. The patient also has blurry vision and ophthalmoplegia on looking peripherally. Mr Wright was recently treated for acute sinusitis and is intermittently experiencing pyrexia.

My main differential would be orbital cellulitis secondary to sinusitis, with differential diagnoses of orbital abscess secondary to conjunctivitis, preseptal cellulitis and HZO.

I would like to refer the patient urgently to ophthalmology, and in the meantime order a computed tomography (CT) head to confirm the diagnosis. I would also take blood cultures and consider commencing the patient on intravenous antibiotics as per trust guidelines

| General Points | | | |
|---|---|---|---|
| Polite to patient | | | |
| Maintains good eye contact | | | |
| Appropriate use of open and closed questions | | | |

## ? QUESTIONS FROM THE EXAMINER

### Name two complications of orbital cellulitis.

These include loss of vision, subperiosteal abscess, intracranial extension of the infection and sepsis.

### What is the most important distinguishing feature of orbital cellulitis?

Ophthalmoplegia, pain with eye movement and/or proptosis.

### What is the most common cause of orbital cellulitis?

Rhinosinusitis is the most common cause of orbital cellulitis. Other less common causes include dacryocystitis, retained orbital foreign body, periocular trauma and dental infection.

### What is often seen on CT scans in orbital cellulitis?

Inflammation of extraocular muscles, fat stranding and anterior displacement of the globe on CT scans suggest orbital cellulitis. Evidence of rhinosinusitis and complications such as abscesses are sometimes noted.

### What investigations can be used to confirm a diagnosis of GCA?

Temporal artery biopsy remains the gold standard for diagnosis. Other helpful investigations include temporal artery ultrasound, positron emission tomography and high-resolution magnetic resonance imaging.

### Which group of patients are usually affected by cellulitis of the eye?

Paediatric patients, usually under the age of 10 years.

### What classification system is used to categorise different types of orbital cellulitis and how many stages are there?

The Chandler classification is used to divide orbital cellulitis into five different stages.

### What percentage of herpes zoster infections can be accounted for by HZO?

10–20% of herpes zoster infections can be accounted for by HZO.

### What is zoster sine herpete (ZSH)?

ZSH is an atypical manifestation of herpes zoster infection, where there are no cutaneous symptoms, and can present with or without ocular involvement, making the diagnosis more difficult.

### Which nerve is affected in HZO?

The ophthalmic division of the trigeminal nerve (cranial nerve V) is affected in HZO.

## Station 10.6    History: Blurred Vision

### Doctor Briefing

You are a junior doctor in the ED and have been asked to see Claire Reynolds, a 21-year-old woman, who has presented with blurred vision in the right eye. She thought the vision would resolve by itself, but unfortunately it has worsened and now her visual acuity is hand movements in that eye. Please take a history from Miss Reynolds, present your findings and formulate an appropriate management plan.

### Patient Briefing

You have come to the ED today because the vision in your right eye has suddenly reduced over the last day. You realised that your vision was blurry 2 days ago, after you woke up from a student night out. Over the 2 days, the vision in your right eye has been deteriorating so quickly that you are concerned. At the moment, you can only detect hand movements in the right eye and colour vision is reduced. Your left eye is normal. You deny eye pain, change in appearance to the eyes or facial asymmetry.

On specific questioning about your medical background, you have nothing significant but you had the flu a month ago. You do not have any allergies. You do not smoke, but you do drink alcohol.

On specific questioning about head injury, you reveal that 2 nights ago when you were at the club, you were assaulted by someone there and sustained a head injury. You remember hitting your head really hard and you still have a bruise over the right side of your forehead.

You are concerned that you have got a bleed in your brain.

### Mark Scheme for Examiner

#### Introduction

| | | | | | |
|---|---|---|---|---|---|
| Cleans hands, introduces self, confirms patient identity and gains consent for history taking | | | | | |

#### History of Presenting Complaint

| Question | Justification | Answer | Thoughts | | | | |
|---|---|---|---|---|---|---|---|
| How long have you had blurry vision? | Helps to determine if this is acute or chronic | 'It started 2 days ago but worsened today' | Sudden blurred vision suggests an acute event. Rapid deterioration is concerning | | | | |
| Which eye is affected, right, left or both? | If both eyes are affected, consider a neurological event, such as stroke, migraine or space-occupying lesion | 'Just the right eye' | Unilateral causes of blurred vision need to be considered, such as anterior ischaemic optic neuropathy and optic neuritis | | | | |
| How would you describe the blurred vision? | A gradual constant 'fog' suggests corneal decompensation whereas a 'black curtain' could indicate amaurosis fugax or retinal detachment/tear | 'Everything is fuzzy' | Wide differential for non-specific blurred vision | | | | |
| Did anything happen before the blurred vision started? | Preceding events could be the cause; for example, lifting a heavy weight could precipitate a Valsalva-induced vitreous haemorrhage | 'I went out 2 nights ago and was attacked by someone and got hit in the head. I've still got some bruising and swelling over the right side of my forehead' | Head trauma could result in intracranial bleed or traumatic head/brain injury | | | | |

## History of Presenting Complaint

| Question | Justification | Answer | Thoughts | | | | |
|---|---|---|---|---|---|---|---|
| Have you had any trauma to your eyes, including exposure to chemical fumes? | Eye trauma could injure the eyes | 'No' | Less likely to be foreign body or reaction to environmental factors | | | | |
| Have you had any trouble with colour vision? | Reduced colour vision suggests a problem with the optic nerve; for example, optic neuritis and orbital cellulitis | 'Now that you mention it, colours don't seem as sharp in the right eye any more' | Concerning symptom suggesting something sinister | | | | |
| Do you have any pain on eye movement? | Optic neuritis may cause pain on looking in various directions | 'No' | No additional concerns | | | | |
| Have your pupils changed in appearance? | A single large pupil in bright and dark conditions suggests an afferent pathway defect, which can be checked by the swinging-torch test | 'No' | No additional concerns | | | | |
| Have you had any scalp tenderness, jaw claudication, temple tenderness or a one-sided headache? | GCA can be associated with anterior ischaemic optic neuropathy | 'No' | No additional concerns | | | | |

## Past Medical History

| | | | | | | | |
|---|---|---|---|---|---|---|---|
| Are you known to suffer from recurrent eye problems, such as uveitis? | The uveitis masquerade syndromes are a group of ocular diseases that may mimic chronic intraocular inflammation | 'I've never had any issues with my eyes' | No additional concerns | | | | |
| Have you ever been diagnosed with multiple sclerosis (MS)? | Prior diagnosis of MS is a risk factor for optic neuritis due to myelination | 'No' | No additional concerns | | | | |
| Do you have any history of eating disorder? | Nutritional deficit could be a cause for optic nerve problems | 'No' | No additional concerns | | | | |

## Drug History

| | | | | | | | |
|---|---|---|---|---|---|---|---|
| Are you on any medications at the moment, or have any allergies? | Amiodarone, ethambutol, cyanide, isoniazid and triethyltin may cause optic nerve damage | 'I'm on the oral contraceptive pill and have been for years. I don't have any allergies' | No additional concerns | | | | |

## Family History

| Question | Justification | Answer | Thoughts | | | | |
|---|---|---|---|---|---|---|---|
| Are there any diseases that run in the family, especially any problems regarding poor vision? | Significantly reduced vision in the family may suggest Leber's hereditary optic neuropathy | 'No' | No additional concerns | | | | |

## Social History

| Question | Justification | Answer | Thoughts | | | | |
|---|---|---|---|---|---|---|---|
| Do you smoke? | Smoking can increase the risk of optic neuropathy | 'No' | No additional concerns | | | | |
| Do you drink alcohol? | Alcohol is no longer considered to cause toxic optic neuropathy, but nutritional deficiencies can cause optic neuropathy | 'Only when I go out, say every 2 weeks' | Unlikely to suffer from nutritional deficiencies secondary to alcoholism | | | | |
| Have you had any travels abroad? | Rule out infectious diseases, such as Lyme disease, tuberculosis (TB) and syphilis | 'I've only been to France, almost 10 years ago' | No additional concerns | | | | |
| Are you working? | Certain occupations are at high risk of eye injuries | 'No, I am a student' | No occupational concerns | | | | |
| How would you describe your diet? | Vitamin $B_1$, $B_2$, $B_6$, $B_{12}$ and folic acid deficiency could be a cause of optic nerve problems | 'I eat a healthy and balanced diet' | No additional concerns | | | | |

## Systems Review

| Question | Justification | Answer | Thoughts | | | | |
|---|---|---|---|---|---|---|---|
| Have you had any recent infections? | If the immune system is compromised, the patient may acquire postviral optic neuritis | 'I had a cold for a week a month ago' | Consider postviral optic neuritis | | | | |
| Do you suffer from a chronic cough? | This may be associated with TB, sarcoidosis and vasculitis | 'No' | No additional concerns | | | | |
| Have you had any muscle or limb weakness? | Screening for symptoms of MS | 'No' | No additional concerns | | | | |
| Have you had any weight loss, fatigue or night sweats? | These suggest a systemic disease, such as vasculitis, which may increase the risk of anterior ischaemic optic neuropathy | 'No' | No additional concerns | | | | |

## Systems Review

| Question | Justification | Answer | Thoughts | | | | | |
|---|---|---|---|---|---|---|---|---|
| Have you experienced any problems with your skin, joints or bowels? | Screening for systemic diseases | 'No more than usual' | No additional concerns | | | | | |

## Finishing

| Question | Justification | Answer | Thoughts | | | | | |
|---|---|---|---|---|---|---|---|---|
| Is there anything else that you would like to tell me about? | May identify useful information that has been missed and help to build rapport with the patient | 'No, I've told you everything' | Take the time to explain what will happen from here | | | | | |
| Do you have any questions? | Allows any final concerns to be addressed | | | | | | | |

## Present Your Findings

Miss Reynolds is a 21-year-old student who has presented with blurry vision in the right eye. It began 2 days ago, after she was assaulted and sustained a head injury. Her right vision has been rapidly deteriorating, and now she can only detect hand movements. Her left vision is unaffected. She also had a cold a month ago.

My main differential would be traumatic axonal injury, with differential diagnosis of postviral optic neuritis.

I would like to refer the patient urgently to ophthalmology for a more thorough examination of the globe and deeper structures behind the eyes, to ensure that they are all intact. In the meantime, I will also organise a head CT scan.

## General Points

| | | | | |
|---|---|---|---|---|
| Polite to patient | | | | |
| Maintains good eye contact | | | | |
| Appropriate use of open and closed questions | | | | |

## ❓ QUESTIONS FROM THE EXAMINER

### Name some examples of visual auras that are associated with migraines.

Typically, if a patient suffers from migraines with aura, they may report scotomas, seeing zigzag patterns or flashing lights.

### What are the functions of the rod and cone cells in the retina?

Rod cells are highly sensitive to light and are therefore vital in night vision, while cone cells function best in bright light and are essential in acute and colour vision. It is thought that there are three types of cone cells – each detecting wavelengths of one of the primary colours: red, blue and green.

### What is the meaning of 'achromatopsia'?

Total loss of visual colour perception.

### Which are the two main charts used to assess visual acuity?

The Snellen chart and the logarithm of the minimum angle of resolution (logMAR) chart.

## What happens to an image after it has passed through the lens and reaches the retina?

Upon reaching the retina, a formed image is inverted and reversed, so upper visual space information is projected to the lower retina and lower visual space information is projected to the upper retina.

## Where in the brain might a lesion be if it is resulting in contralateral homonymous superior quadrantopia?

A lesion at the temporal lobe.

## Where do optic radiations synapse?

In the primary visual cortex.

## On average, how long does it take for a corneal ulcer to heal?

A corneal ulcer is a medical emergency and requires urgent treatment, after which it usually heals within 2–3 weeks.

## If a contact lens wearer presents with a dendritic ulcer, what must you exclude first?

*Acanthamoeba* keratitis.

## When are infants in the UK screened for cataracts?

All newborn babies are offered a physical examination within 72 h of birth, and then again at the newborn baby examination between 6 and 8 weeks. Both examinations include an assessment of the eyes, most importantly looking for the presence of the red reflex, which if absent, could indicate congenital cataracts or other pathologies.

## Station 10.7    Examination: Ophthalmic

### Doctor Briefing

You are a junior doctor in the emergency department (ED) and have been asked to see Keri Whalen, a 67-year-old woman, who has presented with a constantly watery eye with mild irritation. She is otherwise fit and well. Please perform a relevant eye examination on Mrs Whalen and present your findings. You are not required to complete fundoscopy for this station.

### Patient Briefing

You have come to the ED because your eyes are feeling extremely uncomfortable. There is a constant irritation in your left eye, and it is constantly watery, but there is no pain (headache or eye pain). This started yesterday and is getting progressively worse.

You have not been particularly sensitive to light. There has been no purulent discharge, just an excessive amount of tears. Your vision remains unaffected. You have not had any recent trauma to either eye and have never had any ophthalmic procedures.

You have never had this feeling before, and generally have not had any problems with your eyes. You are slightly short-sighted but you do not wear contact lenses or glasses.

You are concerned that there is something stuck in your eyes because you were gardening yesterday and it was really windy, therefore you are worried that something may have blown into your eye when you were cutting the plants.

### Mark Scheme for Examiner

#### Introduction

| | | | | | |
|---|---|---|---|---|---|
| Washes hands, introduces self, confirms patient identity and gains consent for examination | | | | | |
| Asks about pain | | | | | |
| Ensures a chaperone is present | | | | | |
| Appropriately exposes the patient whilst keeping dignity at all times | | | | | |

#### General Inspection

| What are you looking for or examining? | Justification | Thoughts | | | |
|---|---|---|---|---|---|
| General well-being | On initial glance does the patient look well/unwell/in pain? | The patient looks well and does not appear to be in any pain or distress | | | |
| Obvious clues | Look for facial asymmetry and scars (especially near the eyes) that may suggest previous ophthalmic procedures, and drooping of the eyes, which could be ptosis | No other obvious signs on inspection | | | |
| Surroundings | Note any reading aids (glasses or magnifying glasses) or cane for people who are blind | The patient does not have any reading aids with her. She is holding onto a handkerchief, which she uses to wipe her left eye occasionally | | | |

**Eye Examination**

| What are you looking for or examining? | Justification | Thoughts | | | | |
|---|---|---|---|---|---|---|
| Examine the pupils | Inspect the pupil for size and shape. Compare the two eyes | On inspection, both pupils appear normal and symmetrical | | | | |
| | Check that both pupils are reactive to light (direct and consensual) and test accommodation. Compare the two eyes | Both pupils are equal and reactive to light and constrict as expected on accommodation | | | | |
| | It is important to check for a relative afferent pupillary defect (RAPD) using the swinging-torch test. If this is positive, it could indicate optic nerve dysfunction to the afferent nerve pathway | There is no RAPD | | | | |
| Examine the eyelids | Look for lumps, scars, hypo- or hyperpigmentation and oedema. Compare the two eyes | There are no eyelid abnormalities | | | | |
| | It is important also to look at the eyelids from above and the sides, for any evidence of proptosis. Compare the two eyes | There is no evidence of proptosis | | | | |
| Examine the conjunctiva | Note the colour of the conjunctiva and if there is any leukoplakia. Also note any cysts, thickening or symblepharon (traction bands). Compare the two eyes | The left conjunctiva appears mildly erythematous (diffused), but the right conjunctiva appears normal. This could suggest inflammation of the left eye. There are no corneal masses | | | | |
| Examine the cornea | Describe the appearance of the cornea, noting any haziness, foreign body or neovascularisation on the corneal surface. Compare the two eyes | Bilateral corneas appear clear. In the upper temporal quadrant of the left cornea, there is a very small black opacity, that could be a foreign body. In general, her left eye is also more watery than the right eye | | | | |
| Examine the anterior chamber | Check for clarity and describe anything that may be obstructing your view, such as hyphema or keratic precipitates | There was no abnormality in the anterior chamber | | | | |
| Assess visual acuity | Using the Snellen chart, check the visual acuity of each eye separately with a pinhole to assess macular function. Compare the two eyes | The best-corrected visual acuity in both eyes is 6/6 | | | | |
| Assess visual fields | Test all eight meridians of the visual field, for both eyes separately, to assess the patient's peripheral vision. Compare the two eyes | Visual fields were normal in both eyes | | | | |

## Eye Examination

| What are you looking for or examining? | Justification | Thoughts | | | | | |
|---|---|---|---|---|---|---|---|
| Assess eye movements | Using the 'H technique', test the patient's eye movement, looking for any nystagmus, diplopia or eye pain on movement. Compare the two eyes | Bilateral eye movements were normal and there was no evidence of ophthalmoplegia, nystagmus or diplopia | | | | | |

## Finishing

| | | | | | | | |
|---|---|---|---|---|---|---|---|
| Remove your gloves and wash hands | Complying with hand hygiene is vital | No additional concerns | | | | | |

## Present Your Findings

Mrs Whalen is a 67-year-old woman who presented with a watery and irritated left eye. On examination she looks comfortable at rest. Her left conjunctiva appeared mildly erythematous and watery, compared to the right eye. I also noted a black opacity in the upper temporal quadrant of the left conjunctiva. The rest of the eye examination was unremarkable.

I feel the most likely diagnosis is a foreign body in the left eye, with the differential diagnoses being dysfunctional tear syndrome/dry-eye syndrome or viral conjunctivitis.

To complete my examination, I would like to examine Mrs Whalen fully by testing for colour blindness using the Ishihara chart and examining the eyes using an ophthalmoscope, and under a slit lamp with epithelial staining

## General Points

| | | | | |
|---|---|---|---|---|
| Polite to patient | | | | |
| Maintains good eye contact | | | | |
| Clear instruction and explanation to patient | | | | |

## ❓ QUESTIONS FROM THE EXAMINER

### In which part of the optic tract might there be a lesion in a patient presenting with bilateral hemianopia?

A lesion in optic chiasm may result in bilateral hemianopia.

### If you notice xanthelasma around the eyes, what might this suggest about the patient?

It usually indicates high cholesterol level and a certain extent of hyperlipidaemia.

### Approximately what percentage of patients with Graves' disease will develop thyroid eye disease, and what is a known risk factor for it?

Roughly 25% of patients with Graves' disease will develop thyroid eye disease, and smoking increases their risk.

### What is the first page of the Ishihara chart usually used for?

The first page is usually used as the 'test plate', as it does not assess the patient's colour vision, but instead assesses contrast sensitivity. Only if the patient is able to read this test plate would you move on to test the rest of the Ishihara plates.

### What is the meaning of 'scotoma'?

'Scotoma' refers to a central area of absent or reduced vision, surrounded by areas of normal peripheral vision.

**What is the name of a formal assessment tool that can be completed to assess the patient's central visual field accurately?**

The Amsler grid is used to detect metamorphopsia or scotoma involving the central visual field.

**How many components or layers does the tear film have, and what are they called?**

The tear film consists of three components or layers, including the innermost mucus layer, the aqueous layer and the uppermost lipid layer.

**What is Schirmer's test used for?**

Schirmer's test is used to determine if the tear glands are producing enough tears to keep the eyes adequately moist, primarily to diagnose dry-eye syndrome.

**What is the difference between entropion and trichiasis?**

Entropion is a condition where the eyelid is incorrectly turned inwards towards the eye, causing many of the eyelashes to rub along the cornea. Trichiasis occurs when an eyelash incorrectly grows inwards towards the cornea.

**How many extraocular muscles exist and what are their names?**

There are six extraocular muscles – superior rectus, inferior rectus, medial rectus, lateral rectus, superior oblique and inferior oblique.

## Station 10.8   Practical Skill: Fundoscopy Technique

### Doctor Briefing

You are a junior doctor in the ED. You have been asked to see Thomas Grey, a 72-year-old man who has presented with painless loss of vision in his right eye. Please complete fundoscopy on Mr Grey and present your findings.

### Patient Briefing

You have come to the ED because you woke up this morning and were unable to see properly from your right eye. You hit your head a week ago when you tripped and fell on to the floor from standing. Since then, you have also noted flashes and floaters in your right vision. Now you describe the visual loss as being similar to a black curtain spreading across your field of vision, starting from the side to the centre.

Your left eye is completely normal. You are not experiencing any eye pain or discomfort, and there is no discharge from either of your eyes. You have not noticed any eye redness and have not had any recent trauma to the eyes.

You are known to be severely short-sighted and must wear glasses all the time. You have no other significant past medical or ophthalmic history.

You are very concerned that you have a bleed in your brain from when you fell over a week ago.

### Mark Scheme for Examiner

#### Introduction

Washes hands, introduces self and confirms patient identity

Gains consent for the examination, clearly explaining to the patient the close proximity of the examination

Asks about pain

Ensures a chaperone is present

Sets up the room appropriately, by dimming the lights and consider dilating the pupils

Correctly adjusts the settings of the fundoscope

#### General Inspection

| What are you looking for or examining? | Justification | Thoughts | | | | |
|---|---|---|---|---|---|---|
| General well-being | On initial glance does the patient look well/unwell/in pain? | The patient looks well | | | | |
| Obvious clues | Look for facial asymmetry and scars (especially near the eyes) that may suggest previous ophthalmic procedures, and drooping of the eyes, which could be ptosis | No other obvious signs on inspection | | | | |
| Surroundings | Note any reading aids (glasses or magnifying glass) or use of a cane for people who are blind | The patient does not have any reading aids or a cane | | | | |

**Fundoscopy**

| What are you looking for or examining? | Justification | Thoughts | | | | | |
|---|---|---|---|---|---|---|---|
| Examine for the red eye reflex | In a normal eye, this should be present | The red eye reflex was present in the left eye but absent from the right eye | | | | | |
| Examine the optic disc | Locate the optic disc and comment on the colour, contour, size of the disc and cup size | The optic discs in both eyes were of normal colour, contour and size. Bilateral cup sizes were also within normal limits | | | | | |
| Examine the retinal vessels | Follow the course of the vessels from the optic disc towards the periphery, commenting on any colour abnormality, increased tortuosity or narrowing of the vessels | The retinal vessels on the peripheral edge of the right eye appear dark red and tortuous. Retinal vessels of the left eye appear normal | | | | | |
| Examine the macula | Comment on any deposits found in the macula, such as drusen, macular haemorrhages, pigmentation, exudates and cotton-wool spots | It is evident that on the peripheral edge of the right macula there is a large area that appears grey and opaque, which could be a sign of a detached retina | | | | | |
| Examine the peripheral retina | Comment on any retinal deposits, haemorrhages or chorioretinal atrophy | The normal choroidal pattern is also absent, suggesting a potential retinal detachment | | | | | |

**Finishing**

| | | | | | | | |
|---|---|---|---|---|---|---|---|
| Remove your gloves and wash hands | Complying with hand hygiene is vital | No additional concerns | | | | | |

**Present Your Findings**

Mr Grey is a 72-year-old man who presented with painless loss of vision in his right eye. On examination he looks comfortable at rest. Both optic discs appear normal, but the red reflex was absent from his right eye. The peripheral edge of his right eye also revealed a grey and opaque macula, with loss of normal choroidal pattern. The retinal vessels here also appeared dark red and tortuous.

I feel the most likely diagnosis is retinal detachment, with the differential diagnoses being posterior vitreous detachment, choroidal detachment or vitreous haemorrhage.

I would like to refer Mr Grey to ophthalmology urgently for a full examination using a slit lamp or indirect ophthalmoscopy, because the field of view from a direct ophthalmoscopy is too narrow to rule out a retinal detachment. I would also like to check the patient's blood pressure, serum glucose and cholesterol levels, to rule out hypertensive and diabetic retinopathy respectively

**General Points**

| | | | |
|---|---|---|---|
| Polite to patient | | | |
| Maintains good eye contact | | | |
| Clear instruction and explanation to patient | | | |
| Throughout the examination, uses the correct hand to hold the ophthalmoscope (depending on which of the patient's eyes is being examined) | | | |

## ❓ QUESTIONS FROM THE EXAMINER

**Give three examples of topical eyedrops that are used for pupillary dilation.**

These include tropicamide, cyclopentolate, phenylephrine, atropine and adrenaline.

**Which two muscles control pupil size?**

The sphincter pupillae and the dilator pupillae muscles control the size of the pupil. When the sphincter pupillae contract, the pupil constricts and when the dilator pupillae contract, the pupil dilates.

**What are the different indications for using the cobalt blue filter and the red-free filter?**

The cobalt blue filter is usually used to look for corneal abrasions or ulcers after application of fluorescein dye, whereas the red-free filter looks at the centre of the macula and other blood vessels in more detail.

**What is a gonioscopy used for?**

It is an instrument that is used to measure the drainage angle between the iris and the cornea.

**Name three potential causes of a painless red eye.**

A painless red eye could be caused by conjunctivitis, subconjunctival haemorrhage, episcleritis and dry eyes.

**Name three potential causes of a painful red eye.**

A painful red eye could be caused by scleritis, uveitis, corneal abrasion, corneal ulcer, acute angle closure glaucoma (AACG) and foreign bodies.

**Name two causes of an absent red reflex in adult and children respectively.**

Absence of the red reflex in adults can be due to cataracts, vitreous haemorrhage or retinal detachment. Absence of the red reflex in children can be due to congenital cataracts, retinal detachment, vitreous haemorrhage or retinoblastoma.

**What is the primary surgical treatment for proliferative diabetic retinopathy?**

Proliferative diabetic retinopathy can be treated surgically via panretinal photocoagulation.

**What is the blood supply to the optic nerve?**

The optic nerve is supplied by the internal carotid artery, posterior ciliary arteries and the central retinal artery.

**How many layers does the retina have and what are their names?**

The retina is organised into three primary layers, including the photoreceptive layer, the bipolar cell layer and the ganglion cell layer.

# Prescribing

## Outline

## Station 11.1    Acute Left Ventricular Failure

### Doctor Briefing

You are the junior doctor covering a cardiology ward overnight. The nurses fast bleep you to see John Smith, an 85-year-old man, who has become acutely breathless and is coughing up frothy pink sputum. An echocardiogram performed on this admission showed severe left ventricular dysfunction. He had been written up for intravenous (IV) fluids overnight (1 L IV sodium chloride 0.9% over 8 h), since he was deemed to be dehydrated. You have made a presumptive diagnosis of acute left ventricular failure. Please formulate an appropriate management plan and complete the drug chart provided, including the prescription of fluids, regular, as required (PRN) and once-only medications, as appropriate.

### Patient Briefing

You came into hospital 2 days ago because you are waiting to get your pacemaker fitted, which you should be getting tomorrow. You've been asked not to eat or drink anything, but you are thirsty and dehydrated; therefore one of the doctors prescribed you some fluids through your veins.

About 1 h ago, you sudden became very short of breath. Then you started coughing. Fifteen minutes ago, you brought up some frothy pink sputum, so you alerted one of the nurses. Your breathing is getting progressively worse, and you have to prop yourself up to be able to catch your breath.

You are really scared because it feels like you are drowning, and you are worried that you are going to die.

### Patient Details

| Name | John Smith |
|---|---|
| Date of birth | 12/02/1937 |
| Hospital number | 1202350034 |
| Weight | 75 kg |
| Height | 1.82 m |
| Consultant | CAP |
| Hospital/ward | WGH/53 |

| Current medications | Ramipril 5 mg twice a day (BD)<br>Spironolactone 100 mg once a day (OD)<br>Memantine 5 mg OD<br>Paracetamol 1 g four times a day (QDS)<br>Lansoprazole 15 mg OD<br>Glyceryl trinitrate (GTN) 2 puffs PRN |
|---|---|
| Allergies | None |
| Admission date | 11/05/2019 |

## Mark Scheme for Examiner

### Completing the Drug Chart

| Drug Chart Task | Justification | | | | | |
|---|---|---|---|---|---|---|
| Correctly writes patient information:<br>• Name<br>• Date of birth<br>• Hospital number<br>• Weight<br>• Age<br>• Consultant<br>• Ward<br>• Admission date | This is part of vital routine hospital documentation. Weight is important, and several medications require a current weight to calculate dosage | | | | | |
| Completes allergy box, including signing and dating | No medication should be prescribed until you know the patient's allergies | | | | | |
| Prescribes correctly appropriate oxygen therapy:<br>• Drug name<br>• Route<br>• Target saturations | It is important to prescribe oxygen to ensure that it is being used correctly. Prescribe high-flow oxygen via 60% Venturi mask, to maintain saturations at 94–98% | | | | | |
| Stops the IV fluids | The IV infusion has very likely precipitated the onset of acute heart failure secondary to fluid overload. You must remember to treat the underlying cause | | | | | |
| Prescribes correctly appropriate diuretic:<br>• Drug name<br>• Route<br>• Dose | Prescribe loop diuretic IV; for example, furosemide 40 mg. Later you need to consider inserting a urinary catheter to monitor fluid input and output strictly | | | | | |
| Prescribes correctly appropriate analgesia:<br>• Route<br>• Dose | In this case, it would be appropriate to prescribe morphine 1–10 mg IV and GTN spray. If morphine is prescribed, then also prescribe an antiemetic, for example, metoclopramide, as nausea and vomiting are common side effects | | | | | |
| Prescribes correctly regular medications | The person admitting the patient into hospital should be responsible for prescribing all the patient's regular medication and checking it is appropriate for him to continue to take them | | | | | |
| Considers venous thromboembolism (VTE) prophylaxis | Choice of VTE prophylaxis can vary based on patient factors and local trust guidelines | | | | | |

## General Points

Polite to patient

Clear, legible writing on the drug chart using black ink

## Correct Prescription Chart

Name: John Smith

Date of birth: 12/02/1935

Hospital number: 1202350034

Weight: 75 kg

Age: 85 years

Consultant: CAP

Known allergies:
No known drug allergies

Signature: Date:
C. Price    11/05/19
C. PRICE

## Once-Only Medications

| Date | Time | Medicine (Approved Name) | Dose | Route | Prescriber – Sign and Print | Time Given | Given By |
|------|------|--------------------------|------|-------|-----------------------------|------------|----------|
| 11/05/19 | 2000 | Furosemide | 40 mg | IV | C. Price  C. PRICE | | |
| 11/05/19 | 2000 | GTN spray | 2 puffs | Sublingual | C. Price  C. PRICE | | |
| 11/05/19 | 2000 | Morphine (titrate to pain) | 1–10 mg | IV | C. Price  C. PRICE | | |
| 11/05/19 | 2000 | Metoclopramide | 10 mg | IV | C. Price  C. PRICE | | |

| Start | | Route | | | | Stop | |
|-------|--|-------|--|--|--|------|--|
| Date | Time | Mask (%) | Prongs (L/min) | Prescriber – Sign and Print | Administered by | Date | Time |
| 11/05/19 | 2000 | Venturi (60) | | C. Price  C PRICE | | | |

## Venous Thromboembolism Prophylaxis

VTE Risk Assessment:

Yes [ ]

Prophylaxis not required [ ]

Contraindicated [X]

Comment:

Hold until medical review tomorrow

Signature: C. Price  C. PRICE

Date: 12/09/19

| | Date: → Time: ↓ | | | | | | | |
|--|--|--|--|--|--|--|--|--|
| Drug: | | | | | | | | |
| Dose:  Freq:  Route: | | | | | | | | |
| Start:  Stop/review: | | | | | | | | |
| Signature: | | | | | | | | |

## Regular Medications

| | | | Date: → Time: ↓ | | | | | | | | | |
|---|---|---|---|---|---|---|---|---|---|---|---|---|
| Drug: Ramipril | | | 02 | | | | | | | | | |
| Dose: 5 mg | Freq: BD | Route: Oral | 06 | | | | | | | | | |
| | | | ⑩ | | | | | | | | | |
| Start: 12/09/19 | Stop/review: | | ⑭ | | | | | | | | | |
| Signature: C. Price C. PRICE | | | 18 | | | | | | | | | |
| Indication: Hypertension | | | 22 | | | | | | | | | |
| Drug: Spironolactone | | | 02 | | | | | | | | | |
| Dose: 100 mg | Freq: OD | Route: Oral | ⑥ | | | | | | | | | |
| | | | 10 | | | | | | | | | |
| Start: 12/09/19 | Stop/review: | | 14 | | | | | | | | | |
| Signature: C. Price C. PRICE | | | 18 | | | | | | | | | |
| Indication: Ascites | | | 22 | | | | | | | | | |
| Drug: Memantine | | | 02 | | | | | | | | | |
| Dose: 5 mg | Freq: OD | Route: Oral | ⑥ | | | | | | | | | |
| | | | 10 | | | | | | | | | |
| Start: 12/09/19 | Stop/review: | | 14 | | | | | | | | | |
| Signature: C. Price C. PRICE | | | 18 | | | | | | | | | |
| Indication: Dementia | | | 22 | | | | | | | | | |

## Regular Medications

| | | | Date: → | | | | | | | | | | |
|---|---|---|---|---|---|---|---|---|---|---|---|---|---|
| | | | Time: ↓ | | | | | | | | | | |
| Drug: Paracetamol | | | 02 | | | | | | | | | | |
| Dose: 1 g | Freq: QDS | Route: Oral | (06) | | | | | | | | | | |
| | | | (12) | | | | | | | | | | |
| Start: 12/09/19 | Stop/review: | | 14 | | | | | | | | | | |
| Signature: C. Price  C. PRICE | | | (18) | | | | | | | | | | |
| Indication: Back pain | | | (24) | | | | | | | | | | |
| Drug: Lansoprazole | | | 02 | | | | | | | | | | |
| Dose: 15 mg | Freq: OD | Route: Oral | 06 | | | | | | | | | | |
| | | | (10) | | | | | | | | | | |
| Start: 12/09/19 | Stop/review: | | 14 | | | | | | | | | | |
| Signature: C. Price  C. PRICE | | | 18 | | | | | | | | | | |
| Indication: Duodenal ulcer | | | 22 | | | | | | | | | | |

## PRN Medications

| | | | Date: → | | | | | | | | | | |
|---|---|---|---|---|---|---|---|---|---|---|---|---|---|
| | | | Time: ↓ | | | | | | | | | | |
| Drug: Glyceryl trinitrate | | | | | | | | | | | | | |
| Dose: 2 puffs | Freq: PRN | Route: SC | | | | | | | | | | | |
| | | | | | | | | | | | | | |
| Start: 11/05/19 | Stop/review: | | | | | | | | | | | | |
| Signature: C. Price  C. PRICE | | | | | | | | | | | | | |
| Indication: Angina | | | | | | | | | | | | | |

## Fluid Prescriptions

| Date | Fluid | Additive | Volume | Route | Rate | Signature | Given | Batch |
|------|-------|----------|--------|-------|------|-----------|-------|-------|
| 12/09/19 | 0.9% Sodium chloride | None | 1 L | IV | Over 8 h | C. Price  C. PRICE | STOPPED DUE TO FLUID OVERLOAD 12/09/19 C. Price (C. PRICE) | |

## ❓ QUESTIONS FROM THE EXAMINER

### What are the STOPP criteria?

STOPP stands for Screening Tool of Older Persons' potentially inappropriate Prescriptions. These are criteria used to review medication regimes in elderly patients, with the aim of reducing the incidence of medication-related adverse events from polypharmacy and inappropriate prescribing.

### What are the START criteria?

START stands for Screening Tool to Alert doctors to the Right Treatment. They are similar to the STOPP criteria, in that it is also a tool used to review medication regimes in elderly people.

### What is the PRISCUS list?

It is a list of medications that carry an increased risk of side effects when given to elderly patients.

### What is the site of action of loop diuretics and what is their mechanism of action?

They are antagonists of sodium/chloride/potassium co-transporters, which are located in the thick ascending limb of the loop of Henle in the renal tubule.

### How many types of diuretics are there and what are they?

Typically, diuretics are divided into three groups – loop diuretics, thiazide diuretics and potassium-sparing diuretics.

### What are Kerley B lines seen on a chest X-ray and what do they indicate?

Kerley B lines are horizontal lines seen in the periphery of the lungs, usually at the lung bases. They are perpendicular to the pleural surface and extend out to it. If seen, they suggest thickened subpleural interlobar septa, often due to pulmonary oedema.

### What is Cheyne–Stokes respiration?

It is an abnormal pattern of breathing, characterised by episodes of apnoea or periods of paused breathing.

### Describe what the hepatojugular reflex is and name some causes.

Hepatojugular reflex is distension of the neck veins, due to a firm pressure applied over the liver. It can be present in heart failure, cardiac tamponade, tricuspid regurgitation and constrictive pericarditis.

### Why should angiotensin-converting enzyme (ACE) inhibitors be avoided in pregnancy?

They can adversely affect fetal and neonatal blood pressure control and renal function. There have also been reports of skull defects and oligohydramnios.

### Name three main causes of heart failure.

Coronary heart disease, hypertension, cardiomyopathy, arrhythmias, heart valve disease, endocrinology problems (such as diabetes or hyperthyroidism) and congenital heart disease.

## Station 11.2   Acute Myocardial Infarction

### Doctor Briefing

You are the junior doctor covering the acute receiving unit overnight. The nurses fast bleep you to see Perry Terrant, an 80-year-old man, who has been admitted with acute severe chest pain. You have made a presumptive diagnosis of acute myocardial infarction. Please formulate an appropriate management plan and complete the drug chart provided, including the prescription of fluids, regular, PRN and once-only medications as appropriate.

### Patient Briefing

You have come into hospital because at midday you started experiencing severe central chest pain. It feels like a heavy weight has been placed on your chest and you are also finding it slightly difficult to breathe. You are feeling a bit nauseous but have not vomited.

An electrocardiogram (ECG) has been performed; your doctor says it has shown that you are having a heart attack, and therefore you need to be commenced on some medications.

You are really worried that you are going to die from this heart attack and the pain is getting worse; you judge the severity to be 10/10.

### Patient Details

| Name | Perry Terrant |
|---|---|
| Date of birth | 12/03/1940 |
| Hospital number | 1203408558 |
| Weight | 85 kg |
| Height | 1.75 m |
| Consultant | CAP |
| Hospital/ward | WGH/54 |
| Current medications | Allopurinol 100 mg OD<br>Amlodipine 5 mg OD<br>Esomeprazole 20 mg OD<br>Gliclazide 30 mg OD<br>Alendronic acid 10 mg OD<br>Citalopram 10 mg OD<br>Co-careldopa 25/100 mg three times a day (TDS) |
| Allergies | Penicillin (rash) |
| Admission date | 03/10/2019 |

### Mark Scheme for Examiner

#### Completing the Drug Chart

| Drug Chart Task | Justification | | | | | |
|---|---|---|---|---|---|---|
| Correctly writes patient information:<br>• Name<br>• Date of birth<br>• Hospital number<br>• Weight<br>• Age<br>• Consultant<br>• Ward<br>• Admission date | This is part of vital routine hospital documentation. Weight is important and several medications require a current weight to calculate dosage | | | | | |

## Completing the Drug Chart

| Drug Chart Task | Justification | | | | | |
|---|---|---|---|---|---|---|
| Completes allergy box, including signing and dating | No medication should be prescribed until you know the patient's allergies | | | | | |
| Prescribes correctly appropriate oxygen therapy:<br>• Route<br>• Target saturations | It is important to prescribe oxygen to ensure that it is being used correctly. Prescribe high-flow oxygen via 60% Venturi mask, to maintain saturations at 94–98% | | | | | |
| Prescribes correctly appropriate analgesia:<br>• Drug name<br>• Route<br>• Dose | The patient is in severe pain and requires immediate analgesia. Start with morphine 2.5–10 mg IV initially, then titrate to pain. If morphine is prescribed, then also prescribe an antiemetic, for example, metoclopramide, as nausea and vomiting are common side effects | | | | | |
| Prescribes antiplatelet therapy | Prescribe a loading dose of aspirin 300 mg to be chewed, and another antiplatelet such as clopidogrel 300 mg, ticagrelor 180 mg or prasugrel 60 mg (depending on local guidelines) | | | | | |
| Prescribes nitrate | This is typically prescribed as a GTN sublingual spray. If chest pain persists, consider a nitrate infusion | | | | | |
| Prescribes correctly regular medications:<br>• Drug name<br>• Route<br>• Dose<br>• Frequency and timing<br>• Start dates (and review dates if applicable) | The person admitting the patient into hospital should be responsible for prescribing all the patient's regular medication and checking it is appropriate for him to continue to take them | | | | | |
| Considers VTE prophylaxis | Choice of VTE prophylaxis can vary based on patient factors and local trust guidelines | | | | | |

## General Points

| | | | | | | |
|---|---|---|---|---|---|---|
| Polite to patient | | | | | | |
| Clear, legible writing on the drug chart using black ink | | | | | | |

## Correct Prescription Chart

Name: Perry Terrant

Weight: 75 kg

Known allergies:
No known drug allergies

Date of birth: 12/03/1940

Age: 80 years

Hospital number: 1203408558

Consultant: CAP

Signature: Date:
C. Pratt    03/10/19
C. PRATT

## Once-Only Medications

| Date | Time | Medicine (Approved Name) | Dose | Route | Prescriber – Sign and Print | Time Given | Given By |
|------|------|--------------------------|------|-------|------------------------------|------------|----------|
| 03/10/19 | 2200 | Aspirin | 300 mg | Oral | *C. Pratt*<br>C. PRATT | | |
| 03/10/19 | 2200 | Clopidogrel | 300 mg | Oral | *C. Pratt*<br>C. PRATT | | |
| 03/10/19 | 2200 | GTN spray | 2 puffs | Sublingual | *C. Pratt*<br>C. PRATT | | |
| 03/10/19 | 2200 | Morphine (titrate to pain) | 1–10 mg | IV | *C. Pratt*<br>C. PRATT | | |
| 03/10/19 | 2200 | Ondansetron | 4 mg | IV | *C. Pratt*<br>C. PRATT | | |

## Oxygen Therapy

| Start | | | Route | | | Stop | |
|-------|------|----------|--------------|------------------------------|-----------------|------|------|
| Date | Time | Mask (%) | Prongs (L/min) | Prescriber – Sign and Print | Administered by | Date | Time |
| 03/10/19 | 2200 | Venturi (60) | | *C. Pratt*<br>C. PRATT | | | |

## Venous Thromboembolism Prophylaxis

| VTE Risk Assessment: | Comment: |
|---|---|
| Yes [ ] | Hold until medical review tomorrow |
| Prophylaxis not required [ ] | Signature: *C. Pratt* C. PRATT |
| Contraindicated [X] | Date: 03/10/19 |

| | Date: → Time: ↓ | | | | | | | |
|---|---|---|---|---|---|---|---|---|
| **Drug:** | | | | | | | | |
| **Dose:** **Freq:** **Route:** | | | | | | | | |
| | | | | | | | | |
| **Start:** **Stop/review:** | | | | | | | | |
| **Signature:** | | | | | | | | |

## Regular Medications

| | Date: → Time: ↓ | | | | | | | | | | | |
|---|---|---|---|---|---|---|---|---|---|---|---|---|
| Drug: Allopurinol | 02 | | | | | | | | | | | |
| Dose: 100 mg   Freq: OD   Route: Oral | 06 | | | | | | | | | | | |
| | ⑩ | | | | | | | | | | | |
| Start: 03/10/19   Stop/review: | 14 | | | | | | | | | | | |
| Signature: C. Pratt  C. PRATT | 18 | | | | | | | | | | | |
| Indication: Gout prophylaxis | 22 | | | | | | | | | | | |
| Drug: Amlodipine | 02 | | | | | | | | | | | |
| Dose: 5 mg   Freq: OD   Route: Oral | 06 | | | | | | | | | | | |
| | ⑩ | | | | | | | | | | | |
| Start: 03/10/19   Stop/review: | 14 | | | | | | | | | | | |
| Signature: C. Pratt  C. PRATT | 18 | | | | | | | | | | | |
| Indication: Hypertension | 22 | | | | | | | | | | | |
| Drug: Esomeprazole | 02 | | | | | | | | | | | |
| Dose: 20 mg   Freq: OD   Route: Oral | 06 | | | | | | | | | | | |
| | ⑩ | | | | | | | | | | | |
| Start: 03/10/19   Stop/review: | 14 | | | | | | | | | | | |
| Signature: C. Pratt  C. PRATT | 18 | | | | | | | | | | | |
| Indication: Peptic ulcer disease | 22 | | | | | | | | | | | |

## Regular Medications

| | | Date: → | | | | | | | | | | | | | |
|---|---|---|---|---|---|---|---|---|---|---|---|---|---|---|---|
| | | Time: ↓ | | | | | | | | | | | | | |
| Drug: *Gliclazide* | | 02 | | | | | | | | | | | | | |
| Dose: 30 mg | Freq: OD | Route: Oral | 06 | | | | | | | | | | | | | |
| | | | ⑩ | | | | | | | | | | | | | |
| Start: 03/10/19 | Stop/review: | 14 | | | | | | | | | | | | | |
| Signature: *C. Pratt* C. PRATT | | 18 | | | | | | | | | | | | | |
| Indication: *Diabetes* | | 22 | | | | | | | | | | | | | |
| Drug: *Alendronic acid* | | 02 | | | | | | | | | | | | | |
| Dose: 10 mg | Freq: OD | Route: Oral | 06 | | | | | | | | | | | | | |
| | | | ⑩ | | | | | | | | | | | | | |
| Start: 03/10/19 | Stop/review: | 14 | | | | | | | | | | | | | |
| Signature: *C. Pratt* C. PRATT | | 18 | | | | | | | | | | | | | |
| Indication: *Osteoporosis* | | 22 | | | | | | | | | | | | | |
| Drug: *Citalopram* | | 02 | | | | | | | | | | | | | |
| Dose: 10 mg | Freq: OD | Route: Oral | 06 | | | | | | | | | | | | | |
| | | | ⑩ | | | | | | | | | | | | | |
| Start: 03/10/19 | Stop/review: | 14 | | | | | | | | | | | | | |
| Signature: *C. Pratt* C. PRATT | | 18 | | | | | | | | | | | | | |
| Indication: *Depression* | | 22 | | | | | | | | | | | | | |

## Regular Medications

| | | | Date: → | | | | | | | | | | | |
|---|---|---|---|---|---|---|---|---|---|---|---|---|---|---|
| | | | Time: ↓ | | | | | | | | | | | |
| Drug: Co-careldopa | | | ⦿02 | | | | | | | | | | | |
| Dose: 25/100 mg | Freq: TDS | Route: Oral | ⦿06 | | | | | | | | | | | |
| | | | 10 | | | | | | | | | | | |
| Start: 03/10/19 | Stop/review: | | ⦿14 | | | | | | | | | | | |
| Signature: C. Pratt C. PRATT | | | 18 | | | | | | | | | | | |
| Indication: Parkinson's disease | | | ⦿22 | | | | | | | | | | | |

## PRN Medications

| | | | Date: → | | | | | | | | | | | |
|---|---|---|---|---|---|---|---|---|---|---|---|---|---|---|
| | | | Time: ↓ | | | | | | | | | | | |
| Drug: Glyceryl trinitrate | | | | | | | | | | | | | | |
| Dose: 2 puffs | Freq: PRN | Route: SC | | | | | | | | | | | | |
| Start: 11/05/19 | Stop/review: | | | | | | | | | | | | | |
| Signature: C. Price C PRICE | | | | | | | | | | | | | | |
| Indication: Angina | | | | | | | | | | | | | | |
| Drug: Morphine | | | | | | | | | | | | | | |
| Dose: 1–10 mg | Freq: PRN | Route: IV | | | | | | | | | | | | |
| Start: 11/05/19 | Stop/review: | | | | | | | | | | | | | |
| Signature: C. Price C. PRICE | | | | | | | | | | | | | | |
| Indication: Angina | | | | | | | | | | | | | | |

## ? QUESTIONS FROM THE EXAMINER

### What does DAPT stand for and when is it typically used?

DAPT stands for dual antiplatelet therapy, which is often used for secondary prevention of coronary artery disease.

### What are the precursors to platelets?

They are derived from megakaryocytes in the bone marrow.

### How do P2Y12 inhibitors prevent platelet aggregation?

They prevent binding of adenosine diphosphate to a certain platelet receptor, which then inhibits activation of the glycoprotein IIb–IIIa complex, therefore preventing platelet aggregation.

### What is the drug action of ondansetron?

It is a specific $5HT_3$-receptor antagonist that blocks $5HT_3$ receptors in the intestinal tract and in the central nervous system.

### Why should ondansetron be avoided in the first trimester of pregnancy?

Ondansetron use during the first trimester is associated with a small increased risk of congenital abnormalities such as orofacial clefts.

### What is the principal pharmacological action of GTN?

It is a vasodilating agent and activates relaxation of vascular smooth muscle, therefore leading to dilation of both arterial and venous beds.

### Define drug absorption.

It is transportation of the unmetabolized drug from the site of administration to the body circulation system. This can happen through passive (most common), active and facilitated diffusion.

### Define drug distribution.

It is the disbursement of an unmetabolised drug as it moves through the body's blood and tissues.

### What are Beers criteria?

These were developed by the American Geriatric Society, with the aim of improving outcomes in the care of older adults > 65 years of age, designed to reduce older adults' drug-related problems, such as exposure to inappropriate medications.

### If a new left bundle branch block is seen on an ECG, which coronary arteries have been affected?

A new left bundle branch block due to ischaemia is the result of an occluded proximal left anterior descending artery or the left main artery.

## Station 11.3    Exacerbation of Chronic Obstructive Pulmonary Disease (COPD)

### Doctor Briefing

You are the junior doctor working in acute medical admissions and are asked to see Mary Finn, a 78-year-old woman with a history of COPD, who is currently breathless. She normally controls her COPD with inhalers alone and has no home nebulisers or long-term oxygen therapy. She also reports a worsening cough productive of green sputum. The patient is acutely dyspnoeic with an audible wheeze and some use of accessory muscles. The nurses are concerned about carbon dioxide retention and so have given oxygen at 2 L/min via nasal cannulae. You have made a presumptive diagnosis of exacerbation of COPD. Please formulate an appropriate management plan and complete the drug chart provided, including the prescription of fluids, regular, PRN and once-only medications as appropriate.

### Patient Briefing

You have been brought into hospital by your daughter as you are very breathless and unable to walk as far as usual. You are coughing more than usual and producing green sputum. You usually control your COPD with inhalers alone and have no home nebulisers or long-term oxygen therapy. You are finding it difficult to breathe and have been using the pursed-lip breathing you were taught by your doctor. You noticed an audible wheeze yesterday.

On questioning you still smoke around 10 cigarettes a day despite cutting down and trying to quit.

You are concerned you have pneumonia and are worried that you are currently unable to look after yourself while ill.

### Patient Details

| | |
|---|---|
| Name | Mary Finn |
| Date of birth | 12/05/1942 |
| Hospital number | 1205427431 |
| Weight | 65 kg |
| Height | 1.72 m |
| Consultant | RE |
| Hospital/ward | NGH/18 |
| Current medications | Seretide 250 inhaler 2 puffs BD<br>Salbutamol inhaler 2 puffs PRN<br>Levothyroxine 50 mcg OD<br>Allopurinol 100 mg OD<br>Omeprazole 20 mg OD |
| Allergies | Ibuprofen (peptic ulcer) |
| Admission date | 12/09/2019 |

### Mark Scheme for Examiner

#### Completing the Drug Chart

| Drug Chart Task | Justification | | | | |
|---|---|---|---|---|---|
| Correctly writes patient information:<br>• Name<br>• Date of birth<br>• Hospital number<br>• Weight<br>• Age<br>• Consultant<br>• Ward<br>• Admission date | This is part of vital routine hospital documentation. Weight is important and several medications require a current weight to calculate dosage | | | | |

## Completing the Drug Chart

| Drug Chart Task | Justification | | | | | |
|---|---|---|---|---|---|---|
| Completes allergy box, including signing and dating | No medication should be prescribed until you know the patient's allergies | | | | | |
| Prescribes correctly appropriate oxygen therapy:<br>• Route<br>• Target saturations | If the patient has oxygen saturations <88%, then begin oxygen therapy, aiming for oxygen saturations at 88–92%. Deliver using a Venturi mask corresponding to the flow rate of oxygen required | | | | | |
| Prescribes correctly appropriate bronchodilators:<br>• Drug name<br>• Route<br>• Dose<br>• Considers oxygen or air-driven nebuliser | Deliver nebulised salbutamol (5 mg/4 h) and ipratropium (500 mcg/6 h) | | | | | |
| Prescribes correctly appropriate steroid treatment:<br>• Drug name<br>• Route<br>• Dose | Prescribe IV hydrocortisone 200 mg and oral prednisolone 30 mg. Patients should continue treatment for 7–14 days | | | | | |
| Prescribes correctly appropriate antibiotics:<br>• Drug name<br>• Route<br>• Dose<br>• Considers allergies<br>• Considers if stat dose is required | Antibiotic choice varies according to local policy and depending on the patient's allergies. Check if the patient has already taken a course of antibiotics for the current infection and consider cultures | | | | | |
| Prescribes correctly appropriate fluid | Patients with hypovolaemia, such as patients with sepsis, require IV fluids. Consider prescribing fluids as infection is indicated. It is important to exclude heart failure as the cause of dyspnoea before prescribing fluids | | | | | |
| Prescribes correctly regular medications:<br>• Drug name<br>• Route<br>• Dose<br>• Frequency and timing<br>• Start dates (and review dates if applicable) | The person admitting the patient into hospital should be responsible for prescribing all the patient's regular medication and checking it is appropriate for her to continue to take them. Ensure regular inhalers are withheld while the patient is on nebulisers | | | | | |
| Considers treatment options if there is no response to initial treatment | IV aminophylline may be used if the patient does not respond to nebulisers and steroids. A dose of 500 mcg/kg/h should be delivered following a loading dose of 250 mg over 20 min | | | | | |
| Considers VTE prophylaxis | Choice of VTE prophylaxis can vary based on patient factors and local trust guidelines | | | | | |

## General Points

| | | | | | | |
|---|---|---|---|---|---|---|
| Polite to patient | | | | | | |
| Clear, legible writing on the drug chart using black ink | | | | | | |

## Correct Prescription Chart

Name: Mary Finn

Date of birth: 12/05/1942

Hospital number: 1205427431

Weight: 65 kg

Age: 78 years

Consultant: RE

Known allergies:
Ibuprofen (respiratory distress)

Signature:    Date:
R. Edmond    12/09/19
R. EDMOND

## Once-Only Medications

| Date | Time | Medicine (Approved Name) | Dose | Route | Prescriber – Sign and Print | Time Given | Given By |
|---|---|---|---|---|---|---|---|
| 12/09/19 | 1600 | Salbutamol (driven with oxygen) | 5 mg | Neb | R. Edmond R. EDMOND | | |
| 12/09/19 | 1600 | Ipratropium bromide (driven with oxygen) | 500 mg | Neb | R. Edmond R. EDMOND | | |
| 12/09/19 | 1645 | Amoxicillin | 500 mg | Oral | R. Edmond R. EDMOND | | |
| 12/09/19 | 1645 | Prednisolone | 30 mg | Oral | R. Edmond R. EDMOND | | |
| 12/09/19 | 1800 | Enoxaparin | 20 mg | SC | R. Edmond R. EDMOND | | |

## Oxygen Therapy

| Start | | Route | | | | Stop | |
|---|---|---|---|---|---|---|---|
| Date | Time | Mask (%) | Prongs (L/min) | Prescriber – Sign and Print | Administered by | Date | Time |
| 12/09/19 | 1600 | Venturi (60) | | R. Edmond R. EDMOND | | | |

## Venous Thromboembolism Prophylaxis

| VTE Risk Assessment: | Comment: |
|---|---|
| Yes [X] | Signature: R. Edmond  R. EDMOND |
| Prophylaxis not required [ ] | Date: 12/09/19 |
| Contraindicated [ ] | |

| | Date: → Time: ↓ | | | | | | | |
|---|---|---|---|---|---|---|---|---|
| Drug: Enoxaparin | | | | | | | | |
| Dose: 20 mg | Freq: OD | Route: SC | | | | | | |
| Start: 13/09/19 | Stop/review: | | | | | | | |
| Signature: R. Edmond R. EDMOND | | | | | | | | |

## Regular Medications

| | | Date: → | | | | | | | | | | | | |
|---|---|---|---|---|---|---|---|---|---|---|---|---|---|---|
| | | Time: ↓ | | | | | | | | | | | | |
| Drug: Seretide 250 (salmeterol 25 micrograms/fluticasone 250 micrograms) | | 02 | | | | | | | | | | | | |
| Dose: 2 puffs | Freq: BD | Route: Inh | (06) | | | | | | | | | | | |
| | | | 10 | | | | | | | | | | | |
| Start: 12/09/19 | Stop/review: | | (14) | | | | | | | | | | | |
| Signature: R. Edmond R. EDMOND | | 18 | | | | | | | | | | | | |
| Indication: COPD | | 22 | | | | | | | | | | | | |
| Drug: Levothyroxine | | 02 | | | | | | | | | | | | |
| Dose: 50 mcg | Freq: OD | Route: Oral | (06) | | | | | | | | | | | |
| | | | 10 | | | | | | | | | | | |
| Start: 12/09/19 | Stop/review: | | 14 | | | | | | | | | | | |
| Signature: R. Edmond R. EDMOND | | 18 | | | | | | | | | | | | |
| Indication: Hypothyroidism | | 22 | | | | | | | | | | | | |
| Drug: Allopurinol | | 02 | | | | | | | | | | | | |
| Dose: 100 mg | Freq: OD | Route: Oral | 06 | | | | | | | | | | | |
| | | | (10) | | | | | | | | | | | |
| Start: 12/09/19 | Stop/review: | | 14 | | | | | | | | | | | |
| Signature: R. Edmond R. EDMOND | | 18 | | | | | | | | | | | | |
| Indication: Gout prophylaxis | | 22 | | | | | | | | | | | | |

**Regular Medications**

| | | | Date: → | | | | | | | | | | | |
|---|---|---|---|---|---|---|---|---|---|---|---|---|---|---|
| | | | Time: ↓ | | | | | | | | | | | |
| Drug: Omeprazole | | | 02 | | | | | | | | | | | |
| Dose: 20 mg | Freq: OD | Route: Oral | 06 | | | | | | | | | | | |
| | | | (10) | | | | | | | | | | | |
| Start: 12/09/19 | Stop/review: | | 14 | | | | | | | | | | | |
| Signature: R. Edmond R. EDMOND | | | 18 | | | | | | | | | | | |
| Indication: Gastro-oesophageal reflux disease | | | 22 | | | | | | | | | | | |
| Drug: Amoxicillin | | | 02 | | | | | | | | | | | |
| Dose: 500 mg | Freq: TDS | Route: Oral | (06) | | | | | | | | | | | |
| | | | 10 | | | | | | | | | | | |
| Start: 12/09/19 | Stop/review: | | (14) | | | | | | | | | | | |
| Signature: R. Edmond R. EDMOND | | | 18 | | | | | | | | | | | |
| Indication: COPD exacerbation | | | (22) | | | | | | | | | | | |
| Drug: Prednisolone | | | 02 | | | | | | | | | | | |
| Dose: 30 mg | Freq: OD | Route: Oral | 06 | | | | | | | | | | | |
| | | | (10) | | | | | | | | | | | |
| Start: 12/09/19 | Stop/review: | | 14 | | | | | | | | | | | |
| Signature: R. Edmond R. EDMOND | | | 18 | | | | | | | | | | | |
| Indication: COPD exacerbation | | | 22 | | | | | | | | | | | |

## PRN Medications

| | Date: →<br>Time: ↓ | | | | | | | | | | | | |
|---|---|---|---|---|---|---|---|---|---|---|---|---|---|
| Drug: Salbutamol | | | | | | | | | | | | | |
| Dose:<br>2 puffs | Freq:<br>PRN | Route:<br>Inh | | | | | | | | | | | |
| Start:<br>12/09/19 | Stop/review: | | | | | | | | | | | | |
| Signature:<br>R. Edmond<br>R. EDMOND | | | | | | | | | | | | | |
| Indication: COPD | | | | | | | | | | | | | |

## ? QUESTIONS FROM THE EXAMINER

### Why is oxygen delivered via Venturi mask in patients with COPD?

To allow controlled delivery of oxygen. Excessive oxygen delivery may lead to carbon dioxide retention in some COPD patients, as patients rely on hypoxia to drive breathing, leading to hypercapnic respiratory failure. Oxygen saturations should therefore be maintained at 88–92%.

### Should a doctor wait until it is known if a patient retains carbon dioxide before starting oxygen therapy?

No, hypoxia is a greater risk for patients than hypercapnia so oxygen therapy should be started in hypoxic patients. An arterial blood gas should be conducted within an hour in patients starting oxygen therapy or when there are changes in oxygen therapy.

### What percentage of oxygen delivery should be given in COPD patients without carbon dioxide retention?

28–40%. Arterial blood gas should however be repeated to monitor for carbon dioxide retention.

### What might you see on a patient that would alert you that they may have an allergy?

Across most National Health Service hospital, it is standard that patients who have allergies are given a red wrist band to wear, with the aim of reminding healthcare professionals that they have an allergy.

### What are the most common types of drug errors?

According to an investigation carried out by the General Medical Council, the most common drug errors are omission (either as an inpatient or on discharge), incorrect dosing (wrong frequency or dose) and duplication.

### Why is it important to offer smoking cessation support before prescribing home oxygen therapy?

Oxygen is highly flammable, so it is a risk to the patient to have home oxygen therapy while smoking and hence it is important to offer cessation so patients can access this therapy if required.

### How might other healthcare professionals be involved in the care of a patient with COPD?

Physiotherapists can assist in teaching techniques to clear sputum.

### Define 'drug interaction'.

It is an interaction between a drug and another substance that prevents the drug from performing as expected.

### What else should you document with the allergy status?

If patients say that they are allergic to something, you should always ask what happens when they ingest it, and document their reaction in the allergy box.

### What is important to remember when rewriting a drug chart?

It is important to file and clearly write that the new chart has been re-written (including the date) and indicate that the old chart cannot be used (for example, by drawing a big X over the pages). This is to avoid drug errors and potential duplication of medication.

## Station 11.4    Exacerbation of Asthma

### Doctor Briefing

You are the junior doctor in the medical assessment unit. The nurse asks you to see Mark McDonald, a 28-year-old male who has a background of asthma and has become breathless. You have made a presumptive diagnosis of exacerbation of asthma. Please formulate an appropriate management plan and complete the drug chart provided, including the prescription of fluids, regular, PRN and once-only medications as appropriate.

### Patient Briefing

You have known asthma, diagnosed when you were a child; your asthma has been well controlled for the last 5 years. You have felt a tightness in your chest over the past few days and have a productive cough with thick, green sputum. Your breathing has become faster and more difficult over the last 3 h, and is not resolving upon taking your salbutamol reliever inhaler. You have taken 10 puffs of your salbutamol inhaler as described in your asthma plan, but you are still straining to breathe and are unable to talk in full sentences. You can also hear an audible expiratory wheeze when you are breathing.

On specific questioning, you have one previous hospital admission relating to your asthma, which was about 2 years ago, but no previous intensive therapy unit (ITU) admissions.

You are concerned that you will need to be admitted to ITU and be put on a ventilator.

### Patient Details

| | |
|---|---|
| Name | Mark McDonald |
| Date of birth | 25/03/1992 |
| Hospital number | 2503920145 |
| Weight | 83 kg |
| Height | 1.86 m |
| Consultant | MJS |
| Hospital/ward | RIE/45 |
| Current medications | Salbutamol 2 puffs PRN |
| Allergies | Penicillin (facial swelling, breathlessness) |
| Admission date | 15/09/2019 |

### Mark Scheme for Examiner

**Completing the Drug Chart**

| Drug Chart Task | Justification | | | | | |
|---|---|---|---|---|---|---|
| Correctly writes patient information:<br>• Name<br>• Date of birth<br>• Hospital number<br>• Weight<br>• Age<br>• Consultant<br>• Ward<br>• Admission date | This is part of vital routine hospital documentation. Weight is important and several medications require a current weight to calculate dosage | | | | | |
| Completes allergy box, including signing and dating. | No medication should be prescribed until you know the patient's allergies | | | | | |

## Completing the Drug Chart

| Drug Chart Task | Justification | | | | | | |
|---|---|---|---|---|---|---|---|
| Prescribes correctly appropriate oxygen therapy:<br>• Route<br>• Target saturations | It is important to prescribe oxygen to ensure that it is being used correctly. Prescribe oxygen via a non-rebreathe bag to maintain saturations at 94–98% | | | | | | |
| Prescribes correctly appropriate bronchodilators:<br>• Drug name<br>• Route<br>• Dose<br>• Considers oxygen or air-driven nebuliser | 5 mg nebulised salbutamol (or 10 mg terbutaline) should be first-line. The nebuliser should be oxygen-driven if oxygen saturation is <94% | | | | | | |
| Prescribes correctly appropriate steroid treatment:<br>• Drug name<br>• Route<br>• Dose | Prescribe 100 mg hydrocortisone IV or 40–50 mg prednisolone orally (PO). Consider if the patient is able to swallow tablets currently. It is important to note that time for the drug to act is similar for both IV and oral administration unless the patient has gastrointestinal malabsorption | | | | | | |
| Considers the severity of the acute asthma exacerbation and considers additional therapies.<br>• Route<br>• Dose<br>• Escalation required | Consider adding nebulised ipratropium bromide 0.5 mg every 6 h in cases of severe/life-threatening exacerbations according to the National Institute for Health and Care Excellence (NICE) guidelines | | | | | | |
| Prescribes correctly appropriate analgesia:<br>• Drug name<br>• Route<br>• Dose | Following the World Health Organization (WHO) analgesia ladder, paracetamol orally should always be the first line | | | | | | |
| Prescribes correctly regular medications | The person admitting the patient into hospital should be responsible for prescribing all the patient's regular medication and checking it is appropriate for her to continue to take them. Ensure regular inhalers are withheld while the patient is on nebulisers | | | | | | |
| Considers VTE prophylaxis | Choice of VTE prophylaxis can vary based on patient factors and local trust guidelines | | | | | | |

## General Points

| | | | | | | | |
|---|---|---|---|---|---|---|---|
| Polite to patient | | | | | | | |
| Clear, legible writing on the drug chart using black ink | | | | | | | |

## Correct Prescription Chart

| Name: Mark McDonald | Weight: 83 kg | Known allergies:<br>Penicillin (facial swelling/breathlessness) |
|---|---|---|
| Date of birth: 25/03/1992 | Age: 28 years | |
| Hospital number: 2503920145 | Consultant: MJS | Signature: Date:<br>M. Slack ~ 15/09/2019<br>M. SLACK |

## Once-Only Medications

| Date | Time | Medicine (Approved Name) | Dose | Route | Prescriber – Sign and Print | Time Given | Given By |
|------|------|--------------------------|------|-------|------------------------------|------------|----------|
| 15/09/19 | 1100 | Salbutamol (driven with oxygen) | 5 mg | Neb | M. Slack<br>M. SLACK | | |
| 15/09/19 | 1100 | Prednisolone | 40 mg | Oral | M. Slack<br>M. SLACK | | |
| 15/09/19 | 1115 | Ipratropium (driven with oxygen) | 250 micrograms | Neb | M. Slack<br>M. SLACK | | |

## Oxygen Therapy

| Start | | | | Route | | Stop | |
|-------|--|--|--|-------|--|------|--|
| Date | Time | Mask (%) | Prongs (L/min) | Prescriber – Sign and Print | Administered by | Date | Time |
| 15/09/19 | 1100 | Non-rebreathe mask | 15 L/min | M. Slack<br>M. SLACK | | | |

## Venous Thromboembolism Prophylaxis

| VTE Risk Assessment: | Comment: |
|----------------------|----------|
| Yes [X] | Review on ward round |
| Prophylaxis not required [ ] | Signature: M. Slack  M. SLACK |
| Contraindicated [ ] | Date: 15/09/19 |

| | Date: →<br>Time: ↓ | | | | | | | |
|--|--|--|--|--|--|--|--|--|
| Drug: Enoxaparin | | | | | | | | |
| Dose:<br>20 mg | Freq:<br>OD | Route:<br>SC | | | | | | |
| Start:<br>15/09/19 | Stop/review: | | | | | | | |
| Signature:<br>M. Slack<br>M. SLACK | | | | | | | | |

## Regular Medications

| | Date: → | | | | | | | | | |
|---|---|---|---|---|---|---|---|---|---|---|
| | Time: ↓ | | | | | | | | | |
| Drug: Prednisolone | 02 | | | | | | | | | |
| Dose: 40 mg   Freq: OD   Route: Oral | 06 | | | | | | | | | |
| | ⑩ | | | | | | | | | |
| Start: 15/09/19   Stop/review: | 14 | | | | | | | | | |
| Signature: M. Slack   M. SLACK | 18 | | | | | | | | | |
| Indication: Asthma | 22 | | | | | | | | | |
| Drug: Ipratropium | 02 | | | | | | | | | |
| Dose: 250 micrograms   Freq: TDS   Route: Neb | ⑥ | | | | | | | | | |
| | 10 | | | | | | | | | |
| Start: 15/09/19   Stop/review: | ⑭ | | | | | | | | | |
| Signature: M. Slack   M. SLACK | 18 | | | | | | | | | |
| Indication: Asthma | ㉒ | | | | | | | | | |

## PRN Medications

| | Date: → | | | | | | | | | |
|---|---|---|---|---|---|---|---|---|---|---|
| | Time: ↓ | | | | | | | | | |
| Drug: Salbutamol | | | | | | | | | | |
| Dose: 2 puffs   Freq: PRN   Route: Inh | | | | | | | | | | |
| | | | | | | | | | | |
| Start: 12/09/19   Stop/review: | | | | | | | | | | |
| Signature: M. Slack   M. SLACK | | | | | | | | | | |
| Indication: Asthma | | | | | | | | | | |

## ❓ QUESTIONS FROM THE EXAMINER

### What monitoring is important if prescribing an aminophylline infusion?

Cardiac and renal function monitoring, as side effects of aminophylline can include tachycardia and arrhythmias.

### Describe what is meant by diurnal variation, and how this may be investigated when initially diagnosing asthma.

Symptoms vary throughout the day, with worse symptoms and a lower peak flow in the morning due to the varying levels of cortisol. Diurnal variation may be observed by asking a patient to complete a peak flow diary.

### What is the mechanism of action of salbutamol and the potential side effects?

Salbutamol is a beta-2 receptor agonist. Side effects include arrhythmias, headaches, hypokalaemia, palpitations, tremor and nausea.

### Name three common triggers of asthma attacks.

Tobacco smoke, house dust mites, mould, pollen, pets, strong odours and sprays, exercise/strenuous activity.

### In 'seasonal asthma', when is the commonest time for asthma to flare up?

Some people have asthma that only flares up at certain times of the year, typically during hayfever season or when it is cold.

### Name two possible causes of adult-onset asthma.

Occupational asthma, smoking, obesity and female hormones and stressful life events have been suggested to cause adult-onset asthma.

### To what class of drug does terbutaline belong and what are its indications?

Terbutaline is a beta-agonist, like salbutamol. It is indicated in the treatment of asthma and other conditions associated with reversible airway obstruction.

### Define pharmacokinetics, and what are its four steps?

Pharmacokinetics is the study of what the body does to the drug. The four steps are absorption, distribution, metabolism and excretion.

### Define pharmacodynamics.

Pharmacodynamics is the study of what the drug does to the body.

### What is the use of the Medication Appropriateness Index (MAI)?

The MAI is used to assess the appropriateness of a medication prescribed by a healthcare professional. A higher MAI score may increase the risk of hospitalisation.

## Station 11.5   Hyperkalaemia

### Doctor Briefing

You are the junior doctor in the medical assessment unit and you have been asked to see Peter Jones, an 82-year-old patient, who has been admitted from the emergency department (ED) with a 3-day history of vomiting and dehydration. You are asked to chase his bloods and review him overnight. The patient's vomiting has settled with intramuscular (IM) cyclizine but he feels thirsty. His regular medications are aspirin, ramipril, bisoprolol, co-amilofruse, simvastatin and spironolactone. You have made a presumptive diagnosis of hyperkalaemia. Please formulate an appropriate management plan and complete the drug chart provided, including the prescription of fluids, regular, PRN and once-only medications as appropriate.

### Patient Briefing

Three days ago, you started with pain in the lower abdomen on the left-hand side. You have never had pain like this before. You have been feeling flushed, nauseated and generally unwell. You have also noticed that you have had episodes of diarrhoea and loose stool.

You have previously had a heart attack and have known heart failure.

You are concerned because you don't know why the pain is so bad and just want some painkillers.

### Patient Details

| | |
| --- | --- |
| Name | Peter Jones |
| Date of birth | 22/06/1938 |
| Hospital number | 2206381254 |
| Weight | 65 kg |
| Height | 1.73 m |
| Consultant | MJK |
| Hospital/ward | RIE/14 |
| Current medications | Aspirin 75 mg OD<br>Ramipril 5 mg BD<br>Bisoprolol 10 mg OD<br>Co-amilofruse 5/40 mg OD<br>Simvastatin 40 mg nocte (ON)<br>Spironolactone 25 mg OD |
| Allergies | Erythromycin (rash) |
| Admission date | 10/09/2019 |

### Mark Scheme for Examiner

#### Completing the Drug Chart

| Drug Chart Task | Justification | | | | | |
| --- | --- | --- | --- | --- | --- | --- |
| Correctly writes patient information:<br>• Name<br>• Date of birth<br>• Hospital number<br>• Weight<br>• Age<br>• Consultant<br>• Ward<br>• Admission date | This is part of vital routine hospital documentation. Weight is important and several medications require a current weight to calculate dosage | | | | | |

## Completing the Drug Chart

| Drug Chart Task | Justification | | | | |
|---|---|---|---|---|---|
| Completes allergy box, including signing and dating | No medication should be prescribed until you know the patient's allergies | | | | |
| Prescribes correctly appropriate analgesia:<br>• Drug name<br>• Route<br>• Dose<br>• Signature and date | Following the WHO analgesia ladder, paracetamol should always be the first line | | | | |
| Prescribes correctly appropriate antiemetic:<br>• Drug name<br>• Route<br>• Dose<br>• Signature and date | Remember that if your patient is vomiting, it may be hard for him to take tablets, therefore alternative routes should be written up | | | | |
| Prescribes correctly regular medications:<br>• Drug name<br>• Route<br>• Dose<br>• Frequency and timing<br>• Start dates (and review dates if applicable) | The person admitting the patient into hospital should be responsible for prescribing all the patient's regular medication and checking it is appropriate for him to continue to take them | | | | |
| Prescribes correctly medications for cardiac stabilisation | 10% calcium chloride or calcium gluconate should be prescribed if there are ECG changes associated with myocardial instability. They should be given intravenously in 1-mL aliquots to resolution of ECG changes. You must titrate the dose to ECG if available, because if either is given in excess, it can lead to cardiac arrest | | | | |
| Prescribes correctly medications to reduce serum potassium level | Nebulised salbutamol 5 mg and 10 units of Actrapid in 50 mL 50% dextrose (or equivalent) intravenously can help to drive some of the extracellular potassium into cells. If opting for the latter, then you should also prescribe a slow infusion of 10% dextrose to avoid hypoglycaemia (this will need to be prescribed in the fluid section) | | | | |
| Prescribes correctly appropriate fluid | IV fluid is warranted for rehydration and to treat hypovolaemia. Initially you can prescribe a fluid bolus of 500 mL 0.9% sodium chloride, and further fluid prescriptions will be determined by the patient's response | | | | |
| Prescribes correctly appropriate oxygen therapy:<br>• Route<br>• Target saturation | It is important to prescribe oxygen to ensure that it is being used correctly | | | | |
| Prescribes correctly regular medications:<br>• Drug name<br>• Route<br>• Dose<br>• Frequency and timing<br>• Start dates (and review dates if applicable) | The person admitting the patient into hospital should be responsible for prescribing all the patient's regular medication and checking it is appropriate for him to continue to take them | | | | |

## Completing the Drug Chart

| Drug Chart Task | Justification | | | | | | |
|---|---|---|---|---|---|---|---|
| Discontinues any inappropriate medications | You must remember to stop anything that may worsen the condition. Ramipril, spironolactone and co-amilofruse need to be stopped due to hyperkalaemia and acute kidney injury (AKI). Bisoprolol needs to be stopped due to hypotension | | | | | | |
| Considers treatment options if there is no response to initial treatment | You may need to repeat some of the treatment options mentioned above if the patient is not responding at all, or not at the desired rate | | | | | | |
| Considers VTE prophylaxis | Choice of VTE prophylaxis can vary based on patient factors and local trust guidelines | | | | | | |

### General Points

| | | | | | | | |
|---|---|---|---|---|---|---|---|
| Polite to patient | | | | | | | |
| Clear, legible writing on the drug chart using black ink | | | | | | | |

## Correct Prescription Chart

Name: Peter Jones

Date of birth: 22/06/1938

Hospital number: 2206381254

Weight: 65 kg

Age: 82 years

Consultant: MJK

Known allergies:
Erythromycin (rash)

Signature: Date:
M. Khan    10/09/19
M. KHAN

## Once-Only Medications

| Date | Time | Medicine (Approved Name) | Dose | Route | Prescriber – Sign and Print | Time Given | Given By |
|---|---|---|---|---|---|---|---|
| 10/09/19 | 2040 | Calcium gluconate 10% (titrate to ECG) | 1–10 mL | IV | M. Khan M. KHAN | | |
| 10/09/19 | 2050 | Salbutamol (driven in air) | 5 mg | Neb | M. Khan M. KHAN | | |

## Oxygen Therapy

| Start | | | Route | | | Stop | |
|---|---|---|---|---|---|---|---|
| Date | Time | Mask (%) | Prongs (L/min) | Prescriber – Sign and Print | Administered by | Date | Time |
| 10/09/19 | 2040 | | 2 L/min | M. Khan M. KHAN | | | |

## Venous Thromboembolism Prophylaxis

| VTE Risk Assessment: | Comment: |
|---|---|
| Yes [X] | Review on ward round once all bloods back and full assessment performed |
| Prophylaxis not required [ ] | Signature: *M. Khan* M. KHAN |
| Contraindicated [ ] | Date: *10/09/19* |

| | | | Date: → | | | | | | | |
|---|---|---|---|---|---|---|---|---|---|---|
| | | | Time: ↓ | | | | | | | |
| Drug: Enoxaparin | | | | | | | | | | |
| Dose: 20 mg | Freq: OD | Route: SC | | | | | | | | |
| Start: 10/09/19 | Stop/review: | | | | | | | | | |
| Signature: *M. Khan* M. KHAN | | | | | | | | | | |

## Regular Medications

| | | | Date: → | 10/9 | | | | | | |
|---|---|---|---|---|---|---|---|---|---|---|
| | | | Time: ↓ | | | | | | | |
| Drug: Aspirin | | | 02 | | | | | | | |
| Dose: 75 mg | Freq: OD | Route: Oral | 06 | | | | | | | |
| | | | ⑩ | | | | | | | |
| Start: 10/09/19 | Stop/review: | | 14 | | | | | | | |
| Signature: *M. Khan* M. KHAN | | | 18 | | | | | | | |
| Indication: Secondary prevention of acute coronary syndrome (ACS) | | | 22 | | | | | | | |
| Drug: Ramipril | | | 02 | | | | | | | |
| Dose: 5 mg | Freq: BD | Route: PO oral | 06 | | | | | | | |
| | | | ⑩ | | | | | | | |
| Start: 10/09/19 | Stop/review: | | 14 | | | | | | | |
| Signature: *M. Khan* M. KHAN | | | ⑱ | | | | | Stopped due to hyperkalaemia and acute kidney injury 20/11/19 *M. Khan* (M. KHAN) | | |
| Indication: Secondary prevention of ACS | | | 22 | | | | | | | |

## Regular Medications

| Drug: Bisoprolol | | | Date: → Time: ↓ | | | | | | | | |
|---|---|---|---|---|---|---|---|---|---|---|---|
| | | | 02 | | | | | | | | |
| Dose: 10 mg | Freq: OD | Route: Oral | 06 | | | | | | | | |
| | | | (10) | | | | | | Stopped due to hypotension 20/11/19 M. Khan (M. KHAN) | | |
| Start: 10/09/19 | Stop/review: | | 14 | | | | | | | | |
| Signature: M. Khan M. KHAN | | | 18 | | | | | | | | |
| Indication: Secondary prevention of ACS | | | 22 | | | | | | | | |

| Drug: Co-amilofruse 5/40 | | | | | | | | | | | |
|---|---|---|---|---|---|---|---|---|---|---|---|
| | | | 02 | | | | | | | | |
| Dose: 1 sachet | Freq: OD | Route: Oral | 06 | | | | | | | | |
| | | | (10) | | | | | | Stopped due to hyperkalaemia and acute kidney injury 20/11/19 M. Khan (M. KHAN) | | |
| Start: 10/09/19 | Stop/review: | | 14 | | | | | | | | |
| Signature: M. Khan M. KHAN | | | 18 | | | | | | | | |
| Indication: Secondary prevention of ACS | | | 22 | | | | | | | | |

| Drug: Simvastatin | | | | | | | | | | | |
|---|---|---|---|---|---|---|---|---|---|---|---|
| | | | 02 | | | | | | | | |
| Dose: 40 mg | Freq: ON | Route: Oral | 06 | | | | | | | | |
| | | | 10 | | | | | | | | |
| Start: 10/09/19 | Stop/review: | | 14 | | | | | | | | |
| Signature: M. Khan M. KHAN | | | 18 | | | | | | | | |
| Indication: Secondary prevention of ACS | | | (22) | | | | | | | | |

| Drug: Spironolactone | | | | | | | | | | | |
|---|---|---|---|---|---|---|---|---|---|---|---|
| | | | 02 | | | | | | | | |
| Dose: 25 mg | Freq: OD | Route: Oral | 06 | | | | | | | | |
| | | | (10) | | | | | | Stopped due to hyperkalaemia and acute kidney injury 20/11/19 M. Khan (M. KHAN) | | |
| Start: 10/09/19 | Stop/review: | | 14 | | | | | | | | |
| Signature: M. Khan M. KHAN | | | 18 | | | | | | | | |
| Indication: Moderate heart failure | | | 22 | | | | | | | | |

## Fluid Prescriptions

| Date | Fluid | Additive | Volume | Route | Rate | Signature | Given | Batch |
|------|-------|----------|--------|-------|------|-----------|-------|-------|
| 10/09/19 | 10% Dextrose | 10 units of insulin (Actrapid) | 250 mL | IV | Over 30 min | M. Khan M. KHAN | | |

## ❓ QUESTIONS FROM THE EXAMINER

### Explain why prolonged tourniquet time during venipuncture may lead to inaccurate serum potassium results.

It can lead to a decrease in pH caused by localised production of lactic acid from surrounding muscles.

### Name three drugs that can precipitate hyperkalaemia.

Potassium-sparing diuretics (for example, spironolactone, amiloride), non-steroidal anti-inflammatory drugs (NSAIDs), ACE inhibitors, angiotensin receptor blockers, beta-blockers and aspirin.

### What is pseudohyperkalaemia?

It refers to a falsely raised serum or plasma potassium concentration. The in vitro (measured) potassium concentration is above the upper limit of the reference range when the in vivo (actual) value is within the range.

### Name five foods that are rich in potassium.

Bananas, avocados, nuts, dried fruits (for example, prunes, raisins, dates), potatoes and cooked spinach or broccoli.

### Which condition should you consider if a patient's blood results revealed hyponatraemia and hyperkalaemia, and what investigation would be helpful?

You should consider Addison's disease, for which you should measure cortisol level at 9 a.m.

### What are patiromer calcium and sodium zirconium cyclosilicate?

They are both oral potassium exchange agents that are usually commenced in secondary care. They are non-absorbed cation exchange polymers that act as a potassium binder in the gastrointestinal tract.

### How do you correctly cease a medication on the drug chart?

You need to draw a zigzag/wiggly line across all of the boxes corresponding to that medication, to the end of the chart. Clearly write 'STOP' in the box and state the reason(s) why. Lastly, remember to sign and date your alteration.

### Why are decimal points discouraged on drug charts?

Many incidences and 'near-miss' events have been a result of difficulty understanding drug doses that contain decimal points; for example, it is better to write 3 mg than 3.0 mg. Decimal points are known to cause medication errors!

### How do you withhold certain doses on a drug chart, without crossing out the entire medication?

You can put a cross in the box that corresponds to the dose that you want to stop. This would indicate to the nurse that this dose cannot be given, but it would not affect any subsequent doses. You can do this for as many doses as required.

### Name three potential causes of hypokalaemia.

Hypokalaemia can be caused by loop or thiazide diuretics, vomiting and diarrhoea, refeeding syndrome, hypomagnesaemia, Conn's syndrome, renal tubular acidosis, burns and hyperhidrosis.

## Station 11.6   Bowel Obstruction

### Doctor Briefing

You are the junior doctor working on a general surgical ward and are asked to see William McDonald, an 80-year-old man, who has presented with abdominal pain, severe nausea and vomiting. He is an average-sized man, who is confused and looks dehydrated. On closer questioning, you discover that he has not had a bowel motion for the last 5 or 6 days. His past history is remarkable for ischaemic heart disease. He is on aspirin, simvastatin, ramipril and atenolol for a previous myocardial infarction, and other medications. You have made a presumptive diagnosis of bowel obstruction. Please formulate an appropriate management plan and complete the drug chart provided, including the prescription of fluids, regular, PRN and once-only medications as appropriate.

### Patient Briefing

You have come into hospital because over the past few days you have experienced some pain in your lower abdomen and have reduced appetite. Today it's been especially bad, with severity 10/10. You have also been feeling nauseous all morning and have vomited on three occasions.

On specific questioning, you've come to realise that you haven't been able to open your bowels for just under a week. Your abdomen does appear to be slightly more distended than normal all over.

Your medical background consists of ischaemic heart disease and a previous heart attack.

You are concerned because you cannot stop vomiting and the abdominal pain seems to be worsening.

### Patient Details

| | |
|---|---|
| Name | William McDonald |
| Date of birth | 07/06/1940 |
| Hospital number | 0706401225 |
| Weight | 70 kg |
| Height | 1.78 m |
| Consultant | DNA |
| Hospital/ward | WGH/27 |
| Current medications | Aspirin 75 mg OD<br>Ramipril 5 mg BD<br>Atenolol 25 mg OD<br>Co-amilofruse 5/40 mg OD<br>Atorvastatin 80 mg OD<br>Metformin 500 mg OD<br>Movicol 2–4 sachets PRN |
| Allergies | Penicillin (rash) |
| Admission date | 10/09/2019 |

## Mark Scheme for Examiner

### Completing the Drug Chart

| Drug Chart Task | Justification | | | | | |
|---|---|---|---|---|---|---|
| Correctly writes patient information:<br>• Name<br>• Date of birth<br>• Hospital number<br>• Weight<br>• Age<br>• Consultant<br>• Ward<br>• Admission date | This is part of vital routine hospital documentation. Weight is important and several medications require a current weight to calculate dosage | | | | | |
| Completes allergy box, including signing and dating | No medication should be prescribed until you know the patient's allergies | | | | | |
| Prescribes correctly appropriate analgesia:<br>• Drug name<br>• Route<br>• Dose<br>• Signature and date | The patient is in severe pain, and you must help to get it under control to alleviate the patient's symptoms | | | | | |
| Prescribes correctly appropriate antiemetic:<br>• Drug name<br>• Route<br>• Dose<br>• Signature and date | Remember that if your patient is vomiting, it may be hard for him to take tablets; therefore alternative routes should be written up. Metoclopramide is prokinetic and could therefore cause severe pain and even perforation of obstructed bowel by stimulating peristalsis | | | | | |
| Prescribes correctly appropriate fluid | IV fluid is warranted for rehydration, to treat hypovolaemia and to replace electrolytes. Initially you can prescribe a fluid bolus of 500 mL 0.9% sodium chloride, and further fluid prescriptions may be required as maintenance fluid. With this patient, there is some concern about fluid overload. However, with clinical evidence suggestive of shock, he is likely to be in a large negative fluid balance, therefore it's unlikely that you would cause fluid overload so quickly in this case as a substantial amount of fluid would be required to do so | | | | | |
| Prescribes correctly appropriate oxygen therapy:<br>• Route<br>• Target saturation | It is important to prescribe oxygen to ensure that it is being used correctly | | | | | |
| Prescribes correctly regular medications:<br>• Drug name<br>• Route<br>• Dose<br>• Frequency and timing<br>• Start dates (and review dates if applicable) | The person admitting the patient into hospital should be responsible for prescribing all the patient's regular medication and checking it is appropriate for him to continue to take them.<br>This patient may potentially require surgery very soon, therefore must be placed on 'nil by mouth' until told otherwise. This means that the oral route is not available, and an alternative route must be considered | | | | | |
| Discontinues any inappropriate medications | The patient has impaired renal function; therefore medications such as ACE inhibitors, metformin, atenolol, and statin need to be withheld | | | | | |
| Considers VTE prophylaxis | Choice of VTE prophylaxis can vary based on patient factors and local trust guidelines | | | | | |

## General Points

| | | | | |
|---|---|---|---|---|
| Polite to patient | | | | |
| Clear, legible writing on the drug chart using black ink | | | | |

## Correct Prescription Chart

Name: William McDonald

Date of birth: 07/06/1940

Hospital number: 0706401225

Weight: 70 kg

Age: 80 years

Consultant: DNA

Known allergies: Penicillin (rash)

Signature: Date:
D. Akin    10/09/2019
D. AKIN

## Once-Only Medications

| Date | Time | Medicine (Approved Name) | Dose | Route | Prescriber – Sign and Print | Time Given | Given By |
|---|---|---|---|---|---|---|---|
| 10/09/19 | 1400 | Morphine (titrate to pain) | 1–10 mg | IV | D. Akin D. AKIN | | |
| 10/09/19 | 1400 | Cyclizine | 50 mg | IV | D. Akin D. AKIN | | |
| 10/09/19 | 1400 | Paracetamol | 1 g | IV | D. Akin D. AKIN | | |

## Oxygen Therapy

| Start | | Route | | | | Stop | |
|---|---|---|---|---|---|---|---|
| Date | Time | Mask (%) | Prongs (L/min) | Prescriber – Sign and Print | Administered by | Date | Time |
| 10/09/19 | 1400 | Nasal cannula | 4 L/min | D. Akin D. AKIN | | | |

## Venous Thromboembolism Prophylaxis

VTE Risk Assessment:

Yes [ ]

Prophylaxis not required [ ]

Contraindicated [X]

Comment:

Signature: M. Slack   M. SLACK

Date: 20/11/19

| | | Date: → Time: ↓ | | | | | | | | | |
|---|---|---|---|---|---|---|---|---|---|---|---|
| Drug: | | | | | | | | | | | |
| Dose: | Freq: | Route: | | | | | | | | | |
| | | | | | | | | | | | |
| Start: | | Stop/review: | | | | | | | | | |
| Signature: | | | | | | | | | | | |

**Regular Medications**

| | | | Date: → | | | | | | | | | |
|---|---|---|---|---|---|---|---|---|---|---|---|---|
| | | | Time: ↓ | | | | | | | | | |
| Drug: Aspirin | | | 02 | | | | | | | | | |
| Dose: 75 mg | Freq: OD | Route: Oral | 06 | | | | | | | | | |
| | | | ⑩ | | | | | | | | | |
| Start: 20/11/19 | Stop/review: | | 14 | | | | | | | | | |
| Signature: M. Slack M. SLACK | | | 18 | | | | | | | | | |
| Indication: Secondary prevention of ACS | | | 22 | | | | | | | | | |
| Drug: Ramipril | | | 02 | | | | | | | | | |
| Dose: 5 mg | Freq: BD | Route: Oral | 06 | | | | | | | | | |
| | | | ⑩ | | | | | | | | | |
| Start: 20/11/19 | Stop/review: | | 14 | | | | | | | | | |
| Signature: M. Slack M. SLACK | | | ⑱ | | | | | | | | | |
| Indication: Secondary prevention of ACS | | | 22 | | | | | | | | | |
| Drug: Atenolol | | | 02 | | | | | | | | | |
| Dose: 25 mg | Freq: OD | Route: PO | 06 | | | | | | | | | |
| | | | ⑩ | | | | | | | | | |
| Start: 20/11/19 | Stop/review: | | 14 | | | | | | | | | |
| Signature: M. Slack M. SLACK | | | 18 | | | | | | | | | |
| Indication: Secondary prevention of ACS | | | 22 | | | | | | | | | |

## Regular Medications

| | Date: → | | | | | | | | |
|---|---|---|---|---|---|---|---|---|---|
| | Time: ↓ | | | | | | | | |

| Drug: Atorvastatin | 02 | | | | | | | |
|---|---|---|---|---|---|---|---|---|
| Dose: 80 mg / Freq: OD / Route: Oral | 06 | | | | | | | |
| | ⑩ | | | | | | | |
| Start: 20/11/19 / Stop/review: | 14 | | | | | | | |
| Signature: M. Slack / M. SLACK | 18 | | | | | | | |
| Indication: Secondary prevention of ACS | 22 | | | | | | | |

| Drug: Metformin | 02 | | | | | | | |
|---|---|---|---|---|---|---|---|---|
| Dose: 500 mg / Freq: OD / Route: Oral | 06 | | | | | | | |
| | ⑩ | | | | | | | |
| Start: 20/11/19 / Stop/review: | 14 | | | | | | | |
| Signature: M. Slack / M. SLACK | 18 | | | | | | | |
| Indication: Diabetes | 22 | | | | | | | |

| Drug: Movicol | 02 | | | | | | | |
|---|---|---|---|---|---|---|---|---|
| Dose: 1 sachet / Freq: BD / Route: Oral | 06 | | | | | | | |
| | ⑩ | | | | | | | |
| Start: 20/11/19 / Stop/review: | 14 | | | | | | | |
| Signature: M. Slack / M. SLACK | ⑱ | | | | | | | |
| Indication: Constipation | 22 | | | | | | | |

## Fluid Prescriptions

| Date | Fluid | Additive | Volume | Route | Rate | Signature | Given | Batch |
|---|---|---|---|---|---|---|---|---|
| 10/09/19 | Hartmann's solution | None | 500 mL | IV | Over 20 min | *D. Akin*<br>D. AKIN | | |
| 10/09/19 | Hartmann's solution | None | 500 mL | IV | Over 20 min | *D. Akin*<br>D. AKIN | | |
| 10/09/19 | Hartmann's solution | None | 1000 mL | IV | Over 20 min | *D. Akin*<br>D. AKIN | | |

## ❓ QUESTIONS FROM THE EXAMINER

### What do tympanic bowel sounds suggest?

Tympanic bowel sounds means that the sound is 'drum-like'. It is produced by percussion over air-filled structures.

### Define postoperative paralytic ileus.

It refers to constipation and intolerance to oral intake secondary to non-mechanical factors that disrupt the normal gut motility pattern, following surgery.

### What is the most common site of intestinal atresia?

The duodenum.

### Describe the typical abdominal pain experienced in intestinal obstruction.

Normally it is a colicky abdominal pain, focusing at the central or lower abdomen (though it could affect any part of the abdomen). It also usually happens in conjunction with increased peristaltic activity.

### What is adhesiolysis?

It is the surgical procedure that removes abdominal adhesions, which are most commonly a result of previous abdominal surgery.

### What is the difference between complete and partial bowel obstruction?

Complete obstruction is characterised by the failure to pass either stool or flatus whereas in partial obstruction, the patient presents with signs of obstipation but continues to pass gas or stool to some extent.

### What is peristalsis and what stimulates it in the large intestine?

Peristalsis is defined as involuntary movements of longitudinal and circular muscles causing wave-like contractions. It mainly occurs in the digestive gastrointestinal tract, such as the oesophagus, stomach and intestines.

### Describe what the 'Dance sign' is and what it might be a characteristic of.

It is a feeling of emptiness on palpation of the right lower quadrant and may suggest intussusception.

### What is the difference between general sale list (GSL) medications, prescription-only medications (POMs) and pharmacy medications (P medicines)?

GSL are medications that do not need to be used under professional supervision and generally are sold as over-the-counter medications. POMs can only be used under the supervision of a prescribing healthcare professional and can only be obtained with a valid prescription. A P medicine is only available under the supervision of a pharmacist and is only sold in a pharmacy.

### What is the formulation of a drug? Name two examples.

The formulation of a drug is the 'form' that you would like the medication to be in and it describes in what way the medication will be administered to the patient. For instance, tablets, capsules, solution, inhaler, intramuscular injection, subcutaneous injection, infusion, cream or pessary.

## Station 11.7   Abdominal Sepsis

### Doctor Briefing

You are the junior doctor working on a general surgical admissions unit. Your next patient is a 43-year-old woman, Miss Jennifer Williams, who has presented with a 3-day history of worsening left iliac fossa pain and vomiting. She has had some loose stools over the last couple of days. She has a background of diverticular disease and asthma. She is clearly in pain. You have made a presumptive diagnosis of abdominal sepsis. Please formulate an appropriate management plan and complete the drug chart provided, including the prescription of fluids, regular, PRN and once-only medications as appropriate.

### Patient Briefing

Three days ago, you started with pain in the lower abdomen on the left-hand side. You have never had pain like this before. On questioning, you have been feeling flushed, nauseated and generally unwell. You have also noticed that you have had episodes of diarrhoea and loose stool.

Your medical background consists of diverticular disease and asthma.

You are concerned because you don't know why the pain is so bad and just want some painkillers.

### Patient Details

| | |
|---|---|
| Name | Jennifer Williams |
| Date of birth | 12/05/1977 |
| Hospital number | 0706401225 |
| Weight | 70 kg |
| Height | 1.62 m |
| Consultant | MHS |
| Hospital/ward | WGH/27 |
| Current medications | Seretide 250 inhaler 2 puffs BD<br>Salbutamol inhaler 2 puffs PRN<br>Desogestrel 75 mcg OD<br>Simvastatin 10 mg ON |
| Allergies | Erythromycin (rash) |
| Admission date | 20/11/2019 |

### Mark Scheme for Examiner

#### Completing the Drug Chart

| Drug Chart Task | Justification | | | | | |
|---|---|---|---|---|---|---|
| Correctly writes patient information:<br>• Name<br>• Date of birth<br>• Hospital number<br>• Weight<br>• Age<br>• Consultant<br>• Ward<br>• Admission date | This is part of vital routine hospital documentation. Weight is important and several medications require a current weight to calculate dosage | | | | | |

## Completing the Drug Chart

| Drug Chart Task | Justification | | | | | | |
|---|---|---|---|---|---|---|---|
| Completes allergy box, including signing and dating | No medication should be prescribed until you know the patient's allergies | | | | | | |
| Prescribes correctly appropriate analgesia:<br>• Drug name<br>• Route<br>• Dose<br>• Signature and date | Following the WHO analgesia ladder, paracetamol should always be the first line | | | | | | |
| Prescribes correctly appropriate antiemetic:<br>• Drug name<br>• Route<br>• Dose<br>• Signature and date | Remember that if your patient is vomiting, it may be hard for her to take tablets, therefore alternative routes should be written up | | | | | | |
| Prescribes correctly regular medications:<br>• Drug name<br>• Route<br>• Dose<br>• Frequency and timing<br>• Start dates (and review dates if applicable) | The person admitting the patient into hospital should be responsible for prescribing all the patient's regular medication and checking it is appropriate for her to continue to take them | | | | | | |
| Prescribes correctly appropriate antibiotics:<br>• Drug name<br>• Route<br>• Dose<br>• Considers allergies<br>• Considers if stat dose is required | Antibiotic choice varies according to local policy and depending on the patient's allergies | | | | | | |
| Prescribes correctly appropriate fluid | A hypotensive patient will require fluid challenges as well as maintenance fluid. If a patient is stable and only nil by mouth, she may only need maintenance fluid | | | | | | |
| Prescribes correctly appropriate oxygen therapy:<br>• Route<br>• Target saturations | It is important to prescribe oxygen to ensure that it is being used correctly | | | | | | |
| Considers VTE prophylaxis | Choice of VTE prophylaxis can vary based on patient factors and local trust guidelines | | | | | | |

## General Points

| | | | | | | | |
|---|---|---|---|---|---|---|---|
| Polite to patient | | | | | | | |
| Clear, legible writing on the drug chart using black ink | | | | | | | |

## Correct Prescription Chart

Name: Jennifer Williams

Date of birth: 12/05/1977

Hospital number: 0706401225

Weight: 70 kg

Age: 53 years

Consultant: MHS

Known allergies:
Erythromycin (rash)

Signature: Date:
M. Slack   20/11/2019
M. SLACK

## Once-Only Medications

| Date | Time | Medicine (Approved Name) | Dose | Route | Prescriber – Sign and Print | Time Given | Given By |
|------|------|--------------------------|------|-------|------------------------------|------------|----------|
| 20/11/19 | 1430 | Morphine (titrate to pain) | 1–10 mg | IV | M. Slack M. SLACK | | |
| 20/11/19 | 1430 | Cyclizine | 50 mg | IV | M. Slack M. SLACK | | |
| 20/11/19 | 1430 | Paracetamol | 1 g | IV | M. Slack M. SLACK | | |
| 20/11/19 | 1430 | Piperacillin and tazobactam | 4.5 g | IV | M. Slack M. SLACK | | |

## Oxygen Therapy

| Start | | Route | | | | Stop | |
|-------|---|-------|---|---|---|------|---|
| Date | Time | Mask (%) | Prongs (L/min) | Prescriber – Sign and Print | Administered by | Date | Time |
| 20/11/19 | 1430 | Venturi (60) | | M. Slack M. SLACK | | | |

## Venous Thromboembolism Prophylaxis

VTE Risk Assessment:

Yes [ ]

Prophylaxis not required [ ]

Contraindicated [X]

Comment:

Signature: M. Slack M. SLACK

Date: 20/11/19

| | Date: → Time: ↓ | | | | | | | |
|---|---|---|---|---|---|---|---|---|
| Drug: | | | | | | | | |
| Dose: Freq: Route: | | | | | | | | |
| | | | | | | | | |
| Start: Stop/review: | | | | | | | | |
| Signature: | | | | | | | | |

## Regular Medications

| | | | Date: → Time: ↓ | | | | | | | | | |
|---|---|---|---|---|---|---|---|---|---|---|---|---|
| Drug: Seretide 250 (salmeterol 25 micrograms/fluticasone 250 micrograms) | | | 02 | | | | | | | | | |
| Dose: 2 puffs | Freq: BD | Route: Inh | (06) | | | | | | | | | |
| | | | 10 | | | | | | | | | |
| Start: 20/11/19 | Stop/review: | | (14) | | | | | | | | | |
| Signature: M. Slack M. SLACK | | | 18 | | | | | | | | | |
| Indication: Asthma | | | 22 | | | | | | | | | |
| Drug: Desogestrel | | | 02 | | | | | | | | | |
| Dose: 75 mcg | Freq: OD | Route: Oral | 06 | | | | | | | | | |
| | | | (10) | | | | | | | | | |
| Start: 20/11/19 | Stop/review: | | 14 | | | | | | | | | |
| Signature: M. Slack M. SLACK | | | 18 | | | | | | | | | |
| Indication: Contraception | | | 22 | | | | | | | | | |
| Drug: Simvastatin | | | 02 | | | | | | | | | |
| Dose: 10 mg | Freq: ON | Route: Oral | 06 | | | | | | | | | |
| | | | 10 | | | | | | | | | |
| Start: 20/11/19 | Stop/review: | | 14 | | | | | | | | | |
| Signature: M. Slack M. SLACK | | | 18 | | | | | | | | | |
| Indication: Hypercholesterolaemia | | | (22) | | | | | | | | | |

## Regular Medications

| | | | Date: → | | | | | | | | | |
|---|---|---|---|---|---|---|---|---|---|---|---|---|
| | | | Time: ↓ | | | | | | | | | |
| Drug: *Tazocin* | | | 02 | | | | | | | | | |
| Dose: 4.5 g | Freq: TDS | Route: IV | (06) | | | | | | | | | |
| | | | 10 | | | | | | | | | |
| Start: 20/11/19 | Stop/review: | | (14) | | | | | | | | | |
| Signature: *M. Slack* M. SLACK | | | 18 | | | | | | | | | |
| Indication: *Intra-abdominal sepsis* | | | (22) | | | | | | | | | |

## PRN Medications

| | | | Date: → | | | | | | | | | |
|---|---|---|---|---|---|---|---|---|---|---|---|---|
| | | | Time: ↓ | | | | | | | | | |
| Drug: *Salbutamol inhaler* | | | | | | | | | | | | |
| Dose: 2 puffs | Freq: PRN | Route: INH | | | | | | | | | | |
| Start: 20/11/19 | Stop/review: | | | | | | | | | | | |
| Signature: *M. Slack* M. SLACK | | | | | | | | | | | | |
| Indication: *Asthma* | | | | | | | | | | | | |

## Fluid Prescriptions

| Date | Fluid | Additive | Volume | Route | Rate | Signature | Given | Batch |
|---|---|---|---|---|---|---|---|---|
| 20/11/19 | 0.9% Sodium chloride | None | 500 mL | IV | Over 20 min | *M. Khan* M. KHAN | | |

## ❓ QUESTIONS FROM THE EXAMINER

**Define 'diverticulum'.**

A diverticulum is an outpouching of the colonic wall that typically forms a 'pocket'.

**What is a volvulus?**

A condition where a portion of intestine twists on its mesentery, causing obstruction. Most commonly occurs in the sigmoid colon or caecum.

**What is intussusception?**

A condition, more commonly seen in children, where a portion of intestine invaginates into another, causing obstruction.

**Is an erect chest X-ray a useful investigation when assessing someone with an acute abdomen?**

Yes, because it can exclude a perforation. However, it can be difficult to interpret in a patient who is postoperative from laparoscopic surgery as you would expect a small volume of gas to be in the abdominal cavity.

**Can nurses prescribe on the drug chart?**

Yes, certified nurse prescribers are allowed to prescribe specific medication (usually medicines commonly used in their specialty).

**Can you cross off medication on a drug chart?**

Yes, this is commonly done. It is important to sign and date when you cross off a medication, and it is good practice to document why it was stopped in the medical notes.

**Do patches have to be prescribed on a drug chart?**

Yes. Any medication, whatever the preparation, needs to be prescribed on the correct drug chart.

**If a medication is changed from three times a day to twice a day, do you have to rewrite the drug?**

Yes, any changes to a medication would warrant a new prescription for the intended frequency, and the old prescription to be crossed off. You cannot simply put a line through the time that you no longer need the medication to be given at.

**Can alcohol be drunk when taking antibiotics?**

Ideally, patients should not drink alcohol when they are on antibiotics, as it can exacerbate side effects such as nausea and dizziness. This is especially the case when taking metronidazole and/or tinidazole.

**At what weight, and why, should paracetamol be prescribed with caution?**

Paracetamol dose needs to be reduced (from 1 g every 4–6 h to 15 mg/kg every 4–6 h) for an adult weighing less than 50 kg. There is a risk of paracetamol overdose and liver toxicity.

## Station 11.8   Acute Upper Gastrointestinal Bleed

### Doctor Briefing

You are the junior doctor on call and are bleeped to see Steve Smith, a 65-year-old patient, who is having haematemesis. He was admitted directly from the medical outpatient clinic yesterday as he 'was yellow' and had a scan of his abdomen yesterday. He has never vomited blood before, and he does not get indigestion. You see him as he is vomiting frank blood into a sick bowl. He is alert but is slurring his speech and tells you that he was sitting in bed when he vomited 30 min ago. He has vomited repeatedly since then. You have made a presumptive diagnosis of acute upper gastrointestinal bleed. Please formulate an appropriate management plan and complete the drug chart provided, including the prescription of fluids, regular, PRN and once-only medications as appropriate.

### Patient Briefing

You have come into hospital because your wife told you that you looked unwell and that you appear 'yellow' in colour. You have also been getting abdominal pain on and off, but it has not been anything significant. Your appetite has been maintained, and you have not vomited. However, just now while you were sat up in bed, you vomited a large amount of fresh red blood. Since then, you have kept bringing up small amounts of blood. You are slightly confused – you know your personal details such as name and date of birth, but you do not know the date, nor do you recognise where you are. You're also quite drowsy and your speech has begun to slur.

Your medical background includes high cholesterol and chronic constipation. On specific questioning, you drink regularly and smoke socially.

You are concerned because this is the first time it has happened, and it looks like a lot of blood in the sick bowl.

### Patient Details

| | |
|---|---|
| Name | Steve Smith |
| Date of birth | 01/03/1955 |
| Hospital number | 0103551252 |
| Weight | 65 kg |
| Height | 1.73 m |
| Consultant | MJK |
| Hospital/ward | RIE/209 |
| Current medications | Atorvastatin 10 mg ON<br>Lactulose 15 mL BD |
| Allergies | Nil |
| Admission date | 13/09/2019 |

### Mark Scheme for Examiner

**Completing the Drug Chart**

| Drug Chart Task | Justification | | | | | |
|---|---|---|---|---|---|---|
| Correctly writes patient information:<br>• Name<br>• Date of birth<br>• Hospital number<br>• Weight<br>• Age<br>• Consultant<br>• Ward<br>• Admission date | This is part of vital routine hospital documentation. Weight is important and several medications require a current weight to calculate dosage | | | | | |

## Completing the Drug Chart

| Drug Chart Task | Justification | | | | |
|---|---|---|---|---|---|
| Completes allergy box, including signing and dating | No medication should be prescribed until you know the patient's allergies | | | | |
| Prescribes correctly appropriate fluid | This patient is haemodynamically unstable and requires rapid IV fluid resuscitation. You should begin by giving fluid boluses and reassess after each bag. Clearly indicate on the prescription chart if two bags of fluid should be given simultaneously | | | | |
| Prescribe blood transfusion | This is often prescribed on a separate prescription chart. If the patient has capacity, then you should gain consent, but if he does not have capacity, you may act in the patient's best interests in this life-threatening situation | | | | |
| Prescribes correctly appropriate oxygen therapy:<br>• Route<br>• Target saturation | It is important to prescribe oxygen to ensure that it is being used correctly. Aim for oxygen saturation > 94% | | | | |
| Discontinues any inappropriate medications | Consider stopping any medications that increase the risk of bleeding; for example anticoagulants, antiplatelet agents, NSAIDs and selective serotonin reuptake inhibitors | | | | |
| Considers VTE prophylaxis | Choice of VTE prophylaxis can vary based on patient factors and local trust guidelines | | | | |

## General Points

| | | | | |
|---|---|---|---|---|
| Polite to patient | | | | |
| Clear, legible writing on the drug chart using black ink | | | | |

## Correct Prescription Chart

| Name: Steve Smith | Weight: 70 kg | Known allergies:<br>No known drug allergies |
|---|---|---|
| Date of birth: 01/03/1955 | Age: 65 years | |
| Hospital number: 0103551252 | Consultant: MJK | Signature: Date:<br>M. Khan  13/09/2019<br>M. KHAN |

## Oxygen Therapy

| Start | | | Route | | | Stop | |
|---|---|---|---|---|---|---|---|
| Date | Time | Mask (%) | Prongs (L/min) | Prescriber – Sign and Print | Administered by | Date | Time |
| 13/09/19 | 2100 | Nasal cannula | 2 L/min | M. Khan<br>M. KHAN | | | |

## Venous Thromboembolism Prophylaxis

| VTE Risk Assessment: | Comment: |
|---|---|
| Yes [ ] | Signature: *M. Khan* M. KHAN |
| Prophylaxis not required [ ] | Date: 13/09/19 |
| Contraindicated [X] | |

| | Date: → Time: ↓ | | | | | | | | | |
|---|---|---|---|---|---|---|---|---|---|---|
| Drug: | | | | | | | | | | |
| Dose:    Freq:    Route: | | | | | | | | | | |
| | | | | | | | | | | |
| Start:    Stop/review: | | | | | | | | | | |
| Signature: | | | | | | | | | | |

## Fluid Prescription

| Date | Fluid | Additive | Volume | Route | Rate | Signature | Given | Batch |
|---|---|---|---|---|---|---|---|---|
| 13/09/19 Venflon 1 | 0.9% Sodium chloride | None | 500 mL | IV | Over 15 min | *M. Khan* M. KHAN | | |
| 13/09/19 Venflon 2 | 0.9% Sodium chloride | None | 500 mL | IV | Over 15 min | *M. Khan* M. KHAN | | |

## ❓ QUESTIONS FROM THE EXAMINER

### Name three medications with a narrow therapeutic window.

Warfarin, theophylline, phenytoin, carbamazepine, digoxin, lithium and clozapine.

### What is the difference between licensed and unlicensed doses?

Licensed doses have been approved by regulators who have assessed the evidence for the product at a particular dose for a specific indication. Unlicensed or 'off-licence' doses have not been approved by regulators, and the evidence for use at that particular dose for the specific indication has not been assessed.

### As per NICE guidelines, what is the daily maintenance fluid requirement of water?

25–30 mL/kg/day.

### As per NICE guidelines, what is the daily maintenance fluid requirement of sodium, potassium and chloride?

1 mmol/kg/day of each electrolyte.

### As per NICE guidelines, what is the daily maintenance fluid requirement of glucose?

50–100 g of glucose to limit starvation ketosis.

### Name three sources that could contribute to ongoing fluid or electrolyte loss.

Vomiting loss, nasogastric tube loss, diarrhoea, stoma output loss, biliary drainage loss, blood loss, sweating, fever, dehydration and urinary loss.

**How long do you apply pressure to the distal digit to assess capillary refill time (CRT) and what CRT length suggests poor peripheral perfusion?**

Pressure should be applied for 5 s, and then released to assess for CRT properly. A CRT greater than 2 s suggests poor peripheral perfusion.

**Define 'major haemorrhage'.**

It is variously defined as loss of more than one blood volume (approximately 70 mL/kg) within 24 h, or 50% of total blood volume in less than 3 h, or bleeding more than 150 mL/min.

**What are the three rarest blood types?**

AB negative, AB positive and B negative blood groups are the least common.

**In patients who are actively bleeding secondary to an acute upper gastrointestinal bleed, what should the platelet count be maintained at?**

Platelet count should be greater than $50 \times 10^9$/L.

## Station 11.9 Diabetic Ketoacidosis (DKA)

### Doctor Briefing

You are the junior doctor on the medical admissions unit and are seeing Janet Smith, an 18-year-old woman, who has come in with shortness of breath, abdominal pain and vomiting. She is too confused to give you much history, but her mother tells you that she has recently been unwell with diarrhoea and has been passing large amounts of urine. You have made a presumptive diagnosis of DKA. Please formulate an appropriate management plan and complete the drug chart provided, including the prescription of fluids, regular, PRN and once-only medications as appropriate.

### Patient Briefing

You are Janet's mother, Hayley. Janet has been off school for a few days because she's been really tired and has been having diarrhoea. You have also noted that she has been drinking a lot of water and passing large amounts of urine, even in the middle of the night, which is not normal for her. This morning she complained of abdominal pain, and then by the afternoon she was breathless and vomiting, which is why you've brought her into hospital.

Janet does not suffer from any medical conditions.

You are concerned because you do not know what's going on and your daughter appears very unwell.

### Patient Details

| | |
|---|---|
| Name | Janet Smith |
| Date of birth | 01/04/2001 |
| Hospital number | 0104920045 |
| Weight | 64 kg |
| Height | 1.70 m |
| Consultant | CAP |
| Hospital/ward | WGH/53 |
| Current medications | Nil |
| Allergies | Penicillin (rash) |
| Admission date | 06/12/2019 |

### Mark Scheme for Examiner

#### Completing the Drug Chart

| Drug Chart Task | Justification | | | | | |
|---|---|---|---|---|---|---|
| Correctly writes patient information:<br>• Name<br>• Date of birth<br>• Hospital number<br>• Weight<br>• Age<br>• Consultant<br>• Ward<br>• Admission date | This is part of vital routine hospital documentation. Weight is important and several medications require a current weight to calculate dosage | | | | | |

## Completing the Drug Chart

| Drug Chart Task | Justification | | | | |
|---|---|---|---|---|---|
| Completes allergy box, including signing and dating | No medication should be prescribed until you know the patient's allergies | | | | |
| Prescribes correctly fixed-rate insulin infusion | Every trust will have its own protocol and chart for the prescription of fixed-rate insulin. This is usually at a rate of 0.1 unit/kg/h. When the DKA has resolved, the insulin may be switched to sliding-scale insulin | | | | |
| Prescribes correctly appropriate fluid | Prescribe a fluid bolus for the patient initially and then reassess fluid status and continue fluid rehydration if indicated. A venous blood gas can provide helpful information about the patient's progression. Remember to send urea and electrolytes and replace potassium if required | | | | |
| Considers prescribing dextrose infusion | If blood glucose level falls below 14 mmol/L, consider the commencement of 10% glucose IV at 100–125 mL/h | | | | |
| Prescribes correctly appropriate oxygen therapy:<br>• Route<br>• Target saturation | It is important to prescribe oxygen to ensure that it is being used correctly | | | | |
| Considers VTE prophylaxis | Choice of VTE prophylaxis can vary based on patient factors and local trust guidelines | | | | |

## General Points

| | | | | |
|---|---|---|---|---|
| Polite to patient | | | | |
| Clear, legible writing on the drug chart using black ink | | | | |

## Correct Prescription Chart

Name: Janet Smith

Date of birth: 01/04/2001

Hospital number: 0104920045

Weight: 64 kg

Age: 18 years

Consultant: CAP

Known allergies:
Penicillin (rash)

Signature: Date:
C. Price    06/12/19
C. PRICE

## Venous Thromboembolism Prophylaxis

| VTE Risk Assessment: | Comment: |
|---|---|
| Yes [X] | Signature: *C. Price*  C. PRICE |
| Prophylaxis not required [ ] | Date: 06/12/19 |
| Contraindicated [ ] | |

| | Date: → Time: ↓ | | | | | | | | | |
|---|---|---|---|---|---|---|---|---|---|---|
| Drug: Enoxaparin | | | | | | | | | | |
| Dose: 20 mg   Freq: OD   Route: SC | | | | | | | | | | |
| Start: 06/12/19   Stop/review: | | | | | | | | | | |
| Signature: C. Price C. PRICE | | | | | | | | | | |

## Once-Only Medications

| Date | Time | Medicine (Approved Name) | Dose | Route | Prescriber – Sign and Print | Time Given | Given By |
|---|---|---|---|---|---|---|---|
| 06/12/19 | 2000 | 50 units Actrapid in 50 mL 0.9% NaCl | See sliding-scale chart | IV infusion | C. Price C. PRICE | | |

## Insulin Prescription

| Blood Glucose (mmol/L) | Insulin Infusion Rate (unit/h = mL/h) | Route | Prescriber – Sign and Print | Time Given | Given By |
|---|---|---|---|---|---|
| >13 | 6 | IV | Signature: C. Price Print name: C. PRICE | | |
| ≤13 | 3 | | | | |
| ≤10 | 2 | | | | |

## Fluid Prescriptions

| Date | Fluid | Additive | Volume | Route | Rate | Signature | Given | Batch |
|---|---|---|---|---|---|---|---|---|
| 06/12/19 | 0.9% Sodium chloride | None | 1 L | IV | 250mL/h | C. Price C. PRICE | | |

## ❓ QUESTIONS FROM THE EXAMINER

### What signs would suggest that a child is dehydrated?

Sunken eyes, dry mucous membranes, tachycardia, tachypnoea, prolonged CRT, reduced skin turgor, pale skin and cold extremities.

### What are the three diagnostic criteria for DKA?

Hyperglycaemia greater than 11 mmol/L or known diabetes, ketonaemia > 3 mmol/L or ketouria > 2+, plus pH < 7.3 and/or bicarbonate < 15 mmol/L (acidosis).

### Name the three main components in the management of DKA.

Fluid resuscitation, fixed-rate insulin IV infusion and potassium replacement.

### Why do you see profound dehydration in DKA?

Insulin deficiency means that glucose cannot be taken up and metabolised, therefore it stays in the blood stream. During DKA, the glucose is filtered by the kidneys in concentrations that exceed the renal reabsorption capacity, resulting in glycosuria. Glycosuria causes a profound osmotic diuresis which then leads to severe dehydration.

### What is the maximum rate of potassium infusion outside of high dependency unit/ITU?

10 mmol/h.

### What is the fluid resuscitation regime in DKA?

1 L of 0.9% sodium chloride over 1 h, 2 h, 2 h, 4 h, 4 h and 6 h consecutively.

### What is the name of the insulin receptor and how many units does it consist of?

It is called tyrosine kinase and it is composed of two alpha subunits and two beta subunits.

### Which organ is responsible for glycogen synthesis?

The liver.

### What is an insulinoma?

It is a rare tumour in the pancreas that is responsible for excessive insulin production and can lead to fatal hyperinsulinaemia and hypoglycaemic episodes.

### What are the two main groups of IV fluids and what is the difference?

Traditionally IV fluids are either crystalloids or colloids. Crystalloids are solutions of small molecules in water and examples include sodium chloride, Hartmann's solution and dextrose. Colloids are solutions of large organic molecules dispersed in another substance and examples include albumin and gelofusine.

## Station 11.10  Discharge Prescribing

### Doctor Briefing

George Smith is a 50-year-old man who was admitted to hospital recently with a right lower-lobe pneumonia. He is now fit for discharge but requires 'to take out' (TTO) prescriptions of his medications. On admission he was septic with hypotension and an AKI, and his ramipril was withheld. His systolic blood pressure has been 110–120 mmHg throughout admission and ramipril has not been restarted yet. He needs a further 3 days of antibiotics following discharge. He is also requiring paracetamol and morphine sulphate modified-release (MR) for pain, with oramorph for breakthrough pain. Please complete the TTO form below using Mr Smith's drug chart and the *British National Formulary* if necessary.

### Patient Briefing

You have been recovering in hospital from a severe chest infection over the last few days. Your doctor has told you that you are now fit enough to go home and has advised that you continue the antibiotics at home for another 3 days and he will give you some painkillers as well. He also said that your kidney function has been deranged, so has temporarily stopped your blood pressure medication.

You are concerned that you will not get enough medications to take home for your infection.

### Patient Details

| | |
|---|---|
| Name | George Smith |
| Date of birth | 22/12/1970 |
| Hospital number | 2212660994 |
| Weight | 81 kg |
| Height | 1.74 m |
| Consultant | RHM |
| Hospital/ward | RIE/207 |
| Current medications | Levothyroxine 125 mcg OD<br>Aspirin 75 mg OD<br>Omeprazole 40 mg OD<br>Ramipril 5 mg OD |
| Allergies | Nil |
| Admission date | 13/01/2018 |

### Mark Scheme for Examiner

#### Completing the Drug Chart

| Drug Chart Task | Justification | | | | | |
|---|---|---|---|---|---|---|
| Correctly writes patient information:<br>• Name<br>• Date of birth<br>• Hospital number<br>• Age<br>• Consultant<br>• Ward<br>• Admission date<br>• Discharge date | You must have the correct patient details to ensure that the patient is collecting the correct medications | | | | | |

## Completing the Drug Chart

| Drug Chart Task | Justification | | | | |
|---|---|---|---|---|---|
| Completes allergy box, including signing and dating | No medication should be prescribed until you know the patient's allergies | | | | |
| Prescribes correctly regular medications:<br>• Drug name<br>• Route<br>• Dose<br>• Frequency and timing<br>• Duration (number of days to be supplied) | The patient will need to continue most of these drugs, except medications that have been changed (added or removed). Remember to prescribe the antibiotics as a short 3-day supply, as the patient has already taken the remainder of the course (7 days in total) | | | | |
| Documents the reasons for changes to regular medications for the primary care doctor | Explains that ramipril had been temporarily withheld due to AKI and hypotension, and to advise primary care physician to review. Explains the reason for adding antibiotics and painkillers | | | | |
| Prescribes correctly 'as required' medications:<br>• Drug name<br>• Route<br>• Dose<br>• Duration (number of days to be supplied) | Oramorph should be prescribed for the patient for break-through pain. The amount supplied should be based on how much the patient has been using it during the time leading up to discharge in combination with your clinical judgement | | | | |
| Prescribes correctly controlled drugs:<br>• Name and address of the patient<br>• Form and strength of the drug<br>• Either the total quantity or the number of dosage units of the drug, written in both words and figures<br>• Dose of the drug<br>• Prescriber's signature with the prescriber's hospital address | Ensures that all the details are present; otherwise the pharmacy will not be able to dispense the controlled drug | | | | |
| Signs and dates the discharge prescription | This must be done so that pharmacy can dispense the medications to the patient | | | | |

## General Points

| | | | | | |
|---|---|---|---|---|---|
| Polite to patient | | | | | |
| Clear, legible writing on the drug chart, using black ink | | | | | |

## Correct TTO Form

| Drug | Dose and frequency | Duration | Pharmacy |
|---|---|---|---|
| Aspirin | 75 mg OD | 28 days (continue long-term) | |
| Omeprazole | 40 mg OD | 28 days (continue long-term) | |
| Levothyroxine | 125 micrograms OD | 28 days (continue long-term) | |
| Paracetamol | 1 g QDS | 14 days (short-term) | |
| Amoxicillin | 500 mg TDS | Three days remaining (7-day course to finish on 20/01/22) | |

| Medication | Change |
|---|---|
| Ramipril 5 mg OD | Currently withheld due to AKI and hypotension. Primary care physician please recheck the renal function and blood pressure in 1 week and restart ramipril if required |
| Amoxicillin 500 mg TDS | For community-acquired pneumonia. Seven-day course to finish 20/01/22 |
| Paracetamol 1 g QDS | For pleuritic chest pain (short-term) |

| Drug | Dose and frequency | Duration | Pharmacy |
|---|---|---|---|
| MST (morphine sulphate modified-release) 10-mg tablets. Please supply 56 (fifty-six) tablets | 10 mg BD | 28 days | |

## ❓ QUESTIONS FROM THE EXAMINER

### Which medications need to be withheld in AKI or chronic kidney disease?

Some drugs that should be withheld when there is renal impairment include metformin, NSAIDs, certain antibiotics (for example, aminoglycosides), opiates and anticoagulants.

### What are controlled drugs?

They are substances that are known to be particularly harmful or open to abuse; therefore they are regulated by both the Misuse of Drugs Act and the Misuse of Drugs Regulations.

### What do the 'schedules' of controlled drugs refer to and how many 'schedules' exist?

There are five schedules. 'Schedules' is the grouping system used by the Misuse of Drugs Act to reflect the different restrictions that apply to the prescription and monitoring of controlled drugs used for medical purposes. Schedule 1 drugs have the tightest controls, whereas schedule 5 drugs have more relaxed measures.

### To which schedule do drugs that are thought to have no therapeutic value belong?

Schedule 1 drugs, such as LSD and ecstasy, are thought to have no therapeutic benefit and are unlawful to possess or prescribe.

### What adverse effect can result from a patient with known renal impairment continuing to take ramipril at a standard or high dose?

Hyperkalaemia and other side effects of ACE inhibitors, such as hypotension, myalgia, palpitations and constipation, are more common in those with impaired renal function.

### What is the maximum daily dose of ramipril that can be prescribed to patients with estimated glomerular filtration rate less than 60 mL/min/1.73$^2$?

5 mg in 1 day.

### Name one contraindication to levothyroxine.

Thyrotoxicosis.

### What types of food might reduce the absorption of levothyroxine?

Dietary fibre, milk, soya products and coffee may decrease the absorption.

### For which conditions should amoxicillin be cautioned in, due to an increased risk of erythematous rashes?

Acute lymphocytic leukaemia, chronic lymphocytic leukaemia, cytomegalovirus infection and glandular fever.

### Which group of patients are at a higher risk of hypersensitivity or anaphylactic reactions to penicillin?

Patients with a history of atopic allergy (asthma, eczema or hayfever) are at risk of anaphylactic reactions to penicillin. Those with a history of anaphylaxis, urticaria or rash immediately after penicillin administration are at risk of immediate hypersensitivity to penicillin.

## Station 11.11    Analgesia

### Doctor Briefing

You are a junior doctor working in the ED and have been asked to see Peter Robinson, a 20-year-old man, who has suffered a traumatic injury to his left leg while playing rugby. He is complaining of severe pain and is unable to weight bear. The orthopaedic surgeon is in theatres and will come to review the patient when he is finished. Please review the history and examination taken by your colleague, formulate an appropriate management plan and complete the drug chart provided.

### Patient Briefing

You were brought into the ED by your rugby coach because you injured yourself during the game this morning. You are experiencing a lot of pain in your left leg and cannot walk on it. Severity is 9 out of 10.

You are concerned because you are in a lot of pain and haven't been given anything to get it under control.

### Patient Details

| | |
|---|---|
| Name | Peter Robinson |
| Date of birth | 10/12/1990 |
| Hospital number | 1012908911 |
| Weight | 83 kg |
| Height | 1.86 m |
| Consultant | MJR |
| Hospital/ward | WGH/SAU |
| Current medications | Nil |
| Allergies | Nil |
| Admission date | 30/05/19 |

### Mark Scheme for Examiner

| **Completing the Drug Chart** | | | | | | |
|---|---|---|---|---|---|---|
| **Drug Chart Task** | **Justification** | | | | | |
| Correctly writes patient information:<br>• Name<br>• Date of birth<br>• Hospital number<br>• Weight<br>• Age<br>• Consultant<br>• Ward<br>• Admission date | This is part of vital routine hospital documentation. Weight is important and several medications require a current weight to calculate dosage | | | | | |
| Completes allergy box, including signing and dating | No medication should be prescribed until you know the patient's allergies | | | | | |

## Completing the Drug Chart

| Drug Chart Task | Justification | | | | |
|---|---|---|---|---|---|
| Prescribes correctly appropriate analgesia:<br>• Drug name<br>• Route<br>• Dose | The patient is in severe pain and requires immediate analgesia while awaiting orthopaedic review. Always check if the patient has been given any analgesia already. Analgesia should be prescribed using the WHO analgesic ladder as a guide. Start at the step most appropriate for the patient's pain. If the pain is not controlled, avoid changing one drug for another of equal potency in the same class; instead move up the ladder until adequate analgesia is reached | | | | |

## General Points

| | | | | |
|---|---|---|---|---|
| Polite to patient | | | | |
| Clear, legible writing on the drug chart using black ink | | | | |

## Correct Prescription Chart

Name: Peter Robinson

Date of birth: 25/03/1990

Hospital number: 1012908911

Weight: 93 kg

Age: 20 years

Consultant: MJR

Known allergies:
No known drug allergies

Signature: Date:
M. Ross    30.5.19
M. ROSS

## Once-Only Medications

| Date | Time | Medicine (Approved Name) | Dose | Route | Prescriber – Sign and Print | Time Given | Given By |
|---|---|---|---|---|---|---|---|
| 30/05/19 | 1700 | Paracetamol | 1 g | Oral | M. Ross<br>M. ROSS | | |
| 30/05/19 | 1700 | Oramorph (morphine sulphate) 10 mg/5 mL | 10 mg | Oral | M. Ross<br>M. ROSS | | |
| 30/05/19 | 1745 | Oramorph (morphine sulphate) 10 mg/5 mL | 10 mg | Oral | M. Ross<br>M. ROSS | | |

## Venous Thromboembolism Prophylaxis

| VTE Risk Assessment: | Comment: |
| --- | --- |
| Yes [X] | Signature: M. Ross   M. ROSS |
| Prophylaxis not required [ ] | Date: 30/05/19 |
| Contraindicated [ ] | |

| | | Date: → | | | | | | | | | | |
| --- | --- | --- | --- | --- | --- | --- | --- | --- | --- | --- | --- | --- |
| | | Time: ↓ | | | | | | | | | | |
| Drug: Enoxaparin | | | | | | | | | | | | |
| Dose: 20 mg | Freq: OD | Route: SC | | | | | | | | | | |
| Start: 13/09/19 | Stop/review: | | | | | | | | | | | |
| Signature: M. Ross M. ROSS | | | | | | | | | | | | |

## ? QUESTIONS FROM THE EXAMINER

### What causes nociceptive pain and how many types are there?

Nociceptive pain arises when tissue injury activates nociceptors, which are sensitive to noxious stimuli. This type of pain can be subdivided into somatic and visceral pain, depending on the location of activated nociceptors.

### What causes neuropathic pain?

It is caused by structural damage and nerve cell dysfunction in the peripheral or central nervous system.

### What is TENS and how does it work?

TENS stands for 'transcutaneous electrical nerve stimulation'. It is a method of analgesia using small electrical impulses being delivered to the affected areas. The aim is that these impulses can reduce the pain signals being transmitted to the spinal cord and brain.

### What is congenital insensitivity to pain and anhidrosis?

It is a rare hereditary condition that inhibits the ability to perceive physically pain and in which the patient is unable to sweat.

### What is the withdrawal reflex?

It is a spinal reflex that causes a part of the body to move away from a painful stimulus, through muscle reactions (contraction or relaxation).

### Define 'allodynia'.

It is the sensation of pain due to a stimulus that does not normally provoke pain.

### What is the proinflammatory cytokine response?

It is the release of proinflammatory cytokines, which are positive mediators of inflammation, due to inflammasome activation. They can contribute to fever, inflammation, tissue destruction, shock and death.

## What is the yellow card scheme?

It is a scheme that has been derived to provide an early warning that the safety of a medication or medical device may require further investigation, through the voluntary reporting of suspected side effects or medical device incidents, by healthcare professionals and the public.

## What is the maximum daily dose of oral ibuprofen that a paediatric patient can take?

30 mg/kg or 1.2 g within 24 h.

## What do the abbreviations JEJ and PEG stand for, in terms of route of drug administration?

JEJ means via jejunostomy and PEG means via percutaneous endoscopic gastrostomy.

## Station 11.12    Prescribing for Paediatrics

### Doctor Briefing

You are a junior doctor working in the ED and have been asked to see James Taylor, a 7-year-old boy who has presented with wheeze and shortness of breath. This is on a background of a sore throat, runny nose, fever and cough. He has a history of asthma and eczema. His medications are Seretide 250, salbutamol inhalers and montelukast. Review the history and examination taken by your colleague, formulate an appropriate management plan and complete the drug chart provided, including the prescription of fluids, regular, PRN and once-only medications as appropriate.

### Patient Briefing

You are Joanne, James' mum. You have brought James to the hospital because he has been unwell for a week, with symptoms of the flu and a sore throat. You were hoping that he'd have recovered by now, but this morning he sounded rather wheezy and was short of breath. He looks tired and isn't like his normal self.

He is known to have asthma and eczema.

You are concerned that your son will need to be admitted to ITU and be put on a ventilator.

### Patient Details

| | |
|---|---|
| Name | James Taylor |
| Date of birth | 22/03/2012 |
| Hospital number | 2203090334 |
| Weight | 28 kg |
| Height | 1.30 m |
| Consultant | PHR |
| Hospital/ward | SJH/Children's Ward |
| Current medications | Seretide 50 Evohaler 2 puffs BD<br>Salbutamol 2 puffs PRN<br>Montelukast 5 mg OD |
| Allergies | Nil |
| Admission date | 26/05/2019 |

### Mark Scheme for Examiner

#### Completing the Drug Chart

| Drug Chart Task | Justification | | | | | |
|---|---|---|---|---|---|---|
| Correctly writes patient information:<br>• Name<br>• Date of birth<br>• Hospital number<br>• Weight<br>• Age<br>• Consultant<br>• Ward<br>• Admission date | This is part of vital routine hospital documentation. Weight is important and several medications require a current weight to calculate dosage | | | | | |

## Completing the Drug Chart

| Drug Chart Task | Justification | | | | | |
|---|---|---|---|---|---|---|
| Completes allergy box, including signing and dating | No medication should be prescribed until you know the patient's allergies | | | | | |
| Prescribes correctly appropriate oxygen therapy:<br>• Route<br>• Target saturations | It is important to prescribe oxygen to ensure that it is being used correctly. Prescribe oxygen via a non-rebreathe bag to maintain saturations at 94–98% | | | | | |
| Prescribes correctly appropriate bronchodilators:<br>• Drug name<br>• Route<br>• Dose<br>• Considers oxygen or air-driven nebuliser | This child is presenting with life-threatening exacerbation of asthma and is hypoxic. Prescribe 5 mg nebulised salbutamol back to back. The nebuliser should be oxygen-driven if oxygen saturation is <94% | | | | | |
| Prescribes correctly appropriate steroid treatment:<br>• Drug name<br>• Route<br>• Dose | Prescribe 100 mg hydrocortisone IV or 40–50 mg prednisolone PO. Route of administration needs to be carefully considered in conjunction with the patient's ability to comply, and you must consider if the patient is able to swallow tablets currently | | | | | |
| Considers the severity of the acute asthma exacerbation and additional therapies:<br>• Route<br>• Dose<br>• Escalation required | Consider adding nebulised ipratropium bromide 500 mcg and 150 mg magnesium sulphate in cases of severe/life-threatening exacerbations according to the NICE guidelines | | | | | |
| Prescribes correctly appropriate analgesia:<br>• Drug name<br>• Route<br>• Dose | Following the WHO analgesia ladder, paracetamol orally should always be the first line | | | | | |
| Considers VTE prophylaxis | Choice of VTE prophylaxis can vary based on patient factors and local trust guidelines | | | | | |

## General Points

| | | | | | | |
|---|---|---|---|---|---|---|
| Polite to patient | | | | | | |
| Clear, legible writing on the drug chart using black ink | | | | | | |

## Correct Prescription Chart

Name: James Taylor

Date of birth: 22/03/2012

Hospital number: 2203090334

Weight: 28 kg

Age: 7 years

Consultant: MHS

Known allergies:
No known drug allergies

Signature: Date:
M. Slack  26/5/19
M. SLACK

## Once-Only Medications

| Date | Time | Medicine (Approved Name) | Dose | Route | Prescriber – Sign and Print | Time Given | Given By |
|---|---|---|---|---|---|---|---|
| 26/5/19 | 1400 | Salbutamol (driven with oxygen) | 5 mg | Neb | M. Slack / M. SLACK | | |
| 26/5/19 | 1400 | Ipratropium bromide (driven with oxygen) | 500 micrograms | Neb | M. Slack / M. SLACK | | |
| 26/5/19 | 1400 | Magnesium sulphate (driven with oxygen) | 150 mg | Neb | M. Slack / M. SLACK | | |
| 26/5/19 | 1430 | Prednisolone | 40 mg | Oral | M. Slack / M. SLACK | | |
| 26/5/19 | 1430 | Paracetamol | 140 mg | Oral | M. Slack / M. SLACK | | |

## Oxygen Therapy

| | | Route | | | | Stop | |
|---|---|---|---|---|---|---|---|
| Date | Time | Mask (%) | Prongs (L/min) | Prescriber – Sign and Print | Administered by | Date | Time |
| 26/5/19 | 1400 | Non-re-breathe mask | 15 L/min | M. Slack / M. SLACK | | | |

## Regular Medications

| | Date: → Time: ↓ | | | | | | | | |
|---|---|---|---|---|---|---|---|---|---|
| Drug: Seretide 250 (salmeterol 25 micrograms/fluticasone 250 micrograms) | 02 | | | | | | | | |
| Dose: 2 puffs    Freq: BD    Route: Inh | (06) | | | | | | | | |
| | 10 | | | | | | | | |
| Start: 26/5/19    Stop/review: | 14 | | | | | | | | |
| Signature: M. Slack / M. SLACK | 18 | | | | | | | | |
| Indication: Asthma | (22) | | | | | | | | |

## Regular Medications

| Drug: Salbutamol | | | Date: → <br> Time: ↓ | | | | | | | | |
|---|---|---|---|---|---|---|---|---|---|---|---|
| | | | 02 | | | | | | | | |
| Dose: <br> 2 puffs | Freq: <br> BD | Route: <br> Inh | 06 | | | | | | | | |
| | | | ⑩ | | | | | | | | |
| Start: 26/5/19 | | Stop/review: | 14 | | | | | | | | |
| Signature: <br> M. Slack <br> M. SLACK | | | 18 | | | | | | | | |
| Indication: <br> Asthma | | | ㉒ | | | | | | | | |
| Drug: Montelukast | | | 02 | | | | | | | | |
| Dose: <br> 5 mg | Freq: <br> ON | Route: <br> Oral | 06 | | | | | | | | |
| | | | 10 | | | | | | | | |
| Start: 26/5/19 | | Stop/review: | 14 | | | | | | | | |
| Signature: <br> M. Slack <br> M. SLACK | | | 18 | | | | | | | | |
| Indication: <br> Asthma | | | ㉒ | | | | | | | | |

## ? QUESTIONS FROM THE EXAMINER

### When you are prescribing maintenance IV fluids for a child, how do you calculate the rate?

In order to prescribe IV fluids for children, you must obtain the patient's weight. For the first 10 kg, they can receive 100 mL/kg/day, then for the second 10 kg, they can receive 50 mL/kg/day. Any subsequent kilogram can be 20 mL/kg/day.

### Diclofenac suppositories are not licensed for use in children under 6 years except for one group of patients. Which group and for which condition?

Suppositories can be used in children over 1 year for juvenile idiopathic arthritis.

### Define the 'neonatal' period.

A newborn infant aged 0–28 days.

### How are body surface area (BSA) estimates calculated and why are they sometimes preferred to body weight for calculation of paediatric doses?

BSA estimates are derived from the patient's body weight, and they can be the preferable choice as many physiological phenomena correlate better with BSA.

## What is the significance of liver development in paediatrics and drug metabolism?

Neonates have a prolonged half-life for most drugs. Significant and rapid maturation of the liver occurs in the first year of life, and the most rapid elimination of drugs is found in school-age children and adolescents. After that, plasma clearance slows as the patient ages.

## Why is ceftriaxone often avoided in infants less than 1 month old?

There is a risk of biliary stasis when ceftriaxone is used in patients younger than 1 month of age, especially if they have jaundice.

## Why is aspirin avoided in children?

Aspirin is linked to Reye's syndrome in children, which can lead to potentially fatal liver failure. However, it is sometimes indicated for conditions such as Kawasaki disease.

## Why is nitrofurantoin contraindicated in infants less than 3 months old?

It is associated with the risk of haemolytic anaemia.

## Why are tetracyclines avoided in those under 12-year-old?

They can cause discoloration of teeth that are still developing.

## With what code do all prescription forms originating in England begin?

FP10.

# Index

Note: Page numbers followed by "*f*" indicate figures, "*b*" indicate boxes, and "*t*" indicate tables.